VERGENCE EYE MOVEMENTS: BASIC AND CLINICAL ASPECTS

VERGENCE EYE MOVEMENTS: BASIC AND CLINICAL ASPECTS

Editors
CLIFTON M. SCHOR, O.D., Ph.D
KENNETH J. CIUFFREDA, O.D., Ph.D

BUTTERWORTHS
Boston • London
Sydney • Wellington • Durban • Toronto

Every effort has been made to ensure that the drug dosage schedules within this text are accurate and conform to standards accepted at time of publication. However, as treatment recommendations vary in light of continuing research and clinical experience, the reader is advised to verify drug dosage schedules herein with information found on product information sheets. This is especially true in cases of new or infrequently used drugs.

Butterworth Publishers
10 Tower Office Park
Woburn, MA 01801

Library of Congress Cataloging in Publication Data
Main entry under title:

Vergence eye movements.

Bibliography: p.
Includes index.
1. Eye—Movements. 2. Eye—Movement disorders.
3. Binocular vision. I. Schor, Clifton, M., 1943–
II. Ciuffreda, Kenneth J., 1947–
QP477.5.V47 1982 617.7′62 82-12988
ISBN 0-409-95032-7

Printed in the United States of America.

To the memory of

Leo B. Ciuffreda, who taught his son that an A – just isn't good enough–KJC

and

Dean Monroe J. Hirsch, who contributed immensely to the visual health professions–CMS.

Contributors

EDITORS

Clifton M. Schor, O.D., Ph.D.
University of California-Berkeley
School of Optometry
101 Optometry Building
Berkeley, California 94720

Kenneth J. Ciuffreda, O.D., Ph.D.
State University of New York
State College of Optometry
100 East 24th Street
New York, New York 10010

CONTRIBUTORS

Nathan Flax, O.D., M.S.
State University of New York
State College of Optometry
100 East 24th Street
New York, New York 10010

Glenn A. Fry, Ph.D.
The Ohio State University
College of Optometry
Columbus, Ohio 43210

J. David Grisham, O.D., M.Sc.
University of California-Berkeley
School of Optometry
Berkeley, California 94720

Henry W Hofstetter, O.D., Ph.D.
2615 Windermere Woods Drive
Bloomington, Indiana 47401

Steven C. Hokoda, O.D.
State University of New York
State College of Optometry
100 E. 24th Street
New York, New York 10010

George K. Hung, Ph.D.
Department of Electrical Engineering
Rutgers University
Piscataway, New Jersey 08901

Ronald Jones, O.D., Ph.D.
Ohio State University
College of Optometry
338 West Tenth Avenue
Columbus, Ohio 43210

Robert V. Kenyon, Ph.D.
Department of Aeronautics and Astronautics
Massachusetts Institute of Technology
77 Massachusetts Avenue
Cambridge, Massachusetts 02139

Andrew E. Kertesz, Ph.D.
Biomedical Engineering Center
Northwestern University
Evanston, Illinois 60201

V. V. Krishnan, Ph.D.
Division of Engineering
San Francisco State University
San Francisco, California 94132

Herschel W. Leibowitz, Ph.D.
Department of Psychology
Pennsylvania State University
University Park, Pennsylvania 16803

Lawrence E. Mays, Ph.D.
Department of Physiological Optics and Neurosciences Program
904 CDLD
University of Alabama in Birmingham
Birmingham, Alabama 35294

Meredith W. Morgan, Jr., O.D., Ph.D.
1217 Skycrest Drive #4
Walnut Creek, California, 94595

Ken Nakayama, Ph.D.
Smith-Kettlewell Institute of Visual Sciences
2232 Webster Street
San Francisco, California 94115

Hiroshi Ono, Ph.D.
Department of Psychology
York University
4700 Keele Street
Downsview, M3J 1P3 Canada

D. Alfred Owens, Ph.D.
Whitely Psychology Labs
Franklin and Marshall College
Lancaster, Pennsylvania 17604

Gill Roper-Hall, D.B.O.T.
Department of Ophthalmology
Washington University
School of Medicine
660 South Euclid Avenue
St. Louis, Missouri 63110

J. James Saladin, O.D., Ph.D.
Ferris State College
College of Optometry
Big Rapids, Michigan 49307

Alan B. Scott, M.D.
Smith-Kettlewell Institute of Visual Sciences
2232 Webster Street
San Francisco, California 94115

John L. Semmlow, Ph.D.
Department of Electrical Engineering
Rutgers University
P.O. Box 909
Piscataway, New Jersey 08854

James E. Sheedy, O.D., Ph.D.
The Ohio State University
College of Optometry
338 West Tenth Avenue
Columbus, Ohio 43210

Lawrence Stark, M.D.
University of California-Berkeley
School of Optometry
Berkeley, California 94720

Christopher W. Tyler, Ph.D.
Smith-Kettlewell Institute of Visual Sciences
2232 Webster Street
San Francisco, California 94115

Contents

Foreword xxiii

Preface xxvii

Acknowledgments xxix

I. Overview of Maddox Vergence Components 1

1. Normal and Abnormal Vergence 3
Lawrence Stark

Normal Control of Vergence 3
Vergence Main Sequence 5
Triadic Role of Vergence 7
Abnormalities of Vergence 11

2. The Maddox Analysis of Vergence 15
Meredith W. Morgan

II. Tonic and Proximal Vergence 23

3. Perceptual and Motor Consequences of Tonic Vergence 25
D. Alfred Owens and Herschel W. Leibowitz

Historical Background 26
Anatomical and Physiological Resting Positions 26
Maddox's Conception of Tonic Convergence 27
Opponent Vergence Mechanisms 29
Evidence for Tonic Vergence 30
Stress Effects 30
Reduced Illumination and Dark Vergence 32
Vergence for Peripheral Stimuli 38
Development of Vergence Eye Movements 40
Tonic Vergence and Accommodation 42
Perceptual Correlates of Tonic Vergence 46
Specific Distance Tendency 47
Gaze Stability and Illusory Motion Perception 51
Oculomotor Adaptation and Tonic Vergence 54
Motor Adaptation 55
Perceptual Adaptation 60
Summary and Conclusions 67

4. Theoretical and Clinical Importance of Proximal Vergence and Accommodation 75
Steven C. Hokoda and Kenneth J. Ciuffreda

Proximal Convergence 76
Proximal Accommodation 82
Convergence and Accommodation as Cues to Distance 84
Association with Binocular Anomalies 86
Proximal Vergence Interactions 90
Modeling of the Vergence System 92

III. Interactions Between Accommodation and Vergence 99

5. Accommodative Vergence and Accommodation in Normals, Amblyopes, and Strabismics 101
Kenneth J. Ciuffreda and Robert V. Kenyon

Overview of Accommodation in Normals 101
Spatial Frequency 107
Eccentricity 112
Overview of Accommodative Vergence in Normals 114
Oculomotor Interaction of Accommodative Vergence in Normals 117
AC/A Ratio 125
Stability 125
Linearity 128

Effects of Age 129
Effects of Orthoptics 132
Effects of Surgery 139
Drug Effects 140
Accommodation and Accommodative Vergence in Amblyopia and Strabismus 143
Accommodation 145
Static Measures of Accommodative Vergence 153
Accommodative Vergence Substituting for Absent Disparity Vergence 155
Amblyopia and Accommodative Vergence 163
Future Directions 163

6. The Near Response: Theories of Control 175
John L. Semmlow and George K. Hung

General Organization of the Near Triad 176
Early Theories of Near Triad Control 176
Early Models of the Near Triad 181
Complete Models of the Near Triad 184
Model Applications 189
Conclusions 192

IV. Disparity Vergence 197

7. Sensory Processing of Binocular Disparity 199
Christopher W. Tyler

History 199
Sensory Consequences of Binocular Disparity 200
Binocular Visual Direction and The Horopter 201
Binocular Visual Direction 201
Corresponding Retinal Points 202
Types of Horopters 204
Significance of the Point Horopter 205
The Point Horopter and Effects of Convergence 205
Fixation at Infinity and Shear of "Vertical" Meridians 205
Point Horopter with Symmetric Fixation in the Visual Plane 207
Point Horopter with Asymmetric Convergence in the Visual Plane 209
Generalized Point Horopter in Asymmetric Convergence 210
Effects of Eye Torsion on the Form of Horopter 210

Empirical Evidence for the Form of the Horopter 212
Vieth-Müller Circle in the Visual Plane 212
Empirical Vertical Horopter 214
Binocular Fusion 216
Classical Theories of Fusion 216
Physiological Basis of Fusion and Diplopia 218
Characteristics of Fusion 220
Retinal Eccentricity, Fusion, and Cyclofusion 220
The Fusion Horopter 221
Spatial Limits 221
Temporal Aspects 223
Spatiotemporal Interactions 224
Evoked Potentials 227
Dichoptic Stimulation 230
Binocular Mixture 230
Binocular Rivalry 231
Binocular Luster 234
Stereoscopic Vision 235
Binocular Disparity 235
Processing Binocular Disparity 236
Precision of Stereoscopic Localization 238
The Three-Dimensional "Fovea" for Stereoacuity 239
Cyclopean Stereopsis 239
Physiological Basis of Stereopsis by Spatial Disparity 243
A Theoretical Framework for Stereopsis 244
Overview 244
Special-Purpose Mechanisms 246
Structure of the Model 247
Outline 248
Local Processes 249
Local/Global Separation 249
Local Cleaning Operations 256
Depth Averaging 257
Specialized Local Stereoscopic Processes 257
Global Processes in Stereopsis 264
Global Lateral Inhibition 264
Global Processing Limitations 268
Specialized Global Stereoscopic Processes 272
Hypercyclopean Perception 275
Vergence 282
Role of Vergence in Stereopsis 282
Role of Vergence in Space Perception 285
Conclusion 287

8. Horizontal Disparity Vergence 297
Ronald Jones

Psychophysical Disparity 298
Measurement of Ocular Vergence 300
Basic Characteristics of Disparity Vergence 300
Relationship Between Disparity and Vergence Amplitude 303
Target Influences on Disparity Vergence 306
Disparity Vergence and Fixation Distance 309
Sensory Stimulus to Disparity Vergence 309
A Scenario for Disparity Vergence Control 313

9. Vertical and Cyclofusional Disparity Vergence 317
Andrew E. Kertesz

Vertical Fusional Response 317
- Definitions 317
- Background 318
- Symmetric Disparity Presentations 319
- Asymmetric Disparity Presentations 321
- Normal and Stabilized Disparity Viewing Conditions 323
- Effect of Stimulus Size and Complexity 326
- Extrafoveal Stimulation 329

Cyclofusional Response 330
- Definitions 330
- Background 330
- Effect of Stimulus Size 333
- Symmetric Disparity Presentation 336
- Asymmetric Disparity Presentation 339
- Strictly Peripheral Stimulation 341
- Cyclofusional Stimulation that Contains Depth Cues 344

Summary 346

10. Model of the Disparity Vergence System 349
V. V. Krishnan and Lawrence Stark

- Descriptive Model of Disparity Vergence System 350
- Measurement of Disparity Vergence 351
- Modeling Approaches 353

Plant Model 354
Model of Disparity Vergence Controller 358
- Nonlinearities in Disparity Vergence System 365
- Directions for Future Modeling 365

11. The Combination of Version and Vergence 373
Hiroshi Ono

Hering's Theory of Binocular Eye Movement 373
A Restatement of Hering's Hypothesis 373
Misinterpretations of Hering's Hypothesis 375
Analysis of Hering's Hypothesis 376
Experimental Results 381
Results Related to the Two-Components Proposition 382
Results Related to the Equal-Components and Additivity Propositions 385
Summary 397

V. Case Analysis of Binocular Disorders, Excluding Strabismus and Central Nervous System Disorders 401

12. Basic Concepts Underlying Graphical Analysis 403
Glenn A. Fry

Hering's Laws of Equal Innervation 404
Relation Between Accommodation and Convergence .. 404
Base-In and Base-Out Blur-Break Ranges 406
Relative Accommodation 409
Negative Fusional Convergence 410
Mechanisms Underlying Fusional Movements 410
Nature of the Tie-up between Accommodation and Accommodative Convergence 410
The Jampel Center 411
Fusional Convergence vs Triad Convergence 413
Convergent Accommodation vs Accommodative Convergence 415
Timing of Accommodation and Accommodative Convergence Responses 416
Proximal Convergence 416
The Spike 417
Base-In and Base-Out Blur-Break Ranges in Different Persons 421
Fusion Reflex 424
The Triad Pupil Response 427
Age and the AC/A Ratio 427
Measurement of Convergent Accommodation 428
Relation of Accommodative Convergence to Convergent Accommodation 429
Patient-to-Patient Variations in the AC/A Ratio 433

Cyclorotation Associated with Convergence 434
Reciprocal Innervation and Comfort 434

13. Graphical Analysis 439
Henry W Hofstetter

History 439
The Coordinates 439
Accommodation and Convergence Units 440
Uses of the Graph 441
Construction and Design 441
Assumptions and Approximations 441
The "Demand" Line 442
Correction of Convergence Measurement Errors 444
Data to be Plotted 447
Blurs, Breaks, and Recoveries 447
Phorias and Other Tests 448
Computation of Stimulus Values 449
Clinical Interpretation 449
Purposes 449
Errors to Consider 450
The Double Parallelogram Model 451
Depth of Focus Effects 452
Blur and Break Interrelationships 452
A Sample Plotting 454
Negative Fusional Convergence Limits 456
Phorias 457
Positive Fusional Convergence Limits 458
The Near Point of Convergence 459
Linearity Considerations and Diagnosis 460
Clinical Criteria of Adequacy 461
Graphical Analysis in Strabismus 461
Orthoptics Specification 462

14. Fixation Disparity and Vergence Adaptation 465
Clifton M. Schor

History 465
Subjective and Objective Measurement 466
Functional Significance of Fixation Disparity 467
Heterophoria 468
Dissociated and Associated Heterophoria 471
Disparity Vergence and Fixation Disparity 472
Horizontal Fixation Disparity 472

Curve Types 473
Vertical Fixation Disparity 473
Panum's Fusional Limit 473
Retinal Eccentricity 474
Adaptation Phenomenon 476
Influence of Prism Adaptation on Curve Type 478
Prism Adaptation and Exposure Duration 481
Fast and Slow Fusional Vergence 484
A Model of Prism Adaptation and Fixation Disparity 485
Computer Simulations 486
Predictions of Fixation Disparity from Modeling 488
Applications to Horizontal and Vertical Fixation Disparity 491
Functional Significance of Prism Adaptation 492
Orthophorization 492
Stability of Binocular Correspondence 492
Maintenance of Hering's Law 494
Clinical Applications of Fixation Disparity 494
Associated Phoria 494
Paradoxical Fixation Disparity 495
Suppression 495
Motor Control Factors 498
Center of Symmetry 499
Accommodative Vergence, Vergence Accommodation, and Fixation Disparity 501
Convergence Accommodation 503
Graphical Analysis of AC/A and CA/C Interactions .. 505
Prism Adaptation Reduces Convergence Accommodation 506
Therapy of Transient and Sustained Disorders 507
Orthoptics 507
Optical Correction with Lenses and Prisms 508
Quantitative Predictions 509
Measurement of the CA/C Ratio 510
Clinical Implication 511
Sensory Disturbances 512
Orthoptics and Curve Type 512

15. Validity of Diagnostic Criteria and Case Analysis in Binocular Vision Disorders 517
James E. Sheedy and J. James Saladin

Phoria and Vergence Analysis 517
Clinical Measurement 517

Normative Clinical Data 518
Clinical Analysis of Normative Data 520
Fixation Disparity Criteria 521
Clinical Measurement of Fixation Disparity 521
Analysis of Fixation Disparity Data 524
Relationship of Fixation Disparity and Phoria-Vergence 529
Relationships of Diagnostic Criteria to Asthenopia 530
Symptoms 530
Arner and Colleagues Study 530
Sheedy and Saladin—First Study 531
Sheedy and Saladin—Second Study 532
Clinical Diagnosis 534
The Problem 534
Fixation Disparity 535
Phoria and Vergence 536
Clinical Treatment 536
Vision Therapy 537
Lenses and Prisms 537
Summary 538

VI. Diagnosis and Treatment of Strabismus 541

16. Kinematics of Normal and Strabismic Eyes 543
Ken Nakayama

Kinematic Laws of Eye Rotation 544
Conventional Coordinate Representation of Listing's Law 546
Implications for Neuromotor Control 547
Why Listing's Law 551
Vergence Eye Movements 553
Clinical Applications of Eye Kinematics 559

17. Surgical Correction of Strabismus 565
Alan B. Scott

Purpose of Surgery 565
Timing of Strabismus Surgery 566
Infantile Strabismus 566
Acquired Childhood Strabismus 567
Acquired Adult Strabismus 567
Physiology of Strabismus Surgery 567
Mechanical Relationships 567
Possible Training of Innervation 568

Recession 568
Resection 568
Effect of the Antagonist 569
Arc of Contact 569
Transposition Operations 572
Complications 576
Alternatives 576

18. Strabismus Diagnosis and Prognosis 579
Nathan Flax

Classification 579
Adaptations 586
Testing 593
Prognosis 595

19. Treatment of Binocular Dysfunctions 605
J. David Grisham

Characteristics of a Vergence Dysfunction 606
Clinical Assessment of Vergence Facility 610
Changing Vergence Dynamics with Orthoptics 612
Principles of Clinical Treatment 614
Prescription of Prism 615
Added Lens Therapy 616
Orthoptics 618
Management of Binocular Insufficiencies 622
Accommodative Insufficiency 623
Heterophoria and Convergence Insufficiency 625
Fusional Vergence Deficiency 627
Nonsurgical Management of Comitant Strabismus and Associated Conditions 629
Optical Management 629
Amblyopia 632
Anomalous Retinal Correspondence 637
Flom Swing Technique 637
Sensory and Motor Fusion Orthoptics 639
Applications of Biofeedback 642

VII. Neurologic Aspects of Vergence Eye Movements 647

20. Neurophysiological Correlates of Vergence Eye Movements 649
Lawrence E. Mays

Innervation of Extraocular Muscles 650
Motoneuron Activity During Saccades 652
Motoneuron Activity During Vergence 653
Functions of Muscle Fiber Types 653
Combining Vergence and Versional Signals 655
Abducens Internuclear Neurons 655
Vergence and Abducens Internuclear Neurons 657
Vergence Signal 659
Cortical Processing of Binocular Disparity 663
Disparity Detectors 663
Other Cortical Areas 664
Corticooculomotor Pathways 665
Overview 666

21. Clinical Dysfunction of the Vergence System 671
Gill Roper-Hall

Control Areas 671
Vergence System 672
Components of the Vergence System 672
Quantitation of Vergence Ability 673
Relationship Between Vergence Ability and Fusion 675
Clinical Disorders Affecting Vergences 676
Differential Diagnosis of True and Pseudovergence Anomalies 678
Classification of Clinical Vergence Dysfunction 679
Convergence Dysfunction 679
Divergence Dysfunction 686
Convergence and Divergence Dysfunction 689
Vertical Vergence Dysfunction 689
Cyclovergence Dysfunction 693
Acquired Fusional Dysfunction 695

Supplementary Glossary of Control System Terminology 699

Name Index 705

Subject Index 713

FOREWORD

Lawrence Stark

The authors considered this book a multi-authored *textbook* from the start and requested the contributing authors to structure their respective chapters, based on their distinguished research and clinical studies of course, but also with pedagogical constraint so as to be accessible to students of vergence and of binocular vision. Indeed, many authors provided historical perspective and guides for future research. All are agreed that in this complex field, future progress will depend on techniques and knowledge derived from a blend of basic research and of clinical insights. The 21 chapters and the appendix have been grouped into seven sections.

Stark introduces the theme of the text, *normal and abnormal vergence*, from a control point of view. Morgan summarizes the Maddox view of vergence. He astutely ascribes the reliance on accommodative vergence to the technology available at that time. Morgan suggests that if Maddox had rearranged his methodology he might have ascribed the "primary" role differently to vergence accommodation.

Owens and Leibowitz begin the section on *tonic and proximal convergence* with a discussion of tonic vergence; its adaptability, e.g. to prisms, and its possible relationship to heterophoria. They believe that perceptual estimates of distance, Gogel's specific distance tendency, are related to the tonic resting level of vergence. They introduce the term dark focus by which they mean the "bias level" of accommodation. Dark focus is not necessarily related to darkness, since empty field and open loop myopia represent similar means to the same end. It is not a focused state of accomodation but, is rather a non-focused setting dependent on vergence and other factors. Hokoda and Ciuffreda review the contribution that proximal vergence makes to vergence and to vergence-accommodation. They conclude that it is a relatively small and variable factor, but that it should be incorporated into future models of the near response.

The section on *interactions between accommodation and conver-*

gence begins with Ciuffreda and Kenyon who review accommodation, accommodative vergence, and the AC/A ratio in normals and in patients with amblyopia and strabismus. They stress recent findings on the role that accommodative-vergence plays compensating for the absence of disparity vergence in these patients. In the next chapter, Semmlow and Hung provide a tour-de-force with their elegant (though still static) model of accommodation and vergence interactions. This model collates many separate experimental results on AC/A and CA/C ratios and provides a consistent platform for the even more exciting work to come.

The *disparity vergence section* begins with Tyler who discusses the afferent side of the disparity vergence system covering such topics as retinal correspondence, the horopter, binocular sensory fusion, and binocular depth processing. His theoretical framework for stereopsis presents a refined and comprehensive model for understanding this elegant neurophysiological mechanism. Jones reviews disparity vergence and suggests that small inputs drive "fusional" vergence while larger inputs drive "disparity" vergence. He defines many of the sensory and motor elements and addresses historical and current research findings. Kertesz proceeds to kinematic aspects of vergence comparing vertical and cyclofusional disparity mechanisms to the classical horizontal system. He reports slower response times for vertical and cyclovergence and frequent violations of Hering's Law for vertical responses. Kertesz emphasizes the importance of a wide field stimulus for cyclovergence and credits Crone with the first objective demonstration of motor cyclovergence; he employed such a wide angle stimulus. Krishnan describes an engineering control model for disparity vergence with a group of systems block diagrams and mechanical circuit element diagrams. These define our physiological knowledge of the biomechanical "plant" consisting of muscle and globe elasticities and viscosities. More hypothetical neurological mechanisms are pictured in terms of integrators, lags, time delays, leaky integrators, and differentiators; a helpful appendix defines these elementary building blocks for dynamical systems. Finally, Ono describes classical studies on the combination of version and vergence by Hering and more recently Yarbus. Hering well understood that Hering's Law applies equally to vergence as to version. Ono then reviews some complexities that modern eye movement studies have documented including violations of Hering's Law and secondary corrections to these violations.

The section on *quantitative analysis of interactions between vergence components* begins with Fry's description of the assumptions underlying the format for graphical representation of vergence components. These assumptions include that there is one kind of accommodation and several forms of vergence, that there are separate mechanisms for convergence and for divergence, and that there is a single brain center for the near triad. He provides evidence supporting some of these assumptions and rejecting others. Hofstetter thoroughly describes the procedure of graphical analysis with specific examples and interpretations for normal binocular vision and strabismus. Schor provides a historical and updated description of disparity vergence adaptation and its interactions with accommodation, fixation disparity, and the various components of vergence. He presents a new form of graphical analysis which allows clinicians to quantify the complex interactions between accommodation and convergence. Sheedy and Saladin describe the use of fixation disparity as an alternative to the classical case analysis of binocular vision. Fixation disparity is interpreted as manifest stress on the disparity vergence system. Forced vergence fixation disparity provides a performance test of the vergence system as it reacts to various optical, sensory, and motor manipulations.

The section on *strabismus* begins with Nakayama's description of kinematics of normal and strabismic eyes. He provides an insightful view of Listing's Law and presents a convincing argument for its basis in neurological control. Scott describes the many complex variables encountered in surgical procedures for the cosmetic and functional correction of strabismus. This shows the solid clinical background that serves as the basis for his recent clinical trials of botulinin toxin to readjust ocular muscles. Flax presents a thorough classification of strabismus including motor alignment direction and angle of deviation, comitance and variability, frequency of deviation, age of onset, and associated sensory anomalies. He considers the effect of each of these variables upon the prognosis for functional correction of strabismus. Grisham reviews the pragmatic nonsurgical therapeutic procedures for rehabilitation of various accommodative and convergence insufficiencies as well as sensory and motor anomalies associated with strabismus.

The section on *neurology* begins with Mays who reviews the neurophysiological correlates of vergence eye movements including the muscle fiber types, the motorneuronal studies of Keller and Robinson and of Schiller, the exclusion of vergence signals from the abducens intranuclear neurons of the medial longitudinal fasciculus, his own work on a candidate "vergence neuron" in the midbrain, (he cautions us about these neurons because of the synkinesis of the triad), and finally, cortical disparity cells. [New work by Jean Buttner-Ennever suggests that the small-celled subgroup of medical rectus neurons near the Edinger-Westphal complex project to orbital, small fibered components of the medical rectus muscle]. Gill Roper-Hall reviews neurologic disorders that may disturb control areas or pathways serving conjugate and disjugate eye movements. This review is supplemented by case reports illustrating clinical disorders affecting vergences. Finally, Professor George Hung and associate provide a helpful supplemental glossary of control system terminology.

The editors, Schor, and Ciuffreda are to be congratulated on the care and patience that attended their efforts. This volume will be appreciated by students, researchers, and clinicians interested in vergence for many years to come.

Preface

The forward placement of the eyes in the head as a result of the phylogenetic development of binocular vision in vertebrates has been made functionally possible by the simultaneous development of vergence eye movements. The function of these disjunctive eye movements is to support depth-finding and range-finding mechanisms. Binocular vision in humans is based on the physiological combination of information processed by the two eyes so that binocular disparate images referenced to the horopter can stimulate stereoscopic depth perception.

Horizontal vergence eye movements provide a means for moving the zero-disparity horopter reference over a range of viewing distances, thereby reducing disparities subtended by objects in space to within the disparity range of quantitative stereoscopic depth perception. The motor control of the vergence system is also used to scale large qualitative disparities into veridical quantitative depth intervals and provide depth constancy independent of viewing distance.

Operation of the highly sophisticated vergence system relies on underlying control mechanisms receiving input from a variety of stimuli. Maddox was the first to address the problem of multiple control mechanisms of vergence in his book titled *The clinical use of prisms.* (1886) He proposed that there was a hierarchy of vergence mechanisms including tonic, accommodative, proximal, and fusional vergence. The first three were thought to operate independently in response to their stimuli (intrinsic innervation, blur, and nearness, respectively). Fusional vergence was believed to correct any remaining vergence error by responding to the residual retinal-image disparity. Maddox's contribution provides the basis for modern-day quantitative analysis of binocular oculomotor disorders.

Since then, the mechanisms of vergence control have been further elucidated. This book describes the elaborate structure supporting the control of vergence eye movements and the anomalies that may result from its breakdown. The chapters are organized into seven sections including (I) overview of Maddox vergence components, (II) tonic and proximal vergence, (III) interactions between accommodation and vergence, (IV) disparity vergence, (V) case analysis of binocular disorders excluding strabismus and CNS disorders, (VI) diagnosis and treatment of strabismus, and (VII) neurologic aspects of vergence eye movements. Most sections begin with basic aspects of the vergence system and conclude with diagnosis and treatment of clinical anomalies.

This book is the combined effort of researchers and clinicians from a variety of backgrounds including optometry, bioengineering, psychology, physiology, ophthalmology, orthoptics, and neurology. The authors provide a comprehensive and up-to-date description of all aspects of the vergence system. The basic chapters provide insight into anomalies of binocular vision by presenting a framework to describe their neural, anatomical and functional characteristics. The clinical chapters provide both a historical perspective and the most current diagnostic and therapeutic methods available for the management of anomalies of binocular vision. This collection represents an indispensable resource to vision care practitioners.

Clifton M. Schor
Kenneth J. Ciuffreda

Acknowledgments

Chapter 3: Perceptual and Motor Consequences of Tonic Vergence, by D. Alfred Owens and Herschel W. Leibowitz.
Preparation of this chapter was supported in part by grants EY-03898 and EY-03276 from the National Eye Institute.

Chapter 4: Theoretical and Clinical Importance of Proximal Vergence and Accomodation, by Steven C. Hokoda and Kenneth J. Ciuffreda.
We thank Drs. Flax, Lewis, Mathews, Schneider and Suchoff for their helpful comments on an earlier version of the manuscript. Preparation of this chapter was supported in part by NIH grant EY03541 to Kenneth J. Ciuffreda.

Chapter 5: Accommodative Vergence and Accommodation in Normals, Amblyopes, and Strabismics, by Kenneth J. Ciuffreda and Robert V. Kenyon.
We thank Drs. S. Hokoda, A. Lewis, and C. Schor for their helpful comments on an earlier version of the manuscript. Preparation of this chapter was supported in part by NIH grant EY03541 to Kenneth J. Ciuffreda.

Chapter 7: Sensory Processing of Binocular Disparity, by Christopher W. Tyler.
My thanks to James Brodale for the graphics, to Maureen Clarke for pro-

gramming the autostereograms, and to Professors I. P. Howard and S. M. Anstis for their comments on the manuscript.

Chapter 8: Horizontal Disparity Vergence, by Ronald Jones.
This chapter was supported by grant RO1 EYO-2532 from the National Eye Institute.

Chapter 9: Vertical and Cyclofusional Disparity Vergence, by Andrew E. Kertesz.
This chapter was supported in part by research grant EY-1055 from the National Eye Institute.

Chapter 11: The Combination of Version and Vergence, by Hiroshi Ono.
I wish to thank my colleagues in Perception at York University and the many others who have been involved in this research and in the preparation of this chapter.

Chapter 14: Fixation Disparity and Vergence Adaptation, by Clifton M. Schor
Preparation of this chapter was supported by NEI grant EY-02573.

Chapter 16: Kinematics of Normal and Strabismic Eyes, by Ken Nakayama.
I wish to thank Drs. Alan Scott and Arthur Jampolsky for patient referral. This chapter was supported by NIH grants 5 RO1 EY-01582 and 5P30-EY-01186, and by the Smith-Kettlewell Eye Research Foundation.

Chapter 17: Surgical Correction of Strabismus, by Alan B. Scott.
This chapter was supported in part by NIH grant EY-01186.

Chapter 20: Neurophysiological Correlates of Vergence Eye Movements, by Lawrence E. Mays.
This chapter was supported by National Eye Institute grants EY-01189 to D. L. Sparks and EY-03463 to L. E. Mays and a core facility grant EY-03039.

Chapter 21: Clinical Dysfunction of the Vergence System, by Gill Roper-Hall.
Grateful thanks are given to Ronald M. Burde, M.D., Professor of Ophthalmology, Neurology, and Neurosurgery, for his help and guidance in the preparation of this chapter, and the time and patience expended in editing the manuscript.

I

OVERVIEW OF MADDOX VERGENCE COMPONENTS

1
Normal and Abnormal Vergence

Lawrence Stark

In this brief introductory chapter is assembled a background of the control aspects of vergence eye movements.

NORMAL CONTROL OF VERGENCE

The vergence mechanism performs under both symmetric and asymmetric target conditions. The symmetric paradigm is classical because of the absence of saccadic and smooth pursuit versional movements (Figure 1.1). Vergence obeys Hering's law (Hering, 1868), with corresponding muscles different from those for versional eye movements. By algebraic addition and subtraction of the efforts of versional and vergence corresponding muscles, the two eyes can be pointed in any direction. The asymmetric experiment has become an important proof of Hering's law (Alpern and Ellen, 1956; Westheimer and Mitchell, 1956). Here an asymmetric target jumps along the line of sight of one eye and produces in the aligned eye a paradoxical versional saccade and an opposite vergence movement that pull the eye off its line of sight and then restore it. Contrast this with the Mueller accommodative vergence experiment. That the controller vergence is highly precise has been accepted since the study of Riggs and Niehl (1960) using their elegant binocular contact lens method. Recent work questioning precision of vergence, especially when the head is also

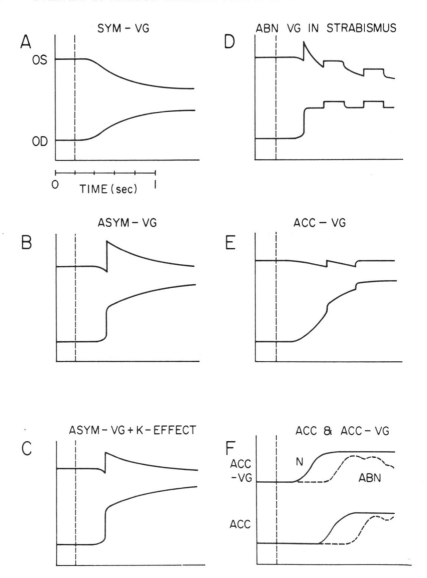

FIGURE 1.1. Vergence eye movements. A) Symmetrical vergence. Vertical dashed line indicates instant of target distance change; upward on ordinate is leftward for left eye, OS, and right eye, OD, time in seconds on abscissa. B) Asymmetrical vergence with target change along axis of left eye. Note initial vergence, then leftward equal saccades, then continuing vergence movements. C) Asymmetrical vergence showing unequal saccades—the sign of the Kenyon effect due to peripheral neuromuscular interaction; initial conditions set by vergence velocity truncated amplitude of oppositely-going saccade. D) Abnormal vergence in a patient with strabismus showing asymmetrical response (like Figure 1.1C)

rotated, has called the Riggs and Niehl result into question (Steinman and Collewijn, 1980), but adequate calibration of the kinematics aspects of this new instrumentation should expose likely experimental artifacts (Larsen and Stark, personal communication, 1981). Kinematic aspects of vergence are of importance since vertical and cyclovergence eye movements occur (Crone and Everhard-Halm, 1975; Hooten et al., 1979).

Control studies by Zuber, Stark (1968) and Krishnan and Stark (1977) (block diagram), following early physiological work by Rashbass, and Westheimer, (1961) have provided explicit bioengineering models (Figure 1.2) for the vergence system as well as a Bode diagram (Figure 1.3) indicating basic frequency response functions. These models will, of course, be corrected and developed by future researchers such as the other contributors to this volume. Finally, the leaky integrator or imperfect memory in vergence and accommodation (Krishnan and Stark, 1975) has a time constant varying from 5 to 15 seconds and allows the vergence system to drift to its phoria position when made "open-loop," as with the cover test maneuver (Krishnan and Stark, 1977) (Figure 1.3).

VERGENCE MAIN SEQUENCE

The dynamics of the vergence movement is apparently not at all limited by the basic dynamic elements of the extraocular muscle system in contrast to the time optimal, very fast saccadic eye movement (Cook and Stark, 1968; Clark and Stark, 1975). (Just recently, Jean Beuttner-Evener has observed a small-celled, presumably slower portion of medial rectus nucleus lying close to the Edinger-Westphal nucleus.) Rather, neurologic control produces a step-envelope of reciprocally innervated, as postulated

to a symmetrical stimulus (compare with Figure 1.1A) and also multiple saccadic intrusions. E) Accommodative vergence showing some vergence in the viewing left eye (in the spirit of Hering's Law but with greatly reduced amplitude) that is corrected by small saccades in response to a developing fixation error. F) Triadic disfacility with slowing of abnormal (ABN) accommodative-vergence (ACC-VG) (dashed lines) as well as accommodation (ACC); compare with normal (N) responses. Normal (N) and abnormal (ABN) accommodative-vergence (upper traces) and normal (solid line) and abnormal (dashed line) accommodation (lower traces). In normal responses accommodation lags accommodative-vergence (400 ms vs 180 ms); both are further delayed in abnormal cases due to central nervous system deficits (not accommodative neuro-muscular delay); note also poorly sustained tonic or dc response. Figure F from Liu JS, Lee M, Jang J, Ciuffreda KJ, Wong JH, Grisham D, Stark L, Objective assessment of accommodation orthoptics. I. Dynamic insufficiency, American Journal of Optometry and Physiological Optics.

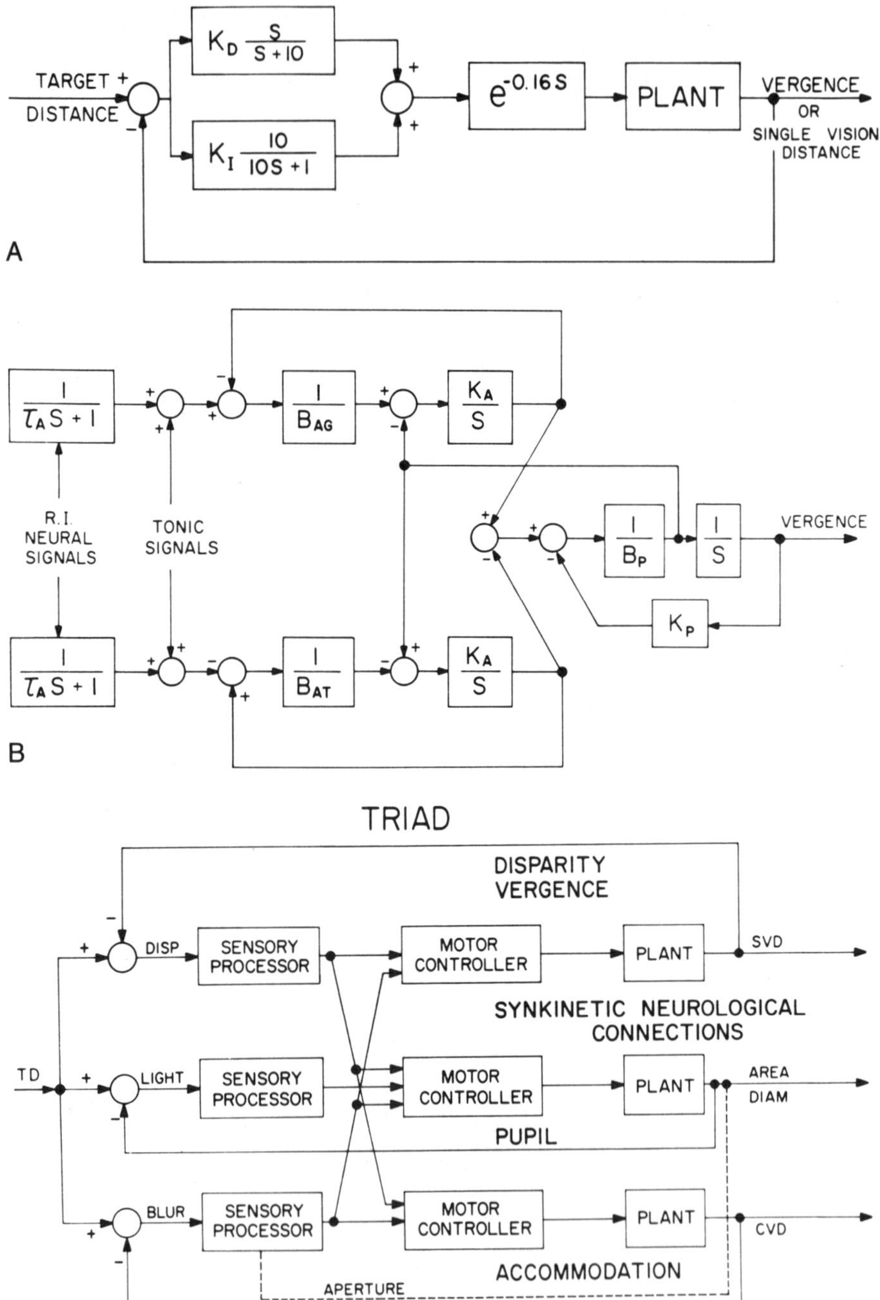
TARGET
DISTANCE
$K_D \frac{S}{S+10}$
$K_I \frac{10}{10S+1}$
$e^{-0.16S}$
PLANT
VERGENCE
OR
SINGLE VISION
DISTANCE
A
$\frac{1}{\tau_A S+1}$
$\frac{1}{B_{AG}}$
$\frac{K_A}{S}$
R.I.
NEURAL
SIGNALS
TONIC
SIGNALS
$\frac{1}{B_P}$
$\frac{1}{S}$
VERGENCE
K_P
$\frac{1}{\tau_A S+1}$
$\frac{1}{B_{AT}}$
$\frac{K_A}{S}$
B
TRIAD
DISPARITY
VERGENCE
DISP
SENSORY
PROCESSOR
MOTOR
CONTROLLER
PLANT
SVD
SYNKINETIC NEUROLOGICAL
CONNECTIONS
TD
LIGHT
SENSORY
PROCESSOR
MOTOR
CONTROLLER
PLANT
AREA
DIAM
PUPIL
BLUR
SENSORY
PROCESSOR
MOTOR
CONTROLLER
PLANT
CVD
ACCOMMODATION
APERTURE
C

by Descartes (Ciuffreda and Stark, 1975), change in motor neuronal firing that results in a quasi-exponential movement lasting approximately 500 msec with a velocity approximately proportional to the amplitude; for example, a 5-degree vergence movement has a 50-degree-per-second velocity. Main sequence data presented (Figure 1.4) have been contributed by Miller (1972), Bahill and Stark (1979), and Kenyon, Ciuffreda, and Stark (1980). The difference between the saccade and the vergence controller signals, acceleration, and velocities can be seen in the model results of Hsu, Bahill, and Stark (1976). Important asymmetric dynamics for convergence and divergence were noted in the experiments of Krishnan and Stark; adjustments of the proportional-integral-differential model enables the model to capture these nonlinear effects (Figures 1.2 and 1.3).

It is important to distinguish between vergence and glissades, the results of pulse step mismatches in saccades (Weber and Daroff, 1972; Easter, 1973; Bahill, Clark, and Stark, 1975; Bahill, Hsu, and Stark, 1978). Glissades are most often monocular and represent dynamic violations of Hering's law (Bahill et al., 1976). Also, glissades do not have the 150- to 200-msec latency between the occurrence of a retinal disparity and the commencement of the binocular disjunctive vergence eye movement. Long-term adaptive changes in vergence dynamics have been described by Carter, Schor, and others and are reviewed in this volume.

TRIADIC ROLE OF VERGENCE

The important synkineses between accommodation and vergence, which also includes the pupil mechanism, has been known for many years (Donders, 1864; Hering, 1868). It is characterized by lower-level motor synkineses or movement together, which is to the greatest extent difficult to be modified. The block diagram (Figure 1.2) that I have used since 1969

FIGURE 1.2. Block diagrams for vergence control. A) Classical PID (proportional-integral-derivative) feedback control model with derivative (K_d) and integral (K_i) paths with their differing time constants; also a time delay of 160 ms; the feedback control is through vision; the plant is detailed in Fig. 1.2B; "s" is the Laplace transform operator. B) Reciprocal innervation (R-I) signals plus tonic signals control the agonist-antagonist pain of muscles; the nonlinear force-velocity relationships (BAG & BAT) are important; other elements include series and parallel elasticities (K_a & K_p) and passive viscosity (B_p). C) Triadic synkinesis between vergence, accommodation and pupil. Note the neurological synkinetic connections. With a disparity error and thus without a target on the fovea the accommodation system cannot act as an error actuated feedback control system and is thus "open loop." Figures A and B are adapted from Krishnan VV, Stark L. A heuristic model for the human vergence eye movement system. Engineers Transactions in Biomedical Engineering, © 1977 IEEE. Reproduced by permission of the publisher.

A

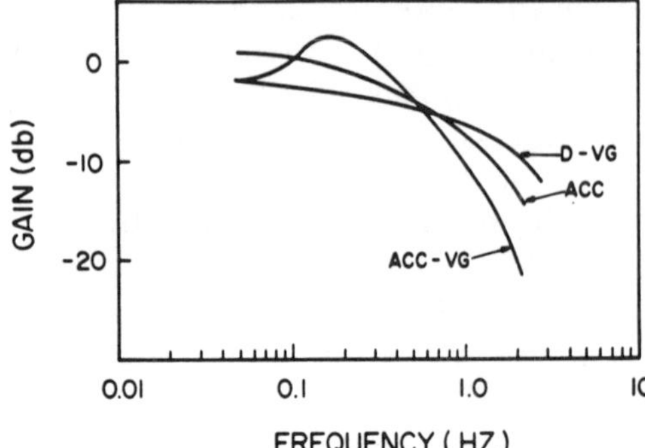
GAIN (db)
0
-10
-20
D - VG
ACC
ACC - VG
0.01
0.1
1.0
10
FREQUENCY (HZ)

B

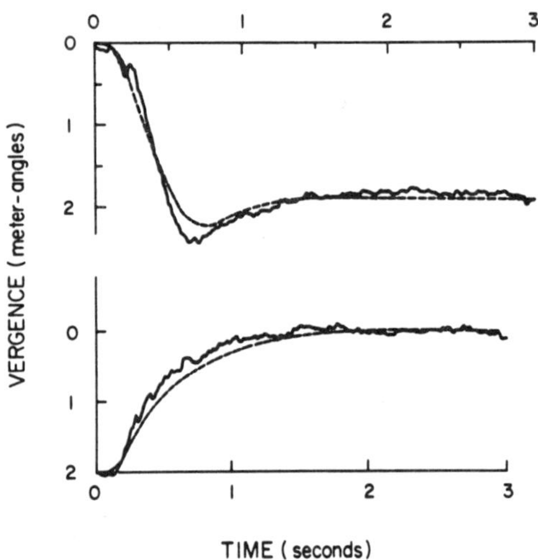
VERGENCE (meter-angles)
0
1
2
3
TIME (seconds)

C

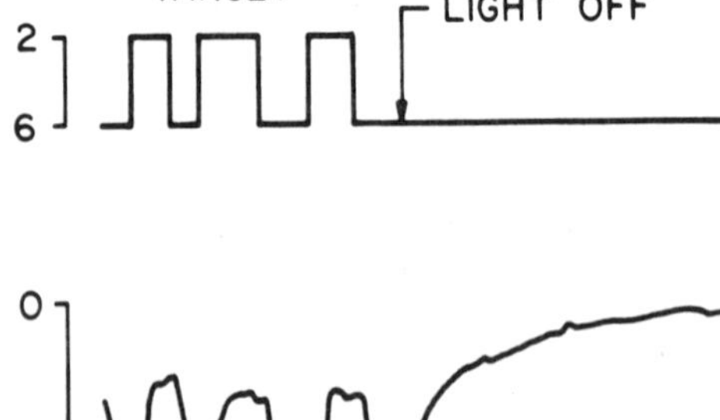
TARGET
LIGHT OFF
2
6
0
6

in teaching the physiological optics of the triad (PO 129) shows these important neurologic interconnections. The zone of single clear binocular vision represents the range within which the dead space of accommodation, increased by pupillary constriction, enables the triadic system to handle noncongruent stimuli (Morgan, 1980; Alpern, 1950). At the edge of the zone of single clear binocular vision, the sensory-visual and oculomotor brain mechanisms have a choice either to accept blur and maintain vergence or to accept disparity and maintain accommodation.

Dynamic triadic responses (Brodkey and Stark, 1967a; 1967b) have been reported by O'Neill and Stark (1968), Yoshida and Watanabe (1969; 1972), and by Krishnan, Phillips, and Stark (1973) (Figure 1.3A); the pupil is also driven both by accommodation (Semmlow and Stark, 1973) and by vergence. This point is substantiated by the results of Marg and Morgan (1949; 1950a, 1950b) who, unfortunately, misinterpreted the extent of vergence synkinetic drive of the pupil by using noncommensurate units. Recent latency data, extending the work of Krishnan, Shirachi, and Stark, (1977), by Myers suggests indirect control of the pupil by synkinetic outflow of the vergence system.

Since the disparity stimulus is not degraded by blurring (Jones and Kerr, 1972), and since the blur stimulus to accommodation is not effective off the fovea (Phillips and Stark, 1977), it seems apparent that when a large disparity occurs, disparity vergence will be the primary optomotor response. When disparity is removed and the target appears on the foveas of both retinas, accommodation can respond to the new value of blur. Of course, vergence accommodation driven synkinetically and almost synchronously with the disparity vergence will have occurred in the interval. While the blur signal is off the foveas, the accommodation system may

←

FIGURE 1.3. Dynamics of vergence. A) Frequency response gain curves for disparity vergence (D-VA); accommodation, ACC; and accommodative-vergence, ACC-VG. The peak in ACC-VG suggest the synkinetic pathway or its synaptic connections contribute additional dynamics in addition to a gain (Reprinted with permission from Vision Research, 13, Krishnan VV, Phillips S, Stark L, Frequency analysis of accommodative vergence and disparity vergence, 1973, Pergamon Press, Ltd.) B) Dynamics of convergence (upper traces) and divergence (lower traces) with excellent fit of I-D model (Figure 1.2A) in dashed lines to experimental data in solid lines with noise; note especially the areas in convergence with measured gains of the model operators. Figure B is adapted from Krishnan VV, Stark L. A heuristic model for the human vergence eye movement system. Engineers Transactions in Biomedical Engineering, © 1977 IEEE. Reproduced by permission of the publisher. C) Leaky integrator in vergence control is demonstrated by the slow divergence (lower trace) with light off (arrow in upper trace); note in contrast rapid control dynamics to target moving between 2 and 6 meter angles (50 and 17 cm) distance. Figure C is adapted from Krishnan VV, Stark L. Integral control in accommodation. Computer Programs in Biomedicine, Elsevier Biomedical Press B.V., 1975. Reprinted by permission of the publisher.

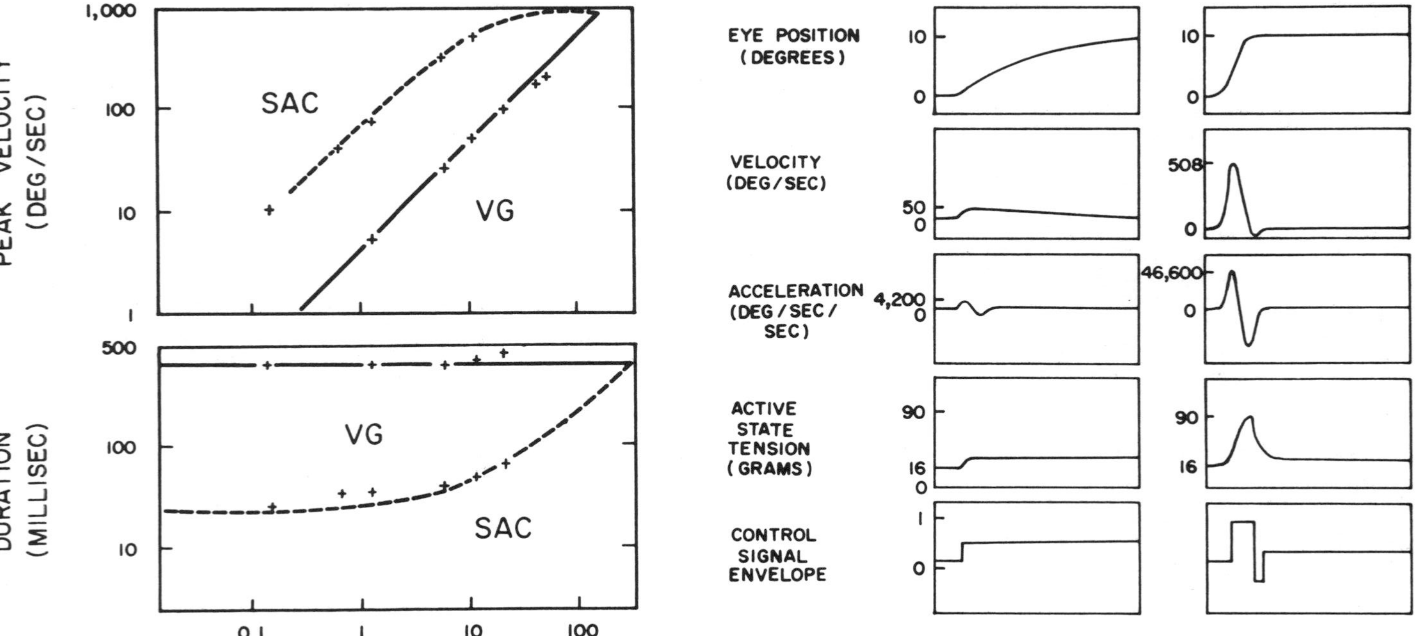

FIGURE 1.4. Dynamical fine structure of vergence eye movements. (A & B) Main sequence with peak velocity-amplitude relationship (A) vergences (VG) and saccades (SAC) and with duration-amplitude relationship (B). Note quasi-linear control behavior of vergence. (C-G) Model responses for vergence (left panel) and saccades (right panel) showing agonist control signal envelopes (G), active state tensims (hypothecated in AV Hill model) (F), acceleration (E), velocity (D) and eye position (C). Note modest values for vergence (left panel) as compared with time optimal dynamics of saccades (right panel). Adapted from Trajectories of saccadic eye movements, Bahill AT, Stark L.

be thought of as "open-loop" (Krishnan and Stark, 1977). This sequence of events is opposed to the Maddox hierarchy concept. See also reviews by Morgan (1980) and Semmlow and Hung (1980).

ABNORMALITIES OF VERGENCE

Disparity is a binocular signal (Stark et al., 1980); it was most interesting to learn that in patients with strabismus and amblyopia, the occurrence of disparity vergence was blocked (Kenyon, Ciuffreda, and Stark, 1980a). (The stimuli in these clinical studies were relatively restricted. We know that wide field stimuli are necessary for cyclovergence (Crone & Everhard-Halm, 1975 and Hooten et al., 1979) and also that increased saccadic latencies occur in amblyopia in the "near periphery", within 8 degrees of the fovea. Thus it may be possible to circumvent the suppression of amblyopia and strabismus and obtain horizontal vergence movements in these patients with wide angle disparity stimuli.) These patients then showed the surprising appearance of accommodative vergence (Kenyon, Ciuffreda, and Stark, 1980a; 1980c) (Figure 1.1D) that acts to keep the nondominant eyes bifixated approximately given the strabismic error (Kenyon, Ciuffreda, and Stark, 1980a). These abnormal responses include two further abnormalities, the occurrence of saccadic intrusions (Ciuffreda, Kenyon, and, Stark, 1979) in strabismus and the Kenyon effect, a peripheral interaction between the ongoing accommodative vergence movement and the very rapid saccade (Figure 1.1C). To achieve the normal, very high velocities of saccades, the eye must not be concomitantly moving in the opposite direction. Such opposing initial velocities degrade the ability of the brief pulse of extraocular muscle force to accelerate the eyeball and produce high-velocity saccades (Kenyon, Ciuffreda, and Stark, 1980b).

The accommodative vergence response is most helpful in diagnosing different types of accommodative disfacility (Liu et al., 1979). Most often the disfacility is due to a deficit in controller signal generation in the central nervous system, even though clinicians may mistakenly attribute it to weakness or slowness of the ciliary muscle. By measuring accommodative vergence, we can demonstrate (Figure 1.1F) that central nervous system lags often do produce this dynamic insufficiency since accommodative vergence is often slowed and delayed as is accommodation.

REFERENCES

Alpern M. The zone of clear single vision at the upper levels of accommodation and convergence. Am J Optom Arch Am Acad Optom 1950;27(10):491–513.

Alpern M, Ellen P. A quantitative analysis of the horizontal movements of the eyes in the experiment. Am J Ophthalmol 1956;42(4):289–96.

Bahill AT, Clark MR, and Stark L. Glissades—eye movements generated by mismatched components of the saccadic motoneural control signal. Math Biosci 1975;26:303–18.

Bahill AT, Ciuffreda KJ, Kenyon R, Stark L. Dynamic and static violations of Hering's law of equal innervation. Am J Optom Physiol Opt 1976;53:786–96.

Bahill AT, Hsu FK, Stark L. Glissadic overshoots are due to pulse width errors. Arch Neurol 1978;35:138–42.

Bahill AT, Stark L. Trajectories of saccadic eye movements. Sci Am 1979;240:84–93.

Brodkey J, Stark, L. Accommodative convergence: an adaptive nonlinear control system. IEEE Trans Systems Sci Cybernet 1967a;SSC-3:121–33.

Brodkey J, Stark L. Feedback control analysis of accommodative convergence. Am J Surg 1967b;114:150–58.

Ciuffreda KJ, Stark L. Descartes law of reciprocal innervation. Am J Optom Physiol Opt 1975;52:663–73.

Ciuffreda KJ, Kenyon RV, Stark L. Saccadic intrusions in strabismus. Arch Opthalmol 1979;97:1673–79.

Clark MR, Stark L. Time optimal behavior of human saccadic eye movement. IEEE Trans. Automatic Control 1975;AC-20:345–48.

Cook G, Stark L. The human eye-movement mechanism: experiments, modelling and model testing. Arch Ophthalmol 1968;79:428–36.

Crone RA, Everhard-Halm Y. Optically induced eye torsion. Albrecht Von Graefes Arch Klin Ophthalmol 1975;196:231–37.

Donders FC. On the anomalies of accommodation and refraction of the eye; with a preliminary essay on physiological dioptrics. London: New Sydenham Society, 1864.

Easter SS. A comment on the "glissade." Vision Res 1973;13:881–82.

Hering E. The theory of binocular vision (1868). Bridgeman B, Stark L, eds, trans. New York: Plenum Press, 1977:1–210.

Hooten K, Myers E, Worrall R, Stark L. Cyclovergence: the motor response to cyclodisparity. Albrecht Von Graefes Arch Klin Ophthalmol 1979;210:65–68.

Hsu FK, Bahill AT, Stark L. Parametric sensitivity analysis of a homeomorphic model for saccadic and vergence eye movements. Comput Programs Biomed 1976;6:108–16.

Jones R, Kerr KE. Vergence eye movements to pairs of disparite stimuli with shape selection cues. Vision Res 1972;12(8):1425–30.

Kenyon RV, Ciuffreda KJ, Stark L. Dynamic vergence eye movements in strabismus and amblyopia: symmetric vergence. Invest. Ophthalmol Vis Sci 1980a;19:60–74.

Kenyon RV, Ciuffreda KJ, Stark L. Unequal saccades during vergence. Am J Optom Physiol Opt 1980b;57:586–94.

Kenyon RV, Ciuffreda KJ, Stark L. An unexpected role for normal accommodative vergence in strabismus and amblyopia. Am J Optom Physiol Opt 1980c;57:566–77.

Krishnan VV, Phillips S, Stark L. Frequency analysis of accommodation, accommodative vergence and disparity vergence. Vision Res 1973;13:1545–53.

Krishnan VV, Shirachi D, Stark L. Dynamic measures of vergence accommodation. Am J Optom Physiol Opt 1977;54:470–73.

Krishnan VV, Stark L. Integral control in accommodation. Comput Programs Biomed 1975;4:237–45.

Krishnan VV, Stark L. A heuristic model for the human vergence eye movement system. IEEE Trans Biomed Eng 1977;BME-24:44–49.

Liu JS, Lee M, Jang J, et al. Objective assessment of accommodation orthoptics. I. Dynamic insufficiency. Am J Optom Physiol Opt 1979;56:285–94.

Marg E, Morgan M, Jr. The pupillary near reflex: the relation of pupillary diameter to accommodation and the various components of convergence. Am J Optom Arch Am Acad Optom 1949;67:1–16.

Marg E, Morgan M, Jr. Further investigation of the pupillary near reflex: the effect of accommodation, fusional convergence, and the proximity factor on pupillary diameter. Am J Optom Arch Am Acad Optom 1950a;96:1–9.

Marg E, Morgan M, Jr. The pupillary fusion reflex. Arch Ophthalmol 1950b;43:871–78.

Miller PJ. Dynamics of voluntary vergence in intermittent exotropia. Master of Science in Mechanical Engineering, Univ Calif Berkeley 1972

Morgan MW. The Maddox classification of vergence eye movements. Am J Optom Physiol Opt 1980;57(9):537–39.

O'Neill WD, Stark L. Triple function ocular monitor. J Opt Soc Am 1968;58:570–73.

Phillips S, Stark L. Blur: a sufficient accommodative stimulus. Doc Ophthalmol 1977;43(1):65–89.

Rashbass C, and Westheimer G. Disjunctive eye movements. J Physiol (London) 1961;159:339–360.

Riggs LA, Niehl EW. Eye movements recorded during convergence and divergence. J Opt Soc Am 1960;50(9):913–30.

Semmlow JL, Hung GK. Binocular interactions of vergence components. Am J Optom Physiol Opt 1980;57(9):559–65.

Semmlow JL, Stark L. Pupil movements to light and accommodative stimulation: a comparative study. Vision Res 1973;13:1087–1100.

Stark L, Kenyon RV, Krishnan VV, Ciuffreda KJ. Disparity vergence: a proposed name for a dominant component of binocular vergence eye movements. Am J Optom Physiol Opt 1980;57:606–09.

Steinman RM, Collewijn H. Binocular retinal image motion during active head rotation. Vision Res 1980;20:415–29.

Weber RB, Daroff RB. Corrective movements following refixation saccades: type and control systems analysis. Vision Res 1972;12:467–75.

Westheimer G, Mitchell AM. Eye movement responses to convergence stimuli. Arch Ophthalmol 1956;55(6):848–56.

Yoshida T, Watanabe A. Analysis of interaction between accommodation and vergence feedback control systems of human eyes. NHK T Broadcasting Sci. Res Labs. 1969;3:72–80.

Yoshida T, Watanabe A. Analysis of the interaction between vergence eye-movement and accommodation. Bull NHK Broadcasting Sci Res Lab 1972;6:29–36.

Zuber BL, and Stark L. Dynamical characteristics of the fusional vergence eye-movement system, IEEE Transactions Systems Science and Cybernetics, 1968;SSC-4:72–79.

2

The Maddox Analysis of Vergence

Meredith W. Morgan

The first complete description of the Maddox classification of vergence eye movements appeared in 1893 in the second edition of his small book, *The clinical use of prisms; and the decentering of lenses.*

Maddox was primarily a clinician writing from clinical experience for the benefit of other clinicians rather than a scientist reporting the results of controlled experiments. As he states in the extract from the preface of the first edition, "The first object [of the book] was to communicate a series of aids to precision in the use of prisms, worked out during several years, which it is hoped will be of some service in this difficult by-way of ophthalmic practice" (p. vii). His thinking was influenced by Donders, Hering, Landolt, von Graefe, LeConte, Stevens, Percival, Prentice, and Risley, as noted on direct references to their publications and concepts, but strangely he makes no reference to Helmholtz. He was familiar with the concepts of relative accommodation (Donders), relative convergence (Donders and Landolt), latent deviations (von Graefe and Stevens), zones of comfort (Donders, Landolt, and Percival) prism diopters[1] (Prentice), and variable prisms (Risley). As Maddox stated, "To prescribe prisms satisfactorily it is necessary to know something of the physiology of convergence, our knowledge of which, however, is still

[1] Although he was familiar with the simplicity and directness of designating vergence movements in prism diopters, he used either degrees or meter angles.

very incomplete. According to Hering's well-proved theory, both eyes move together as though they were a single organ" (p. 83).

Maddox proposed that the total vergence or disjunctive movements required to bifixate any object could be factored into various, more or less independent additive components, each of which was related to the "physiology of convergence," to some identifiable aspect of the stimulus situation, or to both.

> Strictly speaking, there are four elements of convergence, though the first and third are perhaps closely related. The four are: (1) Tonic; (2) Accommodative; (3) Convergence due to "knowledge of nearness", or in other words, "voluntary convergence", for we cannot, without special practice, converge the eyes voluntarily, under ordinary conditions, without doing so by thinking of a near object; (4) fusion convergence. (p. 106)

Tonic vergence, the initial component of vergence, moves the eyes from some undeterminable position of anatomic rest (which Maddox thought would be a position of considerable divergence) to a position in which the object of regard is imaged on the fovea of at least one eye by way of the fixation process. If the object is not located in the midsagittal plane, independent version movement of both eyes will accompany the vergence movement. If the fixated object is at some distance, and if any ametropia has been corrected, the object will be seen clearly. The amount of the tonic vergence induced by the fixation reflex may be exactly right so that the fixated object is imaged on both foveas simultaneously; on the other hand, it may be insufficient or excessive. In these cases reflex or fusional vergence is "added" to tonic vergence to achieve bifoveal fixation.

To determine whether tonic vergence is insufficient or excessive, fusion must be prevented, as it is in the determination of the distance heterophoria. Clinically, the magnitude of tonic vergence cannot be measured since it is not possible to determine the anatomic position of rest. It is possible, however, to determine the degree of insufficiency of tonic vergence (magnitude of any manifest exophoria) or excess (magnitude of any manifest esophoria).

The primary stimulus to tonic vergence is visual—the desire to look at something and the necessity of imaging fixated objects on the fovea. In addition, Maddox identified two essentially nonvisual factors (factors associated with the "physiology of convergence") that could influence the magnitude of tonic vergence. One of these is the tonus exhibited by living, physiologically active, striated muscle. The other factor Maddox called "persistent activity of the converging innervation" (p. 90), which relates to the midbrain control mechanism of the vergence mechanism. The level or magnitude of this persistent activity, Maddox believed, was influenced by factors such as sleep, drowsiness, alcohol, anesthetic agents, and ultimately, by death. In addition, he thought that it was influenced by knowledge of the distance of objects in space and the constant use of some degree of vergence needed for bifixation.

Diplopia will result if tonic vergence does not establish bifoveal fixation. According to Maddox, this disparity would then induce a fusional vergence movement, a "fusional supplement" to tonic vergence to achieve simultaneous bifoveal fixation. While he clearly identifies disparity as the stimulus to fusional supplementary vergence, he hints at a constant use stimulus element to fusional vergence, a conditioned response of sorts. To avoid diplopia, where tonic vergence is inexact (?), "the joint sensations in the brain must all the while be bearing between them the message of continually impending (yet as quickly averted) double vision, by threats of double images, so slight and frequent, that they produce the required effect without our being conscious of their existence" (p. 87).

Thus with ametropia corrected, bifoveal fixation is achieved for distant objects by tonic vergence plus fusional supplementary reflex vergence.

> In near vision, there is an intermediate grade—the accommodative. If one eye be occluded by the hand while vision is directed first to a distant object, and then to a near one, the occluded eye deviates inwards under the hand from an impulse to convergence, which is due chiefly to sympathy with accommodation, but also to the habit of converging where attention is directed to a near object. The second grade of convergence is therefore added on to the first or tonic grade, and its amount depends, of course, on the amount of accommodation in exercise. As a rule, each diopter of accommodation is accompanied by about three-quarters of a meter angle of associated convergence, so that (for) a typical emmetrope, the 4D of accommodation in exercise for vision at a quarter of a meter, are accompanied by 3 m.a. of convergence, leaving a deficit of 1 m.a. to be made up reflexly. . . . (p. 95)

While Maddox stated that the amount of accommodative convergence was a function of the amount of accommodation required for accurate focus, he recognized that it was really the effort of accommodation that determined the amount of accommodative convergence. He noted that the magnitude of accommodative convergence was increased when accommodation was partially paralyzed by atropine and that it was decreased when accommodation was made easier by eserine.

In the fixation of a near object there would be the customary tonic vergence to which would be added accommodative convergence. If these two components were not exact, a fusional supplementary vergence due to disparity would be induced, either positive to make up for any deficiency of tonic plus accommodative convergence, or negative to make up for excess tonic plus accommodative convergence.

In addition to recognizing four components of vergence, Maddox understood that reflex vergence had a relative range that could be determined by finding "the strongest pair of abducting prisms . . . and then the strongest pair of adducting prisms . . . compatible with single distinct vision of an object or type at some chosen distance. . . . The results obtained vary not only according to the peculiarities of the individual, but according to the method pursued. Thus if we test the negative side of the range first, the positive side will be smaller than if we begin with it first. As a rule, the limit of the negative part shows itself by the appearance of diplopia, and the positive part by indistinctness from commencing excess of accommodation" (pp. 111, 122).

Before summarizing my understanding of the Maddox classification of vergence eye movements I wish to quote from a section in his book dealing with the effect of training, since it gives some indication of the basis of his concepts.

> The complex process of coordination of course requires definite cells and groups of cells (centers) for its seat, but the mutual adaptation and correlation of these, quantitatively, seems largely left to be perfected by education. As I have said elsewhere, "Circumstances cannot create a faculty however much they may develop or retard its exercise, but we can conceive that faculties were created with a view to circumstances, and even capable, within limits, of being modified by them". (p. 103)

In summary, Maddox believed that vergence eye movements could be analyzed in terms of additive components. The first one, tonic convergence, moves the eyes from some unknown anatomic position of rest to a relatively more convergent position. This latter position can be determined by the distance phoria measurement with ametropia corrected. The magnitude of tonic vergence is a function of the tonus of the extraocular muscles and the persistent spontaneous activity of the convergence control center, which in turn is a function of various physiological and psychological factors. Any deficit or excess of tonic convergence is compensated by another component of vergence, reflex convergence. The stimulus to reflex vergence is disparity and constant use. A third category is "accommodative-convergence," the magnitude of which is related to the effort of accommodation that is perhaps variable from individual to individual. A fourth type is identified as convergence due to "knowledge of nearness" or "voluntary convergence." Maddox apparently had as much difficulty placing psychic or proximal vergence in his scheme, as have modern investigators (Morgan, 1968). Finally, Maddox proposed that relative vergence was the arithmatic sum of negative and positive reflex vergence.

While it may be true that "circumstances cannot create a faculty," today we suspect that circumstances can alter the manifestation of a faculty. For example, Maddox assumed that fusional vergence was added onto a convergence already established by tonus and accommodation because of the order and circumstances in which he made his determinations. If he had made accommodation unnecessary by having the patient fixate a near object through a pin-hole located before each eye he would have found (if he had been able to make this determination) that the patient accommodated with convergence even though this was unnecessary in the interest of clear vision. Thus if measurement circumstances had been altered, he would have concluded that convergence stimulates accommodation rather than the opposite. In reality, convergence induces accommodation and accommodation induces convergence; neither is solely an independent or a dependent variable. Sensory inputs related to the sharpness of the retinal image and to binocular disparity appear to be processed simultaneously rather than in some serial fashion. Indeed, merely initiating the fixation process from far to near or near to far may institute the correct response. (To some extent Maddox was aware of this.)

While Maddox's analysis may be too simplistic for the scientist, it nevertheless furnishes a model for the clinical analysis of the motor aspects of binocular vision problems that has led to effective therapy. As a clinician, I have found the Maddox analysis much more useful than the Duane-White classification of (1) convergence insufficiency, (2) convergence excess, (3) divergence insufficiency, and (4) divergence excess.[2] The independent variables to be considered in analysis and therapy are not convergence and divergence, but rather (1) tonic vergence, (2) accommodative vergence, (3) reflex or fusional vergence, and (4) the accommodative amplitude. (Fry, 1943 and Morgan, 1968). These are to be considered both qualitatively and quantitatively.

In brief, the clinical application of the Maddox analysis I have used involves the following measurements that are made after correction of any existing ametropia:

1. The magnitude and stability of the heterophoria at a fixation distance between 4 and 6 meters.
2. The magnitude, rapidity, and facility of the relative fusion range at the same fixation distance, paying particular attention to the range opposing the heterophoria.
3. Magnitude and facility of the accommodative amplitude.
4. Magnitude and stability of the heterophoria at a fixation distance between 25 and 40 cm.
5. The change in heterophoria at this same near fixation distance in-

[2] Divergence excess, for example, is due primarily to an insufficiency of tonic vergence associated with a low accommodative convergence.

duced by altering the accommodation by adding plus or minus lenses of known power, usually ± 1.00 diopter (D).

6. Magnitude, rapidity of response, and facility of the relative fusion range at this near fixation distance, particularly the range opposing the heterophoria.

The first determination is a direct measurement of the excess of insufficiency of tonic vergence, and the magnitude of the second represents a measurement of the "capacity" of the vergence system to overcome disparities. From these two determinations, and in light of the facility of reponse, I judge whether the excess or insufficiency of tonic vergence could be a basis for a patient's asthenopia or inadequate visual performance.

The fourth measurement represents the excess or insufficiency of the sum of the tonic, accommodative, and proximal vergences induced by fixation at the near distance used. As at distance, the sixth determination represents a measurement of the capacity of the vergence system to overcome artificially induced disparities. Again as with distance, I make a judgment as to whether the excess of insufficiency of tonic, accommodative, and proximal vergences could be the basis for asthenopia or inadequate visual performance. The facility of response as well as magnitudes must be used in making this judgment.

The fifth finding is a direct measurement of the accommodative vergence per unit of accommodative stimulus. This can be calculated by knowing the patient's interpupillary distance (PD), the heterophoria at distance and at near, and the accommodation required for near fixation distance.[3] A comparison of the gradient and the calculated values should be made to judge the reliability and validity of the various measurements. The calculated value should be somewhat greater because it incorporates proximal vergence, while the gradient measurement does not. Accommodation tends to lag behind the stimulus and thus fixation at near results in a smaller amount of accommodation than that expected for exact focus. This usually makes both the calculated and gradient values too small by some unknown amount. Nevertheless, I expect the calculated value to be only slightly larger than the measured gradient—not more than 1^{Δ} larger.

Measurements of relative accommodation may be made also. They help in judging the reliability and validity of the relative vergences and accommodative vergence measurements.

Several types of therapies can be used either singularly or in combination should the vergence system and its interplay with accommodation cause asthenopia or inadequate visual performance. These therapies are:

[3] $AC/A = PD \text{ in cm} - \dfrac{\textit{tonic vergence—near phoria}}{\textit{fixation distance in diopters}}.$

1. Alter the vergence requirement for bifixation by prescribing prisms.
2. Alter the accommodation requirement by prescribing convex (near only) or concave lens additions to the ametropic correction. This will alter the accommodative vergence.
3. Prescribe orthoptics to increase both range and facility of relative vergence.

In general, prisms for constant wear may be used when the patient has an excess of tonic vergence and a high accommodative vergence (esophoria at both distance and near) or an insufficiency of tonic vergence and a low accommodative vergence (exophoria both at distance and near). The magnitude of the prism should be smaller than the smaller of the two heterophorias. The effect of altering the accommodative demand, usually by prescribing bifocals, is proportional to the magnitude of the accommodative vergence, and therefore the use of added lens power is much more effective when the accommodative convergence/accommodation ratio (AC/A) is 6^{Δ}/1.00 D or greater. Concave lenses have been prescribed for patients with distance exotropia and near exophoria with good results.

Optometric vision training is most effective in younger patients and in those with poor facility of response. In addition, it is a therapy to be used when the magnitude of the relative vergence range is intrinsically low rather than just low with respect to the fusion demand.

REFERENCES

Fry GA. Fundamental variables in relationship between accommodation and convergence. Optom Weekly 1943;34:153–155, 183–185.

Maddox EE. The clinical use of prisms; and the decentering of lenses. Bristol; England: John Wright & Sons, 1893.

Morgan MW. Accommodation and vergence. Am J Optom Arch Am Acad Optom 1968;45:417–54.

II

TONIC AND PROXIMAL VERGENCE

3

Perceptual and Motor Consequences of Tonic Vergence

D. Alfred Owens
Herschel W. Leibowitz

In the absence of visual stimulation, the eyes of an alert individual assume a posture that is intermediate in the functional range of binocular vergence. This intermediate adjustment is referred to as the physiological resting state of the vergence system. It results from continuous tonic innervation of the extraocular muscles that is apparently independent of concurrent visual stimulation, accommodation, and voluntary influences. When the intrinsic tonic innervation is eliminated, as in deep sleep, surgical anesthesia, or death, the eyes return to a divergent anatomic resting state that is determined by mechanical properties of the eyes' suspensory system. Thus tonic innervation can be thought of as a neutral or base-line activity level of the vergence system. It is the starting point for normal vergence responses and it determines the intermediate resting state obtained when there is no visual stimulus, accommodative activity, or voluntary effort to modify vergence.

Tonic vergence has been of interest in a variety of contexts in vision research, ranging from clinical problems of binocular coordination and refraction to psychological studies of space perception and perceptual learning. These diverse viewpoints have introduced different techniques of measurement, terminology, and theory. But despite the diversity of

Preparation of this chapter was supported in part by grants EY-03898 and EY-03276 from the National Eye Institute.

observations and language, several interesting phenomena have emerged as characteristic of tonic vergence. Individuals with ostensibly normal binocular vision exhibit different levels of tonic vergence, and these differences are reflected in systematic biases of both vergence responses and space perception. Evidence indicates that differences in lateral heterophoria, fixation disparity, and distance perception are related to individual differences in tonic vergence. Moreover, the tonic vergence of a given individual can be readily modified through systematic manipulation of the relationship between binocular parallax and fixation distance. This plasticity appears to maintain a relatively stable correspondence between fusional effort and fixation distance. It may serve both to calibrate the effect of vergence on distance perception and to alleviate unusual demands on fusional vergence. The process has important implications for the development of space perception and for adaptation to optical transformations introduced by spectacle lenses or by traumatic or pathological dislocations of the eyeball. Anomalies of this process may well be involved in disorders such as concomitant strabismus and anomalous retinal correspondence.

This chapter provides a brief summary of the evolution of the tonic vergence concept in the context of unidirectional and opponent-process models of vergence eye movements. More recent research on the relationship of tonic vergence to distance perception, fixation disparity, and phoria, with particular attention to the effects of prism adaptation, is discussed with the goal of identifying key issues for further inquiry.

HISTORICAL BACKGROUND

Anatomic and Physiological Resting Positions

Early clinical observations showed that the resting position of the oculomotor system depends on the state of the subject. In deep anesthesia or death, the eyes diverge to a position that is determined by mechanical characteristics of orbital tissues and the eyes' suspensory system. Precise normative values for this anatomic resting position have not been established. Estimates vary from a posture of "slight" divergence (Cogan, 1956; Breinin, 1957) to as much as 68° of divergence (Mann, 1964), with values less than 25° being most frequently cited (Toates, 1974). Abraham (1964) argued on the basis of a comparative analysis of orbital anatomy that the anatomic resting position of humans probably changes over the life span due to changes in the extraocular muscles resulting from convergence activity. He proposed that this position in infants may be 20° more divergent than in adults. Zimmerman, Armstrong, and Scammon (1933) reported that the anatomic resting position is 71° of divergence at birth, suggesting that Abraham (1964) may have underestimated the magnitude of developmental changes.

Maddox's Conception of Tonic Convergence

Maddox (1893) was one of the earliest authors to distinguish between the anatomic and physiological resting positions. He observed that the eyes of alert subjects do not diverge when viewing a distant target with one eye occluded, but rather maintain a parallel or slightly convergent posture. He concluded that this position results from the activity of tonic convergence, which is "due partly to muscular tone and partly to involuntary action of converging innervation" (p. 91).

According to Maddox, all vergence eye movements result from the additive combination of four components of convergence that operate in opposition to the eyes' tendency toward divergence. The three major components—tonic, accommodative, and reflex convergence—are illustrated in Figure 3.1. Here it is evident that Maddox believed tonic convergence is responsible for bringing the eyes from the divergent anatomic resting position to the primary position (angle Ri). Additional convergence to fixate a near target is shown to depend on the added contributions of accommodative convergence and reflex convergence. The latter is now commonly referred to as fusional or disparity convergence (Stark et al., 1980). Maddox's fourth component, voluntary convergence, was attributed to "knowledge of nearness" and was included under the term accommodative convergence.

Maddox recognized that the magnitude of tonic convergence varies among individuals, and he indicated that such differences may influence binocular coordination and may be related to symptoms of ocular discomfort. He claimed that excessive tonic convergence produces latent overconvergence (esophoria), and that deficient tonic convergence produces latent underconvergence (exophoria). To maintain single binocular vision, these tendencies must be compensated by additional reflex (disparity) convergence, which he assumed to be stressful, and hence a potential contributor to eye fatigue, asthenopia, and headaches.

Maddox also observed that tonic convergence can be modified by altering the level of reflex (disparity) convergence required for normal binocular fusion. In a section on the effect of training he reported that:

> . . . if I wear adducting [base-out] prisms, amounting together to 11°d, for ten minutes, the rod test reveals, on their removal, $5\frac{1}{2}°$ of latent convergence as the position of equilibrium for distance instead of my usual convergence of only $\frac{1}{2}°$. In other words, the tonic convergence has been temporarily increased by 5°, and takes a good many minutes to recover its usual dimensions. (p. 102)

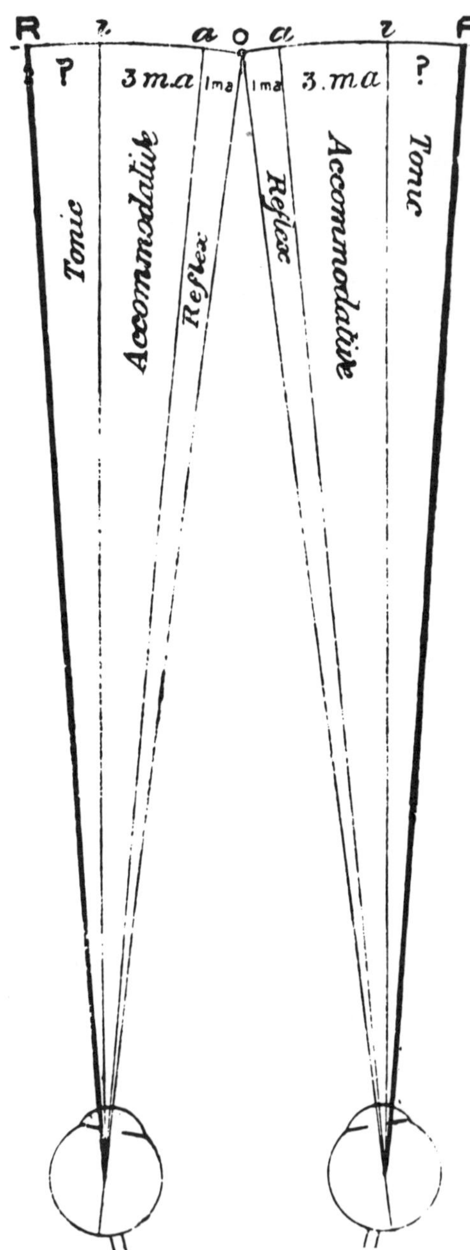

FIGURE 3.1. Schematic representation of the components of convergence taken from Maddox (1893). Tonic convergence is represented by the angle Ri. Reprinted by permission of the publisher, from Maddox EE. *The Clinical Use of Prisms and the Decentering of Lenses*, 2nd edition. Bristol, England: John Wright and Company, 1893.

In addition, he noted that viewing through plus lenses for a few hours reduced his latent divergence for near targets (near exophoria), a change that could also be attributed to increased tonic convergence. Both of these manipulations would initially alter the balance of the three major components of convergence by increasing the demand on reflex (disparity) convergence as compared to the concurrent level of accommodative convergence. Base-out prisms would increase the load on reflex convergence by increasing binocular parallax without changing the accommodative stimulus or accommodative convergence; plus lenses would increase the load on reflex convergence by decreasing the accommodative stimulus and the level of accommodative convergence without changing binocular parallax. The result of both manipulations was an increase in tonic convergence which, according to the additive model, would serve to reduce the effort required of reflex convergence. Thus Maddox's account suggests that changes of tonic convergence may facilitate adaptation to new spectacles and may be an important consequence of visual training.

Opponent Vergence Mechanisms

Subsequent research has confirmed and extended Maddox's observations on individual differences and plasticity of tonic vergence. It has also provided further evidence for relationships among the tonus position, lateral heterophoria, and fixation disparity. However, later research has also led to fundamental revisions of Maddox's model of the vergence system. Most notably, the old unidirectional model of vergence control has been rejected in favor of an opponent-process model.

This theoretical shift followed a prolonged controversy over the existence of an active divergence mechanism. For many years, the accepted view, which was advanced by Maddox, held that only convergent eye movements are active and that divergent eye movements result from passive elastic forces pulling the eyes toward their anatomic resting position. Some authors argued for active divergence on the basis of behavioral evidence, such as the ability to overcome esophoria and the existence of negative fusional reserves; others maintained that these observations could be accounted for more parsimoniously by assuming inhibition of active convergence (reviewed by Toates, 1974). The controversy was eventually resolved in the early 1950s when electromyographic studies of human extraocular muscles demonstrated activity in the lateral recti during divergent eye movements and steady fixation (Björk, 1952; Adler, 1953; Breinin and Moldaver, 1955).

Although the physiological processes controlling vergence are not yet understood, theorists now agree that vergence eye movements are accomplished through the interaction of convergence and divergence activity (Duke-Elder and Wybar, 1973; Burian and von Noorden, 1974;

Toates, 1974). In this context, tonic vergence can be conceptualized as a neutral state, or equilibrium, between resting levels of opposing divergence and convergence mechanisms.

EVIDENCE FOR TONIC VERGENCE

At least four lines of evidence indicate that the physiological resting position of the vergence system corresponds to an intermediate distance. As noted by Maddox and many others, the eyes typically assume a parallel or somewhat convergent posture in the absence of fusable binocular stimuli, yet they return to a divergent posture in deep sleep, anesthesia, and death. Duke-Elder and Wybar (1973) report that clinical observations also show that esotropia tends to increase during fatigue, illness, or emotional arousal. Experimental evidence for a convergent tonus position is provided by studies of the effects of physiological stress, reduced stimulation, and the early development of binocular fixation. Drawing from a wide variety of subject populations and stimulus conditions, this research indicates that the functional range of vergence diminishes whenever visual performance is degraded through stress, impoverished viewing conditions, or immaturity. In all cases, this reduction of binocular range appears to involve increasing overconvergence for distant stimuli and underconvergence for near stimuli. When there is no fusional response, as in darkness, subjects generally maintain an intermediate level of convergence that shows substantial individual differences with an average value of about 120 cm.

Stress Effects

The disruption of fusional eye movements is one of the earliest and most devastating effects of physiological stress on visual performance. This problem is most commonly experienced as diplopia during illness, alcohol intoxication, or following an injury. Several investigations of visual performance under stress, summarized in Table 3.1, indicate that decreased fusional amplitude is the primary effect of hypoxia or alcohol or barbiturates.

In an early study of pilots' vision, Wilmer and Berens (1918) found that hypoxia produced increased esophoria for distant targets, and in many subjects, a recession of the near point of convergence. These findings were later replicated by Adler (1945). Powell (1938) and Colson (1940) found that alcohol intoxication has essentially the same effects on vergence, increasing esophoria at distance and decreasing the maximum level of convergence. A later study by Brecher, Hartman, and Leonard

TABLE 3.1. Evidence for a Bias of Vergence Toward an Intermediate Posture under Conditions of Physiological Stress

Authors and Year	*Condition*	*Number of Subjects*	*Effects on Vergence*
Wilmer and Berens, 1918	Hypoxia	Varied	A) Decreased fusional reserves B) Recession of near point C) More rapid "fatigue" of convergence
Adler, 1945	Hypoxia	8	A) Esophoria at distance B) Increased convergent fusional reserves C) Decreased divergent fusional reserves D) Inconsistent changes of near phoria
Powell, 1938	Alcohol	7	A) Esophoria at 6 m B) Progressive recession of near point
Colson, 1940	Alcohol	21	A) Esophoria at distance B) Little change in convergence reserves C) Loss of divergence reserves
Brecher, Hartman, and Leonard, 1955	Alcohol	14	A) Increased latency of fusion B) Loss of voluntary convergence C) No change in vertical phoria D) Consistent exophoria at 33 cm E) Consistent esophoria at 6 m F) No change in lateral phoria at 56 to 60 cm
Wist, Hughes, and Forney, 1967	Alcohol	9	A) Very low dosages produced esofixation disparity at 7 m
Westheimer, 1963	Barbiturates	—	A) Increased esophoria at 5 m B) Increased exophoria at 33 cm C) Narrowing of the fusional range D) Recession of the near point E) Decreased AC/A ratio
	Amphetamines	—	A) Slightly increased exophoria at 5 m B) Decreased exophoria at 33 cm C) Increased fusional reserves D) Increased AC/A ratio

(1955) replicated these findings and concluded that "the resting position of the eyes at which alcohol does not cause phoria to change is at about 60 cms" (p. 50). Wist, Hughes, and Forney (1967) found that vergence responses are affected even by very low dosages of alcohol. They measured the fixation disparity of nine subjects for a distant foveal stimulus before and after ingestion of only one ounce of whiskey per 150 pounds body weight. Their results showed a statistically significant increase in convergent fixation disparity, ranging from one minute to nearly five minutes of arc for individual subjects.

Westheimer (1963) found that barbiturates have much the same effect as hypoxia and alcohol, while amphetamines tend to induce the opposite response. He reported that moderate dosages of barbiturates produced increased esophoria at 6 m, increased exophoria at 30 cm, decreased fusional range, an increase in the AC/A ratio, and a recession of the near point of convergence.

Since hypoxia and drugs were not observed to affect saccadic eye movements or accommodation, Adler (1945) and Westheimer (1963) both concluded that these stressors selectively influence the central mechanisms controlling vergence. Westheimer also suggested that amphetamines may enhance the activity of the central control mechanisms. According to this view, the accuracy and amplitude of vergence responses depend on the efficiency of central processes. Whenever these processes are depressed, the functional range of binocular vergence progressively diminishes and responses are increasingly biased toward an intermediate distance, which Westheimer estimated to be 60 to 100 cm. Thus the effects of stress on phoria, fixation disparity, fusional reserves, and the AC/A ratio can be interpreted as consequences of a common mechanism, the passive return of vergence to its intermediate tonus position.

Reduced Illumination and Dark Vergence

Several studies (Table 3.2) have shown that vergence is also biased toward an intermediate posture when illumination is reduced and fusable contours are confined to the peripheral visual field.

The earliest quantitative study of vergence in low illumination was conducted by Ivanoff and Bourdy (1954; Ivanoff, 1955). They used a nonius alignment technique to measure vergence responses for a large letter M presented in the lower peripheral field at a wide range of luminances. Vergence responses remained fairly accurate until luminance was reduced to scotopic levels, when increasing fixation disparities began to appear for both near and distant stimuli. Eight of their nine subjects exhibited progressively increasing convergent (eso) fixation disparity for the distant stimulus and simultaneously increasing divergent (exo) fixation disparity

TABLE 3.2. Early Evidence for a Bias of Vergence Toward an Intermediate Distance under Reduced Illumination

Authors and Year	*Conditions*	*Number of Subjects*	*Effects on Vergence*
Ivanoff and Bourdy, 1954	Reduced illumination Periphral stimulus	9	A) Increased esofixation disparity for distant target B) Increased exofixation disparity for near target C) Mean vergence distance in dark = 56 cm
Fincham, 1962	Darkness	10	A) Mean vergence distance = 197 cm
Levy, 1969	Darkness	16	A) Mean convergence in dark = 9.6° or 39 cm

for the near stimulus, finally reaching a fixed intermediate adjustment for both stimuli at the lowest luminance levels. The ninth subject showed a similar decline in the amplitude of vergence, except that this person's responses were progressively biased toward a parallel rather than a convergent posture at the lowest luminances. Individual vergence distances in darkness ranged from 25 cm to 20 m, with an average value of 56 cm (Ivanoff and Bourdy, 1954).

In a later study, Fincham (1962) used infrared photography to measure vergence and accommodation of subjects attempting to "look into distance" in darkness. Consistent with the data of Ivanoff and Bourdy (1954), he found that most subjects assumed a convergent posture in the dark. His results also indicated that vergence in darkness did not correspond to the concurrent level of accommodation. Rather, both responses appeared to fluctuate independently about different intermediate dark positions. The difference between the dark states of vergence and accommodation varied from one subject to another, with vergence corresponding to a greater distance for most of the subjects. The average dark vergence of 10 subjects ranged from 1.9 to −0.8 meter angles (53 cm to divergence), with an overall mean of 0.52 meter angles (197.2 cm); average accommodation in darkness ranged from 1.17 to 0 diopters (85 cm to infinity), with an overall mean of 0.73 diopter (137 cm).

Levy (1969) introduced a third method for estimating the "physiological position of rest" based on measures of the resting direction of gaze for each eye. He used a perimeter to present pairs of briefly flashed monocular stimuli at various positions along the principal meridians in an otherwise dark room. On each trial the subject saw a point of light appear for one second, followed by three seconds of darkness, and then the point of light reappeared for one second. The subject's task was to report the position of the second stimulus as compared with that of the first. Since the two stimuli were always presented at the same point in space, any difference in their apparent position could be attributed to a change in eye position during the dark interval. Levy reasoned that the eye would passively drift toward its resting position when the first light point was extinguished. As a consequence, the second light point would appear to be displaced relative to the first in the direction opposite the eye's drift. For example, stimulus pairs presented above the eye's resting direction would consistently elicit "higher" responses for the second stimulus of the pair, while those presented below the resting direction would consistently elicit "lower" responses, and those presented in coincidence with the eye's resting direction would elicit random directional (or "no change") responses. Levy used a double-staircase technique to measure successively the vertical and horizontal components of each eye's resting position for 16 subjects. The results showed large individual differences with standard deviations ranging from over 9° to nearly 14°. On the average, subjects' gaze deviated downward by 5.85° at rest. They exhibited fairly strong convergence, averaging 9.6°, and no significant vertical phoria in the dark.

Levy's results suggest that tonic vergence corresponds to a closer distance (about 39 cm, assuming an interpupillary distance of 65 mm) than is indicated by the data of Ivanoff and Bourdy (1954) and Fincham (1962). This discrepancy might be due to differences in the subjects' tasks: for Ivanoff and Bourdy, they performed a nonius alignment while viewing a dim peripheral stimulus; for Fincham, they simply looked into the distance in darkness; and for Levy, they judged the relative positions of briefly flashed stimuli. One might speculate that response strategies for the last task introduced some "proximal convergence" in addition to tonic vergence, but further investigation would be necessary to test this possibility. In any case, all three studies showed that vergence assumes an intermediate posture in low illumination or darkness.

Due to the small number of subjects and large intersubject variability, it is not possible to infer normative values for tonic vergence from the data reviewed so far. One should note, however, that the range of mean fixation distances obtained in darkness, (39 to 197 cm) is similar to that obtained under alcohol or barbiturate intoxication, (56 to 100 cm).

More extensive data on vergence in the absence of stimulation have been reported by Owens and Leibowitz (1980). In a study of the relationship between oculomotor adjustments and distance perception in low illumination, they measured the accommodation and vergence of 60 college students in total darkness. Dark vergence measures were taken with a nonius alignment technique under conditions designed to minimize stimuli for binocular fusion and accommodation. As illustrated in Figure 3.2, laser light was used to produce two dichoptic speckle patterns shaped like vertical bars and viewed in a dark field. Over a series of presentations, these bars were flashed at various lateral separations for 125 msec, shorter than the reaction time of either vergence or accommodation (Rashbash and Westheimer, 1961). The dark vergence position was defined according to the position of the dichoptic bars when they appeared to be aligned vertically. The dark focus of accommodation was measured with a laser optometer (Hennessy and Leibowitz, 1972) that was incorporated into the same apparatus. Throughout these measures, the subjects were frequently encouraged to relax and to avoid straining their eyes in any way. The subjects' perceived distance for a fixation point viewed in a dark surround was also measured. (These data are discussed in a later section.)

The distributions of dark focus and dark vergence values are illustrated in Figure 3.3. Dark focus data are given as diopters of accommodation, and the dark vergence data are given as degrees of convergence normalized to an interpupillary distance of 65 mm. These distributions differ in two ways. First, the average values correspond to different dis-

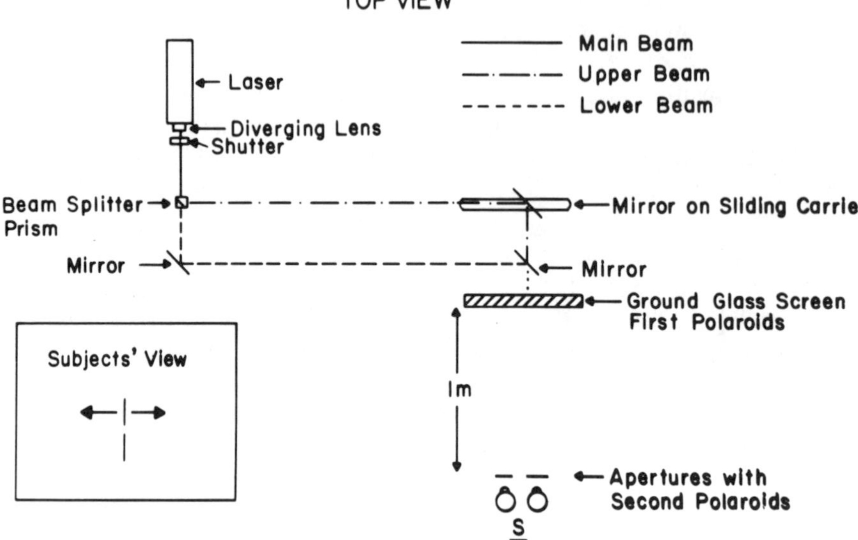

FIGURE 3.2. Schematic diagram of the apparatus used to measure ocular vergence in darkness. Reprinted by permission of the publisher, from Owens DA, Leibowitz HW. Oculomotor adjustments in darkness and the specific distance tendency. Perception and Psychophysics, 1976.

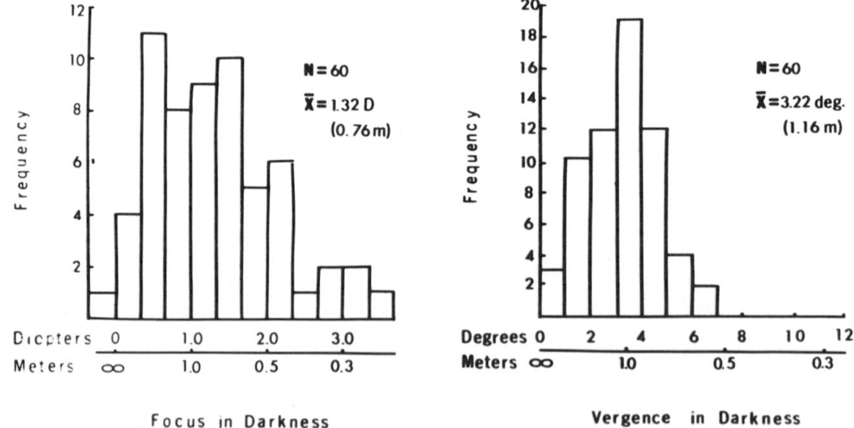

FIGURE 3.3. Frequency distributions of the dark focus of accommodation and dark vergence positions of 60 college-age subjects. The difference between the mean dark focus and dark vergence values is statistically significant ($t = -4.41$, $df = 59$, $P < 0.002$). Reprinted by permission of the publisher, from Owens DA, Leibowitz HW. Accommodation, convergence, and distance perception in low illumination. American Journal of Optometry and Physiological Optics, © (1980), American Academy of Optometry per The Williams & Wilkins Company (agent).

tances. The mean dark focus was 1.32 diopters of accommodation, or 76 cm, while the mean dark vergence was 3.22 degrees convergence, or 116 cm. Second, the dark focus distribution shows greater intersubject variation than the dark vergence distribution. In darkness, refractive states ranged from low hyperopia to an equivalent distance of 28 cm, whereas dark vergence ranged from infinity (parallel axes) to about 50 cm.

Consistent with earlier measures of vergence in low illumination, these data clearly show that most subjects converged to an intermediate distance and that the dark vergence position varies across subjects. Indeed, the average dark vergence distance found by Owens and Leibowitz (1976a; 116 cm) is remarkably similar to the midpoint of the wide range of mean dark vergence distances reported by earlier investigators (118 cm). Moreover, the results presented in Figure 3.3 confirmed Fincham's (1962) report that vergence and accommodation dissociate under low illumination. Although both vergence and accommodation assumed intermediate adjustments in the dark, the average equivalent distances of these adjustments were significantly different. This dissociation is illustrated more clearly as a scatter diagram in Figure 3.4, which compares the dark focus and dark vergence values of individual subjects. If vergence and accommodation maintained their usual correspondence in darkness, the dark focus and dark vergence data should be highly correlated with all the data points clustered tightly along a linear regression line. Contrary to this prediction, the data are widely dispersed with a correlation of only 0.32. For this reason, Owens and Leibowitz (1980) proposed that the dark vergence measures represent the resting or tonus position of the vergence system, unbiased by accommodative or fusional convergence.

Vergence for Peripheral Stimuli

Similar to the effects of reduced illumination, studies of vergence eye movements for peripheral stimuli indicate that fusional responses are also increasingly biased toward an intermediate tonus position as the retinal eccentricity of binocular stimuli increases.

Ogle, Mussey, and Prangen (1949) showed that fixation disparity is generally greater for peripheral than for central stimuli. Using a forced (prism) duction procedure, they obtained fixation disparity curves for two subjects who viewed an acuity chart with a central area containing no fusable contours and ranging in size from 0.75° to 6° of visual angle. For both subjects, increasing the eccentricity of fusable contours resulted in an increase in both convergent and divergent fixation disparities. Ogle and associates attributed the changes in fixation disparity to the increased size of Panum's areas in the periphery. Since the threshold for diplopia,

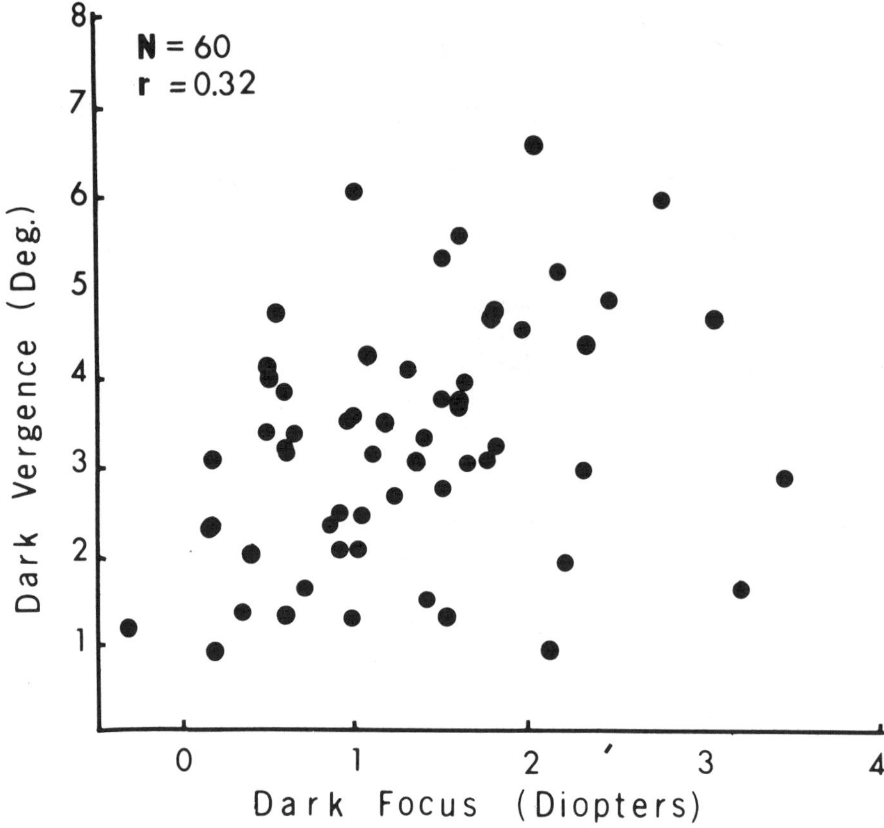

FIGURE 3.4. Scatter diagram illustrating the relation between the dark focus of accommodation and dark vergence of 60 subjects. Reprinted by permission of the publisher, from Owens DA, Leibowitz HW. Accommodation, convergence, and distance perception in low illumination. American Journal of Optometry and Physiological Optics, © (1980), American Academy of Optometry per The Williams & Wilkins Company (agent).

(Mitchell, 1966a,b) increases with retinal eccentricity, increased fixation disparity can be tolerated without disruption of perceptual fusion.

More recently, Francis (1979; Francis and Owens, 1980) measured the accuracy of vergence responses for dim binocular stimuli that were viewed at various retinal eccentricities over distances ranging from 28.5 to 342 cm. Central fixation was maintained with a weak monocular fixation point that would not stimulate accommodation (Owens and Leibowitz, 1975). In one experiment the binocular stimuli consisted of two luminous vertical bars laterally flanking the central fixation point at eccentricities of 2°, 4°, and 8°. In a second experiment the binocular stimuli

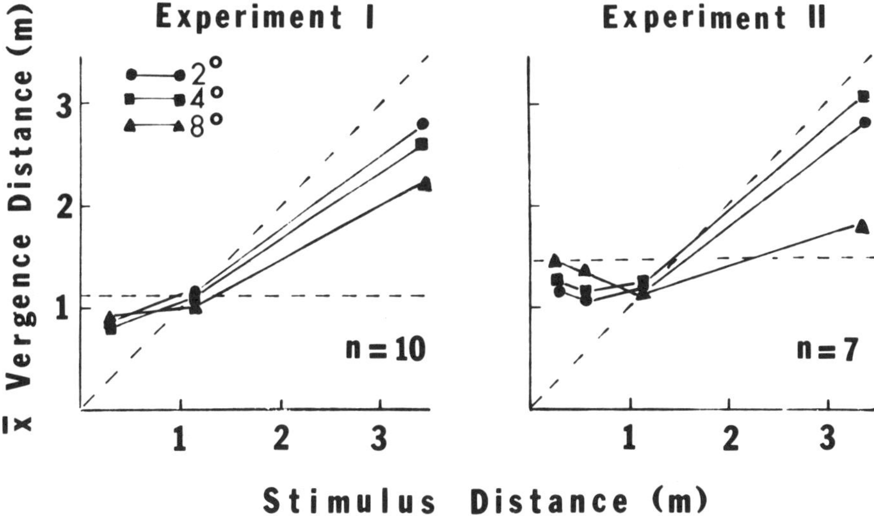

FIGURE 3.5. Vergence responses as a function of distance for binocular stimuli presented at peripheral retinal eccentricities of 2°, 4°, and 8°. The dashed diagonal lines represent accurate vergence, and the dashed horizontal lines represent the average vergence distances in total darkness. Reprinted with permission from Vision Research, Francis EL, Owens DA, The accuracy of convergence for peripheral stimuli, in press, Pergamon Press, Ltd.

were pairs of weaker luminous squares presented at the same eccentricities as the vertical bars of experiment I.

Figure 3.5 shows the mean fixation distances as a function of stimulus distance for each retinal eccentricity in both experiments. The diagonal dashed lines represent accurate vergence response values and the horizontal lines represent the subjects' average vergence position in total darkness. These data show that the mean dark vergence of the 10 subjects in experiment I corresponded to 112 cm and that of the 7 subjects in experiment II corresponded to 148 cm. In both experiments, vergence responses for peripheral stimuli were increasingly biased toward the dark vergence distance as retinal eccentricity increased.

These results confirm the earlier report of Ogle and co-workers (1949) that fixation disparity increases as fusable contours are confined to increasingly peripheral portions of the visual field. Furthermore, they demonstrate that this reduction in the accuracy of vergence is obtained under conditions in which the fusion stimuli are viewed in real space as well as under the more artificial conditions imposed by prism duction tests. Of greatest interest in the present context, Francis' (1979) study shows that, as with reduced illumination, the fixation disparity arising with peripheral stimulation can be characterized as a passive lag of vergence responses toward the subjects' dark vergence or tonus position. The data of individual subjects as well as group means showed that they tended to underconverge for stimuli positioned nearer than the dark vergence distance, to overconverge for stimuli beyond the dark vergence distance, and to remain accurate regardless of retinal eccentricity for stimuli positioned at the dark vergence distance (Francis and Owens, 1980).

Thus the effects of both reduced illumination and increased retinal eccentricity are qualitatively similar to those of hypoxia, alcohol, and barbiturates. When stimulus quality is reduced, the functional range of binocular vergence progressively diminishes as vergence responses are increasingly biased toward an intermediate posture that corresponds, on the average, to a distance of about 120 cm. Similar to the effects of stress, this tendency can be attributed to decreased efficiency of the central mechanisms controlling vergence. Unlike the effects of stress, however, fixation disparity resulting from reduced stimulation is thought to reflect changes in sensitivity to retinal disparity rather than physiological depression of the neural centers controlling vergence. It is well known that both reduced illumination and increased retinal eccentricity increase the size of Panum's fusional areas. That is, greater retinal disparity is necessary to produce diplopia (Mitchell, 1966a, 1966b). Consequently, the effective stimulus for fusional vergence becomes coarser, permitting greater fixation disparity without diplopia. At the same time, these stimulus manipulations also degrade sensitivity to spatial contrast, thus diminishing accommodative responsiveness (Owens, 1980) and, presumably, the strength of accommodative vergence. The overall result is that tonic vergence comes to dominate vergence eye movements as fusional and accommodative vergence become progressively weaker.

This account of the effects of stress and reduced stimulation on binocular vergence is based on studies that tested fewer than a dozen subjects under narrowly defined conditions. While they all indicate that vergence is biased toward an intermediate posture under nonoptimal conditions, the hypothesis that both stress and reduced stimulation produce a bias toward the *same* intermediate tonus position has not been tested. Evidence reviewed in subsequent sections indicates that the level of tonic vergence is strongly affected by unusual fusional demands (e.g., prism adaptation) and by early development. It is possible that some forms of physiological stress also affect the absolute value of the tonus position as well as the overall amplitude of fusional eye movements.

Development of Vergence Eye Movements

Recent studies of the development of binocular fixation in human infants have revealed interesting parallels with the effects of stimulus degradation on vergence responses of adults. Based on photographic records of corneal reflections, at least two investigations have shown that newborns adjust their vergence in the appropriate direction for changes in the distance of fixated stimuli. The accuracy of these responses appears to be limited, however, in much the same way as that of adults for peripheral, dimly illuminated stimuli.

Slater and Findley (1975) photographed the eye positions of 12 newborns ranging from 1 to 8 days of age, who viewed two vertical rows of lights at distances of 10 and 20 inches. All infants changed convergence in the appropriate direction when the distance of the stimulus was changed. The mean change in vergence was 2.6 degrees, within one-half degree of the appropriate change. Although on the average newborns converged by approximately the correct amount, repeated measures of single subjects showed that vergence was not stable but rather tended to waver between overconvergence and underconvergence, resulting in standard deviations of 2° and 2.3° for the 20-inch and 10-inch distances, respectively. Even greater fluctuations of convergence were found in a second experiment in which 11 newborns were tested with stimulus distances of 5 and 10 inches. While these infants also converged reasonably accurately for the 10-inch distance, their responses for the 5-inch distance were highly variable, and in most cases, showed *less* convergence than for the 10-inch distance.

A later study by Aslin (1977) used motion-picture photography to evaluate vergence responses to dynamic stimuli of infants one to six months old. In his first experiment, one-, and two-, and three-month old infants viewed a luminous cross as it approached or receded over a distance range of 15 to 57 cm. Consistent with the findings of Slater and Findley (1975), all age groups exhibited vergence eye movements in the appropriate direction. On trials in which the stimulus approached the subject, the youngest infants tended to underconverge, lagging behind the stimulus, while the older infants showed increasingly rapid and accurate vergence movements. In a second experiment, Aslin tested the vergence responses of infants three, four and one-half, and six months old for small changes of binocular parallax (2.5° and 5°) induced by prisms. The results showed that consistent responses for such small vergence stimuli were not obtained until six months of age. Thus the available evidence indicates that the vergence system is active, although with only limited range and accuracy, in the newborn, and that its amplitude, speed, and precision improve gradually over at least the first six months of life.

Aslin (1981) proposed that the development of accurate binocular fixation depends on concomitant improvement in the infants' sensitivity to retinal disparity. Consistent with other aspects of binocular development (Aslin and Dumais, 1980) he suggested that the disparity threshold for diplopia (Panum's area) is quite large for young infants and gradually decreases with development. Consequently, older infants require increasingly accurate vergence adjustments to maintain perceptual fusion. Aslin explains the fixation disparity frequently exhibited by young infants as reflecting a general tendency of the vergence system to lag toward its resting position by an amount limited by the extent of Panum's area.

In support of this hypothesis, Aslin and Jackson (1981) found that the dark vergence position of infants corresponds to the same distance range as their most accurate vergence responses. They used infrared photography to measure the vergence position in total darkness of 18 infants ranging in age from 5 to 20 weeks. After correcting their measures for the difference between the infants' visual and optical axes (angle alpha), they concluded that the average dark vergence was 7.4° convergent, corresponding to an average fixation distance of 35 cm. Although they noted large differences among subjects, only one infant showed a dark vergence distance greater than one meter. A subsequent study of 24 infants between 3 and 36 months of age replicated the finding that most converged to distances of less than one meter in the dark (Aslin, Dobson, and Jackson, 1982). In addition, simultaneous measures of the infants' refractive states, obtained with photorefraction, showed no significant correlation between the dark vergence posture and the dark focus of accommodation. This finding suggests that, as with adults, the accommodation and vergence systems of young infants may dissociate in the absence of visual stimulation.

It is interesting to note that the average dark vergence of infants appears to be considerably more convergent than that of adults. This difference is particularly impressive when one recalls that the anatomic resting position of infants is probably significantly more divergent (Abraham, 1964; Mann, 1964), implying that the magnitude of tonic convergence is much greater in infants than in adults. This inference agrees with an earlier claim by Adler (1953) that the prevalence of concomitant esotropia in infants and children is related to their "normally excessive" levels of tonic convergence. Although the data base is still small, the findings of Aslin and Jackson (1981) provided the first empirical support for Adler's hypothesis. Further investigation of the nature of developmental changes in dark vergence may well reveal new insights regarding the etiology of strabismus as well as the basic processes controlling vergence eye movements.

Tonic Vergence and Accommodation

The research reviewed so far indicates that vergence eye movements are biased toward an intermediate level of convergence under a variety of conditions, including hypoxia, alcohol and barbiturate intoxication, low illumination, stimulation of only the peripheral retina, and infancy. Based on this evidence we have proposed that the average tonus position of adults is about 3 degrees of convergence, corresponding to a fixation distance of about 120 cm (Figure 3.3).

This conclusion may be puzzling to readers with a clinical background. Most clinical estimates of tonic vergence indicate that the so-called fusion-free position corresponds to nearly parallel visual axes (Maddox, 1893; Hebbard, 1952). Indeed, deviations from this parallel position of orthophoria are generally considered anomalous, if not pathological. This discrepancy between clinical and experimental estimates of tonic vergence is probably due to an important difference in the conditions of measurement. For the most part (excluding studies of stress), experimental measures were taken in total darkness or with only very weak (scotopic or peripheral) stimuli. In contrast, clinical estimates of tonic vergence are usually based on measures of lateral phoria taken with monocular fixation of a bright accommodative stimulus. This latter approach assumes that when viewing a distant target, accommodation is relaxed and therefore should not give rise to accommodative vergence, but a growing body of evidence indicates that this assumption is not warranted (Leibowitz and Owens, 1978).

Rather than resting at infinity as predicted by classical theory (Helmholtz, 1962; Fincham, 1937; Walls, 1942), measures of accommodation in the absence of contoured stimuli indicate that the resting focus corresponds to an intermediate distance. Figure 3.6 illustrates the focus in total darkness of 220 college students who were either emmetropic or wearing their normal spectacle corrections. Similar to the data shown in Figure 3.3, these measures, obtained with a laser optometer, show that the average *dark focus* corresponds to a distance of 67 cm (1.5 D myopic) and varies widely among observers. Other research has shown that subjects assume this same intermediate focus when viewing a bright, empty field or an interference pattern produced by laser light (Leibowitz and Owens, 1975a, 1975b) and when viewing through an optical instrument or pinhole pupils (Hennessy, 1975; Hennessy et al., 1976). Also, when two stimuli are superimposed optically at different distances, subjects tend to focus involuntarily for the one lying closer to the distance of their dark focus (Owens, 1979). Thus accommodation is passively biased toward an intermediate focus in at least three general conditions: (1) when the stimulus is degraded, as with low illumination or contrast; (2) when the quality of the retinal image is independent of focus, as with small pupils or images formed by optical interference; and (3) when the eye has the "option" of focusing either of two superimposed stimuli lying at different distances.

These findings have revitalized an old theory, proposed independently by a number of earlier investigators (Cogan, 1937; Luckiesh and

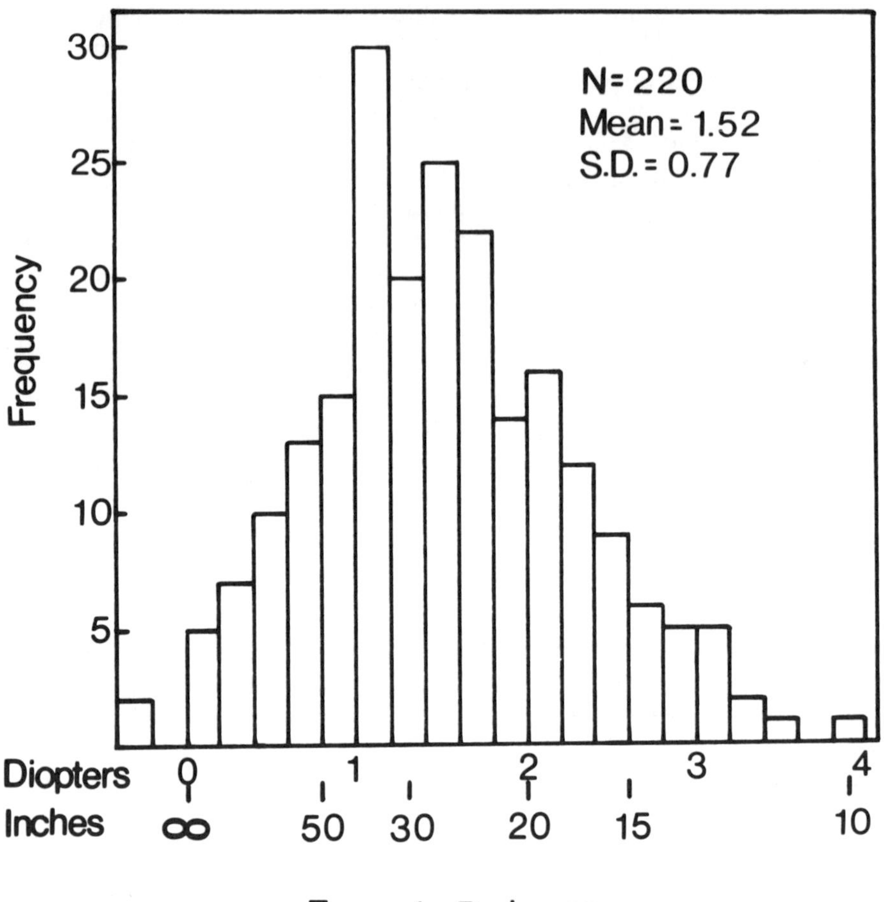

FIGURE 3.6. Frequency distribution of the dark focus of accommodation for 220 college-age subjects. Reprinted by permission of the publisher, from Leibowitz HW, Owens DA. New evidence for the intermediate position of relaxed accommodation. Documenta Ophthalmologica, 1978.

Moss, 1940; Morgan, 1946, 1957; Siebeck, 1953; Schober, 1954; LeGrand, 1967), that the resting state of accommodation corresponds to an intermediate distance rather than to the far point of the eye's focusing range. Similar to the opponent-process theory of vergence control, this view holds that accommodation involves dual focusing mechanisms. In addition to positive accommodation, which serves to focus near stimuli and is determined by parasympathetic innervation, the theory posits a negative accommodation mechanism that serves to focus distant stimuli and is determined by sympathetic innervation. The intermediate resting state (or dark focus) is thought to represent the neutral balance point between these opponent processes.

Returning now to the discrepancy between clinical and experimental estimates of tonic vergence, the dual-process model of accommodation implies that distant fixation targets used in most tests of lateral phoria stimulate a negative accommodative response. The negative accommodation elicited by a stimulus positioned beyond the distance of the subject's dark focus may well induce *accommodative divergence*. While this possibility has not yet been tested experimentally, if confirmed it would provide a simple explanation for the difference between dark vergence and distance phoria. Moreover, assuming that accommodative activity is minimal in darkness, it follows that accommodative vergence is minimal, and therefore dark vergence should represent a more valid measure of tonic vergence than is obtained with conventional measures of lateral phoria.

Further inquiry is necessary, however, to rule out the possibility that vergence and accommodation interact in darkness. As illustrated clinically by the AC/A and CA/C ratios, vergence and accommodation normally exhibit a synergistic relationship. Stimulation of either response is generally accompanied by a proportional change in the same direction by the other response (Fincham and Walton, 1957). Both vergence and accommodation appear to maintain continued "resting innervation" in darkness, and it is possible that the synergism found with adequate stimulation also continues in the absence of visual stimuli. If this were the case, dark vergence could be due to accommodative as well as to tonic activity.

Results from three studies reviewed above (Fincham, 1962; Owens and Leibowitz, 1980; Aslin et al., 1982) have shown that the dark vergence and dark focus positions are only weakly correlated (e.g., Figure 3.4). These data indicate that an individual's dark vergence cannot be predicted on the basis of his or her dark focus, suggesting that vergence and accommodation are dissociated in darkness. However, they do not prove the dissociation. As pointed out by a colleague, comparisons such as that in Figure 3.4 do not take into account individual differences in the AC/A ratio. Subjects with identical dark focus values but different AC/A ratios could exhibit different levels of accommodative convergence in darkness, yielding different dark vergence postures and weakening the statistical correlation between dark vergence and dark focus. Thus to test whether dark vergence is influenced by accommodation, one should consider subjects' AC/A ratios as well as their dark focus.

Bohman and Saladin (1980) tested this possiblity in a study of the relationship between night myopia and accommodative convergence. They reasoned that if the normal synergy of accommodation and convergence is maintained under low illumination, subjects ought to show accommodative convergence that is determined by their particular dark focus (night myopia) and AC/A ratio. Their results indicated that vergence in darkness was not so systematically related, a finding consistent with the assumption that dark vergence is determined by tonic rather than accommodative innervation.

Another strategy to determine whether vergence and accommodation dissociate in darkness would be to look for correlated variations of dark vergence and dark focus over time. Evidence that the dark states fluctuate in synchrony would suggest synergism, while evidence that they fluctuate independently would support the hypothesized dissociation. Unfortunately, continuous records of accommodation and vergence taken simultaneously in darkness have not been reported. There is evidence from steady-state measures however, that dark vergence can be selectively modified without inducing a concomitant change in dark focus. Studies of perceptual adaptation to prisms and lenses (reviewed in a later section) show that dark vergence and distance perception in low illumination are correlated, and they covary as a result of oculomotor adaptation. In contrast, the dark focus of accommodation is neither correlated with perceived distance nor influenced by oculomotor adaptation (Owens and Leibowitz, 1980).

In summary, the available evidence indicates that (1) adjustments of vergence and accommodation are only weakly correlated in darkness, (2) a given individual's dark vergence cannot be predicted accurately from his or her dark focus and AC/A ratio, (3) perceived distance is related to dark vergence and unrelated to the dark focus, and (4) oculomotor adaptation selectively affects dark vergence and distance perception without affecting the dark focus. The most parsimonious interpretation of these findings is that vergence and accommodation assume independent resting or tonus states in the absence of adequate stimulation. Further research will be necessary to establish the generality of this interpretation. If it is correct, then dark vergence can be considered to reflect the subject's level of tonic vergence independent of accommodative vergence.

PERCEPTUAL CORRELATES OF TONIC VERGENCE

Perhaps the oldest literature on vergence and accommodation concerns their role in the perception of distance (reviewed by Boring, 1942). Early in the seventeenth century Descartes proposed that both oculomotor responses may determine the apparent distance of fixated objects. Less than a century later, Berkeley presented a theory of how these responses could become associated with distance perception through experience. In later years, pioneers of vision research including Wundt, Hillebrand, and Baird, conducted experiments to quantify the effects of vergence and accommodation on perceived distance, size, and stereoscopic depth. Reviews of this extensive research can be found in the literature on visual perception (Lie, 1965; McCready, 1965; Foley and Richards, 1972; Kaufman, 1974; Foley, 1980). While the processes underlying space perception are not completely understood, recent studies indicate that at least under low illumination, tonic vergence plays a key role in localizing objects as well as in determining the accuracy of vergence eye movements.

Specific Distance Tendency

One of the recurrent findings of research on space perception is that under low illumination most observers tend to underestimate the distance of far objects and to overestimate the distance of near objects (Grant, 1942; Foley, 1980). This phenomenon has been studied intensively by Gogel and colleagues. Using a variety of innovative techniques for assessing perceived distance, they determined that in the absence of contextual cues objects tend to be localized at an intermediate distance. Gogel referred to this perceptual bias as the *specific distance tendency* and proposed that it represents a fundamental metric for visual space perception (Gogel, 1969, 1977a, 1978; Gogel and Tietz, 1973).

Measurement of the specific distance tendency requires systematic elimination of all other distance cues. For this reason they measured the apparent distance of simple unfamiliar targets, such as a luminous circle or point, under reduced stimulus conditions. In general, under normal, brightly lit conditions, perceived distance was found to be determined by the interaction of oculomotor adjustments and the adjacent surroundings of the stimulus. As the situation was impoverished by eliminating surrounding objects, surfaces, motion parallax, and binocular parallax, perceived distance was found to be progressively biased toward an intermediate distance that varied from one subject to another.

Gogel and co-workers conducted a number of experiments to establish that the specific distance tendency is not an artifact of verbal or other cognitive response biases. Based on this work, they have proposed that the most accurate measure of the specific distance tendency is provided by an indirect method that relies on illusory motion as an index of perceived distance. With this procedure, the subject moves his or her head laterally while viewing a stationary monocular light point presented in darkness. The subject does not know that the light's position is fixed and is asked to report any apparent motion of the light point that is concomitant with head motion. Gogel (1976, 1977b) has shown that illusory motion is seen concomitant with head movements whenever the perceived distance of a target is different from its actual physical distance. When its actual distance is either farther or nearer than its apparent distance, the stimulus appears to move in the same or opposite direction, respectively, as the head motion. Such concomitant motion is not reported when the physical and perceived distances are equivalent. Thus by varying the position of a stimulus until no concomitant motion is reported, one can measure the specific distance tendency without asking the subject to make any deliberate judgments of distance. Using this method, Gogel and Teitz (1973) found the specific distance tendency of 60 subjects to range from approximately 30 cm to over 8 m with an average value of approximately 2 m.

Evidence that accommodation and vergence are biased toward intermediate resting states under impoverished conditions raised the possibility that the specific distance tendency is related to the observer's concurrent oculomotor adjustments. While Gogel and colleagues had demonstrated that the specific distance tendency is independent of stimulus factors, they had not examined its possible relation to accommodation or vergence. Considering the extensive evidence for oculomotor effects on perception under richer stimulus conditions, it seemed plausible that these adjustments might also influence perception in the absence of normal stimulation.

To test this possibility, Owens and Leibowitz (1976b) compared accommodative responses and perceived distance for a single point of light viewed in a dark surround. A laser optometer was used to measure accommodation in total darkness and while viewing the light point at 0.5 and 4 m, and the head-motion technique described above was used to measure perceived distance. The results indicated that the light point was not an effective stimulus for accommodation, and that both accommodation and perceived distance corresponded to intermediate distances regardless of the actual distance of the stimulus. However, as illustrated in Figure 3.7, there was no correlation between the dark focus of individual subjects and the perceived distance of the light point ($r = 0.19$; $p > 0.05$). This finding implied that accommodation had little effect on distance perception under low illumination, but the role of convergence remained uncertain.

A second experiment compared the perceived distance of the light point with the position of vergence in darkness. Again, perceived distance was measured with the head-motion technique, and dark vergence was evaluated with the nonius alignment procedure (Figure 3.2). The results are illustrated in Figure 3.8 as a scatter diagram showing the relationship between individual subjects' dark vergence values and their perceived distance for the light point. To facilitate comparisons, all data have been converted to equivalent vergence angles for a standard interpupillary distance of 65 mm. In an effort to minimize variance unrelated to distance perception, the lateral heterophoria of each subject was measured with near and distant fixation, and the average of those measures was sub-

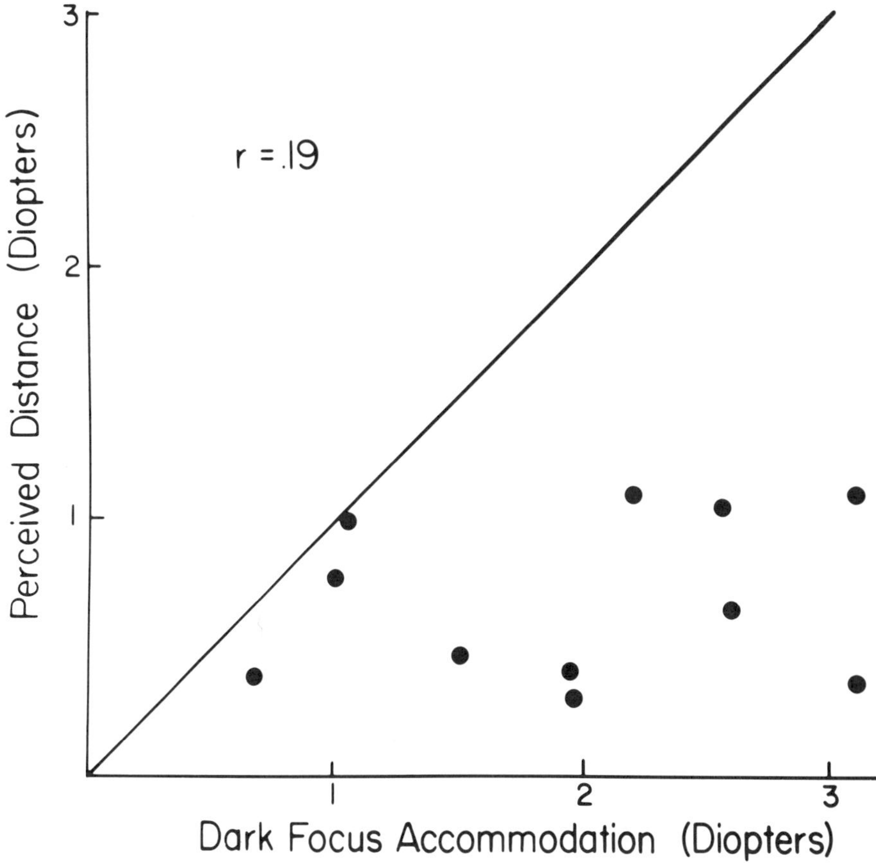

FIGURE 3.7. Scatter diagram showing the relation between the dark focus of accommodation and the perceived distance of a single point of light viewed in darkness. Reprinted by permission of the publisher, from Owens DA, Leibowitz HW. Oculomotor adjustments in darkness and the specific distance tendency. Perception and Psychophysics, 1976.

tracted from the subject's dark vergence value. As shown in Figure 3.8, corrected dark vergence values were found to be significantly correlated with perceived distance ($r = 0.76$; $p < 0.01$). A similar comparison of perceived distance with dark vergence *before* normalizing the data for phoria produced a somewhat weaker but still statistically significant correlation ($r = 0.56$; $p < 0.05$).

These results imply that the perceived distance of a weak stimulus viewed in the dark can be predicted from the observer's dark vergence value. They do not necessarily imply that dark vergence determines the

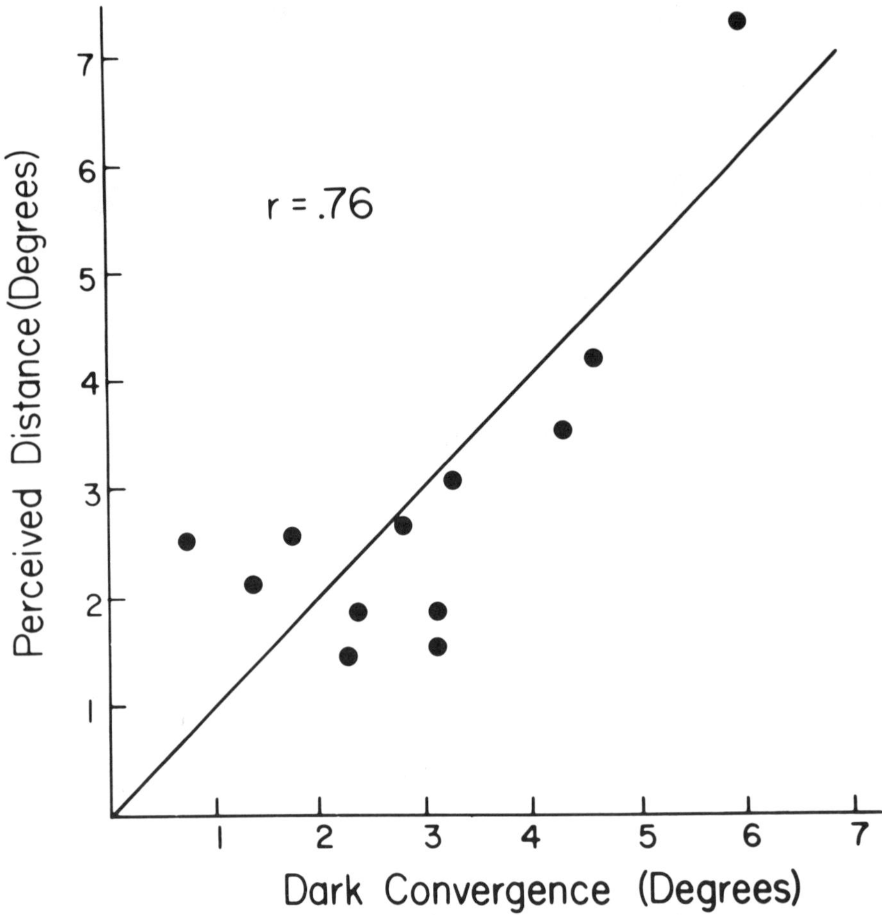

FIGURE 3.8. Scatter diagram showing the relation between the dark vergence and the perceived distance of a single point of light in darkness. Reprinted by permission of the publisher, from Owens DA, Leibowitz HW. Oculomotor adjustments in darkness and the specific distance tendency. Perception and Psychophysics, 1976.

specific distance tendency however, since correlational data do not justify the inference of causal relations. The same data might be interpreted as indicating that the specific distance tendency determines dark vergence, or that both are determined by a third, unspecified variable or process. In any case, the evidence clearly indicates that under low illumination, vergence is more important than accommodation for distance perception. This conclusion lends further support to the notion that vergence and accommodation do not maintain their normal correspondence in darkness.

Gaze Stability and Illusory Motion Perception

The head-motion procedure developed by Gogel for measuring perceived distance raises a fundamental question regarding the mechanisms of motion perception under impoverished stimulus conditions. The correlation between dark vergence and the distance at which the light point appeared stationary during head movements suggested that tonic vergence might also play a role in illusory motion. Our colleague, Robert B. Post, has recently proposed an explanation for this phenomenon.

Post's (1981) argument follows from an analysis of the processes by which gaze is normally stabilized during head and object motion. Two anatomically distinct systems subserve this vital function. An older gaze-stability system developed early in evolution. It is mediated by midbrain structures consisting of two neural loops that have no direct conscious consequences. One loop responds primarily to vestibular activity, although other input from the neck and body may also contribute. Its function is to initiate compensatory eye movements that maintain gaze stability during movements of the head and body. The visual loop serves the same function but is activated by contours in the visual field (optokinetic nystagmus, OKN). This older system is the primary means of image stabilization in nonfoveated animals. A newer system, referred to as the pursuit system, developed later in conjunction with the evolution of the fovea. Its primary function is to track moving objects. Unlike the older system, the pursuit system does have conscious perceptual consequences. Specifically, the effort involved in pursuit eye movements produces an efferent motion signal (efference copy or corollary discharge) that gives rise to the sensation of object movement and accounts for normal motion perception when tracking a moving object even though there is no retinal image motion.

The pursuit system may also be activated when the older system fails to maintain gaze stability. This activation of the pursuit system to prevent loss of fixation is responsible for the apparent movement of a fixated light when the light and the head undergo equal and simultaneous accelerations in the dark (oculogyral and oculogravic illusions) (Whiteside et al., 1965). In this case, the vestibular input initiates a slow-phase nystagmic movement opposite to the acceleration. Since the fixated light is stationary with respect to the observer, this vestibuloocular reflex (VOR) would result in a loss of fixation, so that a pursuit eye movement in the opposite direction (i.e., the direction of acceleration) is required to maintain fixation. In effect, the observer is making a pursuit effort, which is normally associated with moving objects, for a stationary (retinal) stimulus. This generates an efferent motion signal that results in an illusory motion of the light in the direction of the pursuit effort. Thus this phenomenon may be viewed as the result of a failure of the "old" gaze stability

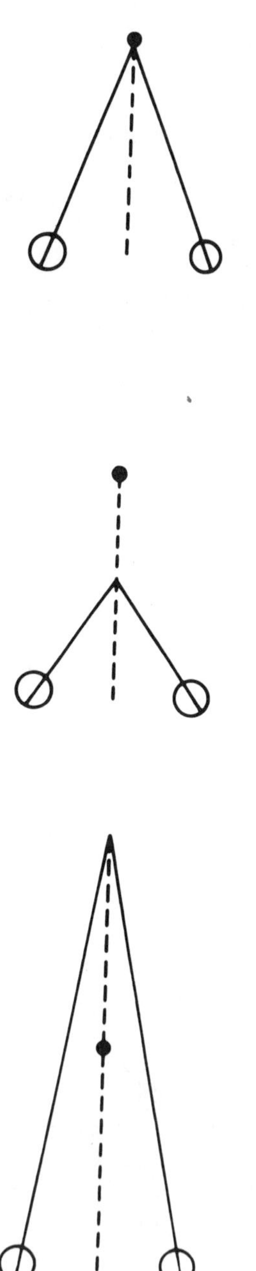

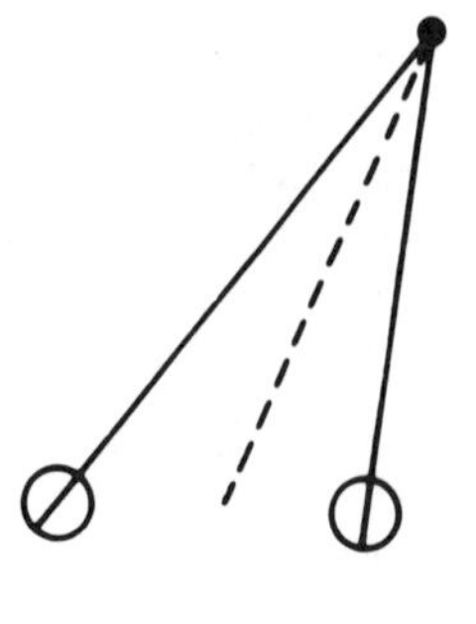

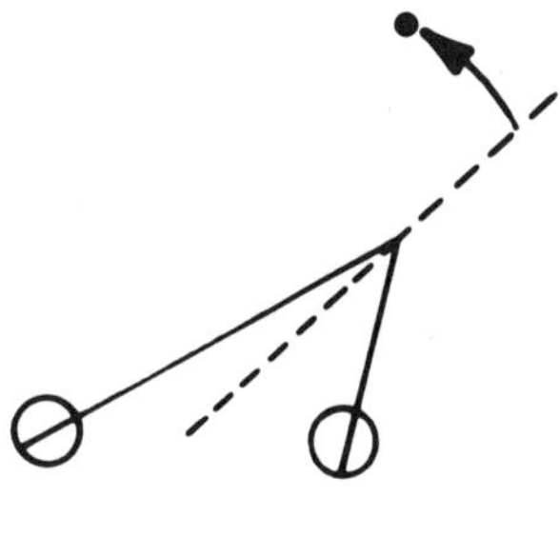

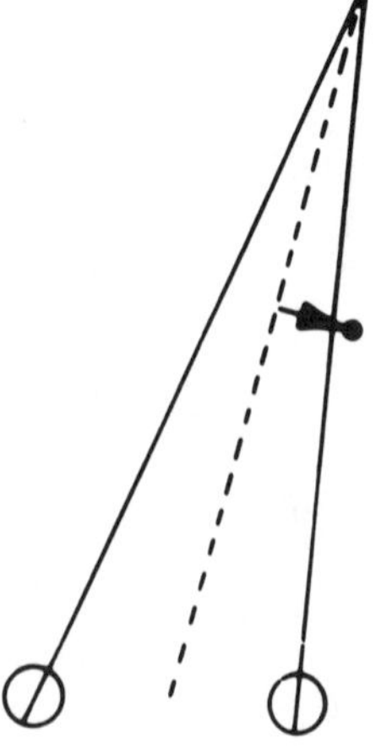

systems necessitating activation of the "new" pursuit system. Activation of the pursuit system to oppose reflexive eye movements (resulting from the older system) is referred to as nystagmus suppression. The efferent activity associated with this effort may be the basis for a number of illusory motion phenomena.

While this may seem paradoxical, the anatomic and functional separation of these two systems is well established in the literature and was elegantly demonstrated in an experiment by Brandt, Dichgans, and Büchele (1974). A subject seated inside a rotating striped drum will report, after 5 or 10 seconds, a compelling sensation of body rotation in a direction opposite to that of the drum. This phenomenon is referred to as circular vection and is typically accompanied by optokinetic nystagmus with the slow phase in the same direction as drum rotation. If, however, the subject views a small mirror so that the central visual field is stimulated by stripes moving in the direction opposite to those in the peripheral field, nystagmus immediately shifts to correspond to the central stimulus without affecting the sensation of self-motion. In this situation, the tracking eye movements and the apparent motion of the central stripes are mediated by the pursuit system, while the sensation of circular vection and the after-nystagmus that follows extinction of illumination are mediated by the older system.

The relevance of these gaze stability systems to the head-motion technique for measuring perceived distance is illustrated in Figure 3.9 (Post and Leibowitz, 1982). In the top row, a monocular point of light is placed at the dark vergence distance. Assume that the magnitude of the VOR is determined by the dark vergence position. In this case, translatory movements of the head will initiate compensatory eye movements that are adequate to maintain fixation. In the middle row, however, the point of light is located beyond the dark vergence distance, so that the VOR is too large and, if unopposed, would result in a loss of fixation. Thus a

FIGURE 3.9. Schematic diagram of the contributions of the vestibuloocular reflex (VOR) and the pursuit system in maintaining fixation during head translation to the left. Filled circles indicate the location of a monocular visual target. Solid lines represent the convergence distance relative to the distance of the target. (*Upper*) Convergence corresponds to target distance and the VOR is adequate to maintain fixation during movement of the head. (*Middle*) Convergence corresponds to a distance closer than the stimulus. The VOR is excessive so that an opposing effort from the pursuit system, in the direction of the arrow, is necessary to prevent loss of fixation. (*Lower*) Convergence corresponds to a distance greater than the stimulus; the VOR is inadequate and must be supplemented by the pursuit system. Whenever the pursuit system is activated, illusory motion in the direction of the effort results. Reprinted with permission from Vision Research, Post RB, Leibowitz HW, The effect of convergence on the vestibulo-ocular reflex and implications for perceived movement, 1982, Pergamon Press, Ltd.

pursuit effort in the direction *with* the head motion is necessary to cancel the excessive VOR. In line with the functional role of the pursuit system, the stationary light point would appear to move in the same direction as the pursuit effort or with the direction of head motion. When the point of light is located nearer than the dark vergence distance (bottom row), the VOR would be too small, again causing a loss of fixation if unopposed by pursuit effort. In this case, a pursuit effort in the *opposite* direction as the head motion is required to supplement the inadequate VOR. This pursuit effort produces illusory motion in the direction opposite as the head motion.

The hypothesized role of vergence in determining the magnitude of the VOR has been empirically demonstrated by Post and Leibowitz (1982). This mechanism should not be too surprising. Compensatory eye movements associated with linear head translations must be calibrated in some way to correspond to the distance of fixation. In an illuminated environment, fusional vergence and compensatory eye movements are enhanced by visual contours so that there is no need for pursuit effort to maintain fixation, and therefore no concomitant illusory motion. Under impoverished stimulus conditions, vergence responses are biased toward the tonic or dark vergence position (Ivanoff and Bourdy, 1954; Francis and Owens, 1980), and consequently the VOR will be too small for stimuli nearer than the dark vergence distance and too large for stimuli farther than the dark vergence distance. Whenever the VOR does not correspond to the stimulus distance, a supplementary pursuit effort is necessary to maintain fixation; the associated efferent signal gives rise to illusory motion. This is an appealing explanation for illusory concomitant motion because it depends on identifiable oculomotor mechanisms rather than on mentalistic concepts that are so pervasive in the perception literature.

OCULOMOTOR ADAPTATION AND TONIC VERGENCE

The evidence reviewed so far indicates that tonic vergence plays a significant role in both the coordination and the perceptual correlates of vergence eye movements. It biases vergence responses under conditions of physiological stress and reduced stimulation, it appears to be independent of accommodation, and it is involved in the misperception of distance and illusory motion under impoverished conditions. These findings suggest that tonic vergence is a key factor in the neural control and the perceptual consequences of binocular vergence. This view is supported by evidence that tonic vergence is also involved in perceptual and motor adapatation to modifications of the relationship between fusional demands and fixation distance.

Motor Adaptation

The clinical literature suggests that unusual demands on fusional vergence result in subsequent changes in vergence behavior, including transient changes in phoria, fixation disparity, and the limits of the fusional range (fusional reserves). These changes are probably related to a phenomenon frequently encountered by attempts to correct phoria or small tropias with prisms. In many cases, the patient "eats the prism," exhibiting an increased ocular deviation that counteracts the prism correction and thus restores the original phoria or tropia (Carter, 1963; Crone, 1969; Campos and Catellani, 1978). Systematic studies of such effects indicate that they may reflect adaptive changes of tonic vergence. This interpretation implies that tonic vergence depends at least partly on processes of sensory fusion and is thereby an important mechanism of so-called orthophorization (i.e., the general tendency to develop and maintain low levels of heterophoria despite changes in optical demands). It also suggests that anomalies of tonic vergence may be involved in some aspects of concomitant strabismus (Adler, 1953; Campos and Catellani, 1978; Crone and Hardjowijoto, 1979).

As cited earlier, Maddox (1893) reported marked changes in his "tonic convergence" as assessed by measures of phoria, after viewing through base-out prisms or plus lenses. Both of these conditions increased the demands on fusional convergence—the prisms by increasing binocular parallax and the lenses by decreasing accommodative convergence—and in both cases, tonic vergence (phoria) shifted in the direction of increased fusional demands. Maddox felt that such changes are adaptive, serving to relieve unusual stress on fusional vergence.

Later investigators found that using prisms to measure fusional reserves and fixation disparity can produce systematic changes in phoria. Alpern (1946) reported that standard clinical duction tests, which place a greater stress on fusional convergence than fusional divergence, produced increased esophoria at distance in 91% of his subjects and increased esophoria at near (16 inches) in 72%. Morgan (1947) found that successive tests of fusional reserves in either the convergent or divergent direction produced a consistent shift of lateral phoria in the same direction as the prism duction. Other studies have shown that vertical as well as lateral phoria is modified by prism duction tests, that the magnitude of such changes in phoria depends on the rate and the duration of increased fusional demand, and that the change in phoria decays gradually over a period of minutes to hours after removal of the prisms (Ellerbröck, 1950; Vaegan and Pye, 1979; Henson and North, 1980).

In a fascinating series of clinical and experimental observations, Carter (1963, 1965) has shown that prolonged viewing through base-in or base-out prisms induces changes in fixation disparity and fusional reserves as well as in phoria. When opposite-base prisms were first introduced, subjects typically showed an increased lag of vergence responses, failing to compensate fully for the optical deviation. These anomalous fixation disparities disappeared within 5 to 15 minutes of continued viewing through the prisms. At the same time, lateral phoria measured with the prisms in place returned to the original level measured without prisms. With progressive increments of prism power, the fixation disparity and phoria of some subjects adapted to base-in prisms as strong as 10^{Δ} and to base-out prisms as strong as 32^{Δ}. After adaptation, fixation disparity curves and phoria measures taken with the prisms in place appeared to be normal, implying that the actual position of the eyes had shifted as much as 30^{Δ}. Additional duction tests of one subject showed that after adapting to 9^{Δ} base-in prisms, the divergence reserve (measured by introducing *additional* base-in prism power) was within 2^{Δ} of the subject's original base-in breakpoint. That is, the actual divergence of the eyes at the breakpoint increased by 7^{Δ} through adaptation to the base-in prisms. The adaptive changes in fixation disparity and phoria remained stable for as long as several weeks of continuous exposure to the prisms. Following their removal, the aftereffects of adaptation were observed to decay over a period of 15 minutes to 8 hours, depending on the post-adaptation viewing conditions. In general, rapid decay (or readaptation to normal) was obtained for subjects who experienced normal binocular fusion immediately after removal of the prisms, while prolonged after-effects were obtained when normal binocular fusion was prevented through sleep (Carter, 1963) or through diplopia resulting from abrupt removal of high-power prisms (Carter, 1965).

Carter (1965) interpreted these variations of fixation disparity and phoria as reflecting adaptive changes in the"tonicity of motor centers" (p. 149). Similar to Maddox's view, he proposed that the changes in "tonicity" reduce ocular discomfort by relieving unusual stress on fusional vergence. Moreover, based on the slow decay of the aftereffects of prism adaptation when normal binocular fusion was absent following removal of the prisms, he concluded that sensory fusion seemed to be necessary for adaptation and for recovery from its aftereffects. He noted that some subjects are incapable of adaptation to opposite-base prisms and suggested that they may lack normal sensory fusion and may therefore be more susceptible to high heterophoria. Extending this argument, he proposed that:

> . . . with most persons some factor is acting to maintain approximate orthophoria. The adaptation to prism vergence in this experiment may be a manifestation of this basic adaptive mechanism of normal binocular vision. (p. 151)

In summary, the evidence indicates that subjects initially fail to compensate fully for new optical demands on vergence. They generally overconverge when viewing through base-out prisms and to underconverge when viewing through base-in prisms, a tendency most commonly manifested as a change in phoria or fixation disparity. After a short period, however, vergence movements come to compensate fully for the prisms, and at the same time, lateral phoria and fusional reserves return to levels initially observed without prisms. In other words, the subjects behave as though the operating range and limits of their vergence eye movements have changed by a constant angle that compensates rather precisely for the optical transformation.

All of these changes can be explained quite simply if one assumes that tonic vergence represents the resting state of the vergence system, and as a corollary, that the tonus position is the starting point for all vergence responses. According to this view, the unusual fusional demands of prism adaptation somehow induce an adaptive shift of the tonus position. Before this shift occurs, the prisms displace the starting point for fusional responses toward one extreme of the functional range. Consequently, increased fusional effort is necessary to fixate stimuli in one direction from the resting (tonus) position, while decreased effort is necessary to fixate stimuli in the opposite direction from the resting position (e.g., base-out prisms increase the demand on convergence while decreasing the demand on divergence responses). At first this asymmetry of fusional effort is accompanied by anomalous phoria and fixation disparity as vergence responses lag toward the initial tonus position. As adaptation progresses, tonic vergence changes so that the starting point for fusional responses resumes its original position *relative* to the functional range of stimulation. As a result, the fusional effort required to fixate any given distance returns to normal levels, and measures of vergence accuracy, lateral phoria, and fusional reserves regain their original values.

This account identifies tonic vergence as the primary mechanism by which the vergence system adapts to optical transformations of the relation between eye position (vergence angle) and fixation distance. While providing a unitary explanation for a wide variety of adaptation phenomena, it raises a more basic question concerning the processes that determine and modify tonic vergence. Early in this chapter, the tonus position was characterized as the neutral or balance point between opposing convergence and divergence mechanisms. A greatly refined version of this simple model has recently been developed on the basis of new evidence concerning the conditions necessary for adaptation of phoria and fixation disparity.

In studies of the effects of brief exposure to opposite base prisms, Schor (1979a, 1979b) demonstrated that fixation disparity and phoria begin to change within the first minute of observation, and that fusional vergence specifically is necessary for such adaptation to occur. He found that increasing the stimulus for fusional convergence by 3 degrees for only 30 to 60 seconds produced a convergent shift in the observers' phoria. In contrast, an increase of accommodative convergence of the same magnitude and duration, induced by viewing monocularly through a −2.0-D lens, produced no change in phoria. In another experiment, Schor tested the effect of binocularly viewing a target at a distance of 50 cm through +2.0-D lenses for 60 seconds. These lenses decreased accommodation, thereby reducing accommodative convergence. To maintain single vision, the reduced accommodative convergence would have to be compensated by increased fusional convergence. Thus additional fusional convergence activity was required by the positive lenses, even though the vergence posture necessary for sensory fusion was identical with and without the lenses. Viewing through the positive lenses caused an increase in phoria comparable to that following a 3-degree disparity-induced fusional response. These findings imply that accommodative vergence has no effect on phoria, while very brief increases in fusional vergence, stimulated either by retinal disparity or by the need to compensate for accommodative divergence, produces an adaptive change in phoria.

Building on a concept first proposed by Hofmann and Bielschowsky (1900), Schor (1980) has developed a quantitative model that accounts for adaptive changes in fixation disparity and phoria through the activity of two fusional vergence systems. The more familiar system, called fast-fusional vergence, responds immediately to eliminate retinal disparity by initiating the necessary convergence or divergence movement. The second system, slow-fusional vergence, is not directly affected by the stimulus but rather is driven by the effort of the fast-fusional system. When the fast-acting system is forced to respond vigorously (as with prism duction tests, prism adaptation procedures, and sustained near convergence), its output initiates gradually increasing activity in the corresponding slow-acting mechanism. The increased slow-fusional activity serves to reduce the effort required by the fast-fusional system, and it continues to influence vergence posture after the fast-acting response ceases. According to this model there are four rather than two mechanisms of fusional vergence. In addition to the well-known fast convergence and divergence mechanisms, the model posits dual slow-acting opponent mechanisms.

Another interesting feature of Schor's model concerns the control of steady-state vergence. The necessary stimulus both for initiating and for maintaining fast-fusional responses is retinal disparity. Consequently, precise binocular registration eliminates the necessary stimulus for fast fusion. The fast-fusional response then decays causing vergence to drift until retinal disparity reaches a magnitude that stimulates an increasing innervation, which cancels or compensates for the decay of the fast-fu-

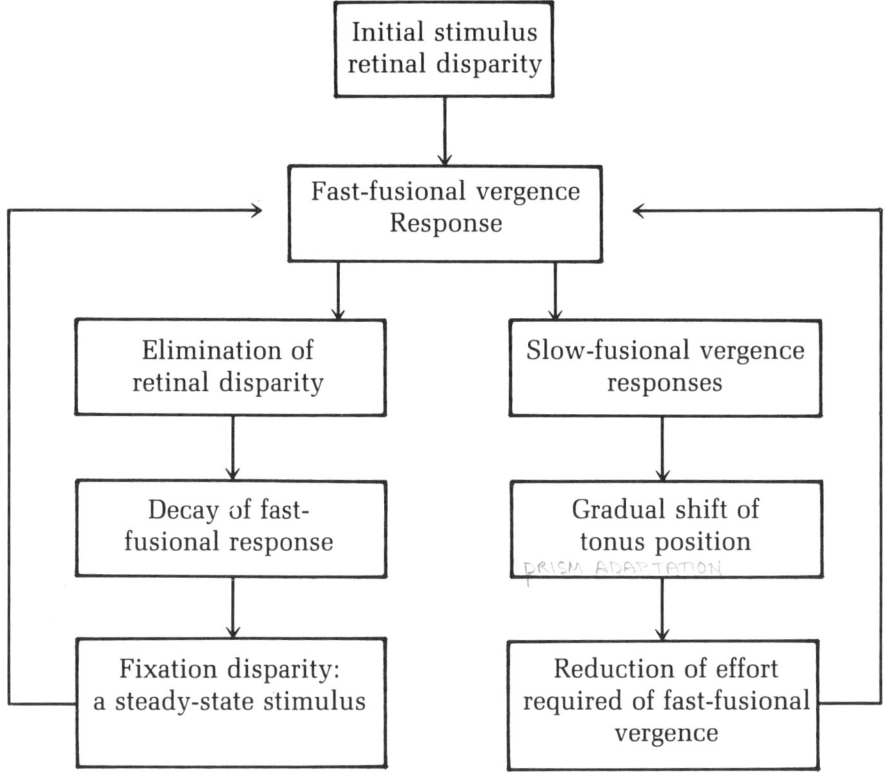

FIGURE 3.10. Schematic representation based on Schor's model of the relationship of fast-fusional vergence, slow-fusional vergence, and fixation disparity.

sional response. This vergence error, generally known as fixation disparity, is then maintained as a constant stimulus to prevent further decay of the fast-fusional response. Thus Schor's model characterizes fixation disparity as a purposeful error. Rather than an anomaly of binocular vergence, fixation disparity provides an error signal that is necessary for sustained fusion. The theoretical relations among fast-fusional vergence, slow-fusional vergence, and fixation disparity are schematically illustrated in Figure 3.10.

Schor's model is particularly interesting in the present context because it suggests heuristic explanations both for the progressive deterioration of vergence accuracy with stress or reduced stimulation, and for the adaptive changes in tonic vergence following unusual fusional demands. Since fixation disparity is the error signal or stimulus for sustained fast-fusional vergence, the model predicts that any condition that either decreases sensitivity to retinal disparity (e.g., low illumination) or increases the stress on vergence control centers (e.g., hypoxia) will result in larger steady-state vergence errors (i.e., fixation disparity). This prediction is consistent with the view presented earlier that any decrease in the efficiency of vergence control will produce an increased lag of vergence responses toward the resting or tonus position. Schor's model also implies that tonic vergence is partly, or perhaps fully, determined by the slow-fusional vergence mechanisms. Strong fusional demands such as those introduced by prisms or lenses require greater effort by the fast-fusional mechanisms and are therefore accompanied by faster decay of the fast-fusional response. This increased decay has two effects: (1) it results in a larger steady-state fixation disparity, which prevents further decay by stimulating additional fast-fusional effort; and (2) the added fast-fusional effort induces increased output from the corresponding slow-fusional mechanism, which supplements and thus relieves the effort required of the fast-fusional mechanism. In effect, unusual stress on the fast-fusional system serves through modulation of the activity of the slow-fusional system to readjust the tonus position so that less fast-fusional effort is required to maintain fusion. Consequently, a smaller error signal is necessary to maintain fusion, and therefore the fixation disparity for steady-state stimuli decreases. In addition, since the slow-fusional response decays slowly, the altered level of tonic innervation continues after the unusual stimulus demands are removed. Thus the altered slow-fusional activity induced by the effort of fast-fusional vergence can account for (1) the gradual reduction of fixation disparity during prism adaptation and (2) the prolonged change in the tonus position (dark vergence) following adaptation to opposite-base prisms.

Perceptual Adaptation

Numerous studies in psychology literature have reported that viewing through opposite-base prisms for a short time produces changes in distance perception that are similar to the effect of prism adaptation on vergence eye movements (Wallach and Frey, 1972; Wallach, Frey, and Bode, 1972; Craske and Crawshaw, 1974; von Hofsten, 1979; Owens and Leibowitz, 1980; Ebenholtz, 1981). Subjects typically misperceive distance when first looking through the prisms, then adapt over the course of 10 minutes or less, regaining normal distance perception. When the prisms are removed they again misperceive distance, but now in the direction opposite to their earlier errors. For example, when first exposed to base-out prisms, subjects tend to under-reach when grasping for objects. Such errors diminish rapidly with experience viewing through the prisms, but when the prisms are removed after adaptation the subjects tend to over-reach. They behave as though the relationship between binocular parallax and distance perception changes to compensate for the changes in fusional eye movements required for clear single vision.

These findings imply that viewing through opposite-base prisms induces some sort of recalibration of the effects of oculomotor adjustments on distance perception. The underlying processes remained unclear, however, because the experimental conditions could have modified accommodation and accommodative vergence as well as fusional vergence. Since most studies of perceptual adaptation neglected to measure oculomotor responses, they could not specify whether perceptual changes were related to the oculomotor effects of prism adaptation.

To clarify this, Owens and Leibowitz (1980) investigated the effects of adaptation to prisms and lenses on accommodation and vergence as well as on distance perception. The dark focus, dark vergence, and perceived distance of 60 subjects were measured before and after wearing adaptation spectacles containing 4^{Δ} base-out prisms and -1.25-diopter lenses for 20 minutes. This combination was selected to assure that vergence and accommodation increased by equal amounts and thus maintained their normal correspondence during adaptation.

The subjects were divided into three groups that performed different tasks during adaptation. One group (walkers) walked through the psychology building and engaged in several activities requiring eye-hand coordination, including table tennis and pitch-and-catch. A second group (riders) did not participate in the perceptual motor tasks, but followed the same path riding in a wheelchair. The third group (readers) remained in one position reading a magazine throughout the adaptation period and were not permitted to use their hands. This variation of adaptation conditions was used because, in a series of now classic experiments, Held (1965) and his colleagues had shown that active experience is an important requisite for perceptual adaptation to laterally displacing prisms. We reasoned that active experience might also be important for adaptation to optically induced depth displacements.

Each subject's accommodation and vergence in darkness and perceived distance of a single point of light were measured immediately before and after the adaptation period. The dark focus of accommodation was measured with a laser optometer, and dark vergence was measured by the nonius alignment technique described earlier (Figure 3.2). No fusional or accommodative stimuli were present during either measurement. Distance perception was assessed by asking the subjects to point from below at the location of a point of light that was presented at various distances on a surface extending from the subject's chin. This target was seen binocularly at 10, 20, 30, and 40 cm in an otherwise dark field. The pointing responses were performed under open-loop conditions in which the subjects were not given visual or verbal feedback about the accuracy of their responses. Each measure was taken at least three times both before and after adaptation; the spectacles were not worn during any of these measures.

A previous experiment (Owens and Leibowitz, 1976b) had shown that under low illumination distance perception is independent of accommodation (Figure 3.7) but is correlated with subjects' dark vergence distance (Figure 3.8). This suggested that accommodation and vergence may be dissociated under reduced stimulus conditions, and that vergence independently affects distance perception. The effects of oculomotor adaptation provided further evidence for the dissociation of vergence and accommodation in darkness and confirmed the priority of vergence as a determinant of perceived distance.

Figure 3.11 summarizes the average dark vergence and dark focus values before and after adaptation for each of the three adaptation conditions. These results show that dark vergence tended to be greater after adaptation than before. That is, it shifted toward increased convergence, the same direction as the increased fusional demand of the adaptation spectacles. This effect was more striking for the walking and riding conditions than for the reading condition. Averaging across all conditions,

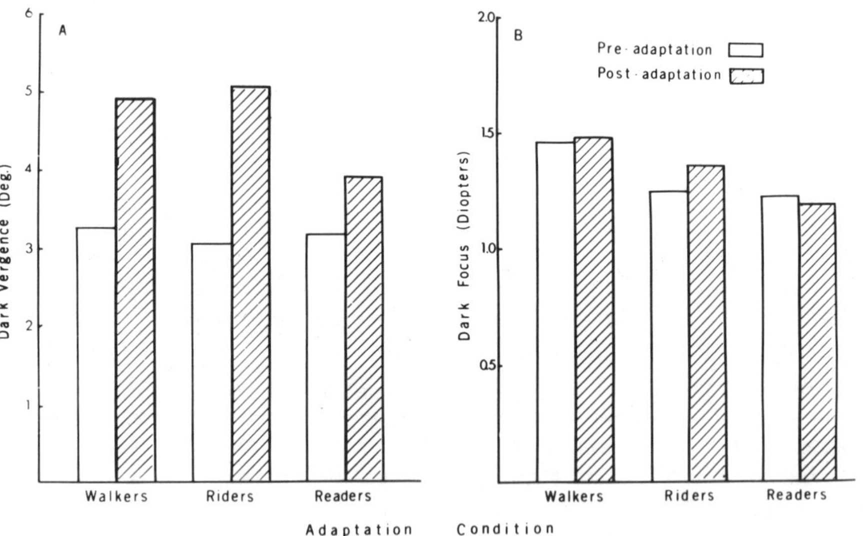

FIGURE 3.11. Mean dark vergence and dark focus values obtained before and after subjects adapted to spectacles containing base-out prisms and negative lenses. Reprinted by permission of the publisher, from Owens DA, Leibowitz HW. Accommodation, convergence, and distance perception in low illumination. American Journal of Optometry and Physiological Optics, © (1980), American Academy of Optometry per The Williams & Wilkins Company (agent).

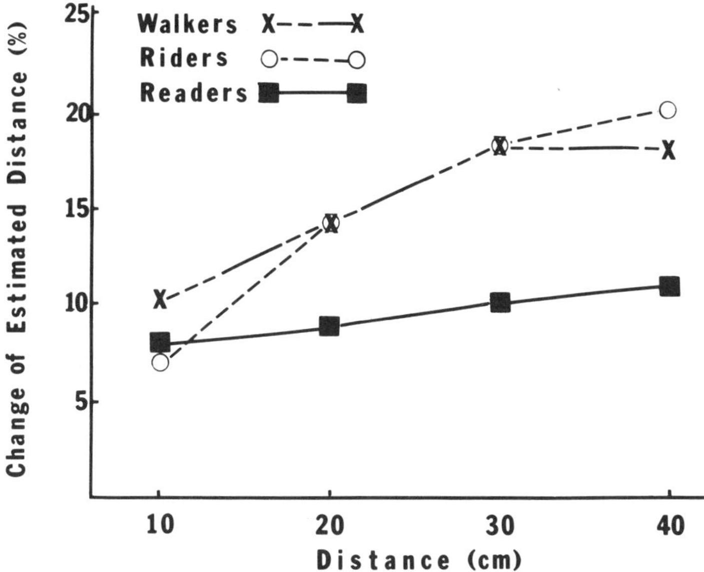

FIGURE 3.12. Mean percentage change in the perceived distance of a point of light following adaptation to spectacles containing base-out prisms and negative lenses. Reprinted by permission of the publisher, from Owens DA, Leibowitz HW. Accommodation, convergence, and distance perception in low illumination. American Journal of Optometry and Physiological Optics, © (1980), American Academy of Optometry per The Williams & Wilkins Company (agent).

the mean dark focus changed by only 2%, which was not significant; however, the change in mean dark vergence was 43%, a highly significant shift.

The effect of oculomotor adaptation on distance perception paralleled its effect on dark vergence. Averaging across conditions, adaptation produced a significant increase in mean perceived distance. The magnitude of this change was greater for the walking and riding groups than for the reading group. These data are presented in Figure 3.12 as the average percentage change in perceived distance as a function of stimulus distance. Comparison of Figures 3.11 and 3.12 suggests that the effects on both perceived distance and dark vergence depend on the activity experienced during adaptation.

These results support the view that convergence is more important than accommodation as a determinant of distance perception. The specific distance tendency was found to be significantly correlated with dark vergence (Figure 3.8) but unrelated to the dark focus of accommodation (Figure 3.7). In darkness, subjects tended to perceive a monocular point of light at a distance corresponding to their dark vergence regardless of their particular dark focus. Moreover, oculomotor adaptation produced similar changes in dark vergence and distance perception, while producing no change in the dark focus of accommodation (Figures 3.11 and 3.12). The correlated adaptation of dark vergence and perceived distance was also evident when comparing the various adaptation conditions separately. The readers who showed the smallest increase in dark vergence also showed the smallest increase in perceived distance; the walkers and riders who showed greater increases in dark vergence also showed greater changes in perceived distance. Thus in accord with Held's (1965) earlier work these results indicate that active interaction with the environment enhances oculomotor and perceptual adaptation to modifications of the relation between fusional responses and fixation distance.

Ebenholtz (1981) has partially replicated and extended these findings in a series of experiments comparing the effects of oculomotor adaptation and sustained convergence on lateral heterophoria and distance perception. He measured lateral phoria and perceived distance while subjects viewed (monocularly and binocularly, respectively) an array of seven points of light presented at distances ranging from 28.4 to 50 cm. These measurements were taken before and after the subjects participated in either of two experimental manipulations: (1) the adaptation paradigm in which they wore spectacles containing 5^{Δ} base-out prisms and −1.5-D lenses for 10 to 15 minutes, or (2) the induction paradigm in which they continuously fixated stimuli nearer than 30 cm for 6 to 15 minutes.

The results showed that both paradigms produced significant aftereffects on perceived distance and phoria, with greater effects produced by adaptation than by induction. Similar to our findings, subjects showed increased perceived distance and a correlated increase of esophoria after prism adaptation. The aftereffect of perceived distance reached asymptotic levels within 15 minutes of exposure to the prisms and lenses. When converted to angular units, the aftereffect of perceived distance was somewhat smaller than that of phoria. The induction paradigm also produced increases in perceived distance and esophoria, but these effects were only about one-third as strong and decayed much more rapidly than those of prism adaptation.

Ebenholtz (1981) suggested that one reason for these smaller aftereffects might be the limited number of contours that were visible during induction. Subjects interacted with a bright normal environment during prism adaptation, but they viewed only an array of seven light points during induction. He proposed that the strength of the aftereffects of both procedures might depend partly on the number of central "disparity detectors" that are activated. The precise role of binocular stimulation is not clear from this experiment, however, because the subjects experienced different activities as well as different visual stimuli.

The importance of fusable binocular stimulation for oculomotor adaptation is indicated more clearly by two preliminary studies that compared monocular and binocular exposure to prisms and lenses while subjects engaged in similar interactions with the environment. Ebenholtz (1981) reports a comparison of the effects of binocular adaptation to base-out prisms and minus lenses on phoria and distance perception with the effects of monocular adaptation to a −1.5-diopter lens. He reasoned that the increased accommodation required by the negative lens would induce accommodative convergence, and that the increased accommodative convergence might produce aftereffects similar to those following the increased fusional convergence induced by binocular viewing through base-out prisms. His results showed that monocular adaptation had no effect on either distance perception or phoria. This finding agrees with the results of an unpublished study conducted by Kleiner, Heffner, and Derbort (1981) in Owens' laboratory. This experiment compared the effects of binocular, monocular, and alternating monocular exposure to adaptation spectacles containing base-out prisms and negative lenses. The results showed that binocular adaptation produced significant aftereffects on dark vergence and fixation disparity, and a substantial shift in distance perception in the expected direction that did not reach statistical significance. In contrast, the monocular and alternating monocular conditions produced no significant effects on any of the dependent measures. Taken together, these preliminary findings suggest that stimulation of fusional vergence during adaptation is essential for perceptual as well as for oculomotor adaptation.

One of the most striking aspects of the perceptual effects of prism adaptation is their similarity to changes in the accuracy of vergence eye movements. When optical transformations are first introduced, both distance perception and vergence accuracy are disrupted. These errors nearly disappear within a period of minutes if the subject is permitted to interact with the surrounding environment and is capable of binocular fusion. For both, errors in the direction opposite to those first observed are found when prisms or lenses are removed following adaptation. Neither perceptual nor motor adaptation has been observed following exposure to optical manipulations that affect only accommodation and accommodative vergence. This finding, in conjunction with the fact that procedures resulting in correlated changes of distance perception and dark vergence have no effect on accommodation, suggests that accommodation is not involved in the relation of vergence to distance perception or in their concomitant adaptation to optical rearrangement. Rather, the available evidence indicates that the necessary condition for both perceptual and motor adaptation is the introduction of unusual demands for fusional vergence activity, as with opposite-base prisms (Carter, 1963, 1965; von

Hofsten, 1979; Owens and Leibowitz, 1980), spherical lenses that alter the requirements for fusional activity by reducing or eliminating the contribution of accommodative vergence (Maddox, 1893; Schor, 1979b), or tasks requiring prolonged fixation of near targets (Ebenholtz and Wolfson, 1975; Ebenholtz, 1981).

The similarity of perceptual and motor adaptation to unusual fusional demands suggests that they involve a common underlying mechanism. Von Hofsten (1976) has proposed a theory of the role of vergence in distance perception, which in combination with the concepts described earlier, allows a simple interpretation of the adaptation phenomena reviewed above. Once again, a key assumption is that the dark vergence position represents the tonic resting state of the vergence system, a posture that involves no activity or "effort" on the part of (fast-)fusional or accommodative mechanisms.

According to von Hofsten (1976), perceived distance is not related directly to the vergence angle of the visual axes, but is dependent on the extent to which a vergence response departs from the physiological resting state. Similar to Post's (1981) explanation of illusory motion perception in terms of "pursuit effort," von Hofsten's theory implies that the perception of distance is influenced by the amount of *vergence effort* required for binocular sensory fusion. In this case, the tonus position would correspond to a "specific" intermediate distance, while increasing convergence effort would be accompanied by proportionately decreasing perceived distance and increasing divergence effort by proportionately increasing perceived distance. Any manipulation that displaces the resting position to correspond to a new distance would alter the effort required to fixate all distances, and therefore would introduce systematic errors of distance perception. In general, a shift of the resting position toward a nearer distance would result in reduced convergence effort and increased divergence effort, with both leading to errors of overestimation. Conversely, a shift of the resting position toward a farther distance would result in increased convergence effort and decreased divergence effort leading to errors of underestimation.

The distance corresponding to the resting position can be changed by optical means or by oculomotor adaptation, and in both cases the effects on perceived distance are consistent with von Hofsten's theory. Consider, for example, the effect of viewing through base-out prisms. The prisms deviate the visual axes in the temporal direction so that initially the subject's dark vergence angle corresponds to a greater distance, and greater convergence effort (or less divergence effort) is required to fixate all stimuli. As a result, the subject initially perceives all stimuli as being closer than reality and under-reaches in open-loop pointing tasks. With continued exposure to the prisms, the misperception of distance decreases and reaching become more accurate. Consistent with von Hofsten's theory, this perceptual adaptation is accompanied by a convergent shift of the dark vergence position. The results illustrated in Figure 3.11 show that the mean dark vergence after removal of base-out prisms was over 1.5 degrees more convergent than measures taken prior to adaptation. This shift in the resting position would reduce the convergence effort required for near stimuli and diminish the tendency to underestimate distance. When the prisms were removed, however, this shift of the dark vergence reference position would result in an anomalous decrease in convergence effort for near stimuli and a concomitant increase in divergence effort for distant stimuli, which would tend to cause the overestimation of distance illustrated in Figure 3.12

SUMMARY AND CONCLUSIONS

Tonic vergence was one of the earliest concepts to emerge from analysis of vergence eye movements. Although the concept has survived for nearly a century, surprisingly little scientific inquiry has been directed toward clarifying its general significance or specific consequences for binocular vision. Even less attention has been paid to the physiological processes responsible for determining and modifying tonic vergence.

This chapter has reviewed a variety of phenomena drawn from the literatures on visual space perception, binocular eye movements, and clinical assessment, which share a common characteristic. They all appear to be related to or result from a systematic bias of the vergence system toward an intermediate adjustment. Perhaps the simplest examples are the effects of physiological stress, which may be induced by hypoxia, alcohol, or barbiturates, and those resulting from reduced sensory feedback due to decreased illumination and eccentric viewing. Both types of manipulations generally result in a progressive bias of vergence toward an intermediate posture that corresponds to the resting or tonus state assumed whenever central control processes are inactive.

A similar explanation has been offered for the development of vergence eye movements in early infancy. Like adults in low illumination, infants exhibit fixation disparities that vary over distance. Their most accurate fixation occurs for intermediate distances similar to the vergence distance found in total darkness. Unlike adults, however, infants' dark vergence posture corresponds to a nearer distance. The available evidence also indicates that vergence accuracy improves greatly over the first six months of life, a time during which sensory mechanisms of binocular vision are rapidly maturing. This concomitant improvement suggests that immature sensory processes may limit the accuracy of fusional vergence in infants resulting in a bias of vergence responses toward the tonus position.

There is evidence that anomalies of space perception under reduced stimulus conditions may also be due to a bias of vergence toward the tonus position. In darkness, the perception of distance and motion are most accurate for stimuli located at the dark vergence distance, and systematic errors are observed when the stimulus distance differs from the dark vergence distance. Distant stimuli are misperceived as being too close, and even though objectively stationary, appear to move in the same direction as the observer's head movements; stationary near stimuli are misperceived as being too far and appear to move opposite any movements of the head. These misperceptions can be explained most simply as resulting from a passive tendency to assume an intermediate vergence posture under impoverished viewing conditions.

This interpretation is consistent with perceptual and motor adaptation to modifications of the relation between fusional vergence and distance. Indeed, research on vergence adaptation has yielded some of the most exciting findings and stimulated development of the most sophisticated theoretical models of tonic vergence. These studies have established that tonic vergence is quite plastic. It readily adjusts to unusual demands on fusional vergence, such as those introduced by opposite-base ophthalmic prisms. Adaptive changes in tonic (dark) vergence are correlated with the recovery of normal vergence accuracy and normal space perception, suggesting that both oculomotor and perceptual adaptation depend on a common process, a "recalibration" of the tonus position of the vergence system. According to this view, the tonus position can be characterized as a range setting. It represents the starting point for all active vergence responses and the reference point for scaling the effects of vergence on space perception. Both perceptual and motor processes are disrupted whenever the tonus position is abruptly displaced (as by prisms) to a new fixation distance. Such displacements initiate an adaptive process that within a period of minutes shifts tonic vergence toward the original fixation distance, restoring the normal operating range and perceptual effects of vergence eye movements. This adaptive process appears to require active involvement of fusional vergence, supporting the theoretical position that tonic vergence depends on "slow"-fusional mechanisms whose activity is modified by "fast"-fusional vergence. Schor's (1980) quantitative model of this interaction may serve as a springboard to a more comprehensive understanding of tonic vergence and its relation to fusional mechanisms. Whatever the ultimate explanation, the adaptability of tonic vergence may be a common factor in such diverse phenomena as perceptual adaptation, orthophorization, and concomitant strabismus.

Finally, it should be emphasized that although the data base is conceptually broad, it is also empirically shallow. The tonic vergence concept is most appealing because it may help to integrate our understanding of phenomena ranging from the diplopia of alcohol intoxication to the adaptation of distance perception to prisms. Unfortunately, there is very little empirical evidence directly comparing the phenomena reviewed here. One of the most important questions for further study is whether the vergence biases observed under conditions of stress and impoverished stimulation, for example, are equivalent. Similarly, the generality of the effects of tonic vergence on the accuracy of fixation should be explored more fully. Of particular interest is the extent to which individual differences in dark vergence are responsible for variations in clinical measures such as lateral heterophoria and fixation disparity. A related and perhaps more challenging question concerns the possible role of tonic vergence in such serious anomalies of binocular vision as concomitant strabismus and anomalous retinal correspondence. Possible interactions between tonic vergence and accommodation should also be studied further.

The role of tonic vergence in space perception raises another set of complex questions. These concern not only the role of vergence, but also its interactions with oculomotor adjustments such as accommodation and the vestibuloocular reflex, and with other determinants of perceived distance and direction such as version eye movements, optical flow patterns, and contextual information. For example, the preceding account of the role of tonic vergence in distance perception does not address the question of what determines the "specific distance" that correlates with the tonus position and serves as the reference value for perceptual effects of active vergence responses. Also, the relative effects of accommodative vergence on perception and their relation to the tonic and fusional vergence components remain to be clarified.

Ultimately, our understanding of vergence behavior and its influence on perception should be correlated with underlying physiological processes. These issues are just beginning to attract active interest in the neuroscience community, and major relationships remain to be discovered. Perhaps the mechanisms of tonic vergence will prove to be more easily identified than other aspects of vergence control. This suggestion follows from the observation that the extraocular muscles are unique among mammalian muscle groups because their fibers are sharply differentiated into fast, or twitch groups and slow, or tonic groups. These groups differ in their structure, innervation, and response characteristics (Bach-y-Rita, 1967; Breinin, 1971; Jampel, 1967). At a superficial level, their differences are parallel to the theoretical distinction between the fast and slow fusional vergence systems. It would be interesting to determine whether this parallel is merely coincidental or whether indeed tonic fibers of the rectus muscles play a special role in tonic vergence.

There is good reason to believe that tonic vergence is a fundamental characteristic of the vergence system. It is a necessary component of the opponent process theory of binocular vergence, and it has proved to be a unifying concept for many phenomena of binocular vergence. Yet it may be the least explored aspect of vergence behavior. Perhaps this review will stimulate investigations to clarify further the nature of tonic vergence and its role in binocular vision.

REFERENCES

Abraham SV. The basic position of rest—convergence and divergence. J Pediatr Ophthalmol 1964;1:9–24.

Adler FH. Effect of anoxia on heterophoria and its analogy with convergent concomitant squint. Arch Ophthalmol 1945;35:227–32.

Adler FH. Pathologic physiology of strabismus. Arch Ophthalmol 1953;50:19–29.

Alpern M. The after-effect of lateral duction testing on subsequent phoria measurements. Am J Optom 1946;23:442–47.

Aslin RN. Development of binocular fixation in human infants. J Exp Child Psychol 1977;23:133–50.

Aslin RN. Oculomotor constraints on binocular vision in infants. Paper presented to the Society for Research in Child Development, April 1981, Boston.

Aslin RN, Dumais ST. Binocular vision in infants: a review and a theoretical framework. Adv Child Devel Behav 1980;15:53–94.

Aslin RN, Jackson RW. Dark vergence in human infants. Paper presented to the Association for Research in Vision and Ophthalmology, May 1981, Sarasota. Abstract in *Invest Ophthal Vis Sci*, 1981, *20*, 47.

Aslin RN, Dobson V, Jackson RW. Dark vergence and dark focus in human infants. Paper presented to the Association for Research in Vision and Ophthalmology, May 1982, Sarasota. Abstract in *Invest Ophthal Vis Sci*, 1982, *22*, 105.

Bach-y-Rita P. Neurophysiology of extraocular muscles. Invest Ophthalmol Vis Sci 1967;6:229–34.

Björk A. Electrical activity of human extrinsic eye muscles. Experientia 1952;8.

Bohman CE, Saladin JJ. The relation between night myopia and accommodative convergence. Am J Optom Physiol Opt 1980;57:551–58.

Boring EG. Sensation and perception in the history of experimental psychology. New York: Appleton-Century-Crofts, 1942.

Brandt T, Dichgans J, Büchele W. Motion habituation: inverted self-motion and optokinetic afternystagmus. Exp Brain Res 1974;21:337–52.

Brecher GA, Hartman AP, Leonard DD. Effect of alcohol on binocular vision. Am J Ophthalmol 1955;39:44–51.

Breinin GM. The position of rest during anesthesia and sleep. Arch Ophthalmol 1957;57:323–26.

Breinin GM. The structure and function of extraocular muscles—an appraisal of the duality concept. Am J Ophthalmol 1971;72:1–9.

Breinin GM, Moldaver J. Electromyography of the human extra-ocular muscles. I. Normal kinesiology; divergence mechanism. Arch Ophthalmol 1955; 54:200–210.

Burian HM, von Noorden GK. Binocular vision and ocular motility. St. Louis: CV Mosby, 1974.
Campos EC, Catellani CO. Further evidence for the fusional nature of the compensation (or "eating up") of prisms in concomitant strabismus. Int Ophthalmol 1978;1:57–62.
Carter DB. Effects of prolonged wearing of prism. Am J Optom 1963;40:265–73.
Carter DB. Fixation disparity and heterophoria following prolonged wearing of prisms. Am J Optom 1965;42:141–52.
Cogan DG. Accommodation and the autonomic nervous system. Arch Ophthalmol 1937;18:739–66.
Cogan DG. Neurology of ocular muscles. 2nd ed. Springfield, Il.: Charles C Thomas, 1956.
Colson ZW. The effect of alcohol on vision: an experimental investigation. JAMA 1940;115:1525–27.
Craske B, Crawshaw M. Adaptive changes of opposite sign in the oculomotor systems of the two eyes. Q J Exp Psychol 1974;26:106–113.
Crone RA. Heterophoria. I. The role of microanomalous correspondence. Albrecht Von Graefes Arch klin exp Ophthalmol 1969;177:52–65.
Crone RA, Hardjowijoto S. What is normal binocular vision? Doc Ophthalmol 1979;47:163–99.
Duke-Elder S, Wybar K. Ocular motility and strabismus. In: Duke-Elder S., ed. System of ophthalmology. Vol 11. London: Kimpton, 1973.
Ebenholtz SM. Hysteresis effects in the vergence control system: perceptual implications. In: Fisher DF, Monty RA, Senders JW, eds. Eye movements: visual perception and cognition. Hillsdale, N.J.: Erlbaum, 1981.
Ebenholtz SM, Wolfson DM. Perceptual aftereffects of sustained convergence. Percept Psychophysics 1975;17:485–91.
Ellerbrock VJ. Tonicity induced by fusional movements. Am J Optom 1950;27:8–20.
Fincham EF. The mechanism of accommodation. Br J Ophthalmol (Monogr Suppl) 1937;8:1–80.
Fincham EF. Accommodation and convergence in the absence of retinal images. Vision Res 1962;1:425–40.
Fincham EF, Walton J. The reciprocal actions of accommodation and convergence. J Physiol (Lond) 1957;137:488–508.
Foley JM. Binocular distance perception. Psychol Rev 1980;87:411–34.
Foley J, Richards W. Effects of voluntary eye movement and convergence on the binocular appreciation of depth. Percept Psychophysics 1972;11:423–27.
Francis EL. Individual dark vergence: its effect on fixation disparity, phoria, and perceived distance. Senior research thesis, Franklin and Marshall College, Lancaster, PA, 1979.
Francis EL, Owens DA. The accuracy of convergence for peripheral stimuli. Paper presented at the Topical Meeting on Recent Advances in Vision, Optical Society of America, April 1980, Sarasota.
Gogel WC. The sensing of retinal size. Vision Res 1969;9:1079–94.
Gogel WC. An indirect method of measuring perceived distance from familiar size. Percept Psychophysics 1976;20:419–29.
Gogel WC. The metric of visual space. In: Epstein W, ed. Stability and constancy in visual perception: mechanisms and processes. New York: Wiley, 1977a.

Gogel WC. An indirect measure of perceived distance from oculomotor cues. Percept Psychophysics 1977b;21:3–11.

Gogel WC. Size, distance, and depth perception. In: Carterette EC, Friedman MP, eds. Perceptual processing, handbook of perception. Vol. 9. New York: Academic Press, 1978:299–333.

Gogel WC, Teitz JD. Absolute motion parallax and the specific distance tendency. Percept Psychophysics 1973;13:284–92.

Grant VW. Accommodation and convergence in visual space perception. J Exp Psychol 1942;31:89–104.

Hebbard FW. Measuring tonic convergence. Am J Optom 1952;29:221–30.

Held R. Plasticity in sensory-motor systems. Sci Am 1965;213:84–94.

Helmholtz H. Handbook of physiological optics. Vol. 1. New York: Dover Publications, 1962.

Hennessy RT. Instrument myopia. J Opt Soc Am 1975;65:1114–20.

Hennessy RT, Leibowitz HW. Laser optometer incorporating the Badal principle. Behav Res Methods Instrumentation 1972;4:237–39.

Hennessy, RT, Iida T, Shiina K, Leibowitz HW. The effect of pupil size on accommodation. Vision Res 1976;16:587–89.

Henson DB, North R. Adaptation to prism-induced heterophoria. Am J Optom Physiol Opt 1980;57:129–37.

Hofmann FB, Bielschowsky A. Über die der Willkür entzogenen Fusionsbewegungen der Augen. Pflügers Arch 1900;80:1–40.

Ivanoff A. Night binocular convergence and night myopia. J Opt Soc Am 1955;45:769–70.

Ivanoff A, Bourdy C. Le comportement de la convergence en nocturne (The behavior of convergence in night vision). Ann Optique Oculaire 1954;3:70–75.

Jampel RS. Multiple motor systems in the extraocular muscles of man. Invest Ophthalmol Visual Sci 1967;6:288–93.

Kaufman L. Sight and mind. New York: Oxford University Press, 1974.

Kleiner K, Heffner P, Derbort J. Convergence as a determinant of egocentric distance perception. Student research project, Franklin and Marshall College, Lancaster, PA, 1981.

LeGrand Y. Form and space vision. Bloomington, Ind.: Indiana University Press, 1967.

Leibowitz HW, Owens DA. Anomalous myopias and the intermediate dark focus of accommodation. Science 1975a;189:646–48.

Leibowitz HW, Owens DA. Night myopia and the intermediate dark focus of accommodation. J Opt Soc Am 1975b;65:1121–28.

Leibowitz HW, Owens DA. New evidence for the intermediate position of relaxed accommodation. Doc Ophthalmol 1978;46:133–47.

Levy J. Physiological position of rest and phoria. Am J Ophthalmol 1969;68:706–13.

Lie I. Convergence as a cue to perceived size and distance. Scand J Psychol 1965;6:109–116.

Luckiesh M, Moss FK. Functional adaptation to near vision. J Exp Psychol 1940;26:352–56.

McCready DW. Size-distance perception and accommodation convergence micropsia—a critique. Vision Res 1965;5:189–206.

Maddox EE. The clinical use of prisms; and the decentering of lenses. 2nd ed. Bristol, England: John Wright & Sons, 1893.
Mann I. The development of the human eye. New York: Grune & Stratton, 1964.
Mitchell DE. A review of the concept of "Panum's fusional areas." Am J Optom 1966a;43:387–401.
Mitchell DE. Retinal disparity and diplopia. Vision Res 1966b;6:441–51.
Morgan MW Jr. A new theory for the control of accommodation. Am J Optom 1946;23:99–110.
Morgan MW Jr. The direction of visual lines when fusion is broken as in duction tests. Am J Optom 1947;24:8–12.
Morgan MW Jr. The resting state of accommodation. Am J Optom 1957;34:347–53.
Ogle KN, Mussey MA, Prangen AdeH. Fixation disparity and the fusional processes in binocular single vision. Am J Ophthalmol 1949;32:1069–87.
Owens DA. The Mandelbaum effect: evidence for an accommodative bias toward intermediate viewing distances. J Opt Soc Am 1979;69:646–52.
Owens DA. A comparison of accommodative responsiveness and contrast sensitivity for sinusoidal gratings. Vision Res 1980;20:159–67.
Owens DA, Leibowitz HW. The fixation point as a stimulus for accommodation. Vision Res 1975;15:1161–63.
Owens DA, Leibowitz HW. Oculomotor adjustments in darkness and the specific distance tendency. Percept Psychophysics 1976b;20:2–9.
Owens DA, Leibowitz HW. Accommodation, convergence, and distance perception in low illumination. Am J Optom Physiol Opt 1980;57:540–50.
Post RB. Stimulus control of circular vection and optokinetic afternystagmus. PhD disseration, Pennsylvania State University, University Park, 1981.
Post RB, Leibowitz HW. The effect of convergence on the vestibuloocular reflex and implications for perceived movement. Vision Res 1982;*22*,461–65.
Powell WH. Ocular manifestations of alcohol and a consideration of individual variations in seven case studies. Aviat Med June 1938;97–103.
Rashbass C, Westheimer G. Disjunctive eye movements. J Physiol 1961;159:339–60.
Schober H. Über die Akkommodationsruhelage. Optik 1954;6:282–90.
Schor CM. The influence of rapid prism adaptation upon fixation disparity. Vision Res 1979a;19:757–65.
Schor CM. The relationship between fusional vergence eye movements and fixation disparity. Vision Res 1979b;19:1359–67.
Schor CM. Fixation disparity: a steady-state error of disparity-induced vergence. Am J Optom Physiol Opt 1980;57:618–31.
Siebeck R. The antagonistic innervation of the ciliary muscle and the rest position of accommodation. Optician December 11, 1953;535–40.
Slater AM, Findley JM. Binocular fixation and the newborn baby. J Exp Child Psychol 1975;20:248–73.
Stark L, Kenyon RV, Krishnan VV, Ciufredda KJ. Disparity vergence: a proposed name for a dominant component of binocular vergence eye movements. Am J Optom Physiol Opt 1980;57:606–609.
Toates FM. Vergence eye movements. Doc Ophthalmol 1974;37:153–214.
Vaegan, Pye D. Independence of convergence and divergence: norms, age trends, and potentiation in mechanized prism vergence tests. Am J Optom Physiol Opt 1979;56:143–52.

von Hofsten C. The role of convergence in visual space perception. Vision Res 1976;16:193–98.

von Hofsten C. Recalibration of the convergence system. Perception 1979;8:37–42.

Wallach H, Frey KJ. Adaptation in distance perception based on oculomotor cues. Percep Psychophysics 1972;11:77–83.

Wallach H, Frey KJ, Bode KA. The nature of adaptation in distance perception based on oculomotor cues. Percept Psychophysics 1972;11:110–16.

Walls GL. The vertebrate eye and its adaptive radiation. Bloomfield, Mich.: Cranbrook Institute of Science, 1942.

Westheimer G. Amphetamine, barbiturates, and accommodation-convergence. Arch Ophthalmol 1963;70:830–836.

Whiteside TDM, Graybiel A, Niven JI. Visual illusions of movement. Brain 1965;88:193–210.

Wilmer WH, Berens C. The effect of altitude on ocular functions. JAMA 1918;71:1394–98.

Wist ER, Hughes FW, Forney RB. Effect of low blood alcohol level on stereoscopic acuity and fixation disparity. Perceptual Motor Skills 1967;24:83–87.

Zimmerman AA, Armstrong EL, Scammon RE. The change in position of the eyeballs during fetal life. Anat Rec 1933;59:109–34.

4

Theoretical and Clinical Importance of Proximal Vergence and Accommodation

Steven C. Hokoda
Kenneth J. Ciuffreda

The influence of perceived distance on convergence has attracted considerable attention. As early as 1893, Maddox, in his classification of vergence eye movements, included convergence due to "knowledge of nearness" (now referred to as proximal vergence) as one of the four components of vergence. Various methods of investigation have been employed in the study of proximal vergence. These have included comparison of instrument and free-space phoria (or tropia) measurements, differences between calculated AC/A ratios (changing the accommodative demand by altering fixation distance) and gradient AC/A ratios (changing the accommodative demand by optical means with constant fixation distance), experimental arrangements encouraging misperception of distance, and infrared photography of eye position with near fixation in the dark. Measurements of proximal vergence are generally expressed as a ratio with change in convergence (in prism diopters) divided by the change in test distance (in diopters). Values fall in the range of $0.5^{\Delta}/D$ to $2.0^{\Delta}/D$. For subjects with normal binocular vision, an inverse relationship with accommodative vergence has been demonstrated; there have also been interactions between proximal and fusional vergence. Increased levels of proximal vergence are found when positive fusional vergence is stimulated and decreased levels with stimulation of negative fusional vergence. In addition, association of abnormal proximal vergence levels in patients with binocular vision anomalies has been found. Proximal vergence is increased in esotropia and divergence excess exotropia and decreased in convergence insufficiency. Orthoptics and lens application may alter proximal vergence. Proximal effects on accommodation probably play a lesser role. Normal patients show minimal influence, while those with binocular dysfunctions show effects that are both more frequent and of greater magnitude. Little consideration has been given to proximal influences in modeling of the vergence and accommodation systems. Since proximal effects can be demonstrated in many individuals with normal binocular vision, particularly on vergence, and they are frequently abnormal in patients with anomalous binocular vision, incorporation of a proximal component into a general quantitative model of the vergence and accommodation systems seems not only warranted but essential. This chapter covers these topics in detail.

PROXIMAL CONVERGENCE

The notion that perceived distance influences convergence explains the differences found between AC/A ratios determined at fixed (gradient method) and multiple (calculated method) test distances. Very high correlations would be expected between the two ratios were these functions solely dependent on accommodative drive to the vergence system. Low correlations have been found, however, between dissociated phoria gradient AC/A ratios and the difference between near and far phorias (Rubie, 1979–80), and between AC/A ratios derived from gradient fixation disparity measures and the difference between near and far associated phorias (Ogle et al., 1967). Such low correlations suggest the influence of an additional variable, namely testing distance, on the near phoria.

With disparity (fusional) vergence open-looped,[1] as is true during dissociated phoria measurements, and accommodation monitored to factor out any AC/A-related change in the angle of deviation, testing distance has been found to affect convergence (Hofstetter, 1942; Morgan, 1944a; Alpern, 1955). Closed-loop disparity vergence testing, as in the measurement of fixation disparity, also shows a distance effect on vergence, although the available data do not exclude accommodative interaction (Ogle and Martens, 1957; Ogle et al. 1967).

[1] By "opening the loop" on the disparity vergence system through prism dissociation or occlusion of an eye, one prevents normal feedback of disparity error. This is in contrast to the more typical situation in which the disparity vergence system is closed-loop and visual feedback regarding disparity error is available.

Evidence for a direct perceptual effect on vergence from perceived distance has been found in investigations using presentations of playing cards varying in size (Alpern, 1958) and overlayed so that perception of the relative distances of the cards was reversed (Morgan, 1962). Both procedures yielded convergence changes independent of accommodation, with increased size or apparent nearness associated with increased convergence.

Consideration of proximal effects on convergence is warranted on the basis of magnitude of response. Table 4.1, an updated and expanded version of a table presented by Knoll (1959), shows a range of values from 0.53^{Δ}/D to 2.03^{Δ}/D, with an average tabulated value of 1.29^{Δ}/D. We will use Knoll's PCT designation, which refers to the ratio of change in proximal vergence to change in test distance (in diopters). In light of the mean gradient stimulus AC/A ratio for this population of $4.04 \pm 1.33^{\Delta}$/D (Morgan, 1944b) and the importance attached to accommodative convergence in the evaluation of binocular function (Morgan, 1968; Borish, 1975), proximal vergence can be a significant entity. It can contribute up to 50% of the total near vergence response under open-looped conditions.

Applying corrections for prism effectivity to gross phoropter phoria findings in determining the actual rotation of the eye (Alpern, 1957;[2] Pratt, 1962), the magnitude of phoria measurements decreases proportionately more at nearer test distances. The net effect would increase any difference between calculated and gradient AC/A ratios, a common method of estimating proximal vergence magnitude. This would result in an increased amount of convergence attributable to proximal factors. For example, in a patient with an interpupillary distance of 60 mm, distance exophoria of 1^{Δ}, near exophoria (40 cm) of 4^{Δ}, and +1.0D gradient value of 8^{Δ} exophoria, there would be a calculated AC/A ratio of 4.8^{Δ}/D and a gradient AC/A ratio of 4.0^{Δ}/D. The difference yields a proximal convergence ratio of 0.8^{Δ}/D. Calculations ignoring corrections for prism effectivity would result in underestimation of the proximal vergence contribution. A two-diopter hyperope, an emmetrope, and a two-diopter myope would have their PCT underestimated by 0.3^{Δ}/D, 0.5^{Δ}/D, and 0.8^{Δ}/D, respectively.

The rate of change of proximal vergence with change in test distance remains unclear. A linear increase in proximal convergence with distance

[2] Alpern's correction factor for prism effectivity (distance in meters) is:

$$\frac{t}{(1 - 0.027\,D)(t + s) + 0.027}$$

t = distance from object to spectacle plane;
D = power of spectacle lens and add (diopters);
s = distance from prism to spectacle plane (assume = 0.035);
0.027 = assumed distance from spectacle plane to center of rotation of eye.

TABLE 4.1. Summary of Proximal Vergence in Past Investigations

Authors and Year	*Subjects*	*Method*	*Accommodative Measurement*	*PCT*
Tait, 1933	18–30 yr n = 200	Zero accommodative level phoria at 33.3 cm minus 6 m phoria and near fusion demand for binocular fixation	Stimulus	$1.87 \pm 2.39^{\Delta}$/D
Hofstetter, 1942	28 young adults	34.5 cm gradient AC/A minus 5 m gradient AC/A Haploscopic measures	Response	$0.73 \pm 0.57^{\Delta}$/D
Morgan, 1944a	20–30 yr n = 50	Near fusion demand for binocular fixation (40 cm minus tonicity, accom-converg, and fusional convergence) Haploscopic measures	Response	$1.2 \pm 0.8^{\Delta}$/D
Morgan, 1950	413 nonpresbyopes	Calculated AC/A (6 m and 40 cm) minus gradient AC/A (+1.00 D at 40 cm)	Stimulus	1.4^{Δ}/D
Shapero and Levy, 1953	24–35 yr $\bar{X}$: 28.5 yr n = 8	Phorias compared across same accommodative demand (0-3 D) for different distances (6 m-33.3 cm); prism effectivity correction	Stimulus	0.87^{Δ}/D
Manas and Schulman, 1954	22 young adults	Calculated AC/A (6 m and 40 cm) minus gradient AC/A (+1.00 D at 40 cm)	Stimulus	$0.53 \pm 1.17^{\Delta}$/D
Alpern, 1955	11 young adults	Zero accommodative level phoria at different distances (5.9 m-20 cm) Haploscopic measures	Response	0.71^{Δ}/D

Ogle and Martens, 1957	19–50 yr $\bar{X}$: 27 ± 2.6 yr n = 28	Calculated AC/A (4.4 m to 14 cm) minus 40 cm gradient AC/A; prism effectivity correction	Stimulus	0.9 ± 0.9^{Δ}/D
	14–72 yr $\bar{X}$: 31 ± 12.8 yr n = 104	Calculated AC/A (associated phorias at 4.4 m and 40 cm) minus fixation disparity derived AC/A at 40 cm; prism effectivity correction	Stimulus	1.52 ± 1.62^{Δ}/D
Hofstetter, 1957	20–27, one 47 yr $\bar{X}$: 22.5 yr n = 21	33.3 cm gradient AC/A minus 6 m gradient AC/A; prism effectivity correction	Stimulus	0.87^{Δ}/D
Ogle et al., (1967)	11–79 yr $\bar{X}$: 32 ± 12 yr n = 256	Calculated AC/A (associated phorias at 2.5 m and 33.3 cm) minus fixation disparity derived AC/A at 33.3 cm; prism effectivity correction	Stimulus	1.81 ± 1.95^{Δ}/D
Franceschetti and Burian, 1970	95 unspecified age	Calculated AC/A minus 40 cm gradient AC/A	Stimulus	2.03^{Δ}/D
Sheedy and Saladin, 1975	22–39 yr n = 13	Zero accommodative level phoria at 40 cm minus distance phoria and near fusion demand for binocular fixation	Stimulus	1.96 ± 1.72^{Δ}/D
Hokoda 1982 (unpublished data)	6–47 yr $\bar{X}$: 28.5 ± 10 yr n = 106	Calculated AC/A (4.5 m and 40 cm); minus gradient AC/A (40 cm)	Stimulus	1.70 ± 1.72^{Δ}/D

(in diopters) was found by Hofstetter (1951) using measures of dissociated phoropter phorias and prism vergence limits. Shapero and Levy (1953) generally found a decreasing rate of change of proximal vergence as test distance decreased. There are several problems with their findings, however. They found gradient (stimulus) AC/A ratios to decrease with closer test distances, although Alpern (1955) found that test distance did not affect the response AC/A ratio. An additional complication arises from a change in experimental procedure. For the three closest test distances the subject held the fixated target, adding an unaccounted but probably important variable. Stern (1953) found significantly greater convergence (two prism diopters) when the target was touched by the subject ($n = 50$) when measuring phorias in a modified mirror stereoscope with fixation at 40 cm. Data from our laboratory (Hokoda and Ciuffreda, unpublished data) also showed small increases in convergence (0.5^{Δ}/D) for calculated stimulus AC/A ratios when the subject held the target. Alpern (1955) used stigmatoscopy[3] to monitor accommodative response as distance effects on proximal vergence were investigated. He expressed proximal vergence as the change in phoria for which the accommodative response was zero diopters as a function of the test distance in diopters. Although mean data for his 11 subjects showed a somewhat linear increase in proximal convergence over the middle test distances, none of the subjects followed this mean response pattern in a regular fashion, and considerable variability and nonlinearity in individual findings were evident. Alpern's zero-accommodation phorias for 2 m to 33.3 cm show more consistency than phorias for distances outside this range, suggesting that proximal convergence may be more reliably determined at intermediate test distances. Evidence for nonlinearity of proximal effects poses problems in describing a rate of change in simple terms. As the PCT designation facilitates comparison between diverse findings, however, we will continue to express proximal vergence in this manner, but keep this limitation in mind.

Instrument and free-space measures of phorias frequently show differences despite keeping the stimulus to accommodation constant. This is assumed to be due to the interaction of awareness of the actual target distance (in the instrument) and convergence. The demonstration of a direct perceptual effect, namely increased convergence resulting from perceived nearness (Alpern, 1958; Morgan, 1962), supports the notion that instrument convergence (as such differences are frequently termed) reflects proximal influences.

Comparison of instrument phoria measurements to free-space measures yields conflicting results. Neumueller (1942) measured phorias in the stereoscope as well as conventional dissociated phoropter phorias in

[3] In stigmatoscopy a small point of light (stigma) is superimposed on an acuity target and adjusted to its smallest diameter while maintaining clarity of the target.

free space. Using his calculations of instrument convergence for the far phoria findings (the difference between free space and stereoscope phorias), we divided this quantity by the 20-cm distance from the stereoscope eyepiece to the far-point target setting (in diopters) to determine PCTs for his subjects (n = 22). The average value was 1.74 ± 1.29$^{\Delta}$/D. This falls within the range of values in Table 4.1, suggesting that similar functions are being measured by the different techniques. In contrast, troposcopic determinations of proximal convergence yielded results that differed significantly from free-space measures. This raises the question as to whether these different techniques are indeed measuring the same function. Franceschetti and Burian (1970) compared two methods of measuring proximal convergence. They determined instrument convergence from the difference between instrument and free-space cover test phorias, as well as PCT from the difference between calculated and gradient AC/A ratios. Comparisons were made between results in a random population (n = 122), members of families with a history of exotropia (n = 42), and members of families with a history of esotropia (n = 74). We then found PCTs for the instrument measures by dividing their average instrument convergence values by the nine-inch fixation distance of the troposcope tube (in diopters) (Thompson, 1952). Table 4.2 summarizes these calculations that show much smaller PCTs for the instrument measures. In addition to the marked differences in average PCT values between the instrument and free-space techniques, frequency histograms presented for instrument-convergence and free-space PCTs indicated that this effect was more than a simple shift in response. The PCTs from free-space measures showed roughly normal distributions in all three groups; PCTs derived from fixation disparity have shown a similar distribution (Ogle et al., 1967). In contrast, troposcopic measures showed a different type of distribution. There was a marked leptokurtosis around zero in all three groups. Thus it is not at all clear that the same influences are involved in these two techniques.

Two factors that may be involved in producing different PCTs when comparing across different measurement techniques are size of the field

TABLE 4.2. Comparison of PCTs by Two Techniques

Population	*Troposcope PCT* ($^{\Delta}$/*D*)	Free Space PCT ($^{\Delta}$/*D*)
Random	0.25	2.03
XT families	—	1.52
ET families	0.25	2.00

Source: Franceschetti and Burian, 1970.

of view and perceived distance. Peripheral retinal areas provide strong fusional stimuli (Burian, 1939), and size of the stimulus field affects fusional vergence ranges (Kertesz, 1981). In light of Hofstetter's (1951) finding that fusional and proximal vergence interact, we cannot discount the possible influence of instrument aperture size on PCT determinations. Thus phoropter measures may be influenced by the small apertures and large surrounding lens banks through which the subject views the target. Furthermore, in none of the studies mentioned was the subject's perceived target distance either reported or measured. Perhaps distance perception varies with different testing conditions. Should this prove to be so, measures of perceived distance may permit comparison of different methods of determining proximal vergence by providing a common reference point.

PROXIMAL ACCOMMODATION

Effects on accommodation of awareness of distance are generally regarded as small, and some even question their existence (Hofstetter, 1942; Morgan, 1944a; Alpern, 1955, 1958). In patients exhibiting binocular dysfunctions, perceived distance does appear to be an important factor in accommodative performance, resulting in reduced or variable responses when change in the stimulus is brought about solely by lenses (Asher, 1952; Ogle et al., 1967; Hokoda and Ciuffreda, 1982).

Instrument myopia, the finding of relatively greater myopia with refractometer measures than with free-space measures (Bradford and Lawson, 1954), is often attributed to proximal factors influencing accommodative response. Challenging the notion of perceived distance effects, Hennessy (1975) presented evidence suggesting that instrument myopia is related to the shift of accommodation toward its resting state. Hennessy and Leibowitz (1971) supported the idea that perceptual factors may still be involved, however. They found that a peripheral aperture that was moved closer to the eye resulted in increased accommodation when both the accommodation and vergence systems were effectively open-looped.

Ittelson and Ames (1950) believed their data provided support for the existence of proximal accommodation. From their experiment in which card size but not card vergence was varied, they concluded that such stimuli affected distance perception and shifted accommodation in the direction of the apparent distance change. Following Ittelson and Ames' arrangement of varying target size to simulate a distance change, Alpern (1958) did not find significant accommodative shifts; however, he did note a trend consistent with a proximal effect. Larger target size, which simulated a closer viewing distance, was associated with increased accommodation. In an experiment by Morgan (1962), subjects monocularly viewed playing cards with size and (apparent) overlay arranged to reverse their perception of relative distances. No significant accommodative shifts were found under these conditions. In all three of these studies, accommodation was measured under closed-loop conditions. As this condition limits the amount of accommodative change that can occur before a secondary blur stimulus appears, open-loop investigations must be performed before a definitive statement can be made regarding distance effects on accommodation.

Visual imagery has been found to induce small changes of accommodation consistent with the direction of the imagined distance. Both static and dynamic changes on the order of 0.5 D have been found with accommodation measured under open-looped conditions when subjects were instructed to "think near" or "think far" (Westheimer, 1957; Malmstrom and Randle, 1976). Distance effects on voluntary accommodation were evident in two of Marg's (1951) seven subjects who were able to exercise more positive voluntary accommodation with closer test distances when instructed to attempt to accommodate for a point closer than the actual target.

Awareness of distance may influence clinical measures of accommodation. Parks (1962) felt that this prevented measurement of the full accommodative amplitude using the minus-lens technique with far fixation. Hokoda and Ciuffreda (1982) compared accommodative amplitude measurements by the push-up and minus-lens techniques at 40 cm and found 0.5 D less accommodation with minus lenses in their small group of normal subjects (n = 5). This was in contrast to the 1.8-D difference measured in the dominant eyes of their amblyopes (n = 10). Asher (1952) has shown a similar distance effect occurring in a number of his subjects, most of whom had binocular dysfunctions associated with asthenopia, while attempting to measure minus-lens gradient AC/A ratios during distance fixation. A relative inability to respond to the lenses was indicated both by decreased accommodative amplitude using minus lenses at far as compared to levels of accommodation attained with near test distances, and by decreased accommodative convergence at far when compared to their respective 20 cm gradient values. Guzzinati (1953) presented data similar to Asher's showing greater occurrence of this distance effect in patients with binocular dysfunctions.

Gradient stimulus AC/A ratio measurements often exhibited nonlinearities when positive lenses were used at near to change the accommodative stimulus (Tait, 1933). Ogle and Martens (1957) reported that 50% of their subjects (n = 28) demonstrated this phenomenon and attributed the result to accommodation being influenced by awareness of actual test distance. They felt that this awareness inhibited greater relaxation of accommodation. In a later work (Ogle et al., 1967) their clinical impression was that these nonlinearities were more commonly found in patients with binocular abnormalities and asthenopia than in normal asymptomatic individuals.

Our clinical experience supports these findings of strong distance effects in patients with binocular dysfunctions. Furthermore, we have found visual imagery helpful in enhancing poor accommodative response to lenses. For example, in a patient with binocular dysfunction and asthenopia, a −3 D lens (well within push-up accommodative amplitude) is interposed during monocular viewing of a distant target. The patient initially remarks that the lens blurs the target. No "reflex" accommodation occurs, nor does the patient have any strategy for clearing the blurred image. With an instruction to "think close, as if the target were within arm's reach," accommodation frequently changes in the appropriate direction, and the target clears.

CONVERGENCE AND ACCOMMODATION AS CUES TO DISTANCE

Related to the influence of perceived distance on the oculomotor adjustment of convergence and accommodation is the extent to which static changes in these two motor systems themselves can be used as cues to distance. There is general agreement that accommodation is an ineffective distance cue, while convergence in the absence of other more salient cues such as overlay, texture gradients, and motion parallax can influence distance judgments to some degree. This is believed to occur primarily through a size-constancy–related mechanism. Size constancy is often explained by the size-distance invariance hypothesis. This states that a given visual angle determines a unique ratio of perceived size to perceived distance (see Epstein, 1977, for a review).[4] Alpern (1969) proposed that a reciprocal relationship exists between proximal vergence and vergence influence on perceived distance and perceived size. This occurs through continued association of the two processes in everyday operation of perceptual constancy. For example, an object approaching an observer maintains the same phenomenal size, although retinal image size constantly increases. Convergence and accommodation also increase in response to the approaching object. Manipulating one element can affect the others. Thus increasing retinal image size under reduced viewing conditions (such as monocular fixation in a dark, empty surround) can result in closer perceived distance and increased convergence (proximal convergence). Similarly, increasing convergence demand can result in decreased perceived distance and smaller perceived size associated with the constant retinal image size.

[4] A simple example of the size-distance invariance hypothesis is provided by Emmert's law, which describes the situation with afterimages (constant retinal size) in which perceived afterimage size varies directly with projected distance (see Hochberg, 1971, for a review). Comparing the perceived size of an afterimage projected on a wall at a distance of 5 feet to projection at 10 feet, one would report a doubling of its size at the farther distance.

Accommodative change has generally been ruled out as influencing distance perception. Heineman, Tulving, and Nachmias (1959) demonstrated that accomodative change was not necessary for change in perceived size of targets subtending a constant visual angle when viewed under reduced conditions at several test distances. These size changes were attributed to convergence change. Alexander (1975), using a cross-modal paradigm to measure tactual judgments of changes in perceived size with minus lenses and monocular viewing, also attributed accommodative convergence micropsia to convergence change as well as to lens minification. Under binocular viewing, lens minification alone accounted for changes in perceived size.

During the clinical assessment of vergences, patients often report changes in size and distance of the target. It appears to get smaller and closer with increasing base-out prism and larger and farther with base-in prism. This has been referred to as the SILO response: smaller-in, larger-out (see Alexander, 1974, for a review). A different response is often reported, however. Hermans (1954) found that with increased convergence under binocular fixation an object could look either closer or farther, although in either case apparent size decreased. Heineman, Tulving, and Nachmias (1959) reported that verbal estimates of distance change were most often in the direction opposite to physical change in target position for their experimental arrangement, even though simultaneous size judgments and convergence changes implied relatively correct registration of distance (closer test distance associated with smaller perceived size and increased convergence for their targets that subtended the same visual angle). These SOLI responses (smaller-out, larger-in) probably reflect the influence of familiar size, for example, assumed or known size of an object (see Epstein, 1967, for a review). Observers expecting distant objects to appear smaller than near objects of the same assumed physical size will bias distance judgments accordingly. Such effects are generally regarded as cognitive or inferential, although evidence for a contributing direct perceptual effect has been described (Wallach et al., 1972).

Certain experimental conditions have shown apparent distance to decrease as convergence level increased (Ono et al., 1971; Ritter, 1977; Foley, 1977; Owens and Leibowitz, 1980). Studies on size and depth constancy indicate that convergence does provide cues to distance for the visual system (Heineman et al., 1959; Wallach and Zuckerman, 1963; Wallach et al., 1972). The presence of SOLI responses with convergence micropsia, however, together with Foley's (1977) findings that different methods of assessing perceived distance can result in different responses, creates problems in evaluating distance perception. The goal of relating proximal vergence to perceived distance requires both the application of consistent measurement techniques and use of some method sensitive to perceived distance yet free of conflicting cognitive factors.

Gogel (1981) presents evidence supporting the use of his head-motion procedure to measure perceived distance free from cognitive factors of familiar size. Subjects monocularly view a target while moving their head from side to side. A stationary object, misperceived in distance, will appear to move from side to side in the direction opposite to the head movement if it is perceived farther and in the same direction if it is perceived closer than the actual test target location. Such perceived target movement can be nulled by physically moving the target from side to side concomitant with head movement. Perceived distance can then be calculated from these manipulations. Gogel found that changes in verbal reports of perceived target distance resulted from biasing size judgments of the fixated target by suggesting it was the same size as some familiar object that the subject was able to view and feel (larger suggested size increasing distance reports, smaller suggested size decreasing distance reports). No effect on distance perception based on the head-motion procedure was found. Perceived lateral movement of the target with head motion was the same despite suggested size manipulations. Thus it appears that Gogel's procedure may allow measurement of perceived distance free from confounding cognitive factors and provide a tool for investigation of the influence of perceived distance on proximal vergence and accommodation. It is of interest that some optometrists (Getz, 1974) believe that vision training should include techniques directed toward equating distance perception in the dominant and nondominant eyes of strabismics and amblyopes. Our preliminary findings using a variation of Gogel's procedure show differences in perceived distance of a fixed target between dominant and nondominant eyes of both. This contrasts with the results on patients with normal binocular vision, which show no difference in distance perception between the eyes.

ASSOCIATION WITH BINOCULAR ANOMALIES

An element arising out of many of the studies on proximal vergence has been the association between abnormal PCTs and binocular vision anomalies. For example, in Morgan's study (1962) where size and apparent overlay of playing cards were used to reverse distance perception, only one of four subjects consistently demonstrated increased convergence with simulated near distance that was not attributable to accommodative convergence. This subject was a constant esotrope. Of Alpern's 11 subjects in an investigation of distance effects on vergence (1955), the individual with the greatest distance effect was a constant esotrope with anomalous correspondence. Another subject showing a strong proximal convergence response had a history of early esotropia that had been corrected. Five others demonstrated relatively consistent proximal effects. Of these, three showed suppression or reduced stereoacuity on clinical measures demonstrating abnormality of binocular vision.

Both abnormally high and low PCTs have been found in patients with binocular dysfunctions. Ogle, Martens, and Dyer (1967) found fixation-disparity–derived PCTs for patients with convergence excess (esophoria greater at near than far) larger (3.6^{Δ}/D, n = 20) than in their mean clinic population (1.81^{Δ}/D, n = 256). In contrast, they found abnormally low PCT values in patients with convergence insufficiency (exophoria greater at near than far). This group's mean PCT was only 1.2^{Δ} per D (n = 81). Cornell (1979–80) presented a case report on one patient with convergence insufficiency. To measure proximal convergence, infrared photography was used to record vergence angle of the eyes as the subject touched and fixated an object in the dark at several near test distances. The patient demonstrated reduced proximal convergence compared to normals (Cornell and Mitchell, 1979–80).

Instrument convergence, the finding of more convergence with haploscopic instrument measures than with free-space measures, is assumed to reflect proximal influences. It is particularly evident in strabismics. Thompson (1952) consistently found relatively more esotropia in the synoptophore than with free-space (cover test) measures in strabismics. Franceschetti and Burian (1970) also compared free-space and instrument measurements. Accommodative esotropes (n = 40) averaged 7.6^{Δ} more esotropia and nonaccommodative esotropes (n = 36) averaged 5.9^{Δ} more esotropia in the synoptophore than in free space. In contrast, their normal population (n = 22) measured only 1.1^{Δ} more relative esophoria in the instrument than with the cover test.

Bifocal treatment of accommodative esotropia sheds some light on proximal convergence (von Noorden et al., 1978). Eighty-four young accommodative esotropes who initially showed some degree of fusion at near were followed for an average of 44 months. Stimulus AC/A ratios were determined by the +3.0 D gradient cover test at 33.3 cm. Following lens therapy subjects fell into four groups based on fusional ability. Using their data, we calculated PCTs (difference between calculated and gradient AC/A ratios determined from cover tests) assuming an average interpupillary distance of 54 mm. Group one (n = 12, 7 received supplemental orthoptic therapy) now demonstrated fusion at far and near without bifocals. The initial PCT averaged 4.9^{Δ}/D and fell to 0.5^{Δ}/D following treatment. Group two (n = 19, 3 received orthoptics) had shown progressive improvement in fusion and reduced lens add for near; they were still under treatment at completion of the study. Average PCT fell from an initial value of 5.8^{Δ}/D to 4.1^{Δ}/D at their last evaluation. Group three (n = 39, 4 received orthoptics) had maintained fusion with bifocals but was still dependent on them, and reduction in the near lens add was not possible; PCTs for this group showed minimal change, decreasing from 5.6$^{\Delta}$/D to 5.3$^{\Delta}$/D. The fourth group (n = 14, 1 received orthoptic therapy) slowly lost fusional ability over time despite the use of maximum lens add (+3.5 D). Furthermore, this group showed an average increase in PCT from an initial value of 4.6$^{\Delta}$/D to a final value of 6.3$^{\Delta}$/D. This last group also showed the smallest gradient AC/A ratio: 4.8$^{\Delta}$/D, as compared to 7.2$^{\Delta}$/D, 7.1$^{\Delta}$/D, and 6.1$^{\Delta}$/D for groups one, two, and three respectively. As plus lenses often poorly control accommodative responses at near (Ogle and Martens, 1957), the +3.0 D gradient technique used here may be underestimating the AC/A ratio. Also, these calculations are based on AC/A ratio determinations made only at the initial examination, therefore conclusions must be tentative. The suggestion remains, however, that these esotropes had high initial PCTs, and it appears that reduction of proximal convergence either plays some role or reflects some process in the recovery of fusional skills.

Patients with divergence excess have also been examined with regard to proximal vergence effects. Ogle, Martens, and Dyer (1967) presented PCT data derived from fixation disparity on seven of these patients (distance exodeviation much greater than at near). The PCT values for the group averaged 3.0$^{\Delta}$/D. This was higher than the mean (1.81$^{\Delta}$/D) for their total clinic population (n = 256). Cooper, Ciuffreda, and Kruger (1982) examined four exotropes with divergence excess, two simulated (near and far deviation approximately equal after 45 minutes of occlusion of the deviating eye), and two true (far deviation 10 or more prism diopters greater than near following prolonged occlusion). Their measurements indicated response AC/A ratios within the normal to high normal range (5.9$^{\Delta}$/D mean). Based on changes in the angle of deviation following occlusion, as well as the different AC/A ratios found for calculated and gradient procedures, they suggested that proximal factors played an important role in patients with true divergence-excess exotropia.

Change in the magnitude of exotropia with change in distance fixation suggests the influence of knowledge or awareness of distance. Burian and Smith (1971) studied a population (n = 105) consisting of divergence-excess exotropes, basic exotropes (similar deviation near and far), convergence-insufficiency exotropes, and consecutive exotropes (surgically treated esotropes now exhibiting an exotropia). For all groups, the strabismic deviation increased (generally three to nine prism diopters) in about 30% of the subjects as fixation distance increased from 20 feet to 100 feet. An AC/A-related change in the exotropia, even as small as three prism diopters, would require an AC/A ratio of 23$^{\Delta}$/D for the 0.13-D change in accommodative stimulus. Such extremely high and grossly nonlinear AC/A ratios suggested by these observations are unlikely. Gradient stimulus AC/A ratios (+3.0 D at 33.3 cm) on the nine patients whose exotropia increased by at least 10 prism diopters (which would require an AC/A ratio of at least 77$^{\Delta}$/D) were less than 4$^{\Delta}$/D in all but two patients, both of whom measured 6.7$^{\Delta}$/D. A more reasonable explanation is suggested based on accommodative stimulus-response data. Generally, some amount of accommodation is present at low stimulus levels (Morgan, 1968), with the magnitude of response perhaps related to awareness of the testing distance. Assuming 1.25 D of accommodation with fixation at 20 feet and an AC/A ratio of 4$^{\Delta}$/D, if fixation at 100 feet resulted in accommodation approximating 0.0 D, a change in the angle of exotropia of five prism diopters would result. Whatever the mechanism, some aspect of awareness of distance is apparently involved in this increase in angle of deviation. Although low PCTs are found in convergence insufficiency, while patients with divergence excess show high PCTs (Ogle et al, 1967), the finding of similar percentages (about 30%) of patients with increased angle of deviation with distant fixation (Burian and Smith, 1971) suggests some degree of commonality of the underlying mechanism(s).

Available data provide some evidence that proximal vergence can be modified by orthoptic therapy. Fixation disparity derived PCT ratios were measured in five patients who underwent orthoptic therapy for binocular dysfunctions (Ogle et al., 1967). Three showed changes in PCT following therapy, increasing by 0.5$^{\Delta}$/D, 1.1$^{\Delta}$/D, and 3.6$^{\Delta}$/D. In Cornell's case report (1979–80) of convergence insufficiency, a program of orthoptic therapy was instituted with improvement of clinical findings (convergence near point, synoptophore vergence ranges, and accommodative amplitude) and alleviation of symptoms. Proximal convergence was assessed by a dark convergence task (described earlier). Initially, convergence on this task was significantly reduced when compared to data on normal patients. On repetition of the task following orthoptic therapy, performance fell within the lower limits of the normal group response. Unfortuantely, no other measures of proximal convergence were described, and it is unclear what relation this type of measurement has with more conventional methods. Recently, Mannen, Bannon, and Septon (1981) found decreased PCTs on a small group of normal subjects (n = 7) following four weeks of base-out vergence training that resulted in increased vergence ranges.

Visual imagery has been used as an aid in strabismus therapy. The term mental effort was introduced by Cantonnet and Filliozat (1938) referring to the role of visual imagery in changing the angle of strabismus. "Thinking far" was used to produce divergence in esotropia, while "thinking near" produced convergence in exotropia. Giles (1949) has further elaborated on the topic and presented case reports of strabismics aided in functional or cosmetic cures through use of the visual imagery approach. Recently, Forrest (1976) discussed the use of visual imagery effects for aiding the extension of base-in prism vergence ranges. Together with the experimental evidence in support of imagery effects on accommodation (Westheimer, 1957; Malmstrom and Randle, 1976), such techniques appear to be useful tools in orthoptic therapy.

PROXIMAL VERGENCE INTERACTIONS

Several researchers have attempted to relate proximal and accommodative vergence. Maddox (1893) postulated an inverse relationship between the two. Hofstetter (1942) found a small negative correlation between them for haploscopic response data, although a later study (Hofstetter, 1951) using accommodative stimulus values did not support this. Morgan (1950) investigated accommodative convergence on a large clinic population (n = 413) and found a linear, inverse relationship between proximal and accommodative vergence. Data derived from fixation disparity measures also showed a small negative correlation between them (Ogle et al., 1967).

An intimate relationship between proximal and fusional (disparity) vergence has been demonstrated by Hofstetter (1951). He found different values of proximal vergence when comparing gradient phorias and vergences taken at 6 m and 33.3 cm. The base-in prism limits gave 0.5^{Δ}/D PCT, phorias showed a PCT of 0.87^{Δ}/D, and the base-out limits yielded 2.53^{Δ}/D PCT. Hofstetter thought that proximal vergence could not simply be added to the other components of vergence, but should be expressed as some proportionality factor modifying fusional vergence. Mannen, Bannon, and Septon (1981) measured similar fusional influences. Based on their orthoptic findings that showed increased positive fusional vergence and decreased PCTs (particularly the base-out PCT), they suggested that proximal vergence may act as a "reserve", supplementing deficient positive fusional vergence in normal subjects having low AC/A ratios. Knoll (1959) proposed the presence of two components to proximal vergence. Based primarily on Hofstetter's finding of fusional interactions (1951), Knoll speculated that in addition to an independent proximal vergence component there existed a separate fusional-proximal vergence function that acts to modify fusional vergence. Additional evidence for interactions occurring between proximal and fusional vergence has been provided by data derived from fixation disparity (Ogle and Martens, 1957). For these data, during which fusional vergence was active, higher PCTs were found. They averaged almost twice the mean PCT calculated from Maddox rod phorias (disparity vergence open-looped), although AC/A ratios (fixation-disparity–derived and gradient) showed very close agreement for the different techniques on the two populations tested. Morgan (1950) believed the association of proximal and fusional vergence to be one of a learned conditioned reflex. For example, to explain the presence of negative PCTs he proposed that high levels of accommodative convergence would necesitate negative fusional movements to maintain fusion. This would establish a conditioned association between relative divergence and proximity.

Although the above evidence could be used to argue against the existence of a separate proximal vergence component, a number of factors do support independent proximal influences on vergence behavior. Hofstetter's study on fusional influences (1951) did not show significant correlation between total near fusional range and proximal vergence. He interpreted this finding as indicating independent origins. Demonstration of a direct perceptual effect on vergence (Alpern, 1958; Morgan, 1962), as well as the presence of high levels of proximal vergence in strabismics lacking normal binocular vision provides evidence that, indeed, a separate proximal vergence component exists.

With regard to learned conditioned reflex associations, Morgan (1960) mentioned the facilitatory role depressed gaze has on convergence. Measuring accommodation and convergence on a tilting haploscope during downward gaze, Knoll (1962) found increased esophoria in the absence of significant increase in accommodation. He speculated that this effect was attributable to a learned association between downward gaze and close working distance.

One might expect that with increasing presbyopia and a decreasing contribution of accommodative convergence as higher near lens adds are employed, the PCT would increase to facilitate single binocular vision. Morgan (1960) believed that proximal vergence was more important than accommodative vergence in presbyopia, and that it gained increasing importance as accommodative amplitude decreased. He did not feel, however, that proximal vergence would increase significantly with age; available data do not indicate a strong trend between them. Sheedy and Saladin (1975) found similar PCTs in presbyopes (n = 10) and nonpresbyopes (n = 13). Shapero and Nadell (1957) found very small increases, no increases, or even decreases in proximal vergence with closer working distances in presbyopic subjects. Ogle, Martens, and Dyer (1967) presented data derived from fixation disparity on 12 presbyopes (aged 52 to 79 years). They found an average PCT of 1.52^{Δ}/D. This was slightly less than their mean clinic population finding (n = 256, 11 to 79 years) of 1.81^{Δ}/D. Although their data suggested decreasing PCTs with increasing age, rank ordering of the presbyopic PCTs by age revealed no significant correlation (*p* greater than 0.05).

It becomes clear that proximal vergence effects are complex, and further experimentation will be needed to understand this important Maddox component. Fusional and accommodative vergence appear to interact with proximal vergence, but different methods of determining the level and magnitude of these interactions results in findings that are not always clearly interrelated. The shape of the curve of proximal vergence as a function of distance remains unclear. Abnormalities of binocular vision are associated with large proximal effects, although here again the underlying mechanisms are not understood. Other factors, such as position of the plane of regard (depressed gaze) and haptic input may influence the measure. Possibly of greatest importance is perceived distance, which shows promise as a key factor in relating many of these findings.

MODELING OF THE VERGENCE SYSTEM

The Maddox (1893) classification of vergence includes disparity ("fusional"), accommodative, tonic, and proximal ("voluntary") vergence,

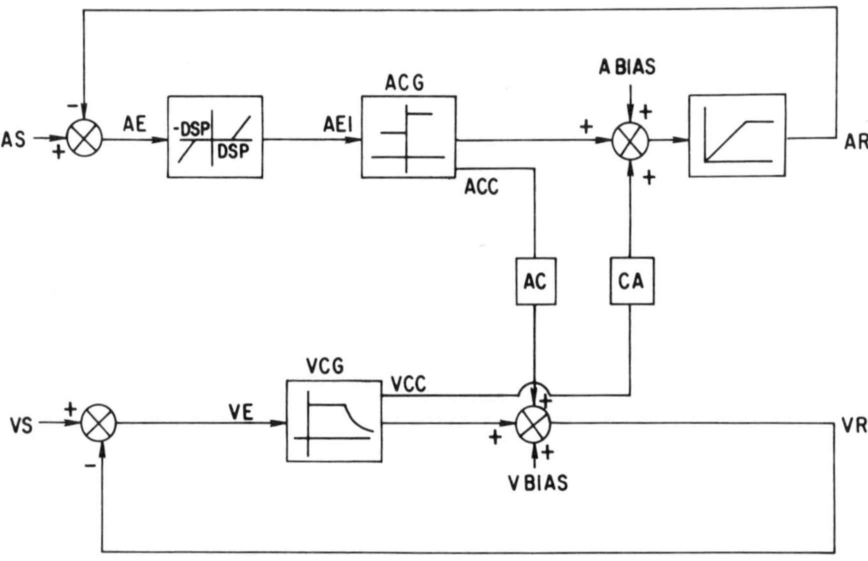

FIGURE 4.1 Overall block diagram of the Hung-Semmlow interactive dual feedback model of the accommodation and vergence systems. AS = accommodative stimulus, AE = accommodative error, DSP = dead space operator or depth of focus, AE1 = output of dead space operator, ACG = accommodative controller gain, ACC = output from accommodative controller, ABIAS = accommodative bias, AR = accommodative response, AC = cross-link gain to vergence system, VS = vergence stimulus, VE = vergence error, VCG = vergence controller gain, VCC = output from vergence controller, VBIAS = vergence bias, VR = vergence response, CA = cross-link gain to accommodation system. For greater detail on the model, see Chapter 6. Reprinted by permission of the publisher, from Hung GK, Semmlow JL. Static behavior of accommodation and vergence: computer simulation of an interactive dual-feedback system. Institute of Electrical and Electronics Engineers Transactions in Biomedical Engineering, © 1980 IEEE.

however, only disparity and accommodative vergence have been incorporated into most models of the vergence eye movement system. This section discusses the components of vergence and summarizes the arguments presented throughout this chapter that make clear the need to include proximal vergence in future models.

Each component of vergence has its own unique stimulus for elicitation of an optimal response. Disparity vergence refers to that component driven by binocular stimuli falling on noncorresponding retinal elements. It is probably the dominant component (Stark et al., 1980). Accommodative vergence refers to the blur-driven component, and it probably plays a major role only when stimuli fall on or near the fovea (Semmlow, 1981). Tonic vergence refers to that component due to tonus of the extraocular muscles derived from baseline neural discharge. Lastly, proximal vergence refers to the component due to awareness of nearness of the stimulus. Proximal vergence has been regarded as small and variable in magnitude, and of being somewhat elusive by nature of its having more of a psychological than physiological basis.

On what grounds should proximal vergence be included in future models of the vergence eye movement system? First, in the normal population, proximal vergence may be as high as 2^{Δ}/D with an average of about 1^{Δ}/D. While this may seem small, relative to the accommodative vergence component the proximal vergence contribution can be substantial. For example, in a patient having 4^{Δ}/D AC/A ratio and 2^{Δ}/D PCT ratio, the proximal vergence contribution equals one-half the accommodative vergence contribution to the total vergence response. This breakdown of vergence components in the clinical population has been discussed by Morgan (1944a). Second, proximal vergence may interact with the other vergence components, so its deletion from a model may account for subtle discrepancies found between experimental and model results. Third, in many patients having binocular vision anomalies such as strabismus, proximal vergence is typically outside normal limits. For example, in divergence-excess exotropia, proximal vergence may be abnormally high, leading to an inflated stimulus AC/A ratio when measured by clincial procedures using distance and near fixation. Based on these arguments, we propose that proximal vergence be included in future models of the vergence system. Once a block diagram is developed based on careful measures and calculations to determine system gain and linearity under a variety of stimulus conditions, modification for inclusion into the Hung-Semmlow vergence model (Figure 4.1) (1980) would seem warranted.[5]

[5] Although Toates' (1974) earlier model of the vergence system was one of the few to incorporate all four components, much of it was descriptive rather than quantitative in nature. Thus we prefer the Hung-Semmlow model.

This quantitative model of the normal system already has disparity and accommodative vergence channels, as well as a vergence bias component that includes tonic vergence (Figure 4.1). Such a comprehensive model would provide for a complete description of the vergence eye movement system for use in theoretical analyses as well as in clinical diagnoses.[6]

REFERENCES

Alexander KR. The foundations of the SILO response. Opt Weekly 1974;65:446–509.

Alexander KR. On the nature of accommodative micropsia. Am J Optom Physiol Opt 1975;52:79–84.

Alpern M. Testing distance effect on phoria measurement at various accommodation levels. Arch Ophthalmol 1955;54:906–15.

Alpern M. The position of the eyes during prism vergence. Arch Ophthalmol 1957;57:345–53.

Alpern M. Vergence and accommodation. I. Can change in size induce vergence movements? Arch Ophthalmol 1958;60:355–57.

Alpern M. Movements of the eyes. In: Davson H, ed. The eye. Vol. 3. 2nd ed. New York: Academic Press, 1969.

Asher H. Stimulus to convergence in normal and asthenopic subjects. Br J Ophthalmol 1952;36:666–75.

Borish IM. Clinical refraction. 3rd ed. Chicago: Professional Press, 1975.

Bradford RT, Lawson LJ. Clinical evaluation of the Rodenstock refractometer. Arch Ophthalmol 1954;51:695–700.

Burian HM. Fusional movements: the role of peripheral retinal stimuli. Arch Ophthalmol 1939;21:486–91.

Burian HM, Smith DR. Comparative measurement of exodeviations at twenty and one hundred feet. Trans Am Ophthalmol Soc 1971;69:188–99.

Cantonnet A, Filliozat J. Strabismus. 2nd ed. London: M. Wiseman, 1938.

Cooper J, Ciuffreda KJ, Kruger PB. Stimulus and response AC/A ratios in intermittent exotropia of the divergence excess type. Br J Ophthalmol 1982; 66:398–404.

Cornell E. The influence of orthoptic treatment on proximal convergence. Aust Orthopt J 1979–80;17:30–32.

Cornell E, Mitchell R. An evaluation of proximal convergence by the use of infrared photography. Aust Orthopt J 1979–80;17:24–29.

Epstein W. Varieties of perceptual learning. New York: McGraw-Hill, 1967.

Epstein W. Historical introduction to the constancies. In: Epstein W, ed. Stability and constancy in visual perception. New York: Wiley, 1977.

Foley JM. Effect of distance information and range on two indices of visually perceived distance. Perception 1977;6:449–60.

[6] Proximal effects on accommodation probably play a lesser role, and omission of a proximal accommodation component in the Hung-Semmlow model would introduce little error for normal binocular systems based on experimental and clinical evidence. Effects are both more frequently encountered and of greater magnitude for subjects with abnormal binocular systems, and may warrant consideration.

Forrest EB. Clinical manifestations of visual information processing. J Am Optom Assoc 1976;47:499–507.

Franceschetti AT, Burian HM. Proximal convergence. In: Strabismus 69. St. Louis: CV Mosby, 1970.

Getz DJ. Strabismus and amblyopia. Duncan, Okla.: Optometric Extension Program Foundation, 1974.

Giles GH. The practice of orthoptics. 2nd ed. London: Hammond, Hammond, 1949.

Gogel WC. The role of suggested size in distance responses. Percept Psychophysics 1981;30:149–55.

Guzzinati GC. Richerche sull' importanza della convergenza prossimale in soggetti ortoforici ed eteroforici. Ann Ottal 1953;79:475–82.

Heineman EG, Tulving E. Nachmias J. The effect of oculomotor adjustments on apparent size. Am J Psychol 1959;72:32–45.

Hennessy RT. Instrument myopia. J Opt Soc Am 1975;65:1114–20.

Hennessy RT, Leibowitz HW. The effect of a peripheral stimulus on accommodation. Percept Psychophysics 1971;10:129–32.

Hermans TG. The relationship of convergence and elevation changes to judgments of size. J Exp Psychol 1954;48:204–208.

Hochberg J. Perception. II. Space and movement. In: Kling JW, Riggs LA, eds. Woodworth and Schlosberg's experimental psychology. 3rd ed. New York: Holt, Rinehart, & Winston, 1971.

Hofstetter HW. The proximal factor in accommodation and convergence. Am J Optom Arch Am Acad Optom 1942;19:67–76.

Hofstetter HW. The relationship of proximal convergence to fusional and accommodative convergence. Am J Optom Arch Am Acad Optom 1951;28:300–308.

Hokoda SC, Ciuffreda KJ. (in press) Measurement of accommodative amplitude in amblyopia. Ophthalmic Physiol Optics.

Hung GK, Semmlow JL. Static behavior of accommodation and vergence: computer simulation of an interactive dual-feedback system. IEEE Trans Biomed Eng 1980;BME-27:439–47.

Ittelson WH, Ames AA. Accommodation, convergence, and their relation to apparent distance. J Psychol 1950;30:43–62.

Kertesz AE. Effect of stimulus size on fusion and vergence. J. Opt Soc Am 1981;71:289–93.

Knoll HA. Proximal factors in convergence. Am J Optom Arch Am Acad Optom 1959;36:378–81.

Knoll HA. The relationship between accommodation and convergence and elevation of the plane of regard. Am J Optom Arch Am Acad Optom 1962;39:130–34.

Maddox EE. The clinical use of prisms. 2nd ed. Bristol, England: John Wright & Sons, 1893.

Malmstrom FV, Randle RJ. Effects of visual imagery on the accommodative response. Percept Psychophysics 1976;19:450–53.

Mannen DL, Bannon MJ, Septon RD. Effects of base-out training on proximal convergence. Am J Optom Physiol Optics 1981;58:1187–93.

Manas L, Shulman P. The variation in the accommodative convergence accommodation (AC/A) ratio upon periodic retesting. Am J Optom Arch Am Acad Optom 1954;31:385–96.

Marg E. An investigation of voluntary as distinguished from reflex accommodation. Am J Optom Arch Am Acad Optom 1951;28:347–56.

Morgan MW. Accommodation and its relationship to convergence. Am J Optom Arch Am Acad Optom 1944a;21:183–95.

Morgan MW. The clinical aspects of accommodation and convergence. Am J Optom Arch Am Acad Optom 1944b;21:301–13.

Morgan MW. A comparison of clinical methods of measuring accommodative convergence. Am J Optom Arch Am Acad Optom 1950;27:385–96.

Morgan MW. Anomalies of the visual neuromuscular system of the aging patient. In: Hirsch MJ, Wick RE, eds. Vision of the aging patient. Philadelphia: Chilton Book Co., 1960.

Morgan MW. Effect of perceived distance on accommodation and convergence. Trans Int Ophthalm Opt Cong, New York: Hafner Pub Co., 1962.

Morgan MW. Accommodation and vergence. Am J Optom Arch Am Acad Optom 1968;46:417–54.

Neumueller J. Proximal convergence and accommodation. Am J Optom Arch Am Acad Optom 1942;19:16–25.

Ogle KN, Martens TG. On the accommodative convergence and the proximal convergence. Arch Ophthalmol 1957;57:702–15.

Ogle KN, Martens TG, Dyer JA. Oculomotor imbalance in binocular vision and fixation disparity. Philadelphia: Lea & Febiger, 1967.

Ono H, Mitson L, Seabrook K. Change in convergence and retinal disparities as an explanation for the wallpaper phenomenon. J Exp Psychol 1971;91:1–10.

Owens DA, Leibowitz HW. Accommodation, convergence and distance perception in low illumination. Am J Optom Physiol Opt 1980;57:540–50.

Parks MN. Etiologic and compensatory factors of comitant horizontal deviations in children. In: Haik GK, ed. Strabismus: symposium of the New Orleans Academy of Ophthalmology. St. Louis: CV Mosby, 1962.

Pratt CB. The variation in phorias with time after dissociation and magnitude of convergence. Am J Optom Arch Am Acad Optom 1962;39:257–63.

Ritter M. Effect of disparity and viewing distance on perceived depth. Percept Psychophysics 1977;22:400–407.

Rubie C. The effect of the AC/A ratio on the difference between distance and near measurements of deviation. Aust Orthopt J 1979–80;17:37–41.

Semmlow JL. Oculomotor response to near stimuli: the near triad. In: Zuber BL, ed. Models of oculomotor behavior and control. Boca Raton, Florida: CRC Press, 1981.

Shapero M, Levy M. The variation of proximal convergence with change in distance. Am J Optom Arch Am Acad Optom 1953;30:403–16.

Shapero M, Nadell M. Accommodation and convergence responses in beginning and absolute presbyopes. Am J Optom Arch Am Acad Optom 1957;34:606–22.

Sheedy JE, Saladin JJ. Exophoria at near in presbyopia. Am J Optom Physiol Opt 1975;52:474–81.

Stark L, Kenyon RV, Krishnan VV, Ciuffreda KJ. Disparity vergence: a proposed name for a dominant component of binocular vergence eye movements. Am J Optom Physiol Opt 1980;57:606–609.

Stern A. The effect of target variation and kinesthesis upon near heterophoria measurements. Am J Optom 1953;30:351–65.

Tait EF. A report on the results of the experimental variation of the stimulus conditions in the responses of the accommodative convergence reflex. Am J Optom 1933;10:428–35.

Thompson DA. Measurements with cover test versus troposcope. Am Orthopt J 1952;2:47–52.

Toates FM. Vergence eye movements. Doc Ophthalmol 1974;37:153–214.

von Noorden GK, Morris J, Edelman P. Efficacy of bifocals in the treatment of accommodative esotropia. Am J Ophthalmol 1978;85:830–34.

Wallach H, Zuckerman C. The constancy of stereoscopic depth. Am J Psych 1963;76:404–12.

Wallach H, Frey KJ, Bode KA. The nature of adaptation in distance perception based on oculomotor cues. Percept Psychophysics 1972;11:110–16.

Westheimer G. Accommodation measurements in empty fields. J Opt Soc Am 1957;47:714–18.

III

INTERACTIONS BETWEEN ACCOMMODATION AND VERGENCE

5

Accommodative Vergence and Accommodation in Normals, Amblyopes, and Strabismics

Kenneth J. Ciuffreda
Robert V. Kenyon

Accommodative vergence refers to a blur-driven change in the horizontal position of the visual axes. This synkinesis between accommodation and vergence was initially described by the German physiologist Mueller in 1826. The theoretical and clinical importance of accommodative vergence is evident in its role as the primary component in the Maddox (1886) hierarchy of vergence control (see Chapter 2). This chapter provides an overview of accommodation and accommodative vergence in normals, reviews critically several important basic and clinical aspects of the AC/A ratio, and discusses accommodation and accommodative vergence function in amblyopia and strabismus.[1]

OVERVIEW OF ACCOMMODATION IN NORMALS

Accommodation refers to the crystalline lens-produced change in dioptric power of the eye. It generally occurs in response to a visual stimulus such

[1] The reader is directed to Fincham (1937), Crane (1966), Ogle et al. (1967), Morgan (1968), Alpern (1969), and Toates (1972) for excellent overviews of the topic of accommodative vergence and accommodation.

as a blurred target to focus and maximize spatial contrast (amplitude and/or gradient) of the retinal image (Fujii et al., 1970; Krishnan et al., 1973). The response is mediated by retinal cones (Campbell, 1954a, 1954b). While blur is a sufficient stimulus for accommodation (Troelstra et al., 1964; Phillips and Stark, 1977), other factors play a role in eliciting the response. If micromovements of the eye are voluntarily inhibited, the accommodative response to a blurred foveal target is not initiated (Fincham, 1951). Chromatic aberration appears to be an important cue for the accommodation system with respect to appropriate change in direction (Fincham, 1951; Campbell and Westheimer, 1959). Although accommodation is believed to be equal in the two eyes (Stoddard and Morgan, 1942; Ogle, 1950; Ball, 1952), some data suggest it may be unequal (0.5 to 1.5 D) during marked asymmetric convergence in normals, with greater accommodation in the eye that would normally have the larger retinal image (Rosenberg et al., 1953). Stripped of all target information except blur, the even-error nature of the accommodation system becomes evident, that is, the system can determine magnitude but not direction of a pure blur change (Troelstra et al., 1964). As target luminance decreases, variability of the accommodation response increases (Alpern, 1958). Decrease in target contrast (Heath, 1956; Bour, 1981) and increase in target velocity (Kellndorfer et al., in preparation) reduce the accommodative response.

Stimulation of the accommodative system by introducing successively larger step changes in stimulus with concurrent measures of the static or steady-state response results in a plot of the accommodative stimulus-response curve (Morgan, 1944a, 1944b; 1968) (Figure 5.1). Stim-

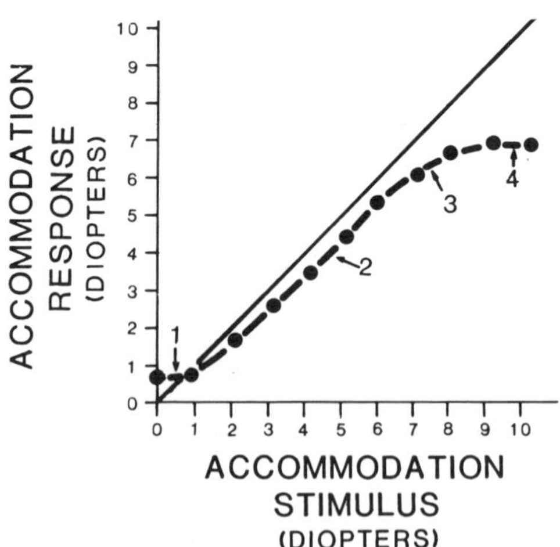

FIGURE 5.1. Static accommodative stimulus-response curve for a normal subject. 1 = initial non-linear region, 2 = linear region, 3 = transitional soft saturation region, and 4 = hard saturation presbyopic region.

uli encompass the entire response range (Morgan, 1968, see especially his Figure 15; Saladin and Stark, 1975), which includes: (1) the initial nonlinear portion of the curve from 0 to 1.5 diopters of accommodative stimulus over which the accommodative response is approximately constant, with mean population values ranging from 0.5 to 1.5 diopters; this response is strongly influenced by the accommodative bias or tonic accommodation level (Hung and Semmlow, 1980); (2) the linear manifest zone over which a change in accommodative stimulus produces a proportional change in accommodative response; this response is typically less than the stimulus, producing the so-called lazy lag of accommodation as a result of control properties of the accommodation system (Toates, 1972) and depth of focus of the eye (± 0.1 to ± 0.5 diopters) (Campbell, 1957; Green et al., 1980) that is inversely related to pupil diameter; (3) the nonlinear transition zone (region of soft saturation) over which further increases in stimulus produce a change in response, but progressively smaller than would be found for the same stimulus change over the manifest zone, and (4) the nonlinear latent zone (region of hard saturation), which defines the amplitude of accommodation, over which still further increases in stimulus fail to produce additional increases in response; however, ciliary body force increases in this zone, but presumed sclerosis of the crystalline lens and capsule impedes further rounding of the lens to increase lenticular dioptric power, that is, functional presbyopia is attained (Saladin and Stark, 1975).

Much information regarding the accommodation system has been gained by study of its dynamics (Kasai et al., 1971), especially with aid of systems analysis. Accommodation is correlated in the two eyes (Campbell, 1960; Clark and Crane, 1978) (Figure 5.2). Accommodative latency is 370 ± 80 msec; the accommodative response approximates an exponential having a time constant[2] of 250 msec and a total response time (latency plus accommodation change) of about 1 second; peak velocity may be as high as 10 diopters per second for a 2-diopter step change; and target information is monitored and responded to continuously (Campbell and Westheimer, 1960). Range nonlinearities are also evident (Shirachi et al., 1978). Some of these values are amenable to change by orthoptic therapy (Liu et al., 1979) (Figure 5.3). Microfluctuations in steady-state accommodation (using power spectrum analysis) show a dominant frequency at 0.5 Hz, and with a large pupil an additional dominant frequency at 2 Hz; these fluctuations increase with increased accommodation (Campbell et al., 1959; Denieul, 1982). These microfluctuations can serve to enhance the accommodative response (Hung et al, 1982). Closed-loop frequency response to sinusoidal variation in dioptric vergence shows the

[2] The time constant refers to the time necessary for a response to change to 63% of its final steady-state value.

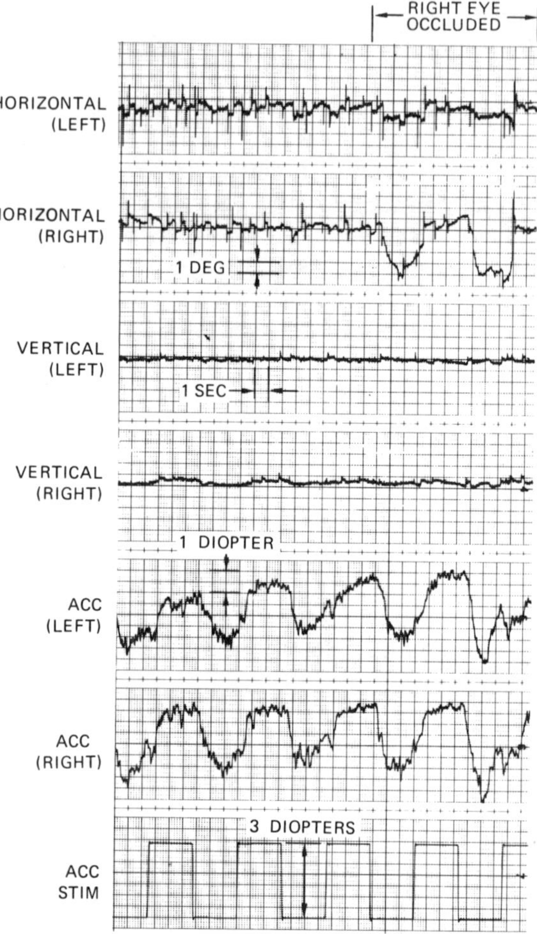

FIGURE 5.2. Binocular responses to simultaneous target movement along the axis of each eye without any change in the lateral position of the target in each eye (i.e., no change in target vergence). Note the accommodative responses, without any vergence response, in the left half of the record and the accommodative vergence responses in the right half of the record when one eye is occluded. The responses shown in the left half of the record probably reflects what is occurring clinically during binocular accommodative rock exercises, as well as during measures of positive and negative relative accommodation. Correlation of accommodation between the two eyes is evident. Reprinted by permission of the publisher, from Clark MR, Crane HD. Dynamic interactions in binocular vision. In: Senders JW, Fisher DF, Monty RH, eds. *Eye Movements and the Higher Psychological Functions*. Hillsdale: Lawrence Erlbaum Associates, Inc., 1978.

[3] The cut-off frequency or −3dB (decibels) point is the final point in a frequency response curve at which the system response drops 3 dB or to 0.707 of its peak value on its way out of the passband.

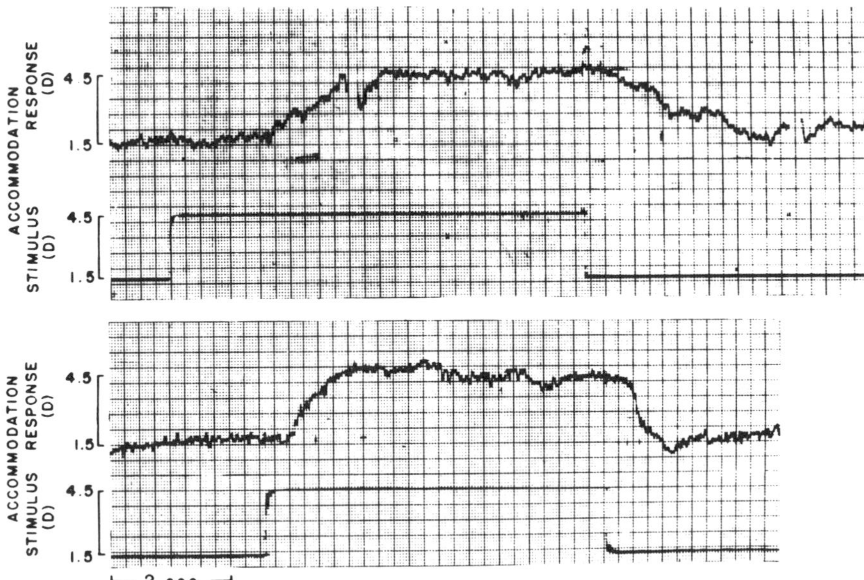

FIGURE 5.3. A Accommodation responses of subject. Upper records show slow response dynamics for positive accommodation and slow, multiphasic response dynamics for relaxation of accommodation before orthoptics training. Bottom records show the patient's improvement after training with faster velocities in both directions of accommodation. Two discontinuous spikes in upper record are blinks. Stimuli are unpredictable step changes between targets set at 1.5 and 4.5 D. B Change of accommodation characteristics in the three subjects as measured weekly through changes in time constants, latencies, and flipper rates during their orthoptics programs. Mean values are plotted for time-constant and latency graphs with standard errors denoted by the error bars. Flipper rates are self-reported by each subject. Reprinted by permission of the publisher, from Liu JS, Lee M, Jang J, Ciuffreda KJ, Wong JH, Grisham D, Stark L. Objective assessment of accommodation orthoptics: dynamic insufficiency. American Journal of Optometry and Physiological Optics, © (1979), American Academy of Optometry per The Williams & Wilkins Company (agent).

response down 3 dB[3] at 0.4 Hz, although a detectable response is still present at 4 Hz (Campbell and Westheimer, 1960; Stark, 1968; Yoshida and Watanabe, 1969). A phase lag is also present that increases with increased frequency of sinusoidal target oscillation. The phase lag is less than expected based on the latency of accommodation, suggesting evidence of a predictor operator (Stark et al., 1967; van der Wildt et al., 1974). The open-loop response for small-step input is about seven times greater than the closed-loop response, and the gain is similarly increased over most of the response range for predictable sinusoidal inputs. This enhanced response is to be expected when the system is open-looped (van der Wildt et al., 1974). With the accommodation system open-looped

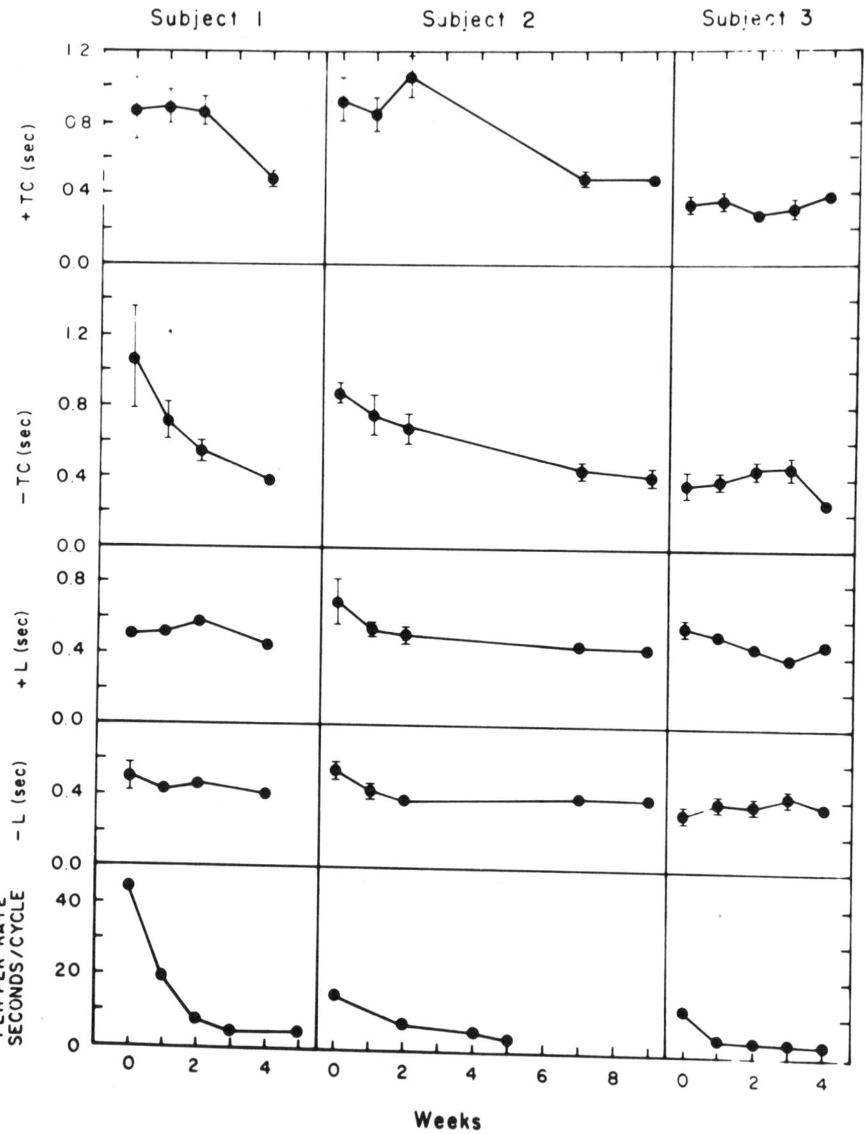

FIGURE 5.3. (*Continued*)

(total darkness, ganzfeld, or pin-hole), the accommodation system response eventually (15 to 40 seconds) approaches a common steady-state level dependent upon one's accommodative bias, although the dynamics under these three conditions differ as shown in Figure 5.4 (Phillips, 1974).

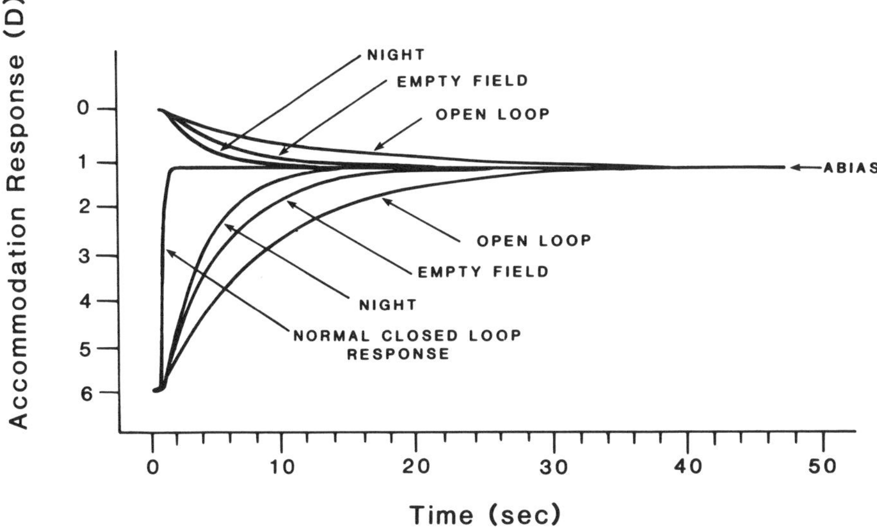

FIGURE 5.4. Dynamics of open-loop accommodation. Accommodative feedback loop opened by having the subject view in total darkness, in a ganzfeld, or through a pin-hole resulting in time constants of 4, 6, and 10 seconds, respectively. This demonstrates how residual information content affects dynamics of response but not final resting level. Reprinted by permission from Phillips SR. Ocular neurological control systems: accommodation and the near response triad. PhD dissertation, University of California, 1974.

Spatial Frequency

The effect of target spatial frequency on the accommodative response has received considerable attention. Phillips (1974) used a haploscope-optometer to measure static accommodative responses as a function of target spatial frequency (target contrast = 63%) for sinusoidal and square-wave gratings in four normal subjects. For sinusoidal gratings, changes of accommodation occurred to gratings from 1 to 25 cycles per degree, although responses were most accurate and easiest to elicit in the midrange of 3 to 10 cycles per degree (Figure 5.5). The similarity in ranges for accuracy of accommodation and sensitivity to contrast suggested an intimate relationship between these two functions. For spatial frequencies less than 1 cycle per degree the contrast gradient was too shallow, and for spatial frequencies greater than 25 cycles per degree it was too fine to provide

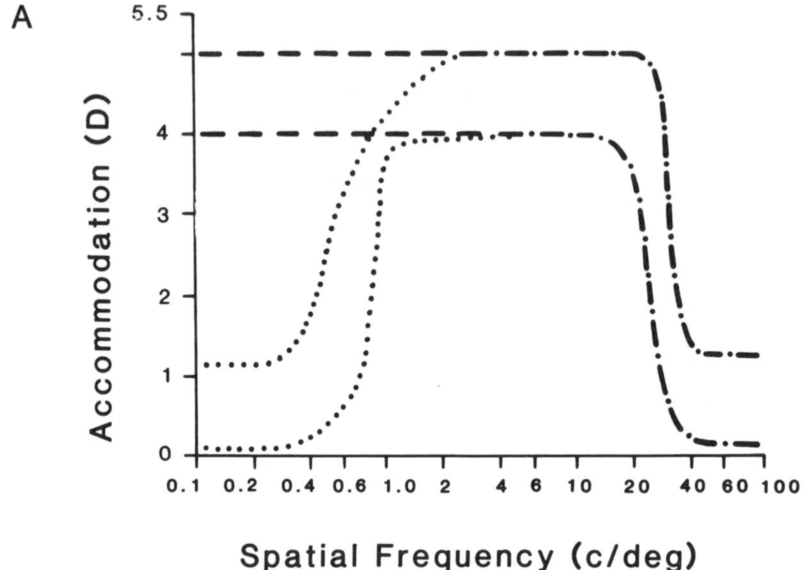

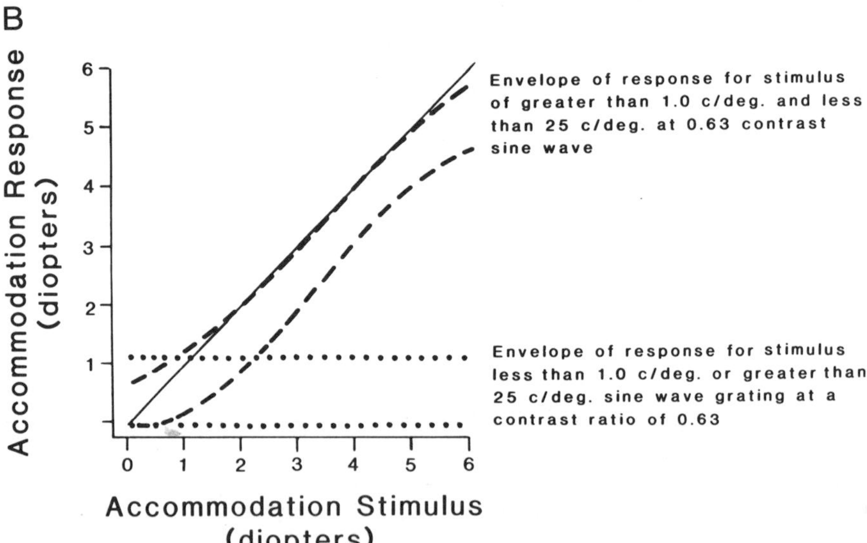

FIGURE 5.5. Accommodative responses as a function of spatial frequency for sinusoidal gratings. A Envelope of accommodative responses to spatial gratings at 5.5 and 0 diopters for three subjects; dashed lines represent envelope of square-wave responses. B Envelope of accommodative responses for sine-wave gratings. C Accommodation responses to the target change from a −6 diopter sphere (DS) star target to a 50% modulation, sinusoidal grating of the spatial frequency and subtense indicated, at a vergence of −2 DS. Responses to five target changes of each type have been superimposed so that the target changes always occurred at

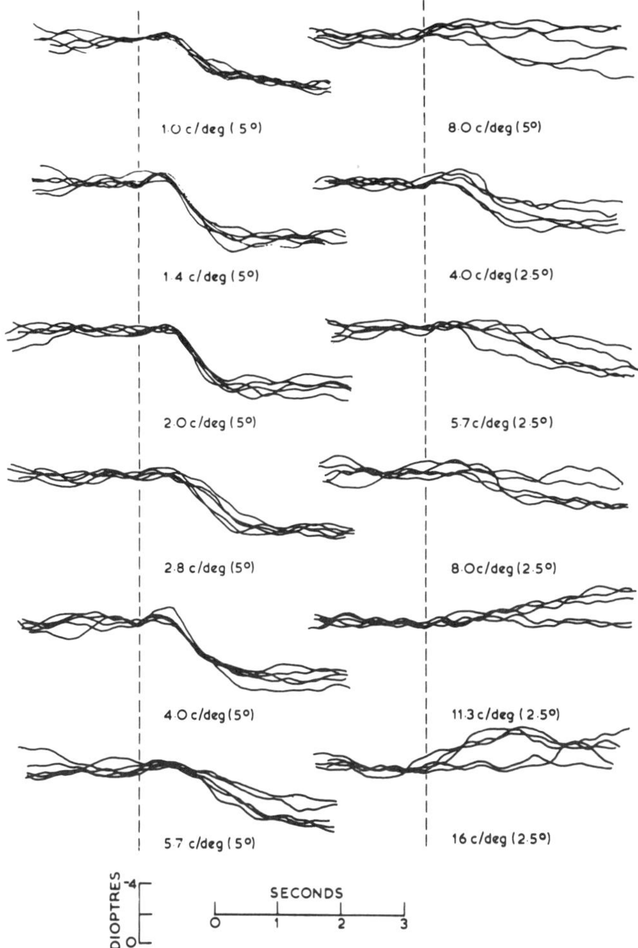

the times indicated by the vertical dash lines. Subject HW 23 years old, 7-mm pupil, accommodative resting state −2 DS. Average field luminance 25 cd/m^2. D Comparison of relative accommodative responsiveness (*continuous lines*) and contrast sensitivity functions (*broken lines*) of four observers for sinusoidal gratings. Spearman rank-order correlations (rho) of the two functions are indicated for each observer. Figures A and B are adapted from Phillips SR. Ocular neurological control systems: accommodation and the near response triad. PhD dissertation, University of California, 1974. Reprinted by permission. Figure C reprinted by permission of the publisher, from Charman WN, Heron G. Spatial frequency and the dynamics of the accommodation response. Optica Acta, 1979. Figure D reprinted with permission from Vision Research, Owens DA, A comparison of accommodative responsiveness and contrast sensitivity for sinusoidal gratings, 1980, Pergamon Press, Ltd.

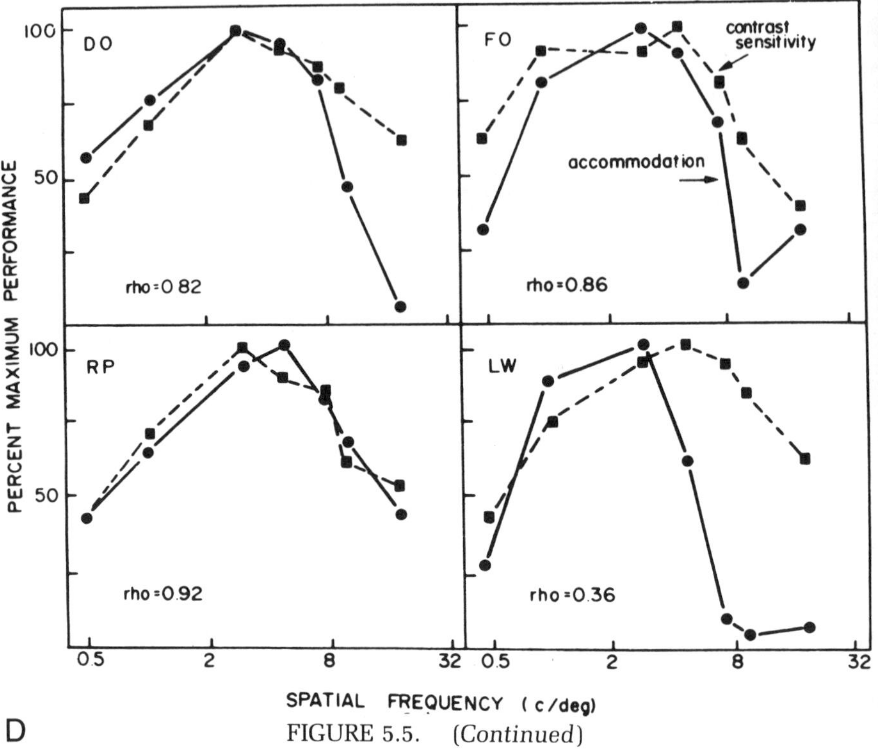

D FIGURE 5.5. *(Continued)*

the requisite blur information to drive the accommodation system. In both instances, accommodation went to its bias level, that is, to the "no stimulus" or empty field level. The high spatial frequency cutoff for accommodation was the same for square-wave gratings as for sinusoidal gratings, suggesting similarity in contrast gradient resolution. For all practical purposes there was no low spatial frequency cutoff effect, as decreasing the spatial frequency of a square-wave grating simply reduces the number of light/dark borders in the field but not the contrast gradient. Phillips also found that the minimum contrast to elicit an accommodative response was 10 times greater than the contrast threshold for visibility of the same grating.

Similarly, Charman and Tucker (1977) using a laser optometer measured static accommodation responses to presentation of single high-contrast (target contrast = 83%) spatial frequency sinusoidal gratings. They found the response to be a function of target spatial frequency as well as target vergence. For target dioptric vergences less than the subject's empty field accommodation level, the response was generally greater than the accommodative stimulus for low spatial frequency gratings, reached a minimum at 5 cycles per degree, and then increased (i.e., overaccommodated) at higher frequencies. For target vergences greater than the subject's empty field accommodation level, the accommodation response increased monotonically with spatial frequency. It was less than the accommodative stimulus for spatial frequencies less than 10 cycles per degree, while it increased and was frequently greater than the accommodative stimulus for spatial frequencies over 10 cycles per degree. The slope of the accommodative stimulus-response curve decreased as target spatial frequency decreased. Of particular interest was the experienced subject's inability to accommodate accurately on a grating of 23 cycles per degree, which was within his resolution capability. This suggested to Charman and Tucker that the accommodation system uses low spatial frequency information as a coarse guide for response, while high spatial frequency information is used to refine the response. That low spatial frequency information guides accommodation has been further suggested by study of accommodation dynamics (Figure 5.5) (Charman and Heron, 1979). They also found no relationship between spatial frequency and accommodation latency or total accommodation response time.

More recently, Owens (1980) attempted to differentiate between the contrast-control and the fine-focus-control hypotheses as the basic mechanism underlying the neurologic control of accommodation. In the former, the accommodation system tries to maximize spatial contrast at the fovea, and thus one would predict accommodation responses to be most accurate in the midrange over which visual sensitivity to contrast is greatest. In the latter, defocus effects are more evident for fine than for gross details, and thus one would predict accommodation responses to be more accurate for high than for low spatial frequencies. Owens measured accommodation stimulus-response curves using a laser optometer and obtained contrast sensitivity functions in four normal subjects. His results were similar to those of Phillips (1974), with accommodation being most accurate and easy to elicit for spatial frequencies in the region of the peak of their respective contrast sensitivity functions (Figure 5.5). This result provides additional evidence in favor of the contrast-control hypothesis. Owens further attributed differences between his findings and those of Charman and Tucker (1977), whose results support the fine-focus-control hypothesis, to the instruction set provided the subjects. Owens advised subjects to view the gratings "naturally, without straining the eye," and thus only "reflex" accommodation was employed; in contrast, Charman and Tucker advised subjects to obtain "best possible" focus, and thus it was speculated that both "reflex" and "voluntary" accommodation components contributed to the response, the combination of which is believed to represent the best possible system performance. If this is indeed true, it suggests that the strategy of the accommodation system, and thus its basic static response, may depend on the task demanded of the individual. Recent results by Bour (1981) confirm the basic findings of Phillips (1974) and Owens (1980).

Eccentricity

Effects of target retinal eccentricity on the accommodation response have been investigated. Whiteside (1957), using thin concentric circles of various angular extents (with no foveal fixation point) as peripheral accommodative stimuli, found that targets 4 degrees or more from the fovea exerted little influence on the static accommodative level (far point of the eye), and thus constituted a poor stimulus to accommodation. Hennessy and Leibowitz (1971) investigated the effects of objects in the near peripheral visual field on the static accommodative response to a defocused foveal spot of light, that is, a poor foveal stimulus to accommodation, located 6 meters away. They found that as a circular aperture with constant angular extent (4 degrees) was moved in discrete steps closer to the subject, small increases in the static accommodative response proportional to aperture distance (but less than the aperture stimulus to accommodation in terms of distance from the subject) were measured. Moreover, when the aperture diameter was reduced to 1 degree so that its border

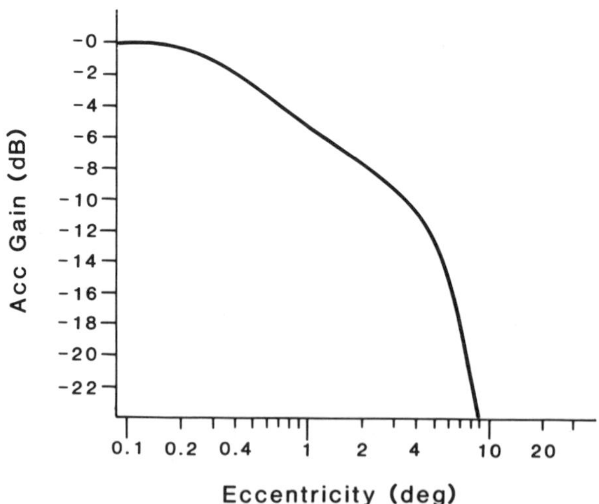

FIGURE 5.6. Plot of effectiveness of defocused target in driving accommodation as a function of retinal eccentricity. A Magnitude of the response has been calculated as a percent of the response to a centrally fixated target. Data averaged from three subjects. B Gain (decibels) also plotted. Reprinted by permission, from Phillips SR. Ocular neurological control systems: accommodation and the near response triad. PhD dissertation, University of California, 1974.

was closer to the fovea, effect of this peripheral stimulus was greater. Besides implications regarding perceptual factors on accommodation (see Chapter 4), the results suggest that a peripheral stimulus to accommodation may influence the static accommodative response in the presence of a degraded foveal stimulus. The influence of the peripheral field on the accommodative state may be used to explain the phenomenon of instrument myopia (Schober et al., 1970).

Phillips (1974) investigated accommodation as a function of target retinal eccentricity using a dynamic optometer (Figure 5.6). He found that the accommodative response could be elicited from the central retinal area, presumably resulting from stimulation of cones within that region. Defining the accommodative response amplitude for direct foveal stimulation as 100%, the accommodative response amplitude declined to 50, 20, and 0% for 1.5, 5, and 10 degrees target retinal eccentricity, respectively. From this he concluded that the vergence system (vergence accommodation) and/or volitional factors (voluntary accommodation) initially drives the accommodation system (during normal binocular viewing) for targets falling greater than 10 degrees from the fovea, while a com-

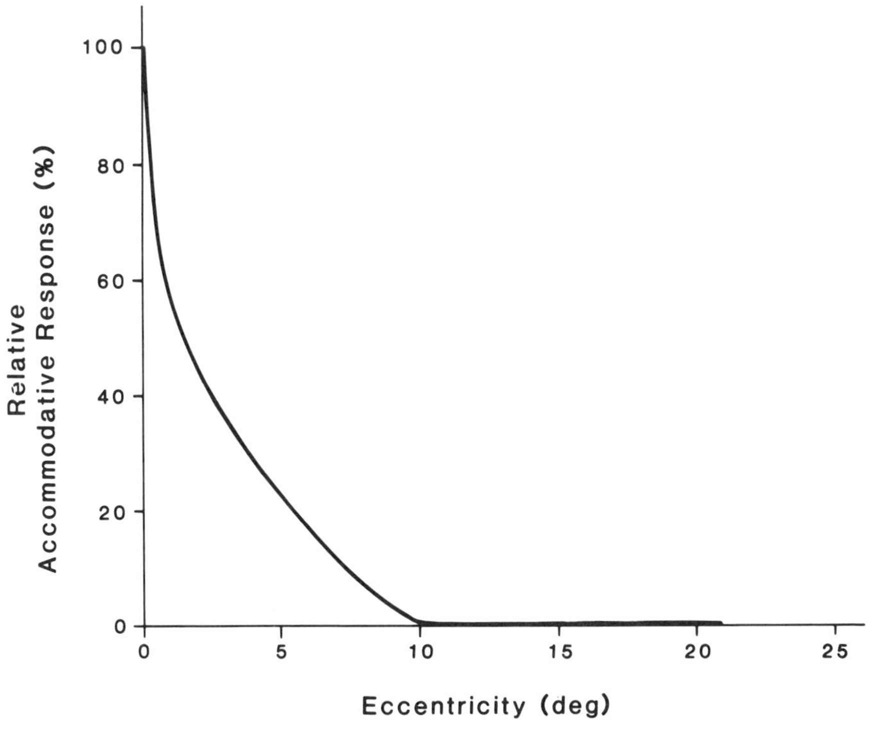

FIGURE 5.6. *(Continued)*

bination of stimulus-driven accommodation (i.e., blur), voluntary accommodation, and vergence accommodation summate to produce the total accommodative response for targets falling less than 10 degrees from the fovea. The situation itself is dynamic, however, and the accommodative contributions coming from these various sources probably combine and change in a complex manner as the targets get closer to the foveas during the ongoing vergence movement. Recent results (Hung, Ciuffreda, and Semmlow, unpublished data) demonstrate that the accommodative response approaches the resting state of accommodation as stimulus eccentricity increases, and thus stimulus effectiveness decreases.

OVERVIEW OF ACCOMMODATIVE VERGENCE IN NORMALS

Accommodative vergence refers to a blur-driven change in the horizontal alignment of the eyes. In the classic example (and conceptually the most

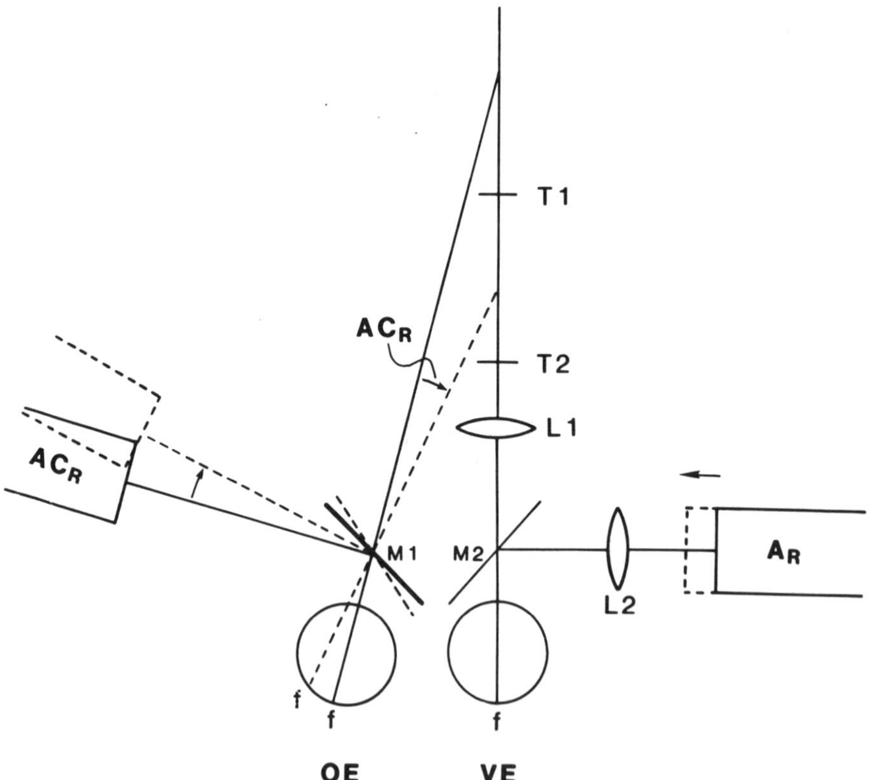

FIGURE 5.7. A Haploscope-optometer used in determination of static response AC/A ratios. Key: f = fovea, OE = occluded eye, VE = viewing eye, M1 = full-silvered mirror, M2 = half-silvered mirror, L1 = stimulus Badal lens, L2 = stigma

simple case due to the monocular nature of the stimulus), a target moved inward along the line of sight of one eye will produce a slow, nasalward rotation in the covered eye (Mueller, 1826)—the first demonstration of the synkinesis between accommodation and vergence. Recent work (Kenyon et al., 1978) shows that binocular accommodative vergence ensues as the subject attempts to clear the blurred monocular stimulus. If a haploscope-optometer (Figure 5.7) is used to measure static accommodation and accommodative vergence responses as increases in target vergence are introduced during the Mueller-type experiment, the amount of change in accommodative vergence (expressed in units of prism diopters) per unit change in accommodation (expressed in units of diopters) results in a measure called the response AC/A ratio (accommodative convergence to accommodation) (Morgan, 1968). Over most of the response range the relationship is approximately linear. Mean population AC/A value is 4.0 ±2.0:1 (Morgan, 1968). The AC/A ratio is one of the most clinically and experimentally used measures in assessment of strabismus and its management (Burian, 1971; Windsor, 1971), especially in light of the presence of accommodative vergence at two months of age (Aslin and Jackson, 1979).

Study of its dynamics has added much to our knowledge of accommodative vergence (Brodkey and Stark, 1967a, 1967b). Latency is approximately 200 msec, although a range from 130 to 300 msec has been reported (Allen, 1953; Yamamoto, 1968, 1970; Krishnan et al., 1977; Kenyon et al., 1978). Accommodative vergence has a peak velocity:amplitude

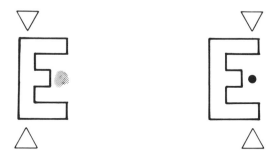

Badal lens, T1 = far target, T2 = near target, A_R = accommodation response, and AC_R = accommodative vergence response. B Subject's view of haploscopically presented targets and portion of free-space targets consisting of reduced Snellen chart (not to scale). *Left* Following a change of target vergence and subsequent accommodative adjustment to clear target blur, the subject sees the focused Snellen letter with one eye, blurred stigma to right of Snellen letter with the same eye, and arrowheads to left of Snellen letter with fellow (left) eye. *Right* Following adjustment of optometer and haploscope arm, the subject sees the focused stigma and arrowhead vertically aligned with stigma. Change in stigma is related to static accommodative response, and change in arrowheads is related to static accommodative vergence response.

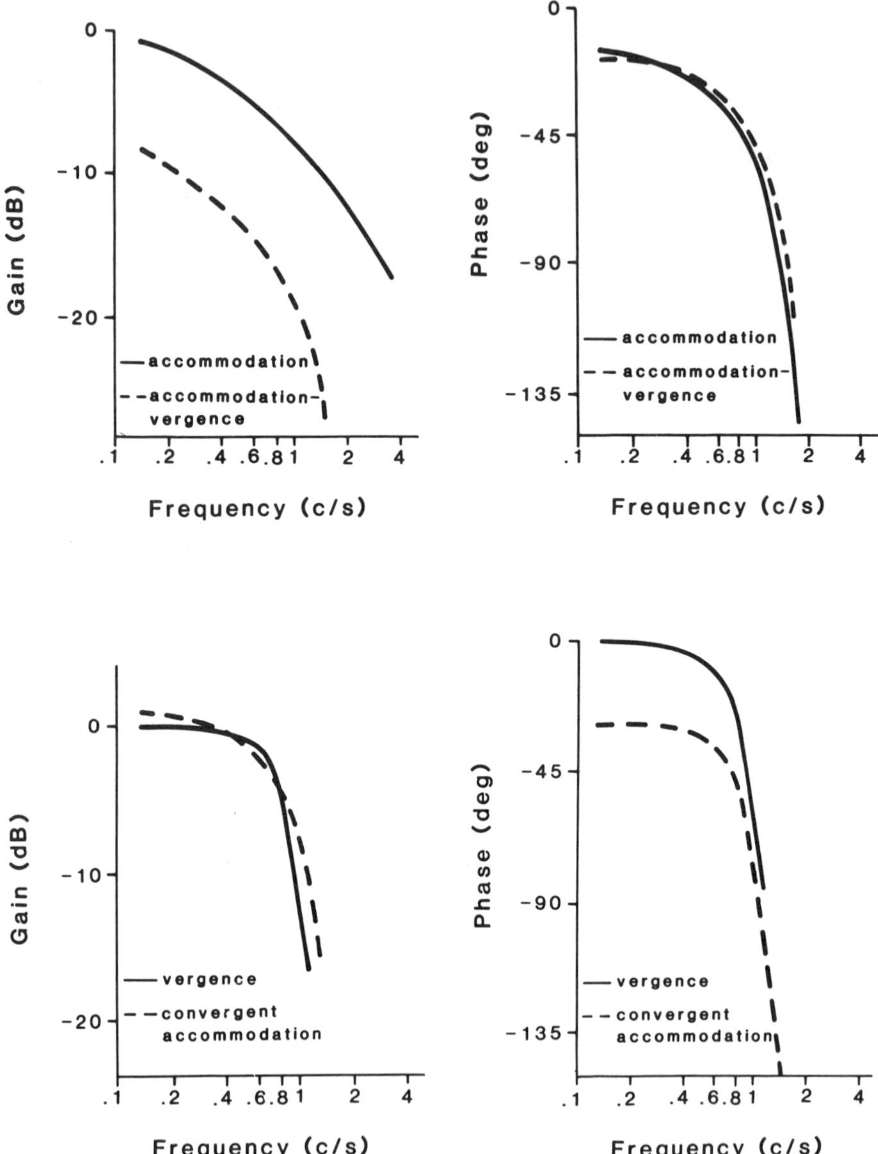

FIGURE 5.8. *Top* Frequency responses of accommodation and of accommodation vergence. Input amplitude 0.85 D (subject WTN). *Bottom* Frequency responses of vergence and convergent accommodation. Input amplitude 3.05 degrees (subject WTN). Adapted from Yoshida T, Watanabe A. Analysis of interaction between accommodation and vergence feedback control systems of human eyes. Bulletin NHK Broadcasting Science Research Laboratories, 1969. Reprinted by permission of the author.

ratio of approximately 5:1; thus a vergence movement of 1 degree would have an associated peak velocity of 5 degrees per second (Kenyon, Ciuffreda, and Stark, unpublished data). Nonlinearities do exist with convergence being slightly faster than divergence (see Chapter 10). Accommodative vergence gain is down 3 dB at 0.3 Hz for nonpredictable inputs with little perceptible response past 1.5 Hz; for predictable inputs a peak in the gain curve greater than unity is evident at 0.2 Hz, suggesting presence of a predictor operator (Krishnan et al., 1973). A phase lag is present for both nonpredictable and predictable sinusoidal inputs that rapidly increases at 1.5 to 2.0 Hz (Krishnan et al., 1973). Based on Wilson's studies on the near triadic response (1973a, 1973b), (1) a midbrain accommodative vergence motor controller with a processing time of 60 msec has been hypothesized, and (2) due to more rapid fall in the gain of accommodative vergence compared to accommodation, less noise is present in the vergence records than in the (simultaneous) accommodation records; this has recently been confirmed by Krishnan, Phillips, and Stark (1973). Frequency response characteristics for accommodation and vergence are summarized in Figure 5.8.

While Maddox (1886) was the first to define the various components of vergence, only recently has attention been directed toward dynamics of these binocular vergence interacting mechanisms (see Chapter 6). Semmlow and Venkiteswaran (1976) have shown that the total dynamic binocular vergence response is a result of disparity vergence (retinal disparity as the input) and accommodative vergence (blur as the input) summing in the "vergence final common pathway." Maddox believed that accommodative vergence acted first as a "coarse" control on the (binocular) vergence response with fusional (disparity) vergence acting as a "supplement" to compensate for inaccuracies in the accommodative-induced vergence change. Contrary to this, Semmlow (1981) believes that inate the possibility of an unequal accommodative vergence control signal of the response; accommodative vergence only plays an important role in the response dynamics as the stimuli approach the fovea where accommodation and accommodative vergence gain are maximum. Recently, Semmlow and Tinor (1978) quantified accommodative vergence gain as a function of retinal eccentricity in normals and showed that it was highest at the fovea and decreased by 50% 4.5 degrees from the fovea (Figure 5.9).

OCULOMOTOR INTERACTION OF ACCOMMODATIVE VERGENCE IN NORMALS

By objectively measuring eye movements, investigators have tried to understand the synkinetic relationship between accommodation and vergence. The first objective recordings of accommodative vergence were per-

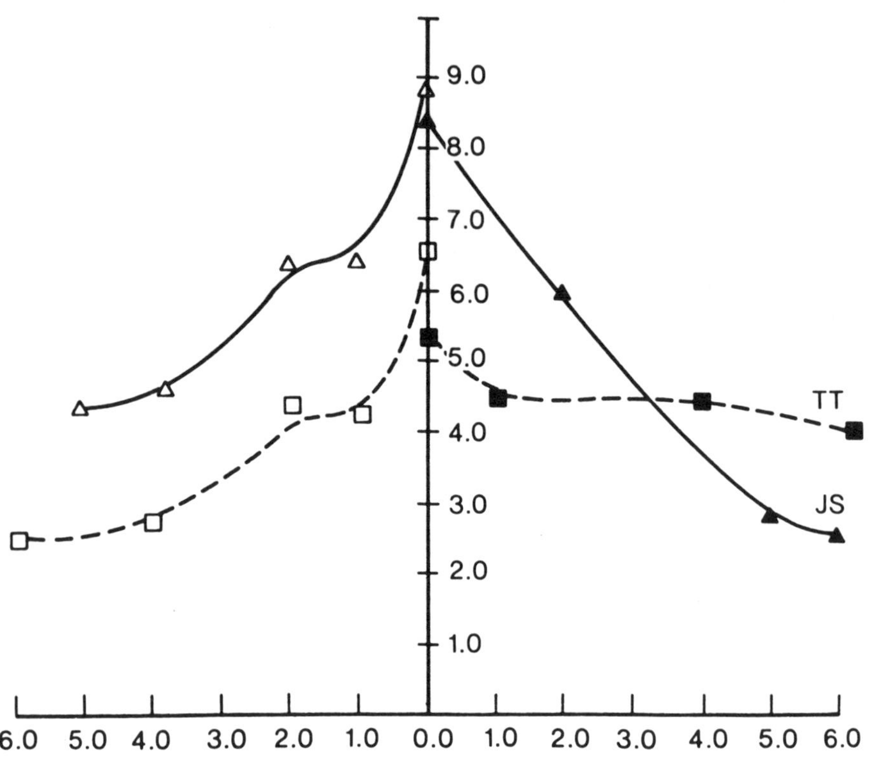

FIGURE 5.9. Variation of accommodative vergence response amplitude for two subjects showing response amplitudes to stimulus positions both right and left of the central fovea. Reprinted by permission of the publisher, from Semmlow JL, Tinor T. Accommodative convergence response to off-foveal retinal images. Journal of the Optical Society of America, 1978.

formed by Alpern and Ellen (1956) using electrooculography (EOG). They reproduced Mueller's (1826) experiment and showed that the covered eye changed position with the stimulus to accommodation, but that the viewing eye remained stationary (Figure 5.10). Since most vergence and versional eye movements adhere to Hering's law (1868) (see also Chapter 11), they explained the steadiness of the viewing eye as resulting from the "predominance of the fixation system." They did not elaborate on this interaction. Subsequent studies did not refute these findings, and in fact, concluded that accommodative vergence was a uniocular response (Robinson, 1966; Brodkey and Stark, 1967; Hermann and Samson, 1967;

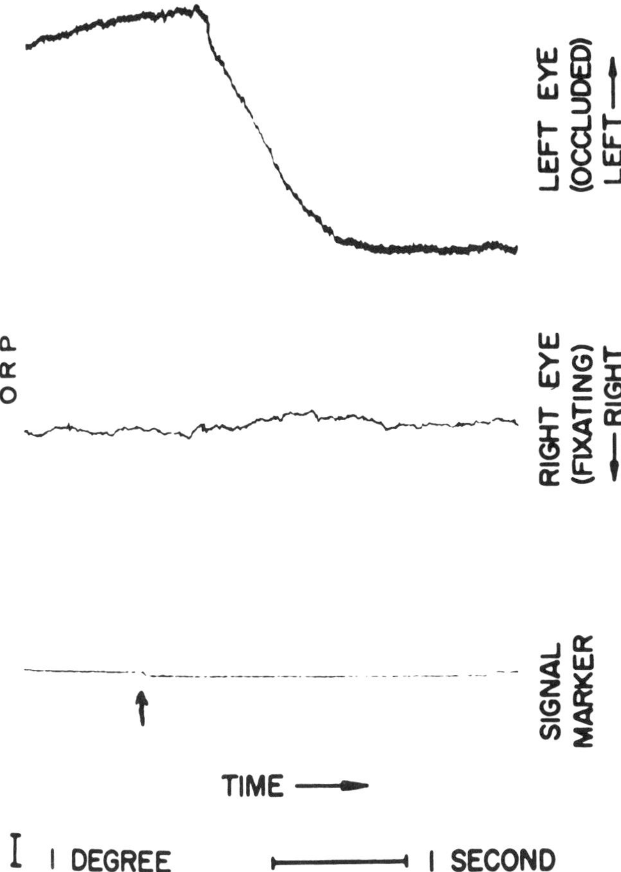

FIGURE 5.10. Record of eye position during accommodative vergence using EOG. Left eye occluded while right eye receives a 5-diopter blur when targets change from 3.4 to 0.18 meters. A clear accommodative vergence appears in the covered eye with little evidence for any response in the viewing eye. Published with permission from the American Journal of Ophthalmology 42:289–296, 1956. Copyright by the Ophthalmic Publishing Company.

Yamamoto, 1968, 1970; Troelstra et al., 1969; Keller and Robinson, 1972; Pickwell, 1972; Keller, 1973; Krishnan et al., 1973).

Only recently has evidence for binocular accommodative vergence emerged. Semmlow and Venkiteswaran (1976) successfully demonstrated binocular vergence to a step change in accommodative stimulus using haploscopically viewed targets at a constant vergence demand. Movements recorded from one eye only showed a smooth movement away and then back to the target (Figure 5.11). The authors assumed that the fellow eye performed the opposite movement and concluded that the initial

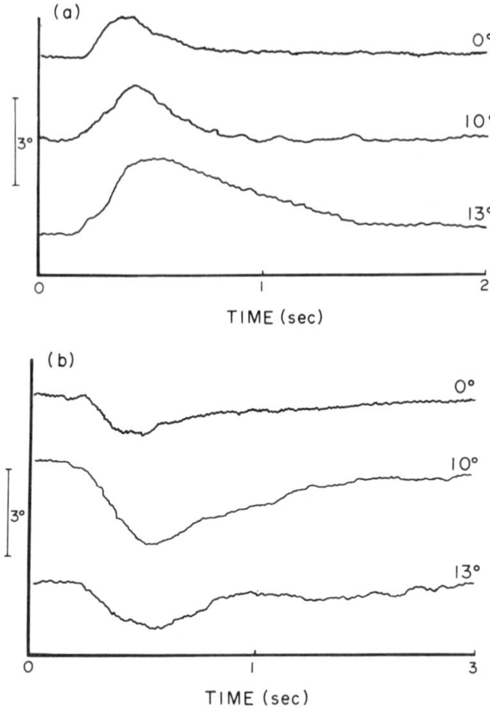

FIGURE 5.11. Vergence movements produced by binocular accommodative stimulation at three levels of constant disparity vergence stimulation (subject JS). A Increasing accommodative stimulation (1-4 diopters), B Decreasing accommodative stimulation (4-1 diopters). Reprinted by permission of the publisher, from Semmlow J, Venkitesvaran N. Dynamic accommodative vergence in binocular vision. Vision Research, 1976.

smooth movement away from the target represented a binocular accommodative vergence response. If the accommodative vergence was disjunctive and equal in each eye, they reasoned a symmetric disparity error would result, and this could be corrected by an opposing symmetric vergence movement. Subsequent smooth return of the eye to the fixation target was interpreted as the symmetric disparity vergence response to this error. Although binocular recordings would have allowed for a stronger argument, their assumption of equal disjunctive accommodative vergence is quite reasonable.

Concurrently and independently, Kenyon, Ciuffreda, and Stark (1978) examined the possibility of a binocular accommodative vergence response during the Mueller paradigm. Since Alpern and Ellen (1956), using the EOG, could find no viewing eye response using this stimulus condition, Kenyon and associates used a low-noise, high-bandwidth infrared reflection monitoring system (Stark et al., 1962) to determine objectively the binocular nature of accommodative vergence. Binocular accommodative vergence movements were found in all responses (n = 415) from five subjects, although the magnitude in each eye was grossly different (Figure 5.12). The average vergence amplitude (excluding saccades) in the viewing eye equalled 0.4° with a range of 0.08° to 1.5°, while in the covered eye vergence averaged 3.5° with a range of 2° to 7°. Thus the viewing eye vergence equalled about 10% of that found in the covered

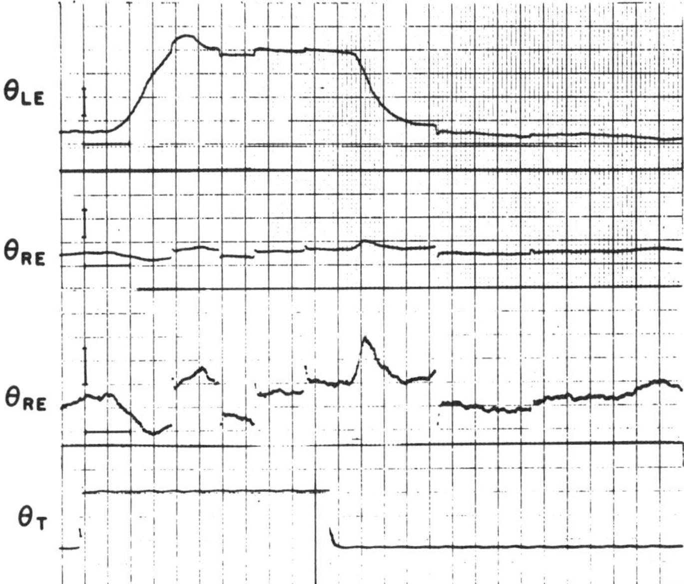

FIGURE 5.12. Binocular accommodative vergence eye movements to an accommodative stimulus of 2 diopters. A The divergence movement shows evidence for a visually triggered smooth pursuit component followed by a corrective saccade. For the following convergence the velocity is reversed and returns the eye to the target without a saccade. B This movement shows both visually triggered smooth pursuit and preprogrammed saccade. Note how the retinal error 200 ms prior to saccade does not equal saccade size. (From Kenyon et al., 1978). Shown from top to bottom as a function of time are covered left eye position, viewing right eye position (gain approximately equal to left eye), viewing right eye (gain greater than left eye), and stimulus onset of middle target denoted by upward deflections and onset of near target (denoted by downward deflections), respectively. Calibration bars represent 0.25° for viewing eye (lower trace), 1° for the covered eye and viewing eye (upper and middle traces) and 400 msec. Leftward movements represented by upward deflections. Reprinted by permission of the publisher, from Kenyon RV, Ciuffreda KJ, Stark L. Binocular eye movements during accommodative vergence. Vision Research, 1978.

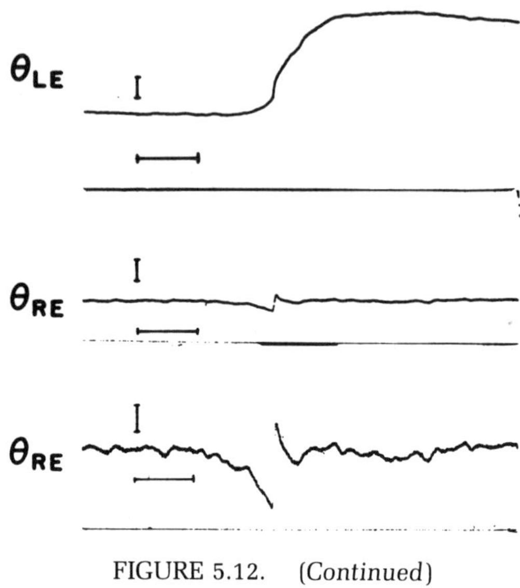

FIGURE 5.12. *(Continued)*

eye, or an average attenuation of accommodative vergence in the viewing eye of 90%. Predictable and nonpredictable target presentations produced similar responses. When the nondominant eye viewed the targets, however, one of two subjects increased the average vergence amplitude in the viewing eye from about 10 to 20% of the covered eye's movement (Figure 5.13). Such a change suggests less precise control of fixation with the nondominant eye.

The apparent discrepancy between Alpern and Ellen (1956), who showed the fixating eye to be stationary, and Kenyon, Ciuffreda, and Stark (1978), who showed accommodative vergence in the fixating eye, can be attributed to the sensitivity of the monitoring instrumentation. The EOG and photocell methods were used simultaneously to monitor the viewing eye during accommodative vergence using the Mueller paradigm (Figure 5.14). Inspection of this record shows a clear response in the photocell trace, but an inconclusive result in the EOG trace. Without the additional photocell information, interpretation of viewing eye vergence in the EOG record is difficult.

The unequal vergence amplitudes during accommodative vergence found by Kenyon's group (1978) seem to contradict Semmlow and Venkiteswaran's (1976) work that suggests an equal accommodative vergence response in each eye. In the latter experiment both eyes viewed a target, and thus a binocular accommodative vergence would create a symmetric disparity error. In the Mueller paradigm only one eye viewed a target, thus binocular accommodative vergence would create velocity and position errors. While the disparity vergence corrections to accommodative vergence response in Semmlow and Venkiteswaran's subjects opposed the movement in both eyes, in the Mueller paradigm the conjugate smooth pursuit and saccades oppose *only* vergence in the viewing eye and add to vergence in the covered eye. Thus one manner in which unequal accommodative vergence amplitudes can be produced is when a disjunctive vergence and a conjugate smooth pursuit and saccadic movements are linearly added to each eye. Evidence for a smooth pursuit component during accommodative vergence is shown in Figure 5.12 by a sharp change

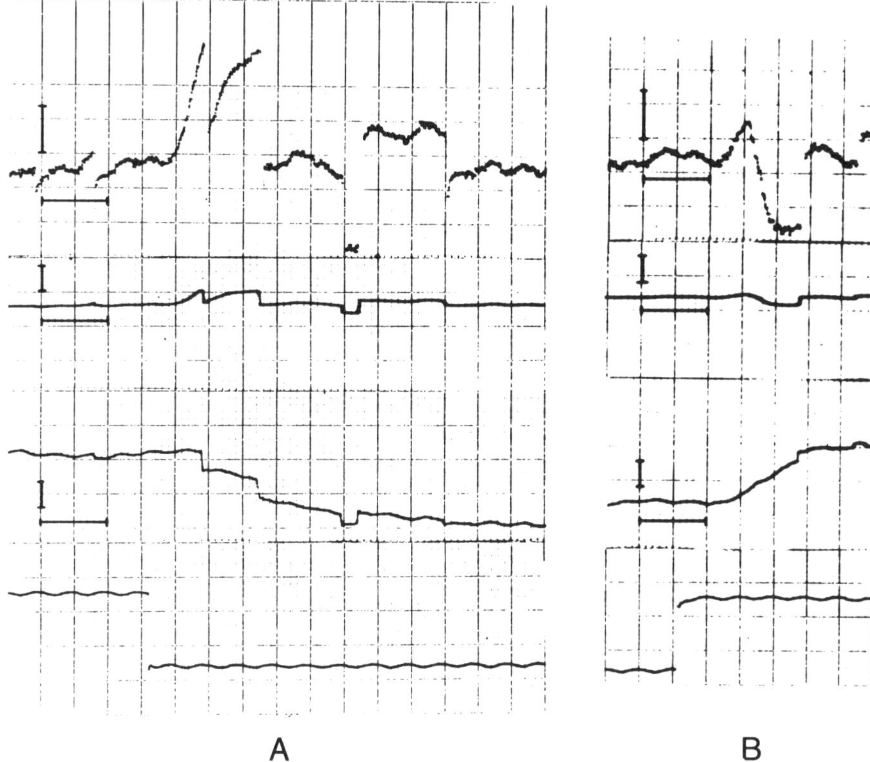

FIGURE 5.13. Binocular accommodative vergence eye movement responses when nondominant left eye viewed a 2-diopter target change. Shown from top to bottom as function of time are left viewing eye position (high gain) and (low gain), right covered eye (gain approximately equal to low gain of left eye), and stimulus (upward deflections denote onset of near target and downward deflections denote onset of middle target), respectively. Calibrations same as previous figure. Note unusual "double" vergence denoted in A and the large vergence response in the viewing eye. Viewing eye vergence amplitudes were smaller when the dominant eye viewed target. Early smooth pursuit component shown in B denoted at the start of the movement. Reprinted by permission of the publisher, from Kenyon RV, Ciuffreda KJ, Stark L. Binocular eye movements during accommodative vergence. Vision Research, 1978.

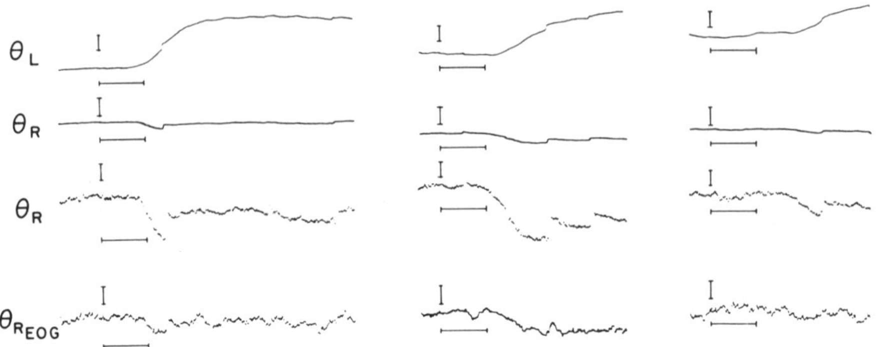

FIGURE 5.14. Binocular eye movements are shown for a normal subject with the dominant right eye viewing a target during divergence. The viewing eye was monitored simultaneously with both photocell and EOG methods; the covered left eye was monitored photoelectrically only. Shown are the position of the covered left eye, the viewing right eye (gain approximately equal to left eye), the viewing right eye (gain four times greater than left eye), and the viewing right eye (EOG method), respectively, from top to bottom as functions of time. Calibration bars represent 0.25° for the viewing right eye (lower two traces), 1° for upper two traces, and 400 msec. Leftward movements are represented by upward deflections. Note clearly observable vergence movement in the viewing right eye monitored with the photoelectric method but only noise and drift in the viewing eye during the same time with EOG recording, demonstrating ineffectiveness of EOG technique for detecting small ocular rotations. Reprinted by permission of the publisher, from Kenyon RV, Ciuffreda KJ, Stark L. Unexpected role for normal accommodative vergence in strabismus and amblyopia. American Journal of Optometry and Physiological Optics, 1980.

in eye velocity 200 msec after the start of vergence in the viewing eye (Kenyon et al., 1978).

If visually-driven smooth pursuit were the only mechanism responsible for the inequalities during accommodative vergence, the vergence amplitudes in each eye would be equal during the 200 msec latency of smooth pursuit. This is not the case; vergence amplitudes in each eye differ significantly during this period (Kenyon et al. 1978). These authors presented evidence suggestive of preprogrammed smooth pursuit occurring at approximately the same time as the vergence, as speculated earlier by Keller (1973). The smooth movements occurring *prior to* vergence in Figure 5.13 strongly suggest the presence of predictive smooth pursuit altering the initial vergence in the viewing eye. While this does not eliminate the possiblity of an unequal accommodative vergence control signal to each eye, it does suggest an alternate way in which these vergence inequalities may be explained by complex oculomotor interactions.

Ono (1981) has recorded binocular accommodative vergence movements of approximately equal amplitude in each eye when the fixation requirements were removed. These and other results (Semmlow and Venkiteswaran, 1976; Kenyon et al., 1978; Rashbass and Westheimer, 1961; Zuber and Stark, 1968) provide us with a picture of a single vergence controller fed by many signals (some visual, some pre-programmed, and others from synkinetically-linked oculomotor systems) whose response is a binocular disjunctive eye movement.

AC/A RATIO

Stability

Manas and Shulman (1954) did not agree with conventional thinking based on earlier clinical test findings that the AC/A ratio was constant, especially in light of its variability being equal to about one-half its mean value. To determine its clinical variability, they measured the stimulus AC/A ratio using the distance/near phoria and plus lens gradient techniques in 22 optometry students over a 7-week period in 20 test sessions. The ratios determined by these two methods were generally correlated, although the average group distance/near phoria value (4.7:1) was greater than the plus gradient value (4.1:1), presumably due to proximal convergence ($\pm 0.25^{\Delta}$/D) (see Chapter 4). Furthermore, the gradient method exhibited about twice the variability of the distance/near phoria method. Based on the stimulus AC/A ratios measured, Manas and Shulman concluded that dispersion of values demonstrated inconstancy of the ratio. They reasoned that since the phoria is not a constant, and the AC/A ratio is based on differences of phoria values, that the AC/A ratio is not constant. A potentially major problem with their study was use of stimulus rather than response AC/A ratios. It is important to note that over time, the distance phoria values were much more stable than the near phoria values, suggesting that variability of the stimulus AC/A ratio was primarily due to variability of the near phoria. Also, variability of the near phoria was probably due to variability of the accommodative response, which was not measured but assumed to equal the stimulus that remained fixed at specified dioptric levels. Errors in measurements and the limit of precision of measurements were not considered, although these factors would indeed contribute to variability of the AC/A ratio. Manas and Shulman also used the plus lens rather than minus lens gradient technique to reduce the stimulus to accommodation, which can result in range nonlinearities of the AC/A ratio (Ogle and Martens, 1957).

Hirsch (1954), in an editorial commentary on the Manas and Shulman (1954) paper, suggested they merely demonstrated that the AC/A ratio has inherent variability, as is true for any repeated set of measurements of a physiological system, and that whether the variability of their data is due to measurement error or to other factors cannot be determined. Hirsch further emphasized that in future research attempting to demonstrate that the AC/A ratio can be changed by some means, such as vision training, one must demonstrate consistent changes greater than the variability of the basic measures taken.

Later, Manas (1955) attempted to develop logical arguments and present some data suggesting inconstancy of the AC/A ratio; however, most of his arguments were either weak or relied on stimulus rather than response AC/A ratio data. Many of the flaws in his discussion have been detailed by Morris (1957). Westheimer (1955a), in response to the Manas paper (1955), indicated that a similar degree of variability was present in his carefully determined (with a haploscope-optometer) response AC/A ratios. Westheimer hoped that future research using better and more precise simultaneous measures of accommodation and accommodative vergence could answer such questions as the stability of the ratio; however, he was not optimistic and believed that more precise measures, especially of accommodation, may be difficult to obtain. In fact, recently Ciuffreda, Cooper and Kruger (unpublished data) determined response AC/A ratios in four normal adult subjects using infrared recording devices and indeed found similar degrees of variability ($\pm 1.5^{\Delta}$/D). Besides measurement errors to account for the variability, it should be recalled that the accommodation and accommodative vergence systems have different frequency-response characteristics, due to different system time delays, which would produce a temporal shift between the continuously recorded responses resulting in increased variability in a point-to-point calculation of the response AC/A ratio; thus 500- to 1000-msec portions of data should be averaged (but these too are subject to error, perhaps ± 0.25 D and $\pm 0.25^{\Delta}$) to help reduce this problem. Morris (1957), following his critique of Manas' paper (1955) and of the Fry (distance/near phoria) and Morgan (plus lens near gradient) clinical methods of determining stimulus AC/A ratios, described what he believed to be a more valid and reliable clinical test. He used the graphic analysis approach (see Chapters 12 and 13) with targets at eight different (real) test distances. His clinical stimulus AC/A ratios (on two patients tested) were greater than the response AC/A ratios determined using a haploscope-optometer. He attributed this to the influence of proximal convergence with his method. Based on extensive testing in patients, Morris concluded that the AC/A ratio was stable using this multipoint graphic analysis approach.

The most scientifically sound study to address the question of the degree of stability of the AC/A ratio was conducted by Flom (1960a). He measured both the stimulus and response AC/A ratios, with a standard clinical refractor and a haploscope-optometer, respectively, in four optometry students at weekly test intervals for 9 to 10 weeks. Accommodative stimuli were 0, 1.5, 2.5, and 3.5 diopters. Statistical techniques were used in data-fitting. The standard deviation of the response AC/A ratio (0.12^{Δ}/D) was less than for the stimulus AC/A ratio (0.18^{Δ}/D) determined by the refractor. Average variability of the AC/A ratios never exceeded 0.25^{Δ}/D, which is quite small. The stability of the response AC/A ratio (Figure 5.15) was determined two ways, and the following was found: (1) there was no significant difference in mean ratios between the first and second halves of the test period; the largest change was 0.68^{Δ}/D; and (2) the AC/A ratio exhibited chance variation over time using the Spearman rank correlation coefficient in relating ratio and trial number. As expected (Alpern et al., 1959), the response AC/A ratio exceeded the stimulus AC/A ratio; the haploscopically determined response AC/A ratio was greater than the refractor stimulus AC/A ratio (by 0.3^{Δ}/D) and the

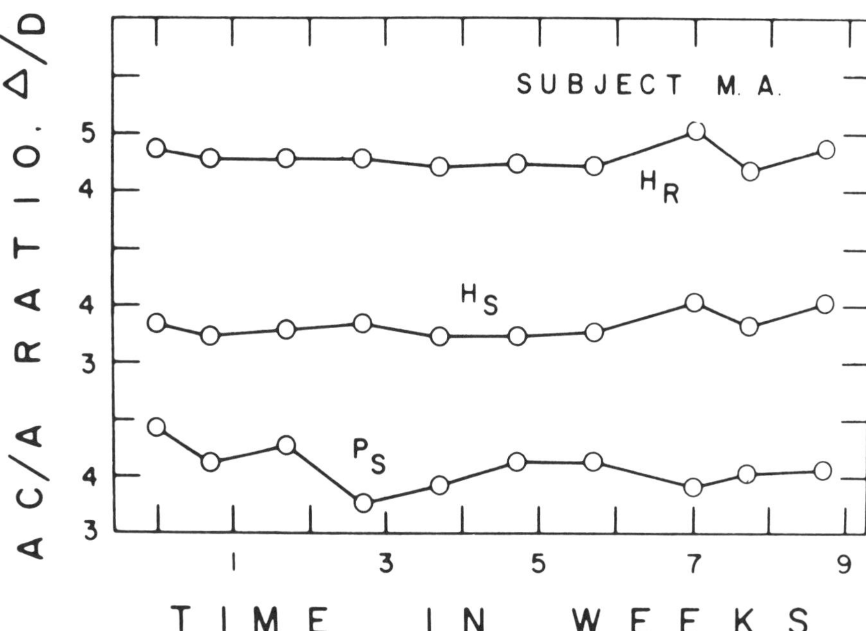

FIGURE 5.15. AC/A ratio plotted as a function of time. Measurements based on accommodative response data with haploscope (H_R), accommodative stimulus data with haploscope (H_S), and accommodative stimulus data with refractor using a Risley prism (P_S). Each circle represents the reciprocal of the slope of the straight line fitted by least squares to 20 data points over an accommodative range of 0 to 3.5 D. Reprinted by permission of the publisher, from Flom MC. On the relationship between accommodation and accommodative convergence, Part II, Stability. American Journal of Optometry and Archives of American Academy of Optometry, © (1960), American Academy of Optometry per The Williams & Wilkins Company (agent).

haploscopically determined stimulus AC/A ratio (by 1.0^{Δ} per D). There was also a high correlation between the response AC/A ratios and the haploscopically determined stimulus AC/A ratios, but not between either of the haploscopically determined AC/A ratios and the refractor stimulus AC/A ratios. Flom concluded that the AC/A ratio was relatively stable and that much of the variability could be explained by random measurement error and biological variation. Stability of the stimulus AC/A ratio was similarly demonstrated by Ogle (1966), who measured it using the fixation disparity method over a six-week period in one subject. Standard deviation of the AC/A ratio was small and quite stable, being about $\pm 0.25^{\Delta}$/D.

Linearity

Westheimer (1955b) investigated the linkage between accommodation and accommodative vergence in two nearly emmetropic, trained observers using a haploscope-optometer to gain additional insight into the question of linearity and stability of the AC/A ratio. Stimuli ranged from +1 to 5 diopters. Precision of measures was at best $\pm 0.25^{\Delta}$ and ± 0.25 D, respectively, for vergence and accommodation. In one subject, the AC/A ratio was nonlinear at each of the two test sessions. The sum of squares was significantly less when the data were fitted with a quadratic rather than a linear expression. In the other subject, the AC/A ratio was nonlinear at only one session. Of interest was the large variability of the measures, having a 95% confidence interval of $\pm 2^{\Delta}$/D. Westheimer suggested that careful statistical studies will be required to answer many of the questions regarding the AC/A ratio.

Ogle and Martens (1957) were interested in the relationship between accommodative and proximal convergence. They measured the stimulus AC/A ratio using the near gradient technique (which measures changes in accommodative vergence only) and the distance/near phoria technique (which measures changes in accommodative vergence that may be contaminated by proximal vergence effects) with targets at several distances. They found a linear relationship between accommodative vergence and accommodative stimulus when real target movement was employed. Nonlinearity of the AC/A ratio was evident in 50% of cases with the gradient technique when plus lenses were used to reduce the stimulus to accommodation. They suggested that only minus lenses should be employed to obtain reliable measures of the AC/A ratio using this method. Later, Martens and Ogle (1959) used the fixation disparity method (Ogle et al., 1949) to measure the stimulus AC/A ratio in 250 patients. Linear AC/A ratios were found in 92% of the cases, with the balance exhibiting some form of nonlinearity. They believed the smaller percentage of patients (8%)

exhibiting nonlinear AC/A ratios in this study as compared to their earlier investigation (50%) (Ogle and Martens, 1957) was due to use of the fixation disparity method, which they believed to be a better clinical procedure than the Maddox rod technique they had used previously.

The most extensive study of the AC/A ratio range nonlinearity was conducted by Alpern, Kincaid, and Lubeck (1959). They used a larger range of stimuli (−4 to +10 D) and smaller incremental changes (0.5 D) than previous investigators. Accommodation and accommodative vergence were measured with a haploscope-optometer in four nonpresbyopic observers. Over the central portion of the response range (+1 to 5 D), a linear relationship was observed among accommodative stimulus, accommodative response, and accommodative vergence response, with nonlinearity evident at either end of this range. (Figure 5.16). Pupil size changes over this linear region were minimal (Alpern et al., 1961).

Flom (1960b) also investigated the linearity of the AC/A ratio. He measured the AC/A ratio with a refractor (stimulus AC/A) and a haploscope-optometer (stimulus and response AC/A) in 12 young adults (8 were receiving orthoptic therapy) over a 12-week period. Stimuli ranged from 0 to either 3.5 diopters (with the refractor) or 6.25 diopters (with the haploscope-optometer). Using a variety of statistical procedures, he found the AC/A ratio to be nonlinear for intermediate stimulus values. He concluded that this nonlinearity, which was small, relatively consistent, and did not exhibit any trend over time, was of no practical significance. Several points deserve comment. First, only two-thirds of the measures for all subjects showed this small but statistically significant nonlinearity. Second, in only 1 of 12 subjects was it found in all techniques employed. Third, the correlation coefficients between convergence and accommodation were extremely high, suggesting only a small degree of nonlinearity (and variability). Last, from the graphs provided it appears that a marked reduction in the degree of nonlinearity would occur if the lowest stimulus level responses had not been included in the calculations. For as clearly demonstrated (Alpern et al., 1959), there is nonlinearity of the AC/A ratio at the lower and higher stimulus levels, but excellent linearity over intermediate (+1 to 5 D) stimulus levels in young adults.

Effects of Age

Although it has been well established and universally accepted that the amplitude of accommodation decreases with age (Donders, 1864; Duane, 1922; Hamasaki et al., 1956; Schapero and Nadell, 1957; Breinin and Chin, 1973) at a rate of approximately 0.4 diopters per year (Hofstetter, 1965), controversy remains regarding the question of change in the AC/A ratio

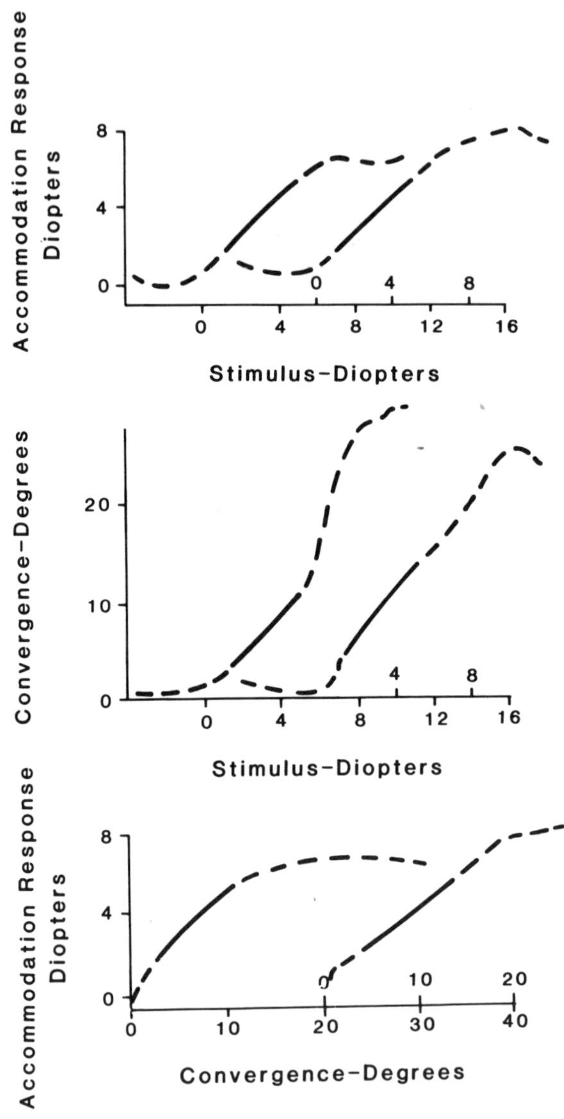

FIGURE 5.16. A Results of the experiment in two observers. The straight lines have been determined statistically. *Top* Relation of accommodation response to accommodation stimulus. *Middle* Relation of the accommodative vergence to the accommodation stimulus. *Lower* Relation of accommodative vergence to accommodation response B Shows relationship between pupil size, accommodation, and accommodative vergence. Figures A and B published with permission from the American Journal of Ophthalmology 52:762–767, 1961; 48:141–148, 1959. Copyright by the Ophthalamic Publishing Company.

with age. In general, results indicate that the stimulus AC/A ratio is either constant or declines slightly with age, while the response AC/A ratio increases with age.

Four population studies using stimulus AC/A methods have been conducted. Using the multilens near gradient technique, Morgan and Peters (1951) found the AC/A ratio in a group of presbyopes (over 45 years of age) to be 3.8 $\pm 2.5^{\Delta}$/D. This was very close to Morgan's (1944b) earlier findings (4.4 $\pm 2.0^{\Delta}$/D) in a group of nonpresbyopes. Davis and Jobe (1957), using an Ortho-rater on 10,000 industrial workers, found the stimulus AC/A ratio to be approximately constant (4.8/1) for ages 18 to 40 years, gradually increase to 5.2/1 at age 47, and then return to the previous lower level at age 50 years. Their report that subjects had difficulty seeing the near target clearly (printed letters) makes the results difficult to interpret,

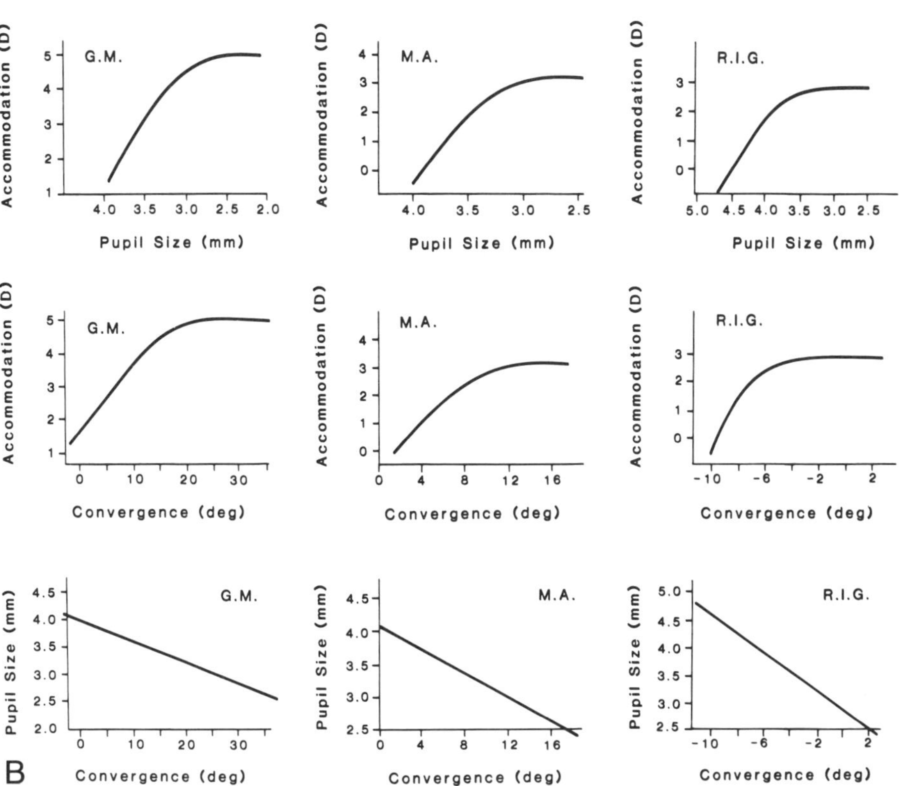

however. Alpern and Hirsch (1960) found a slight decline in stimulus AC/A ratio with age in a large group of clinical patients (n = 1202), going from 5.5/1 at age 10 years to 4/1 at 40 years. Ogle, Martens, and Dyer (1967) found that the AC/A ratios in a small (n = 23) group of presbyopes were similar to those found in nonpresbyopes, although the values were high in a few absolute presbyopes over 60 years of age.

A serious problem common to these studies was the use of stimulus rather than response AC/A ratios. The assumption of equivalence of stimulus and response AC/A ratios may lead to erroneous results (i.e, inflated AC/A ratios) in presbyopes, especially if data points obtained in the transitional accommodative soft saturation region just preceding the amplitude of accommodation (presbyopic hard saturation region) are included in the slope (reciprocal of the AC/A ratio) calculation.

Two studies in which response AC/A ratios were measured have been conducted and provide some evidence that the ratio increases with age. Fry (1959), using himself as the subject and a haploscope-optometer for measurements of accommodation and accommodative vergence, found his response AC/A ratio to increase slightly until age 40 years and thereafter sharply to increase (unfortunately data at only four ages were obtained and used to plot the response function); the AC/A ratio increased from 5.7/1 at age 29 years to 31.5/1^{Δ}/D at age 50 years. The most convincing results in favor of the increase with age are those of Breinin and Chin (1973), who measured and compared stimulus *and* response AC/A ratios in 28 patients ranging from 16 to 60 years of age. Stimulus ratios were approximately constant (perhaps even showing a slight decline) with age, similar to that reported by Alpern and Hirsch (1960). In contrast, when response ratios from these same patients were plotted, there was an increase with age, with this being most prominent past age 40 years. Unfortunately, only seven patients fell into this critical category of over 40 years of age. Similar trends were noted in a longitudinal study of four subjects ages 30 to 40 years over seven to nine years. Results of the Fry (1959) and Breinin and Chin (1973) studies are plotted in Figure 5.17, with similarity of trends being most striking. Further support for an increase in AC/A ratio with age is provided by Fincham (1955), as well as Eskridge (1973), who found the voluntary convergence to accommodation (VC/A) ratio that is highly correlated to the AC/A ratio (Eskridge, 1971) to increase with age in a similar manner (Figure 5.17).

Effects of Orthoptics

The question regarding plasticity or modifibility of the AC/A ratio is one of fundamental importance. From a theoretical point of view it provides insight into the underlying neurologic control of accommodation and

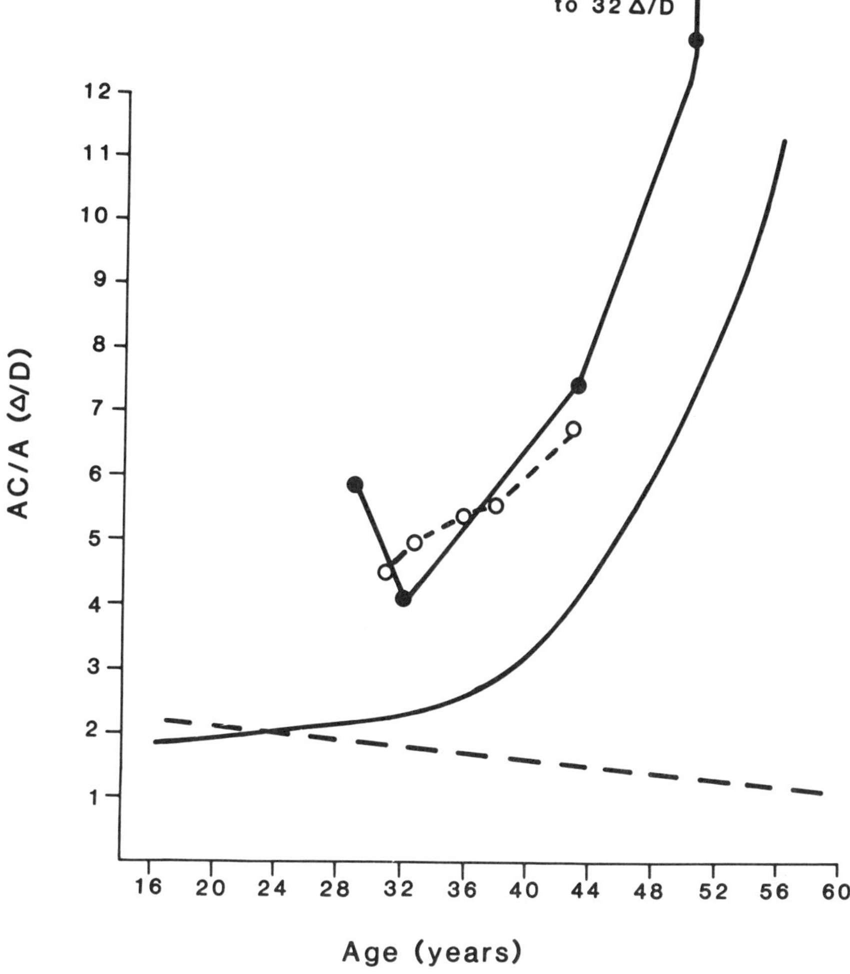

FIGURE 5.17. Plot of AC/A and age. AC/A stimulus (*broken line*) and response (*solid line*) of Breinin and Chin, AC/A response of Fry (*filled circles*), and VC/A response of Eskridge (*open circles*). AC/A response data suggest an increase with age especially after age 40 years.

accommodative vergence. If the ratio is modifiable, is there a critical period during which it is most amenable to change? Does such a modification involve alterations in firing patterns in the normally used pool of neurons or are other neuronal groups in the same or in associated control centers for accommodation and vergence control recruited? Is the effect not central but rather peripheral in origin, such as in the plant (e.g., the ciliary muscle or extrinsic eye muscles)? From a clinical point of view, a positive finding regarding true changes in AC/A ratio could have widespread effect on the treatment of strabismus. At present, optometrists using orthoptics that affect sensory and/or central mechanisms, and ophthalmologists using surgery and/or drugs that affect peripheral mechanisms, treat strabismus with varying degrees of success as defined by cosmetic as well as functional binocular vision criteria. Development of a therapeutic procedure, especially involving noninvasive means that alter the AC/A ratio centrally would be an exceedingly valuable clinical tool; for example, one could use this technique to change a patient with nonrefractive esotropia and a neurologically high AC/A ratio to an orthophore by reducing the ratio. The theoretician and clinician should take note, however, that accommodative vergence under normal binocular viewing conditions does not work alone but rather in a complex interactive manner with disparity vergence and related feedback pathways to assist in the fine focus and bifoveal fixation of an object of interest (see Chapter 6).

There are several reports in the literature that provide insight into the question of modifibility of the AC/A ratio by orthoptics. Lyle and Jackson (1941) calculated the stimulus AC/A ratio using the phoria method in 63 patients. The mean ratios were 4.1 $\pm$2.1 and 5.3 $\pm$1.2$^{\Delta}$/D before and after orthoptic treatment, respectively, showing an increase in average value with a concomitant decrease in variability. In many instances, following treatment large increases in the stimulus AC/A ratio resulted from reduced exophoria at near. In ranking the ease of changing clinical test findings, Morgan (1944b) included distance and near phorias, although he emphasized that any changes were indeed minimal. This suggests that the stimulus AC/A ratio might be altered by orthoptics, but only to a limited extent.

Gibson (1947) presented case results in four nonstrabismic patients receiving orthoptics. Based on the calculated stimulus AC/A ratio using the phoria method, he found that it increased progressively in two patients, slightly increased in one patient, and decreased in another. Heath and Hofstetter (1952) presented detailed clinical findings during the course of 21 months of orthoptics in a six-year-old intermittent, alternating exotrope. Their primary finding was an increase in the fusional recovery range, which probably accounted for the patient's reduction of symptoms associated with near visual tasks. Based on stimulus AC/A ratios using the phoria method, there was a reduction of AC/A during training; however, they believed this to be an apparent rather than true change, being caused by variability of phoria findings early in training and periodic shifting of the zone of single binocular vision due to intermittency of the ocular deviation. A problem with this study was unreliable patient responses, especially early in training. In a preliminary report by Flom (1954), the calculated AC/A ratio was determined in 53 nonstrabismic individuals during vision training. No consistent change of the distance or near phoria, and thus AC/A ratio, was found. When a change was found, test-retest variability was greater than the initial measured change. Flom concluded that any difference in the AC/A ratio was not real, but was a result of a change in accommodative response, a change in proximal convergence, and/or residual fusional convergence present during the test. He also mentioned the preliminary results of Harrigan, who measured response AC/A ratios in 11 subjects receiving vision training. In 10 the response AC/A ratio variability was less than or equal to 0.25^{Δ}/D; in 1 subject, marked changes in the AC/A ratio were measured during and following training, with increases as great as 1.7^{Δ}/D found. Manas (1958) measured stimulus AC/A ratios using the phoria method in 200 clinical patients with binocular vision seeking vision training. Patients were seen for 30-minute training sessions twice a week for six weeks. Conventional version, vergence, and accommodation training were used. He found the mean AC/A ratios to be 4.4 ± 2.6 and $4.9 \pm 2.0^{\Delta}$/D before and after training, respectively, with this 0.5^{Δ}/D change being statistically significant. Thus these results were qualitatively and quantitatively similar to those of Lyle and Jackson (1941) discussed earlier.

Two serious flaws of virtually all these reports were use of stimulus rather than response AC/A ratios and use of the distance/near phoria rather than the multistimulus near gradient technique. The basic problem associated with use of the stimulus AC/A ratio is that accommodative response is not measured but is assumed to equal the accommodative stimulus. While the response AC/A ratio in normals can be estimated by multiplying the stimulus AC/A ratio by 1.08 (Alpern et al., 1959; Alpern, 1969), agreement may be less and variability more in patients having vergence and/or accommodative difficulties (Cooper et al., 1982). Thus during the course of vision training the patient's accommodative response amplitude and accuracy may increase, resulting in reduced exophoria and increased accommodative vergence. If this indeed does occur and the stimulus AC/A ratio is measured, it will give the impression that the true AC/A ratio is increased. The second problem is use of the distance/near phoria technique to determine the stimulus AC/A ratio. This method is affected by proximal convergence (see Chapter 4), which in some cases may be very high, resulting in an inflated AC/A ratio (Breinin et al., 1966). Thus the multilens near gradient technique obviates the proximal factor, which is held constant for all measurements.

A later paper by Flom (1960c) addressed some of these issues. He measured stimulus and response AC/A ratios using phoria and gradient techniques in subjects during the course of orthoptics. His control group consisted of college and optometry students. His experimental group consisted of subjects who had exophoria at near, had poor fusional vergence ranges, and had symptoms related to near work. They received orthoptics treatment three times a week for eight weeks with the goal of improving positive relative convergence. He used the calculated stimulus AC/A ratio (phoria method) in the majority of subjects, but also obtained response AC/A ratios with a haploscope-optometer in a small group. No significant differences in stimulus or response AC/A ratios were found in the control group (n = 24). In one experimental group (n = 87), a statistically significant increase of 0.41^{Δ}/D in stimulus AC/A ratio was found; the follow-up group (n = 11) measured one year later showed some reduction. In another experimental group (n = 8) the orthoptic training interval was divided into two halves, and the mean AC/A ratio for each half across subjects was determined. The response AC/A ratio increased by 0.66^{Δ}/D and the stimulus AC/A ratio increased by 0.32^{Δ}/D, both changes being statistically significant when these two intervals were compared (Figure 5.18). Furthermore, during the entire orthoptic interval, the response AC/A ratio and positive relative convergence progressively increased and were highly positively correlated. For the initial few weeks following termination of treatment, further increases in the response and stimulus AC/A ratios were recorded. One year later, however, both stimulus and response AC/A ratios in five of the subjects returned to the value found just following termination of treatment. From this Flom concluded that the response AC/A ratio could be altered somewhat by orthoptics, but the change was not maintained for long once treatment was terminated. Several points should be noted. First, the increase in stimulus AC/A ratio was in part due to a reduction of the near exophoria. Second, the change in response AC/A ratio was small (0.66^{Δ}/D) and was similar to the stimulus

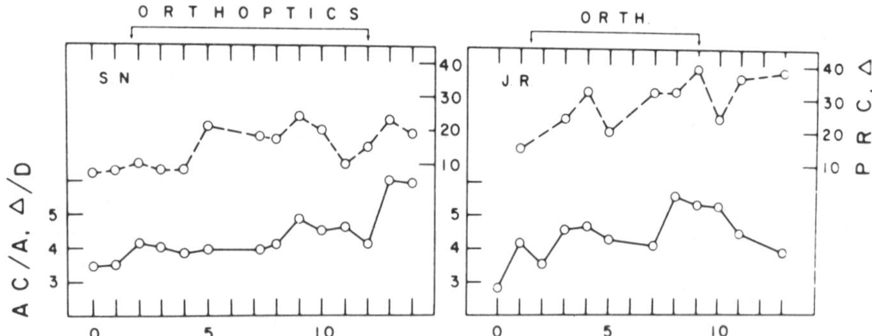

FIGURE 5.18. AC/A ratio and positive relative convergence plotted as a function of time (weeks). AC/A ratio based on accommodative response data obtained with haploscope. Positive relative convergence measured with Risley prisms at 40-cm fixation distance. Reprinted by permission of the publisher, from Flom MC. On the relationship between accommodation and accommodative vergence III. Effects of Orthoptics. American Journal of Optometry and Archives of American Academy of Optometry, © (1960), American Academy of Optometry per The Williams & Wilkins Company (agent).

AC/A ratio change reported by Manas (1958). Third, college students with relatively minor signs and symptoms of triadic dysfunction were used rather than patients exhibiting poor accommodation and/or vergence abilities. It is in these symptomatic patients that the question of modifibility of the AC/A ratio is of prime concern to the clinician. Fourth, preorthoptics AC/A ratios were not recorded.

A related study was conducted by Flom and Takahashi (1962). They investigated the influence of undercorrected (by at least 0.5 D) myopia on the AC/A ratio. In a group ($n = 28$) of undercorrected myopes, stimulus (von Graefe method) and response (haploscope-optometer method) AC/A ratios were determined, with full correction worn immediately after and at least one week following receipt and constant wear of the new prescription. They found the lens-induced near esophoria reduced by 3^{Δ} (reduction was not correlated with degree of undercorrection) with a lesser effect on distance phoria, this resulting in an overall increase in exophoria following a week or so of lens wear. Furthermore, the stimulus AC/A ratios decreased by 0.3^{Δ}/D in the exophores (not a significant change) and 1.0^{Δ}/D in the esophores (a significant change). Most importantly, however, the mean *response* AC/A ratios did not change significantly, although downward trends were the rule. They attributed reductions to reduced positive relative convergence: with the myopia undercorrected, the accommodative stimulus and in turn accommodation and accommodative convergence responses would be reduced. Positive relative convergence would be employed as a supplement to attain accurate bifoveal fixation and fusion at near. Over time this convergence would become conditioned. Now, when the full myopic prescription is suddenly added, the conditioned convergence response persists. In time (approximately one week) it diminishes resulting in a reduction of the AC/A ratio. It would be erroneous to conclude that the AC/A ratio really changed, however, since: (1) the response AC/A ratio remained relatively unchanged and (2) the vergence change was attributed to reduction of the conditioned fusional vergence response rather than any actual change in the response of accommodation and/or accommodative vergence.

Other techniques have been employed to measure and/or modify the AC/A ratio. Ogle, Martens, and Dyer (1967) used the fixation disparity method (Ogle et al., 1949) to determine stimulus AC/A ratios in five patients undergoing standard orthoptics treatment involving vergence and accommodation exercises. Following training, the AC/A ratio was greater in two patients, less in one patient, and equal in the remaining two (Figure 5.19). A problem with this technique is that it results in an indirect, binocular stimulus AC/A ratio that entails complex fixation requirements and stimulus parameters, with these being much different than used for determination of the AC/A ratio using standard clinical techniques. A recent preliminary report by Judge and Miles (1980) indicated that the stimulus AC/A ratio could be markedly increased in normals after only 1 hour of wearing special lenses that effectively doubled the interpupillary distance; decay time was 1.5 hours. The increased esophoria and stimulus AC/A ratio following such lens wear could be explained by a transient fusional aftereffect (Alpern, 1946). To lend credibility to these results careful determinations of response AC/A ratios are essential in a larger group of subjects.

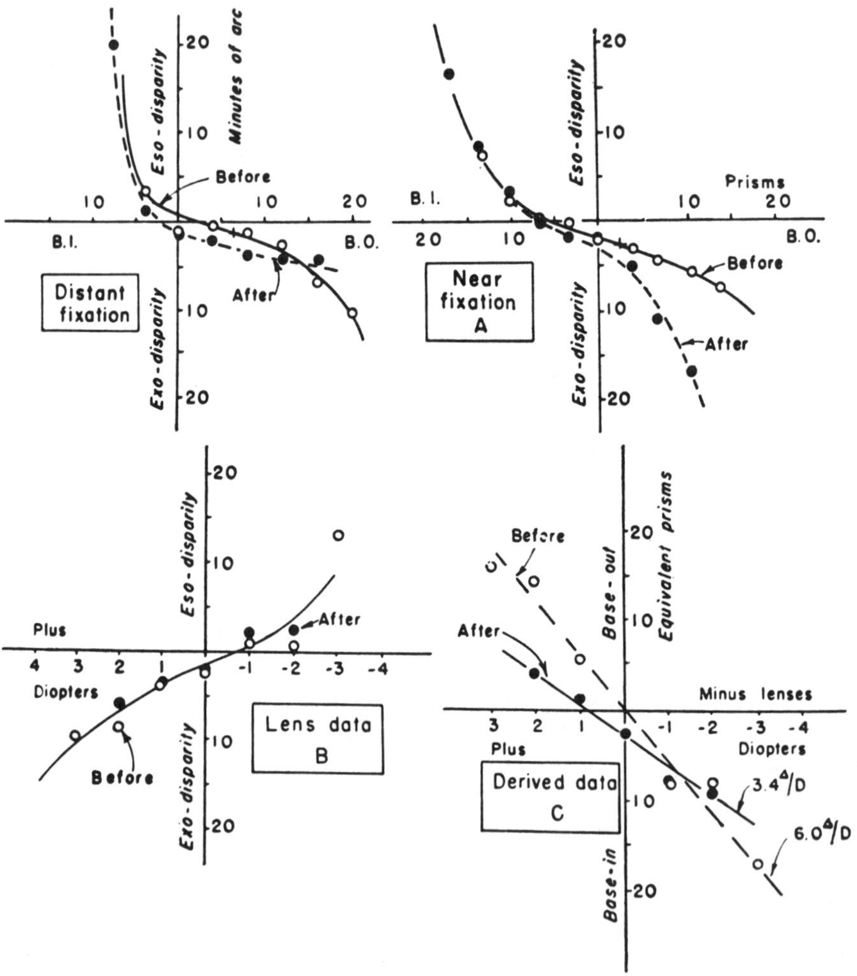

FIGURE 5.19. Fixation disparity data obtained before and after orthoptic exercises showing a change in the stimulus AC/A ratio. Reprinted by permission of the publisher, from Ogle KN, Martens TG, Dyer JA. *Oculomotor Imbalance in Binocular Vision and Fixation Disparity*. Philadelphia: Lea and Febiger, 1967.

Effects of Surgery

Few careful, quantitative studies have been conducted on the effects of extraocular muscle surgery on the AC/A ratio. Ogle and associates (1965, 1967) investigated these effects in patients with either large esophoria or intermittent exotropia. The goal of this surgery was to reduce the deviation mechanically, as well as to shift the fixation disparity curve toward the origin of the graph to reduce the associated phoria. In patients with esophoria both goals were attained; in exotropes only the former was accomplished. In none of the cases was a significant change in the stimulus AC/A ratio recorded as determined by the fixation disparity method. Sears and Guber (1967) reported results on two young children with intermittent, alternating esotropia ($\sim 30^{\Delta}$) at distance and near (Figure 5.20). Stereoacuity was reduced in both patients when fusion prevailed. The multilens near gradient method (Maddox rod) was used to measure stimulus AC/A ratios. Following bimedial rectus recession surgery, there was a

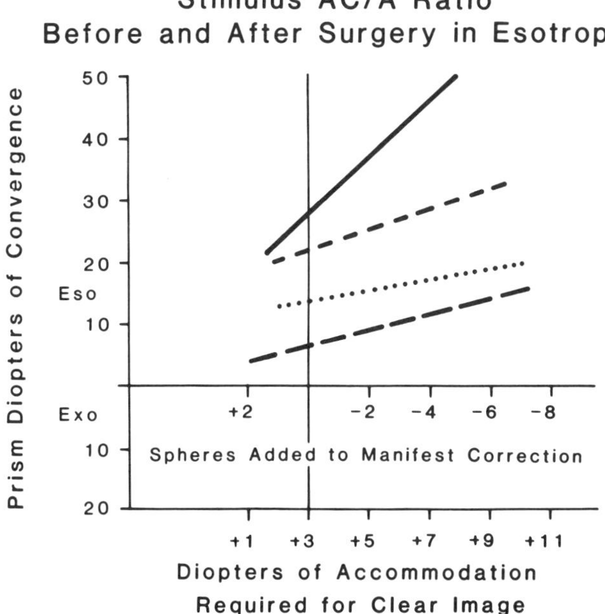

FIGURE 5.20. Plot of accommodation stimulus and accommodative vergence response in one patient. Symbols: solid line = measurements taken prior to any form of therapy, small dashed line = one set of measurements taken after three weeks of phospholine iodide therapy, dotted line = one set of measurements taken two weeks after surgery, large dashed line = measurements made 1, 6, and 12 months after surgery. Published with permission from The American Journal of Ophthalmology 64:872–876, 1967. Copyright by The Ophthalamic Publishing Company.

decrease both in the distance phoria and AC/A ratio. Of particular interest were results comparing the stimulus AC/A ratio as determined with the distance/near phoria and the near gradient procedures. For example, in one patient, using the phoria method it was 10.4^{Δ}/D and 8.7^{Δ}/D before and after surgery, respectively, while with the gradient technique it was 5.0^{Δ}/D and 1.4^{Δ}/D before and after surgery, respectively. These pronounced differences were attributed to proximal convergence effects and/or nonlinear AC/A ratio effects that can be significant and result in erroneous (typically inflated) stimulus AC/A values with the distance/near phoria method (Breinin et al., 1966). These results show that in some patients the stimulus AC/A ratio could be reduced by surgery. It should be emphasized, however, that surgery does not alter the *neural* linkage between accommodation and accommodative vergence, but rather changes the *mechanical* response characteristics of the extraocular muscles, that is, reduces the mechanical advantage of the medial recti. Thus for a given target (blur) input and neural output (to accommodation and vergence) reduced accommodative vergence results.

Drug Effects

The AC/A ratio can be altered by ingestion or topical application of drugs. Ingestion of barbiturates or amphetamines will raise or lower the AC/A (Figure 5.21), respectively, by affecting the central nervous system centers that control accommodation and vergence (Rashbass and Westheimer, 1959; Westheimer, 1963). Westheimer (1963) found that 260 mg of amytal sodium increased accommodative vergence in the covered eye (increased esophoria at distance) for an accommodative stimulus at 5 meters and decreased accommodative vergence (increased exophoria at near) for a stimulus at 33 cm. Also, the near point of convergence receded without a corresponding change in near point of accommodation. These results showed how barbiturates reduce the activity of the vergence but not the accommodative controller. Further evidence to support this hypothesis is that the fusional or disparity vergence range was reduced, response latency increased, and time constant of vergence responses were lengthened by the drug. Thus changes in the AC/A ratio resulted from a depressed response from the vergence controller, whether stimulated by disparity or blur. Cohen and Alpern (1969) found similar results using ethanol. The decrease in AC/A ratio was proportional to the amount of alcohol in the blood; a surprising 5% drop was found with only 0.01 gm per ml blood-alcohol level, which has no known toxic effects. Alcohol had similar results on fusional vergence ranges as barbiturates.

In contrast to barbiturates and alcohol, amphetamine sulfate had a facilitory effect on vergence (Figure 5.21) (Westheimer, 1963). Ingestion

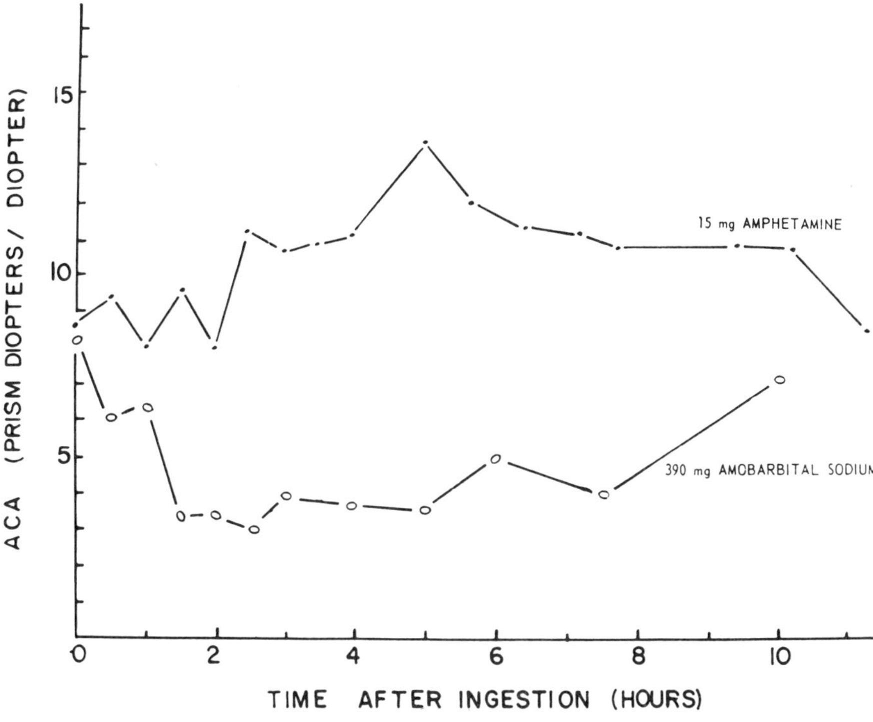

FIGURE 5.21. Changes in AC/A from a subject (age 21, height 6 ft 3 in (190.5 cm), weight 175 lb (79.4 kg) following ingestion of 15-mg racemic amphetamine sulfate (*filled circles*), and in another experiment, 6 grains (390 mg) amobarbital sodium (*open circles*). Reprinted by permission of the publisher, from Westheimer G. Amphetamine, barbiturates, and accommodation convergence. Archives of Ophthalmology, 70:830–836. Copyright 1963, American Medical Association.

of 260 mg amobarbital sodium produced a slight change in accommodative vergence measured in the covered eye toward exophoria at distance, while the accommodative vergence to the 33-cm target decreased the near exophoria. The near points of accommodation and vergence were unchanged and only a slight change in fusional range was noted. Thus amphetamines appeared to tighten the relationship between accommodation and vergence in Westheimer's (1963) subjects, reducing their near exophoria. Effects of the drug on intraocular and extraocular muscle appeared to be minimal, since accommodative amplitude was unimpaired and pupil diameter was constant despite its higher sensitivity to amphetamines than the ciliary muscle's. Thus deficient accommodation, which would result in sensory impairment and increase in accommodative effort, was unlikely. Presence of normal saccades and vestibular nystagmus ruled out changes in vergence response due to drug-induced extraocular muscle deficits.

Topical application of cycloplegic and anticholinesterase drugs causes a rapid increase or decrease in the AC/A ratio, respectively. (Westheimer, 1963; Alpern and Larson, 1960) Alpern and Larson demonstrated increases in the AC/A ratio using 5% eucatropine with 1% hydroxyamphetamine while the subject maintained a constant level of accommodation on a distance target. As the cycloplegic increased its effect, the AC/A ratio increased rapidly (Figure 5.22). This increase is caused by the actions of the accommodation feedback controller's attempt to maintain a clear retinal image. Specifically, the cycloplegic reduces the activation (or effective gain) of the ciliary muscle by blocking the effect of acetylcholine on the motor end plate. Thus to achieve the same accommodative level, the amount of innervation to the ciliary muscle must be increased. This increased accommodative controller effort causes a concurrent increase in the level of accommodative vergence through their synkinetic

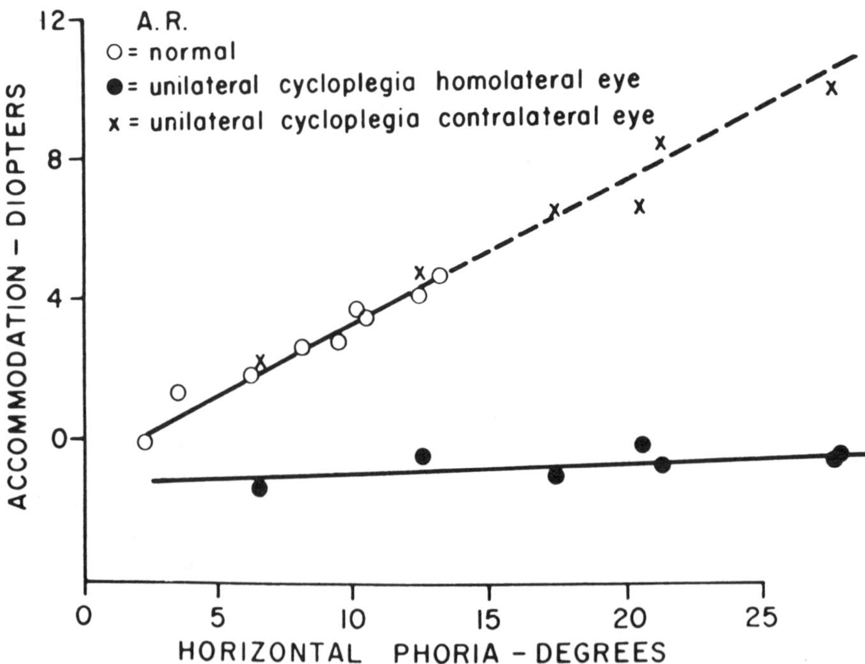

FIGURE 5.22. Influence of cycloplegia on AC/A in both drugged (*filled circles*) and undrugged (*crosses*) eye. The increased innervation to the viewing drugged eye's ciliary muscle is expressed by the sloping line through the undrugged eye's accommodative level with time. Published with permission from the American Journal of Ophthalmology 49:1140–1149, 1960. Copyright by the Ophthalmic Publishing Company.

link. For the same accommodative stimulus an increase in accommodative vergence occurs, producing an increase in the measured AC/A. Alpern and Larson (1960) showed this effect by measuring accommodation in both eyes. Their results (Figure 5.22) showed how the eye treated with cycloplegia had a constant accommodative state, while the covered eye's accommodation increased with time beyond the level found in the other eye. When fixation was changed to the drug-free eye, accommodation levels were again different in each eye, with the drug-free eye having an appropriate accommodation response and the drugged eye having much less. Blocking the action of acetylcholine in the motoneuronal junction in the ciliary muscle by cycloplegic drugs caused the rapid rise in the AC/A ratio with time.

In contrast to the cycloplegic drugs that raised the AC/A ratio, anticholinesterases caused a decrease. Chin and Breinin (1967) showed a decrease in the AC/A ratio when echothiophate iodide was topically administered. This drug inhibits the hydrolyzing effect of acetylcholine by cholinesterase, prolonging the effects of the released acetylcholine. This increased effectiveness of the ciliary muscle innervation reduces the amount of accommodation innervation needed to maintain a clear retinal image for the same accommodative stimulus. This reduced accommodative controller effort causes a concomitant reduction in accommodative vergence through their synkinetic link. For the same stimulus to accommodation, smaller vergence responses are measured and a decrease in the response AC/A ratio is found.

ACCOMMODATION AND ACCOMMODATIVE VERGENCE IN AMBLYOPIA AND STRABISMUS

Amblyopia is an anomaly of monocular vision in which there is reduced visual acuity that cannot be accounted for on the basis of uncorrected refractive error, ocular or neurologic disease, or structural abnormalities in the visual pathways. A common clinical criterion for amblyopia is visual acuity of 20/40 or poorer in one eye and a difference in visual acuity between the two eyes of at least one line (Flom and Neumaier, 1966). Using this criterion, Flom and Neumaier found the prevalence of amblyopia in a general school-age population to be 1.7%. Of course prevalence of amblyopia, ranging from 1% to 5.3% (Burian and von Noorden, 1974), is dependent on visual acuity criterion adopted.

Several vision anomalies may coexist in individuals having amblyopia. Eccentric fixation, an anomaly of monocular vision in which the time-average position of the fovea is off the target of regard, can be regarded as a zero sensorimotor visual direction bias of central origin; it is present in 80% of amblyopic eyes (Brock and Givner, 1952). Strabismus, an anomaly of binocular vision in which the visual axis of one eye fails to intersect the object of interest, may be regarded as a bias (typically neural in origin) in the vergence motor system; it is present in 5% of the population (Flom, unpublished data). In addition, other conditions may occur in association with strabismus. First, diplopia and confusion may result. Since the image of the object of interest now falls on noncorresponding retinal points (i.e., the fovea of one eye and a nonfoveal point in the other eye) that project to different points in visual space, diplopia or double images may be present. As dissimilar images now fall on the fovea of each eye, confusion due to overlapping of these dissimilar images (seen in the same visual direction) may ensue. Second, suppression, the process whereby all or part of the ocular image of one eye is prevented from contributing to the binocular percept, may develop to avoid deleterious effects of diplopia and confusion. Third, anomalous correspondence, in which the two foveas do not correspond, may develop to avoid the effects of diplopic imagery. If the foveas are stimulated either simultaneously or in rapid succession, percepts in two different visual directions will result.

It is well established that many sensory functions are abnormal in amblyopic eyes, such as decreased central visual acuity (Kirschen and Flom, 1978), reduced contrast sensitivity (Hess and Howell, 1977), depressed critical flicker-fusion frequency (Feinberg, 1956; Alpern et al., 1960), and impaired direction sense (Bedell and Flom, 1981). Accommodation, having both *sensory and motor* components, has received relatively little careful attention. Sensory and motor processes involved in converting the blur input into appropriate neural signals to drive both the accommodation and vergence systems may be abnormal in amblyopic eyes.

It is necessary to consider the influence of other factors that may in part adversely affect accommodation and accommodative vergence responses when the amblyopic eye alone receives a blur input. A factor of major importance is eccentric fixation. As Phillips (1974) has demonstrated for accommodation in normals and Semmlow and Tinor (1978) for accommodative convergence in normals, closed-loop gain (ratio of response amplitude to input amplitude) of each system is highest at the fovea and decreases as more eccentric retinal areas are stimulated (Figures 5.6 and 5.9). Decreased gain of accommodation and accommodative vergence might be predicted in an amblyopic eye with eccentric fixation, without the necessity of hypothesizing defective responses resulting from abnormal visual experience, based simply on normal system response characteristics of extrafoveal regions. That retinal cones are involved in the accommodation reflex (Campbell, 1954a) and their density decreases with retinal eccentricity provide further support that reduced accommodation and accommodative vergence response may in part be expected by the presence of eccentric fixation alone. Another factor that may adversely affect accommodation and accommodative vergence is increased amblyopic ocular drift (Ciuffreda, 1977; Ciuffreda et al., 1980). Increased drift amplitude, which may slowly move the eye ± 1.0 degree horizontally to either side of the eccentric fixation point, could produce increased variability of accommodation and accommodative vergence responses, for as mentioned earlier, accommodation and accommodative vergence gain are inversely related to retinal eccentricity of the stimulus, and most amblyopes have eccentric fixation (Brock and Givner, 1952). Increased amblyopic drift velocity, being generally less than 2.5 degrees per second, probably does not degrade visual acuity (Ciuffreda et al., 1980), although it may reduce the contrast (by "smearing") of high spatial frequency suprathreshold target components that would result in reduced accommodative responses (Heath, 1956; Ciuffreda et al., in press). Receptor amblyopia (Enoch, 1959), misalignment of retinal receptors resulting in light striking obliquely and thus being "less efficient" due to the wave guide nature of the receptors, may play a minor role in the loss of visual acuity (Campbell and Gregory, 1960; Green, 1967). Since misaligned receptors do not markedly degrade visual acuity, and slightly less efficient light capture would not result in reduction in target contrast, it appears that receptor amblyopia would not exert a major adverse effect on accommodation. Recent work casts doubt on the existence of receptor amblyopia (Bedell, 1980). Last, optics of the amblyopic eye do not appear to contribute in a major way to accommodation loss, as contrast sensitivity functions are grossly similar when the ocular optics are bypassed (Hess, 1977a, 1977b), and the modulation transfer function in one amblyopic eye was grossly similar to that found in normals (Fankhauser and Rohler, 1967); confirmation of these findings with larger sample sizes is essential before optics and retinal-image smearing effects can be ruled out, however.

ACCOMMODATION

Costenbader, Baier, and McPhail (1948) noted that in some cases of nonparalytic squint, the strabismic deviation was much greater when the amblyopic eye fixated than when the dominant eye fixated (in uncorrected hyperopes with approximately equal refractive error). They believed this was due to the greater accommodative "effort" required for fixation with the amblyopic eye due to its "weakened" accommodation system. The effect of increased accommodative effort (without necessarily producing proportional changes in accommodation) would translate into increased convergence of the eyes due to the synkinesis of accommodation and vergence. Urist (1959) found similar results in some patients with amblyopia and strabismus. He also performed clinical measures of accommodative amplitude in these patients by determining the closest point at which the eye could clearly see small print. He found reduced accommodative amplitude in amblyopic eyes. For example, in one case it was 3 diopters in the amblyopic eye (20/30) and 8 diopters in the dominant eye (20/20). This large difference cannot be explained solely on the basis of difference in visual acuity between the eyes.

Abraham (1961) made clinical estimates of the static accommodative amplitude difference between the eyes, either directly by determining the closest point the patient could see small print clearly, or by inference from near visual acuity measures in former amblyopic patients whose visual acuity in the two eyes was now equal or nearly equal. In the eight patients tested, accommodative amplitude was generally reduced in the previously amblyopic eye. This confirmed his earlier observations of reduced accommodative ability in once-amblyopic eyes (Abraham, 1949, 1952). From this Abraham suggested that visual acuity and accommodative function in the amblyopic eye do not necessarily improve concurrently. Therapy may need to be continued after 20/20 visual acuity is attained. This is similar to a report by Ciuffreda, Kenyon, and Stark (1979), who found some persistence of abnormal eye movements after visual acuity in the amblyopic eye reached 20/20, and suggested that perhaps therapy be continued until eye movements normalized. Abraham also speculated that weakened accommodation may be a factor in the production of strabismus that often accompanies amblyopia. More recently, Keiner (1978) speculated that "uncontrolled accommodation" in the amblyopic eye due to defective ciliary muscle tonus in that eye (producing an "apparent" anisometropia even under cycloplegia) is responsible for the amblyopia and strabismus in certain patients with microstrabismus who exhibit spontaneous recovery in their second or third decade of life. This notion of an accommodative defect under binocular viewing conditions is consistent with the suggestion by Mann (1975) of unequal accommodation as deduced by binocular dynamic retinoscopy.

Otto and Graemiger (1967) performed retinoscopy (without cycloplegia) during visual acuity assessment in young amblyopes with eccentric fixation. They found accommodation to be imprecise and highly variable in the amblyopic eye. Later, Otto and Safra (1974) used a modified, objective, coincidence optometer to measure static accommodation levels at distance and near in patients with high amblyopia (with and without eccentric fixation). Once again, imprecise and highly variable accommodation was found in the amblyopic eye; a large steady-state error persisted and the amount varied in each patient. The accommodative response found in their functional amblyopes with central scotomas was similar to that found in their organic amblyopes with central scotomas. They concluded that the effect of the scotoma on accommodation was the same in both groups. Otto and Safra believed the scotomas were the result of abnormal visual experience that adversely affected the central foveal region, that is, the foveal cones responsible for eliciting the accommodative response (Fincham, 1951; Campbell, 1954a, 1954b). Otto and Safra (1976) later measured static accommodation with their coincidence optometer in normals, in patients having either functional or organic amblyopia, and in patients having either alternating strabismus or a phoria in which suppression occurred intermittently. They again found accommodation in the amblyopic eye to be variable with a large steady-state error present. Otto and Safra believe their results suggest that the unaffected peripheral retina controlled the accommodative response, and that this peripherally generated cone response was inaccurate. In the suppressors (none had amblyopia) they found accommodation to be slightly more variable and not as precise as in normals. They believed this was due to the periodic nature of the functional scotoma in the nondominant eye. The question of variability of accommodation in amblyopic eyes and its influence on the results of psychophysical tests, such as contrast sensitivity, was recently posed by Hess (1977b). In his two amblyopes, contrast sensitivity curves were similar with and without cycloplegia. From this he concluded that (1) accommodative fluctuations had little influence on his measures and (2) an accommodative abnormality did not exist in his amblyopic subjects; however, his results do not provide support for the latter conclusion. Since the majority (almost 80%) of unilateral amblyopes have eccentric fixation (Brock and Givner, 1952) and thus fixate with a nonfoveal retinal region, an error in accommodation due to nonfoveal target stimulation would probably not be as greatly influenced by paralysis of accommodation as it would be by response characteristics of peripheral retinal cones (Phillips, 1974).

Wood and Tomlinson (1974) used a laser optometer to measure accommodative stimulus-response curves in amblyopes. A linear function was found in the amblyopic and dominant eyes. Linear regression analysis demonstrated that the slope of the function was less for the amblyopic eye than the dominant eye. The amblyopic eye responded more than the dominant eye for low stimulus levels (2 to 3 diopters) and less than the dominant eye for high stimulus levels (4 to 7 diopters). Wood and Tomlinson believed their result suggested that there was a loss of contrast sensitivity in the amblyopic eye, especially for high spatial frequencies. Their result in amblyopes was similar to that found by Heath (1956) in normals when targets were optically blurred and thus had low contrast and low spatial frequency content. Results similar to Heath's, and Wood and Tomlinson's, were found by Charman and Tucker (1977) when normal subjects were instructed to accommodate on a target containing several cycles of a single low spatial-frequency sinusoidal grating. From this Charman and Tucker hypothesized that a amblyopic eye, at least with respect to accommodation, has characteristics of a low-pass filter. Recent results on contrast sensitivity in amblyopic eyes confirm this idea for some subjects (Hess and Howell, 1977). Recently, Kirschen, Kendall and Riesen (1981) found slightly increased (almost 0.25 D) accommodative responses during foveation with the amblyopic eye. This suggests that eccentricity of fixation contributes to the increased steady-state accommodative error commonly found in amblyopic eyes.

Work in this area is presently underway by Ciuffreda and colleagues. Ciuffreda (in preparation) measured latencies in one adult with deep amblyopia (20/180) and eccentric fixation (1° superior). While there is ample evidence that eye-hand reaction time (von Noorden, 1961) and saccadic latency (Mackensen, 1958; Ciuffreda et al., 1978a, 1978b) are increased in amblyopic eyes, detailed quantitative analysis of a variety of latencies in amblyopes is not available. It is important, however, in understanding how different afferent pathways are adversely affected in amblyopia in terms of latency. In Ciuffreda's subject, increased latency in the amblyopic eye was evident from measures of saccadic latency, eye-hand reaction time, critical flicker-fusion frequency, and Pulfrich phenomenon, as well as dynamic measures of accommodation. When the dominant eye was stimulated, static and dynamic responses properties of accommodation were within normal limits. With the amblyopic eye stimulated, time constants were normal, latencies were increased, amplitudes were smaller, and variability of responses were greater (Figure 5.23). These results suggest that the accommodation motor controller is normal (since responses were not affected during dominant eye stimulation), but that processing delays reside in early sensory and/or more central areas of the amblyopic pathways.

Recent work in Ciuffreda's laboratory has concentrated on investigating static aspects of accommodation in human amblyopia (Ciuffreda et al., in press). In one study (Ciuffreda et al., submitted) accommodative stimulus-response functions (Figure 5.1) were measured in a group of amblyopes, former amblyopes, strabismics without amblyopia, and normals. From these and other measures taken, the accommodative controller gain (ACG) was computed ($ACG = AR - ABIAS/AE - DSP$; see model configuration in Figure 5.24 for details) (Hung and Semmlow, 1980), and the amblyopic static accommodation system was modeled (Hung et al., 1981; Hung et al., submitted). In normal subjects, slope of the accommodative stimulus-response function and ACG were within normal limits. This was also true for the dominant eye of the amblyopes. In contrast, slope and ACG were reduced in amblyopic eyes, showing reduced accommodative response (or increased steady-state error) over most of the linear response range (Figure 5.25). Effects of eccentricity of fixation in amblyopic eyes were demonstrated, as there was a slight trend toward an increase in interocular difference in both slope and ACG with increase in interocular difference in fixation locus (Ciuffreda et al., submitted). Of

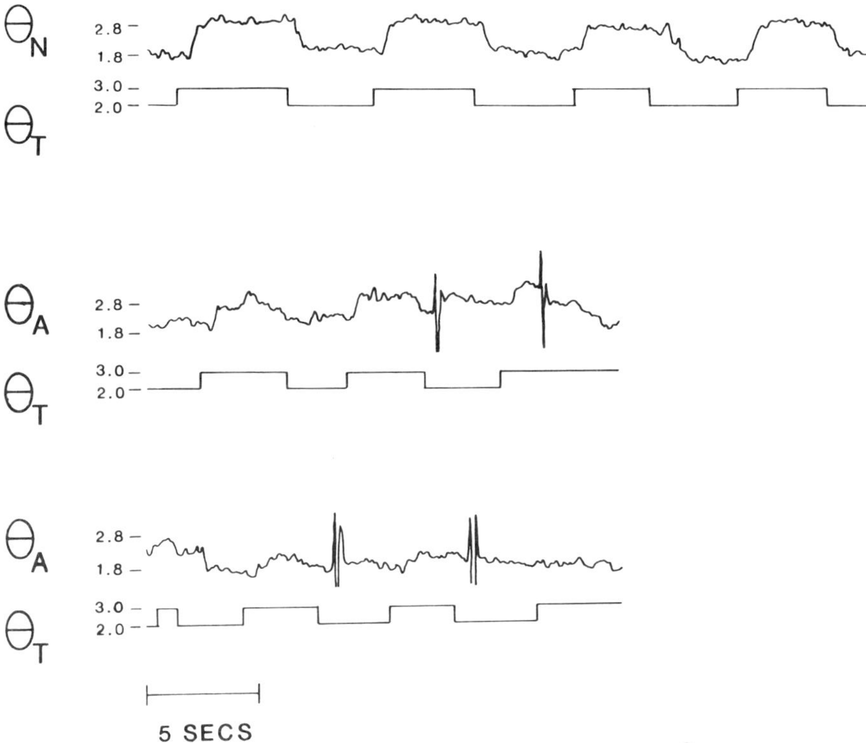

FIGURE 5.23. Dynamic accommodation responses in an adult with deep amblyopia (20/180). Monocular stimulation and recording. Symbols: θ_N = accommodation responses with the dominant eye, θ_A = accommodation responses with the amblyopic eye, and θ_T = target position, all in diopters. Top trace shows normal response dynamics when the dominant eye was stimulated. Middle and lower traces show dynamic responses when the amblyopic eye was stimulated. Note reduced (but with normal peak velocities) or absent responses to step inputs, as well as poor sustaining ability. Accommodation latency increased in the amblyopic eye (600 vs 400 msec). (From Ciuffreda, unpublished data)

interest was the normal and near normal accommodative stimulus-response functions following orthoptic therapy in many of the older amblyopes (Figure 5.26). There sometimes was reduced slope and ACG in the nondominant eyes of strabismics without amblyopia. This suggested that strabismic suppression alone could adversely affect the accommodation system. Similar results were found in formerly amblyopic eyes. This suggested lack of total recovery and/or regression of accommodative function following orthoptic therapy. It is believed that the model parameter ACG can be used in the research environment, in clinical studies, and even in office treatment to assess accommodative function in ambly-

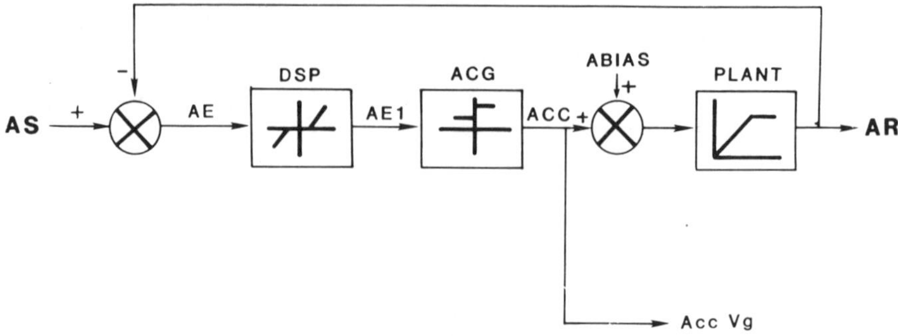

FIGURE 5.24. Block diagram of static model of the accommodative system. Accommodative error (AE) is the difference between accommodative stimulus (AS) and accommodative response (AR). Deadspace (±DSP) reflects depth of focus (DF) of eye. Output (AE1) from deadspace operator goes into accommodative controller which exhibits nonlinear accommodative controller gain (ACG). Output (ACC) from accommodative controller is summed at summing junction and also cross-linked to vergence system (AccVg). Accommodative bias (ABIAS) (accommodative response with disparity vergence and accommodation systems open-looped) also summed here. Output from summing junction goes through a saturation element, which reflects plant saturation of accommodation system, to give accommodative response. Adapted from Hung GK, Semmlow JL. Static behavior of accommodation and vergence: computer simulation of an interactive dual-feedback system. Institute of Electrical and Electronics Engineers Transactions in Biomedical Engineering, © 1980 IEEE.

opia as well as in other conditions in which impaired accommodation occurs (Hung et al., submitted). For example, once depth of focus (±DSP), accommodative bias (ABIAS), and accommodative error (AE) are determined in an individual, accommodative controller gain (ACG) can be read from a graph (Figure 5.27).

Accommodative amplitude in amblyopia has also been studied by Ciuffreda and colleagues. In one investigation (Hokoda and Ciuffreda, in press), the best clinical procedure was determined to assess accommodative amplitude in amblyopic eyes. Using objective dynamic retinoscopy as the standard, they found good agreement using the minus-lens technique, whereas the push-up procedure yielded grossly inflated values (Figure 5.28). These results suggest that either dynamic retinoscopy or the minus-lens procedure be used to obtain accurate, repeatable accommodative amplitude measures in amblyopic eyes. In another study (Ciuffreda et al., submitted) it was found that accommodative amplitude was always reduced in amblyopic eyes when measured accurately. A strong trend was also found for interocular difference in accommodative amplitude to increase as interocular difference in fixation locus increased. Similarly, there was a trend for the ratio of accommodative amplitude (amblyopic:dominant) to decrease as interocular difference in fixation locus increased (Figure 5.29). With respect to orthoptic effects, accommodative amplitude typically increased but did not normalize in amblyopic eyes (Ciuffreda et al., submitted; Selenow and Ciuffreda submitted).

Experiments in progress (Hokoda and Ciuffreda) are concentrating on the effects of target spatial frequency (suprathreshold contrast levels) on the accommodative response in the amblyopic eye. Results thus far clearly demonstrate reduction of static accommodative responses in the

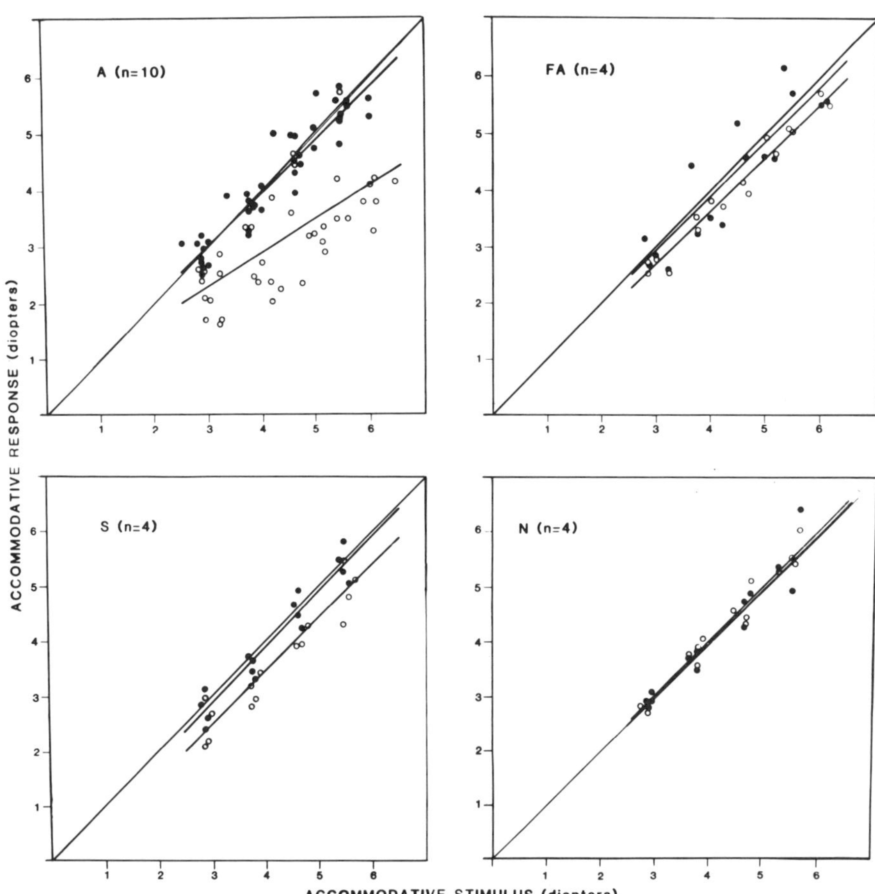

FIGURE 5.25. Accommodative stimulus-response curves in amblyopes (A), former amblyopes (FA), strabismics (S), and normals (N). Symbols: • = dominant eye responses, ○ = nondominant eye responses. Reduced accommodative responses are evident in the amblyopic eyes. There was a statistically significant difference in slope of the linear regression lines in the dominant and amblyopic eyes (t test, $P < 0.05$). No such interocular difference was found in the other three groups (t test, $P > 0.05$).

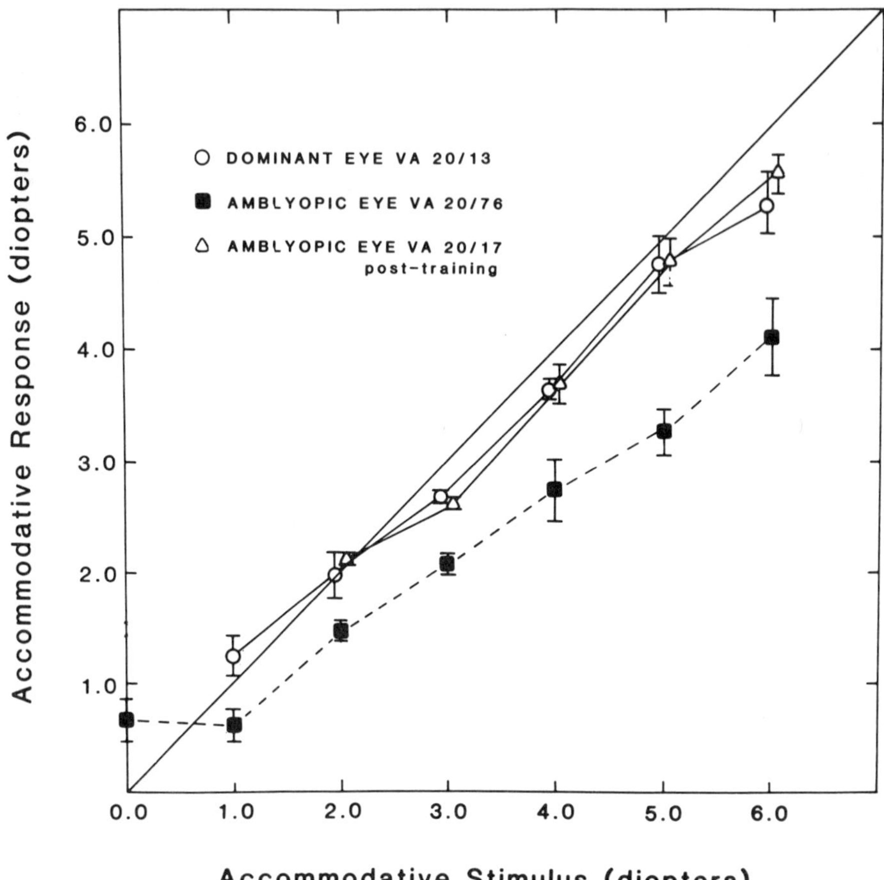

FIGURE 5.26. Accommodative stimulus-response curves in a 12-year-old with strabismic amblyopia, before and after intensive orthoptic therapy. Following therapy, monocular accommodative responses were similar in each eye. $\overline{\chi} \pm 1$ SEM plotted. In dominant eye •, VA = 20/13, ACG = 21, and slope = 0.91; in amblyopic eye before therapy ▪, VA = 20/76, ACG = 7.8, and slope = 0.69; in amblyopic eye after therapy △, VA = 20/17, ACG = 18, and slope = 0.95. Reprinted by permission of the publisher, from Ciuffreda KJ, Hokoda SC, Hung GK, Semmlow JL, Selenow A. Static aspects of accommodation in human amblyopia. American Journal of Optometry and Physiological Optics, in press, American Academy of Optometry per The Williams & Wilkins Company (agent).

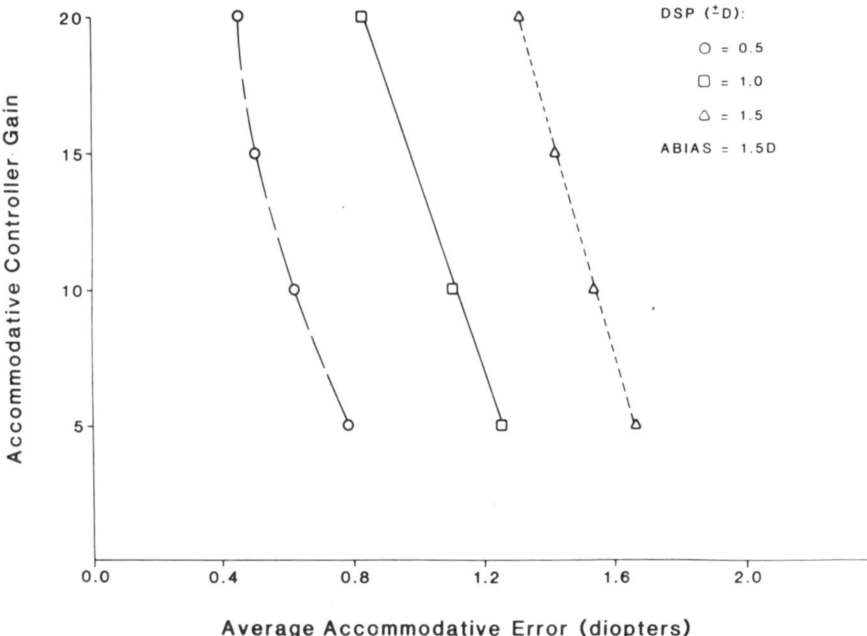

FIGURE 5.27. Computer simulation showing relationship between accommodative controller gain, average accommodative error, and depth of focus for an accommodative bias level of 1.5 diopters.

amblyopic eye with respect to the fellow dominant eye over most of the response range (0.5 to 15 cycles per degree).

Static Measures of Accommodative Vergence

Hofstetter (1946) used a haploscopic technique to measure static response AC/A ratios to determine if the AC/A ratio was innate or learned in individuals with what he considered functionally monocular vision. The finding of normal AC/A ratios (with the dominant eye stimulated) suggested its innate nature. His basic assumption that subjects had congenital strabismus and never had binocular experience was probably incorrect, thus making the results difficult to interpret. Parks (1958) investigated the stimulus AC/A ratio in strabismics by comparing distance and near deviation. Results suggested that 50% of the patients had high AC/A ratios, which could contribute to the production of strabismus, however, actual AC/A values were not provided. Hermann and Samson (1967), in a preliminary study using a photoelectric eye movement technique, attempted to measure accommodative vergence responses in amblyopes and strab-

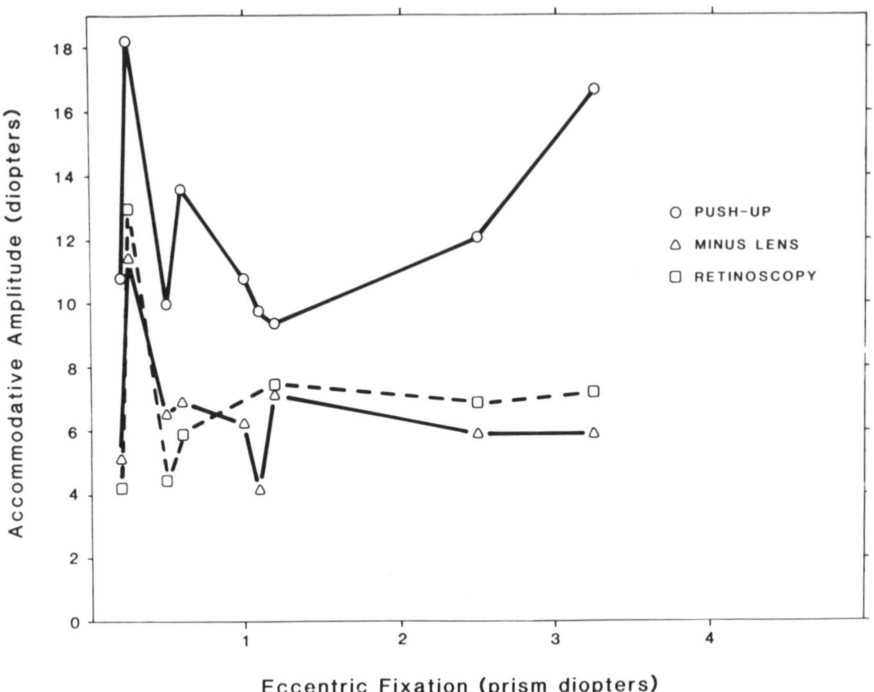

FIGURE 5.28. Accommodative amplitude in the amblyopic eye measured using the push-up, minus-lens, and dynamic retinoscopic techniques. Data of each subject plotted as a function of eccentric fixation in the amblyopic eye. Grossly inflated values evident with the push-up technique.

ismics to determine objective stimulus AC/A ratios with the hope that classification of dynamic accommodative vergence responses (but only with the dominant eye stimulated) would establish surgical strategies in patients with similar static responses but dissimilar dynamic responses. Although a few cases were presented, they never conducted a complete study in which a large number of subjects and a wide range of stimuli were used, nor did they stimulate the amblyopic eye. Recently, Kenyon, Ciuffreda, and Stark (1980) demonstrated in a limited number of subjects that deep amblyopia had a marked effect on the accommodative vergence responses (see next section for complete details).

Cooper, Ciuffreda, and Kruger (1982) investigated accommodation and accommodative vergence in patients with divergence excess (the exodeviation is greater in the distance than at near). A basic question involves the AC/A ratio. Some (Brown, 1971) feel that the AC/A ratio must be very high (13 : 1) in these patients to attain fusion at near. Von Noorden (1969) used standard clinical techniques and found the stimulus AC/A

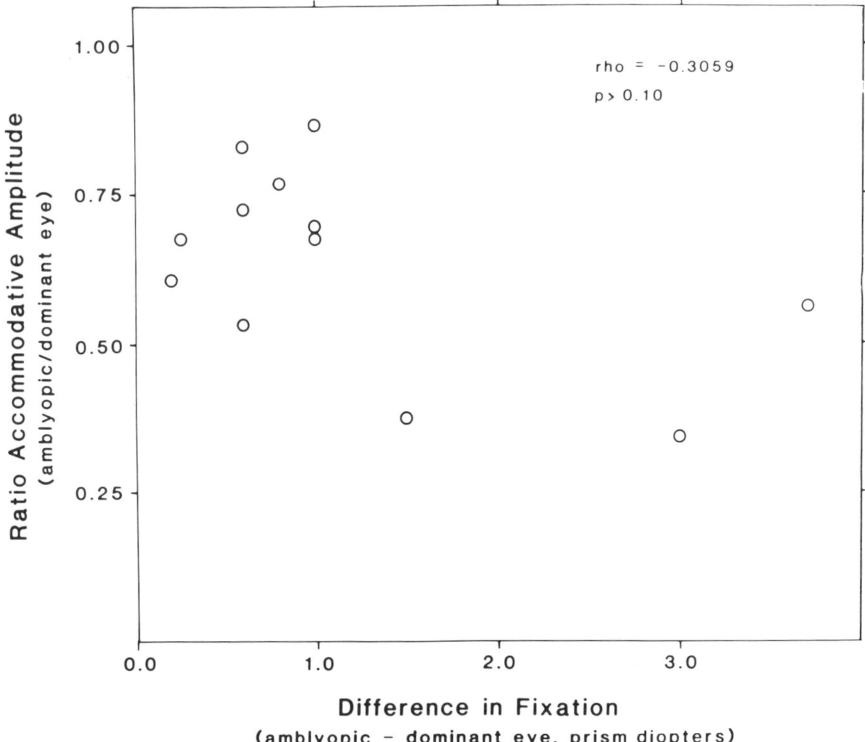

FIGURE 5.29. Ratio of accommodative amplitude between the amblyopic and dominant eyes plotted as a function of interocular difference in fixation locus. There was a trend for this ratio to decrease as difference in fixation (i.e., eccentricity) increased.

ratio to range from 3.3 to 9:1 in these patients. Our findings using infrared methods to monitor continuously and simultaneously accommodation and accommodative vergence (Figure 5.30) and thus obtain objective response AC/A ratios agree with those of von Noorden (1966). Our results demonstrate that the response AC/A ratio is not unusually high in these patients, however, variability of accommodative responses, especially with respect to the dynamic overshoots and frequent accommodation spasms, suggest existence of a dynamic accommodative abnormality in the presence of normal visual acuity.

Accommodative Vergence Substituting for Absent Disparity Vergence

Until recently, vergence eye movements recorded from strabismic and/or amblyopic patients have either been confined to static measures of eye

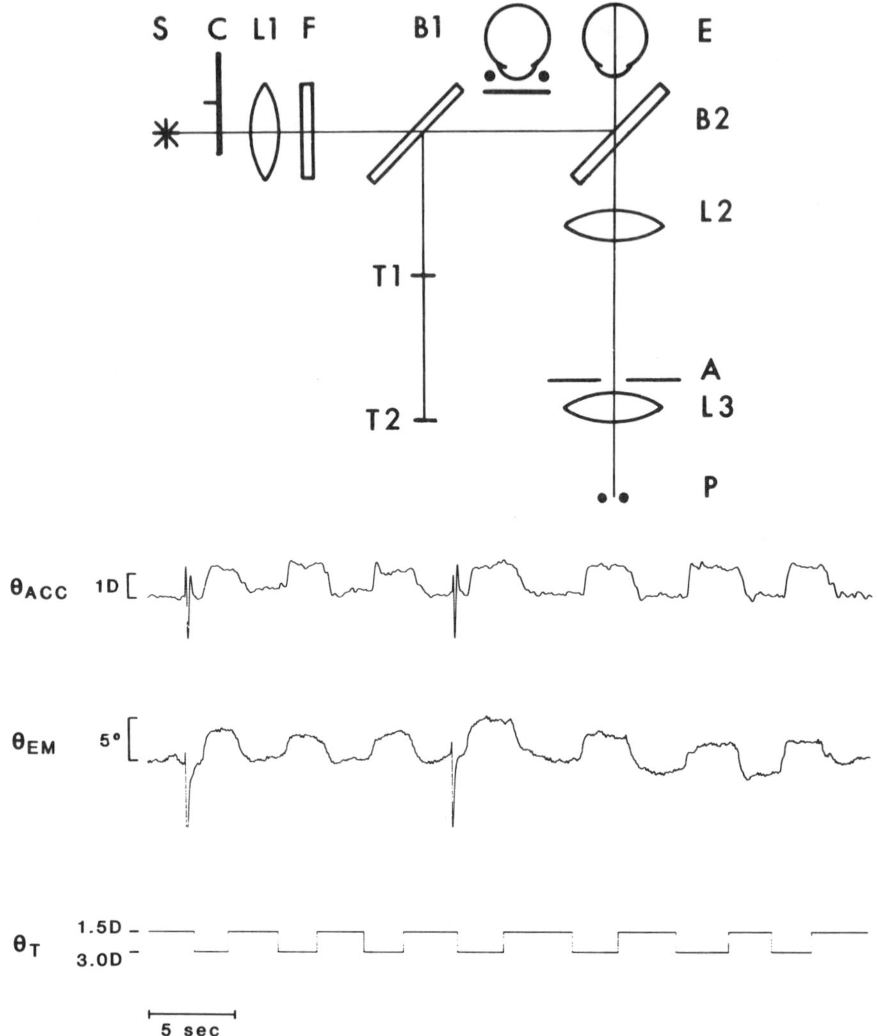

FIGURE 5.30. Response AC/A ratios in intermittent exotropia of the divergent excess type. A Dynamic optometer based on retinoscopic principles having an illumination, recording, and stimulus channel. Symbols: S = light source, C = chopper, L1 = focusing lens, F = infrared filter, B1 and B2 = beam-splitting mirrors, T1 and T2 = targets, L2 and L3 = focusing lenses, A = aperture, P = photocells, E = eyes. Before right eye is an occluder and pair of photodiodes. Accommodation is measured in the viewing left eye and accommodative vergence is measured in the occluded right eye, resulting in dynamic, objective response AC/A ratios. B Responses in a patient. Normal visual acuity in each eye. From top to bottom are accommodation, accommodative vergence, and the stimulus. Reprinted by permission of the publisher, from Cooper J, Ciuffreda KJ, Kruger PB. Stimulus and response AC/A ratios in intermittent exotropia of the divergence excess type. British Journal of Ophthalmology, 1982.

position or inferred from subjective responses (see Burian and von Noorden, 1970, for a comprehensive review). Bielschowsky (1900), Schlodtmann (1900), and Burian (1941) all reported fusional abilities in strabismic patients. Burian (1941), using an elaborate system of projectors and polarizers, haploscopically presented identical images that extended into the periphery of each eye. When these images were made disparate the subject was instructed to report the position of two fiduciary marks in the center of his visual field. Realignment of these marks, which did occur, was interpreted as the result of fusional movements of the eyes. Hallden (1952) found similar results when measuring static eye vergence angles. His measurements were taken at one minute intervals, and he reported that patients took several minutes to realign their eyes. Results similar to Hallden's were recently reported by Bagolini (1976). An alternative interpretation of Burian's result was proposed by Kretschemer (1955) and Mariani and Pasino (1974). They demonstrated how changes in the angle of anomaly could account for the results of Burian's study. Eye position was not measured in any of these studies, however. Furthermore, time course of vergence (several minutes) was much greater than for vergence movements in normals (less than one second) (Westheimer and Mitchell, 1956; Riggs and Neihl, 1960; Rashbass and Westheimer, 1961; Zuber and Stark, 1968).

Only recently have dynamic objective eye movements in strabismic and/or amblyopic patients been measured (Kenyon, 1978; Kenyon et al., 1980a, 1980b, 1981; Schoessler, 1980). Schoessler presented normal and strabismic subjects having anomalous retinal correspondence (ARC) with an asymmetric disparity stimulus using a modified haploscope. With the dominant eye's target stationary at the fovea, the strabismic eye received a change in target position. Vergence responses were reported in all subjects. The direction of vergence changed when the stimulus moved through the patient's ARC point in the nondominant eye and not at the fovea as in normal subjects. This is consistent with the idea of a foveal/nonfoveal binocular zero sensorimotor coordinate correspondence system in ARC rather than a foveal/foveal system as found in normal retinal correspondence (NRC). While eye movements were recorded using a photocell system, the two eye movement channels were subtracted to remove versional components and enhance vergence. Eye movement records were not published, so detailed assessment of the character of the vergence responses was not possible.

Unlike the previous studies that presented targets haploscopically, Kenyon (1978) and colleagues (1980a, 1980b, 1981) introduced vergence stimuli by having subjects fixate targets at different distances. These targets stimulated both vergence and accommodation, providing stimuli similar to those found in everyday viewing. Peripheral retina contributions to vergence were reduced by using small targets of 2° that moved approximately 4° into the periphery. Thus disparities were confined to the foveal and near parafoveal regions. Under conditions in which both target disparity and target distance were randomly changed, altering target disparity and blur, strabismic patients used accommodative vergence instead of disparity vergence to move their eyes to the new target position (Kenyon, 1978; Kenyon et al., 1980a, 1980b, 1981). Comparing normal symmetric vergence movements to patient responses (Figure 5.31), dramatic differences are evident. Instead of a smooth equal disjunctive movement, patients made a saccade to place the dominant eye on the target, followed by an unequal vergence. Patients with intermittent strabismus, constant strabismus with or without amblyopia, and some amblyopes without strabismus showed these abnormal responses (Kenyon, 1978; Kenyon et al., 1980a, 1980b, 1981). Presence of amblyopia alone appeared to have a less dramatic effect than strabismus alone, since amblyopes with 20/40 acuity did not always produce these abnormal responses. Recently, others (Quere, 1979; Quere et al., 1981) reported similar results as well as marked inequality of disparity vergence amplitude in response to symmetric disparity stimuli in amblyopes and strabismics; Pickwell and Hampshire (1981) have provided clinical confirmation.

The results of several additional experiments (Kenyon, 1978) suggested these abnormal vergence responses were driven by accommodation rather than disparity. First, when a patient having strabismus with amblyopia covered the nondominant eye, eye movements did not change. Second, when the normal control had one eye occluded, these responses mimicked the patient's responses under both viewing conditions. Finally, vergence amplitudes in each eye closely matched the amplitude relationship found during accommodative vergence.

Targets aligned along the dominant eye, that is, asymmetric vergence, revealed responses with a similar lack of disparity vergence (Kenyon, 1978; Kenyon et al., 1980b, 1981). In normals, a step change in target distance along the visual axis produced a saccade that distributed the retinal disparity error symmetrically about the foveas of both eyes, followed by an equal vergence (Riggs and Neihl, 1960) (Figure 5.32). Patients' asymmetric vergence responses looked like accommodative vergence (Kenyon et al., 1980b, 1981) (Figure 5.32). Even when targets were aligned along the patient's nondominant eye, the dominant eye made a saccade to the target with a small vergence component, while the axis eye (nondominant) showed a large accommodative vergence response (Figure 5.33). Differences between patient and control responses to asymmetric vergence stimuli, as well as to symmetric vergence stimuli, demonstrated a general lack of disparity vergence in these patients and the consequent use of accommodative vergence under these test conditions.

Based on these experiments, one can begin to consider areas that may be responsible for the abnormal vergence movements. A purely motor dysfunction encompassing the extraocular muscles, oculomotor neurons, or brain stem nuclei is unlikely in these patients, since accommodative

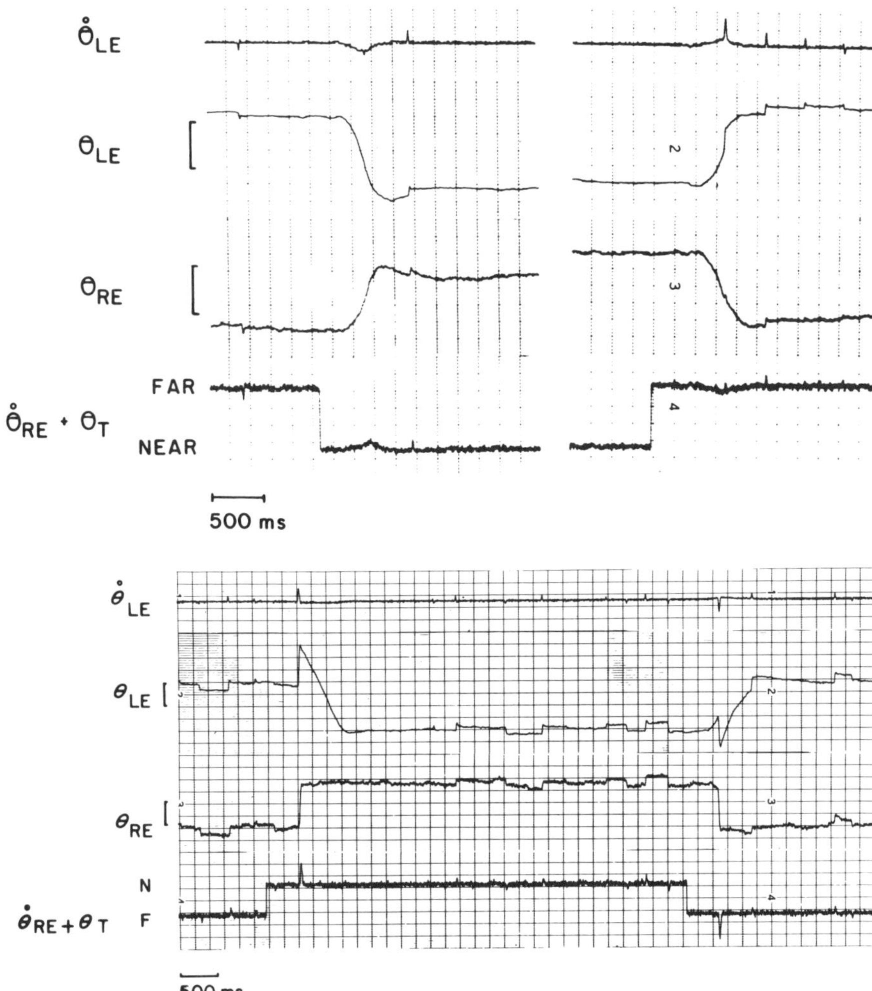

FIGURE 5.31. Symmetric vergence condition with targets along midline. Symbols for all figures unless otherwise noted: θ_{LE} = left eye position; θ_{RE} = right eye position; $\dot{\theta}_{LE}$ = left eye velocity; $\dot{\theta}_{RE} + \theta_T$ = right eye velocity summed with target position. Downward deflections represent rightward movements; calibration bars for position represent 2°, and time markers represent 500 msec. A Control subject shows normal response to symmetric vergence stimuli. B Patient having intermittent strabismus without amblyopia exhibits abnormal response, contrary to normal control subject responses in A. Following target changes, vergence occurs primarily in the strabismic left eye only. Saccade occurring early in response is used to foveate new target with dominant right eye. Same calibrations used in Figures 5.27 through 5.29. Reprinted by permission of the publisher, from Kenyon RV, Ciuffreda KJ, Stark L. Dynamic vergence eye movements in strabismus and amblyopia: symmetric vergence. Investigative Ophthalmology and Visual Science, 19:60–74, 1980.

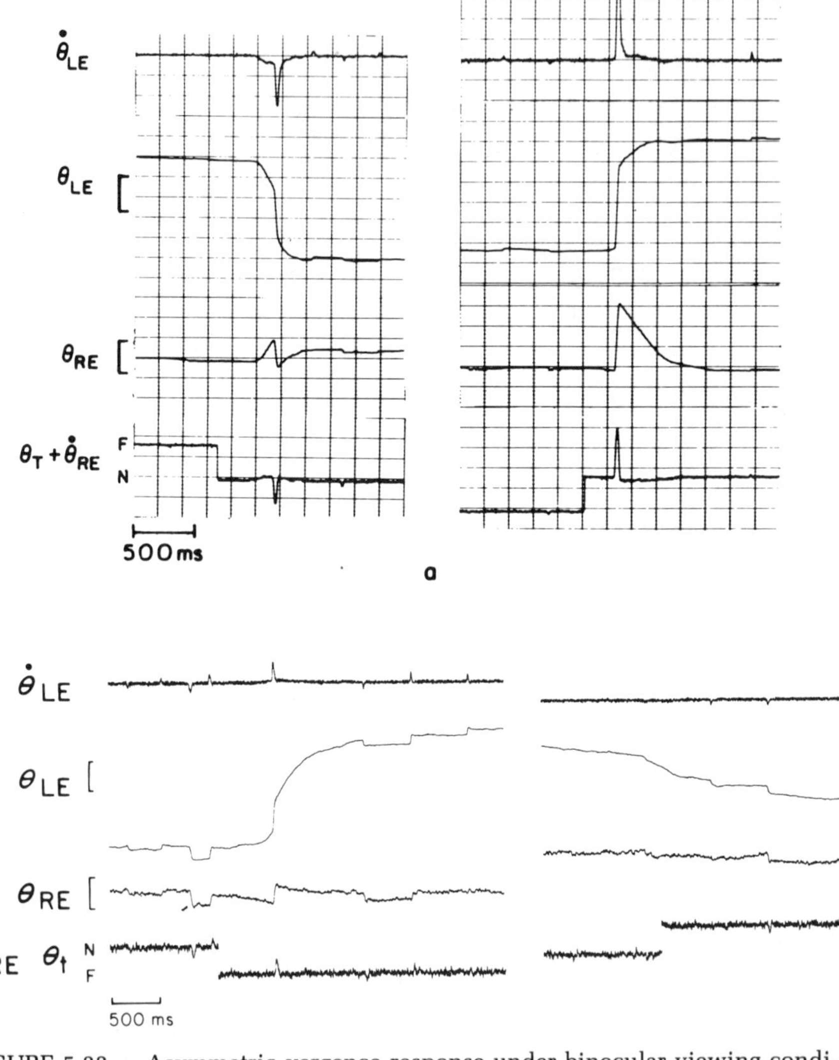

FIGURE 5.32. Asymmetric vergence response under binocular viewing conditions with targets aligned along the dominant eye. A Control subject shows the normal response to asymmetric vergence stimuli: large saccade and vergence place the fovea of each eye on target. Left response is convergence and right response is divergence. B Left intermittent strabismic (exotropia). Normal acuity (20/20) each eye. Response shows lack of equal vergence amplitudes in each eye. Small vergence in the dominant eye, characteristic of accommodation rather than asymmetric vergence responses. Reprinted by permission of the publisher, from Kenyon RV, Ciuffreda KJ, Stark L. Dynamic vergence eye movements in strabismus and amblyopia: asymmetric vergence. British Journal of Ophthalmology, 1981.

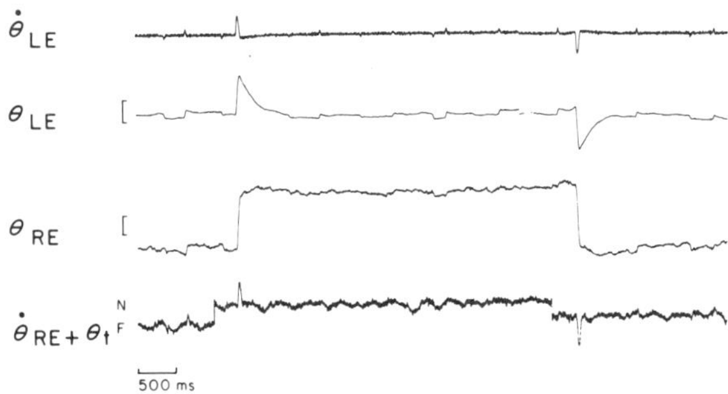

FIGURE 5.33. Asymmetric vergence responses with targets aligned along line of sight of *nondominant* eye. Left intermittent strabismus (exotropia); normal visual acuity (20/20) each eye. Shows large saccades in each eye; vergence amplitudes remain unequal with smaller amplitude in dominant eye. Saccade and vergence serve to place dominant eye on target. Characteristic unequal vergence in dominant eye is shown in this record. Reprinted by permission of the publisher, from Keynon RV, Ciuffreda KJ, Stark L. Dynamic vergence eye movements in strabismus and amblyopia: asymmetric vergence. British Journal of Ophthalmology, 1981.

vergence had normal dynamics and latencies (Kenyon, 1978; Kenyon et al., 1980a, 1980b, 1981). Also, the intermittent nature of these abnormal responses in some patients shows that the basic vergence motor nuclei and controller can still perform disparity vergence movements (Kenyon, 1978; Kenyon et al., 1980b). Higher-level defects are much harder to specify precisely. Suppression is a likely mechanism to block disparity, especially in patients with strabismus having deviations greater than 10 prism diopters (Jampolsky, 1955; Travers, 1938; Pratt-Johnson et al., 1967; Pratt-Johnson and Wee, 1967). Such a suppression mechanism may also block information to disparity processing centers, effectively leaving only information from the dominant eye. Interestingly, Blake and Lehmkuhle (1976) have demonstrated normal grating aftereffects in spite of the presence of suppression associated with strabismus. This suggests that the site for suppression is beyond the site of the grating aftereffect (probably area 17 of the visual cortex). A similar higher-level central site may be responsible for suppression of disparity information used in the control of vergence movements. Reduced visual acuity of the amblyopic eye may also explain the responses from the amblyopes, however, the intermittent nature of abnormal vergence in some patients having amblyopia only suggests that strabismus has a much stronger effect on disparity vergence than does amblyopia (Kenyon, 1978; Kenyon et al., 1980a, 1980b, 1981). Finally, it is possible, although highly speculative, that lack of disparity vergence may be a result of reduced binocular stimulation to corresponding retinal points during childhood. Animal studies that artificially pro-

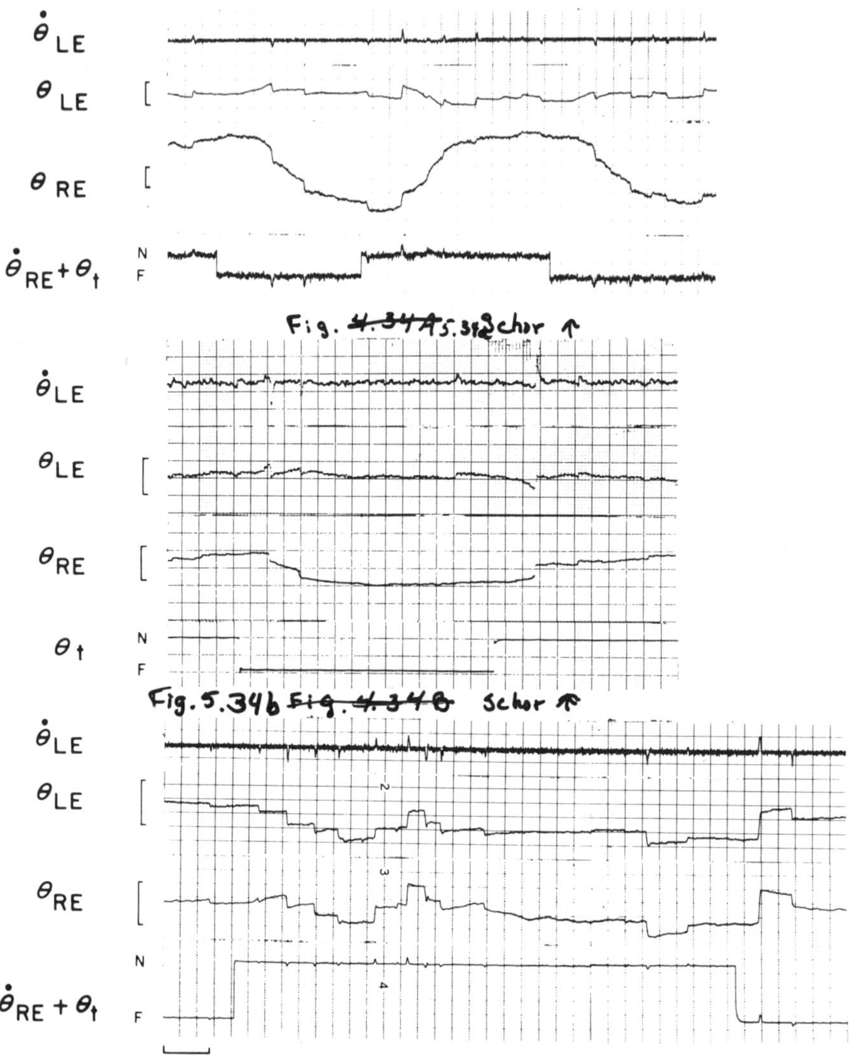

FIGURE 5.34. Accommodative vergence responses with targets aligned along line of sight of *nondominant* eye, with fellow eye covered. Shows effect of deep amblyopia on accommodative vergence. A Left intermittent strabismus (exotropia); normal visual acuity (20/20) each eye. Normal accommodative vergence amplitudes and dynamics in the *nondominant* left eye shown here, similar to that found in the dominant right eye. B Amblyope (20/38) without strabismus. Normal accommodative vergence amplitude and dynamics; similar to dominant right eye responses. C Amblyope (20/400) without strabismus. No discernible normal accommodative vergence response evident when nondominant right eye views target. Reprinted by permission of the publisher, from Kenyon RV, Ciuffreda KJ, Stark L. Dynamic vergence eye movements in strabismus and amblyopia: asymmetric vergence. British Journal of Ophthalmology, 1981.

duce strabismus (and amblyopia) showed a reduction in the number of binocular cortical cells (Hubel and Wiesel, 1965; Ikeda and Tremain, 1977; Baker et al., 1974; Ikeda and Wright, 1974). If cells that code vergence eye movement stimuli are similarly affected, the lack or decreased number of these cells might reduce vergence response capability. Further experiments that record eye movements from strabismic and amblyopic animals may clarify these speculations.

Amblyopia and Accommodative Vergence

Given the reduced visual acuity and contrast sensitivity, as well as eccentric fixation in amblyopes, one would predict reduced accommodation and therefore reduced accommodative vergence. Kenyon (1978) and colleagues (1980b, 1981) have shown reduced accommodative vergence amplitudes when the amblyopic eye alone viewed the accommodative stimulus compared to when the dominant eye viewed the same stimulus. Small to moderate reductions in visual acuity (20/40 to 20/120) had little if any effect on accommodative vergence response in the few patients examined (Figure 5.34). A noticeable drop in accommodative vergence amplitude was found when the visual acuities were less than 20/400. Their study population was not broad enough for them to analyze either a wide range or a large sample of amblyopes. Nevertheless, a pronounced reduction in accommodative vergence occurs in deep amblyopia. Further experiments will be necessary to determine the relationship between degree of amblyopia and/or eccentric fixation and static and dynamic characteristics of accommodative vergence.

FUTURE DIRECTIONS

Although much is known about static and dynamic aspects of accommodation and accommodation vergence in normals, basic information as to the influence and interaction of such factors as ocular aberrations and perceptual components on this blur-driven response remains incomplete. Study of interactions between the accommodation and vergence systems as presently being conducted by Semmlow (1981) should contribute to our knowledge in this area in normal individuals and in patients with binocular vision abnormalities and related asthenopia. Such information will help us understand how these normally complex, and in the case of patients, abnormally functioning systems operate in real-life situations. It may be important to determine which values (for example, the AC/A ratio, CA/C ratio, fixation disparity, and various system dynamics) can be modified by orthoptic therapy and/or play a critical role in development of normal oculomotor triadic responses. Availability of this information could influence the choice of clinical test and treatment plan by excluding, as a result of careful quantitative measures, tests and training procedures that are found to bear little relation to improved visual performance and reduced asthenopia.

The topic of the AC/A ratio is one that hits home to all clinicians, as it traditionally has been and continues to be a primary measure in the evaluation of patients having binocular vision disorders such as strabismus. While many aspects of the AC/A ratio have received considerable attention, with the findings being well accepted, orthoptic and aging effects require additional detailed investigation, especially with respect to clinical implications. The experiment of Flom (1960c) provides us with the most reasonable data showing only a small, transient effect of orthoptic therapy on the response AC/A ratio. Further investigation to include a larger sample of carefully probed normal subjects, and perhaps more importantly, symptomatic patients having frank binocular vision abnormalities, is essential to make a definitive statement on this matter. While the effect of aging on the accommodative amplitude is well documented and accepted by all, our knowledge of its effect on the AC/A ratio remains incomplete and somewhat controversial. Comprehensive longitudinal and cross-sectional studies are needed to clarify this issue. If the response AC/A ratio indeed does increase with age, as many studies suggest, then the manner in which the other vergence and accommodation components interact to achieve and maintain precise focus and bifoveal fixation would provide valuable information regarding such motor system adaptation.

While research in the area of amblyopia and strabismus has been conducted at a frantic pace over the past decade, there has been a paucity of careful investigations related to accommodation and accommodative vergence in these patients. Recent work by Ciuffreda and colleagues (in press) has shown that most amblyopes and some strabismics (without amblyopia) have reduced static accommodative responses when their nondominant eye was tested. Furthermore, orthoptic therapy always improved accommodation in the amblyopic eye. Present work is directed toward a detailed investigation of dynamic aspects of accommodation and accommodative vergence in these patients, including quantification of orthoptic effects on these oculomotor systems. It is hoped that such research will serve not only to assist in our understanding of these anomalous systems and their normal and abnormal development, but in addition, result in improved clinical care.

REFERENCES

Abraham SV. The use of miotics in the treatment of convergent strabismus and anisometropia: a preliminary report. Am J Ophthalmol 1949;32:233–40.

Abraham SV. The use of miotics in the treatment of nonparalytic convergent strabismus. Am J Ophthalmol 1952;35:1191–95.

Abraham SV. Accommodation in the amblyopic eye. Am J Ophthalmol 1961;52:197–200.

Allen MJ. An investigation of the time characteristics of accommodation and convergence of the eyes. Am J Optom 1953;30:393–402.

Alpern M. The after-effect of lateral duction testing on subsequent phoria measurements. Am J Optom 1946;23:442–47.

Alpern M. Variability of accommodation during steady state fixation at various levels of illuminance. J Opt Soc Am 1958;48:193–97.

Alpern M. In: Types of movement, Davson H, ed. The eye. Vol. 3. New York: Academic Press, 1969.

Alpern M, Ellen P. A quantitative analysis of the horizontal movements of the eyes in the experiments of Johannes Muller. I. Methods and results. Am J Ophthalmol 1956;42:289–303.

Alpern M, Hirsch MJ. cited In: Alpern M, Larson BF, Vergence and accommodation. IV. Effect of luminance quantity on the AC/A. Am J Ophthalmol 1960;49:1140–49.

Alpern M, Larson BF. Vergence and accommodation. IV. Effect of luminance quantity on the AC/A. Am J Ophthalmol 1960;49:1140–49.

Alpern M, Flitman DB, Joseph RH. Centrally fixed flicker thresholds in amblyopia. Am J Ophthalmol 1960;40:1194–1202.

Alpern M, Kincaid WM, Lubeck MJ. Vergence and accommodation. III. Proposed definitions of the AC/A ratios. Am J Ophthalmol 1959;48:141–48.

Alpern M, Mason GL, Jardinico RE. Vergence and accommodation. V. Pupil size changes associated with changes in accommodative vergence. Am J Ophthalmol 1961;52:762–67.

Aslin RN, Jackson RW. Accommodative-convergence in young infants: development of a synergistic sensory-motor system. Can J Psychol 1979;33:222–31.

Bagolini B. Sensory anomalies in strabismus. Doc Ophthalmol 1976;41:1–22.

Baker FH, Grigg P, von Noorden GK. Effects of visual deprivation and strabismus on the response of neurons in the visual cortex of monkeys, including studies on the striate and prestriate cortex in the normal animal. Brain Res 1974;66:185–208.

Ball EAW. A study in consensual accommodation. Am J Optom Arch Am Acad Optom 1952;29:561–74.

Bedell HE. Central and peripheral retinal photoreceptor orientation in amblyopic eyes as assessed by the psychophysical Stiles-Crawford function. Invest Ophthalmol Visual Sci 1980;19:49–59.

Bedell HE, Flom MC. Monocular spatial distortion in strabismic amblyopia. Invest Ophthalmol Visual Sci 1981;20:263–68.

Bielschowsky A. Untersuchungen uber das Sehen der Schielender. Albrecht Von Graefes Arch Klin Exp Ophthalmol 1900;50:406.

Blake R, Lehmkuhle SW. On the site of strabismic suppression. Invest Ophthalmol Visual Sci 1976:15:660–63.

Bour LJ. The influence of the spatial distribution of a target on the dynamic response and fluctuations of the accommodation of the human eye. Vision Res 1981:21:1287–1296.

Breinin GM, Chin NB, Ripps H. A rationale for therapy of accommodative strabismus. Am J Ophthalmol 1966;61:1030–37.

Brock FW, Givner I. Fixation anomalies in amblyopia. Arch Ophthalmol 1952;47:775–86.

Brodkey J, Stark L. Accommodative convergence: an adaptive nonlinear control system. Presbyterian St. Lukes Med Bull 1967a;6:30–43.

Brodkey J, Stark L. Feedback control analysis of accommodative convergence. Am J Surg 1967b;114:150–58.

Brown HW. Accommodative convergence in exodeviation. Int Ophthalmol Clin 1971;11:39–45.

Burian HM. Fusional movements in permanent strabismus: a study of the role of central and peripheral retinal regions in the act of binocular vision in squint. Arch Ophthalmol 1941;26:626–52.

Burian HM. Accommodative esotropia. Int Ophthalmol Clin 1971;11:23–26.

Burian HM, von Noorden GK. Binocular vision and ocular motility. St. Louis: CV Mosby, 1974.

Campbell FW. Accommodation reflex. Br Orthopt J 1954a;11:13–17.

Campbell FW. The minimum quantity of light required to elicit the accommodation reflex in man. J Physiol 1954b;123:357–66.

Campbell FW. The depth of field of the human eye. Optica Acta 1957;4:157–64.

Campbell FW. Correlation of accommodation between the two eyes. J Opt Soc Am 1960;50:738.

Campbell FW, Gregory AH. The spatial resolving power of the human retina with oblique incidence. J Opt Soc Am 1960;50:831.

Campbell FW, Westheimer G. Factors influencing accommodation responses of the human eye. J Opt Soc Am 1959;49:568–71.

Campbell FW, Westheimer G. Dynamics of accommodation responses of the human eye. J Physiol 1960;151:285–95.

Campbell FW, Robson JG, Westheimer G. Fluctuations of accommodation under steady viewing conditions. J Physiol 1959;145:579–94.

Charman WN, Heron G. Spatial frequency and the dynamics of the accommodation response. Optica Acta 1979;26:217–28.

Charman WN, Tucker J. Dependence of accommodation response on the spatial frequency spectrum of the observed object. Vision Res 1977;17:129–39.

Chin NB, Breinin GM. Ratio of accommodative convergence to accommodation. Arch Ophthalmol 1967;77:752–56.

Ciuffreda KJ. Eye movements in amblyopia and strabismus. PhD dissertation, School of Optometry, University of California, Berkeley, 1977.

Ciuffreda KJ, Kenyon RV, Stark L. Processing delays in amblyopic eyes: evidence from saccadic latencies. Am J Optom Physiol Opt 1978a;55:187–96.

Ciuffreda KJ, Kenyon RV, Stark L. Increased saccadic latencies in amblyopic eyes. Invest Ophthalmol Visual Sci 1978b;17:697–702.

Ciuffreda KJ, Kenyon RV, Stark L. Different rates of functional recovery of eye movements during orthoptics treatment in an adult amblyope. Invest Ophthalmol Visual Sci 1979;18:213–19.

Ciuffreda KJ, Kenyon RV, Stark L. Increased drift in amblyopic eyes. Br J Ophthalmol 1980;64:7–14.

Ciuffreda KJ, Hokoda SC, Hung GK, Semmlow JL. Accommodative stimulus/response function in human amblyopia. submitted.

Ciuffreda KJ, Hokoda SC. Different rates of functional recovery of the accommodative and related systems in an older strabismic amblyope during the course of orthoptic therapy. submitted.

Ciuffreda KJ, Hokoda SC, Hung GK, Semmlow JL, Selenow A. Static aspects of accommodation in human amblyopia. Am J Optom Physiol Opt in press.

Clark MR, Crane HD. Dynamic interactions in binocular vision. In: Senders JW, Fisher DF, Monty RH, Eye movements and the higher psychological functions. Hillsdale, N.J.: Erlbaum, 1978.

Cohen MM, Alpern M. Vergence and accommodation VI. The influence of ethanol on the AC/A ratio. Arch Ophthalmol 1969;81:518–25.

Cooper J, Ciuffreda KJ, Kruger PB. Stimulus and response AC/A ratios in intermittent exotropia of the divergence excess type. Br J Ophthalmol 1982; 66:398–404.

Costenbader F, Baier D, McPhail A. Vision in strabismus. Arch Ophthalmol 1948;40:438–53.

Crane HD. A theoretical analysis of the visual accommodation system in humans. Stanford Res Inst, Proj 5454 (NASA CR-606).

Davis CJ, Jobe FW. Further studies on the AC/A ratio as measured on the Orthorater. Am J Optom Arch Am Acad Optom 1957;34:16–25.

Denieul P. Effects of stimulus vergence on mean accommodation response, microfluctuations of accommodation and optical quality of the human eye. Vision Res 1982;22:561–69.

Donders FC. On the anomalies of accommodation and refraction of the eye. London: New Sydenham Society, 1864.

Duane A. Studies in monocular and binocular accommodation with their clinical applications. Am J Ophthalmol 1922;5:865–77.

Enoch JM. Receptor amblyopia. Am J Ophthalmol 1959;48:262–74.

Eskridge JB. An investigation of voluntary vergence. Am J Optom Arch Am Acad Optom 1971;48:741–46.

Eskridge JB. Age and the AC/A ratio. Am J Optom Arch Am Acad Optom 1973;50:105–107.

Fankhauser F, Rohler R. The physical stimulus, the quality of the retinal image and foveal brightness discrimination in one amblyopic and two normal eyes. Doc Ophthalmol 1967;23:149–84.

Feinberg I. Critical flicker frequency in amblyopia exanopsia. Am J Ophthalmol 1956;42:472–81.

Fincham EF. The mechanism of accommodation. Br J Ophthalmol (Monogr Suppl 8) 1937;5–80.

Fincham EF. The accommodation reflex and its stimulus. Br J Ophthalmol 1951;35:381–93.

Fincham EF. The proportion of ciliary muscular force required for accommodation. J Physiol 1955;128:99–112.

Flom MC. The use of the accommodative convergence relationship in prescribing orthoptics. Penn Optom 1954;14:3–18.

Flom MC. On the relationship between accommodation and accommodative convergence. II. Stability. Am J Optom Arch Am Acad Optom 1960a;37:517–23.

Flom MC. On the relationship between accommodation and accommodative convergence. I. Linearity. Am J Optom Arch Am Acad Optom 1960b;37:474–82.

Flom MC. On the relationship between accommodation and accommodative vergence. III. Effects of orthoptics. Am J Optom Arch Am Acad Optom 1960c;37:619–32.

Flom MC, Neumaier RW. Prevalence of amblyopia. Public Health Rep, 1966;81:329–41.

Flom MC, Takahashi E. The AC/A ratio and undercorrected myopia. Am J Optom Arch Am Acad Optom 1962;39:305–12.

Fry GA. The effect of age on the AC/A ratio. Am J Optom Arch Am Acad Optom 1959;36:200–303.

Fujii K, Kondo K, Kasai T. An analysis of the human eye accommodation system. Osaka University Technology Reports 925. 1970;20:221–36.

Gibson HW. Clinical orthoptics. London: Hatton Press, 1947.

Green DG. Visual resolution when light enters the eye through different parts of the pupil. J Physiol 1967;190:583–93.

Green DG, Powers MK, Banks MS. Depth of focus, eye size, and visual acuity. Vision Res 1980;20:827–35.

Hallden U. Fusional phenomena in anomalous correspondence. Acta Ophthalmol 1952;37(Suppl 1):1–93.

Hamasaki D, Ong J, Marg E. The amplitude of accommodation in presbyopia. Am J Optom Arch Am Acad Optom 1956:33:3–14.

Heath GG. The influence of visual acuity on accommodative responses of the eye. Am J Optom Arch Am Acad Optom 1956;33:513–24.

Heath GG, Hofstetter HW. The effect of orthoptics on the zone of binocular vision in intermittent extropia—case report. Am J Optom Arch Am Acad Optom 1952;29:12–31.

Hennessy RT, Leibowitz HW. The effect of a peripheral stimulus on accommodation. Percept Psychophys 1971;10:129–32.

Hering E. The theory of binocular vision. In: Bridgeman B, Stark L, eds, trans. New York: Plenum Press, 1977.

Hermann JS, Samson CR. Critical detection of the accommodative convergence to accommodation ratio by photosensor oculography. Arch Ophthalmol 1967;78:424–30.

Hess RF. Eye movements and grating acuity in strabismic amblyopia. Ophthalmic Res 1977a;9:225–37.

Hess RF. Accommodative accuracy in strabismic amblyopia. Aust J Optom 1977b;60:295–98.

Hess RF, Howell ER. The threshold contrast sensitivity function in strabismic amblyopia: evidence for a two-type classification. Vision Res 1977;17:1049–55.

Hirsch MJ. Editorial footnote to Manas and Shulman paper (q.v.). Am J Optom Arch Am Acad Optom 1954;31:395–96.

Hofstetter HW. A longitudinal study of amplitude changes in presbyopia. Am J Optom Arch Am Acad Optom 1965;42:3–8.

Hokoda SC, Ciuffreda KJ. Measurement of accommodative amplitude in amblyopia. Ophthalmic Physiol Opt in press.

Hubel D, Wiesel TN. Binocular interactions in striate cortex of kittens reared with artificial squint. J Neurophysiol 1965;28:1041–59.

Hung GK, Semmlow JL. Static behavior of accommodation and vergence: computer simulation of an interactive dual-feedback system. IEEE Trans Biomed Eng 1980;BME-27:439–47.

Hung GK, Ciuffreda KJ, Semmlow JL. Modeling of human near response disorders. Proceedings of the Ninth Annual Northeast Biomedical Engineering Conference, Rutgers University; New York: Plenum Press, 192–97.

Hung GK, Semmlow JL, Ciuffreda KJ. Accommodative oscillation can enhance average accommodative response: a simulation study. IEEE Trans Syst Man Cybernet 1982; SSC-12:594–98.

Hung GK, Ciuffreda KJ, Semmlow JL, Hokoda SC. Model of static accommodative behavior in human amblyopia. submitted.

Ikeda H, Tremain KE. Different causes for amblyopia and loss of binocularity in squinting kittens. J Physiol 1977;299:26–27P.

Ikeda H, Wright MJ. Is amblyopia due to inappropriate stimulation of the sustained pathways during development? Br J Ophthalmol 1974;58:165–75.

Jampolsky A. Characteristics of suppression in strabismus. Arch Ophthalmol 1955;54:683–96.

Judge SJ, Miles FA. Short-term modification of stimulus AC/A induced by spectacles which alter effective interocular separation. Paper read at Association for Research in Vision and Ophthalmology, May 1980, Orlando, Fla.

Kasai T, Unno M, Fujii K, Sekiguchi M, Shinohara K. Dynamic characteristics of human eye accommodation system. Osaka University Technology Reports 1014. 1971;21:569–86.

Keiner ECJF. Spontaneous recovery in microstrabismus. Ophthalmologica 1978;177:280–83.

Keller EL. Accommodative vergence in the alert monkey: motor unit analysis. Vision Res 1973;13:1565–75.

Keller EL, Robinson DA. Abducens unit behavior in the monkey during vergence movements. Vision Res 1972;12:349–82.

Kellindorfer J, Ciuffreda KJ, Hung GK, Hokoda SC, Semmlow JL. The effect of target velocity on the accommodative response. in prep.

Kenyon RV. Vergence eye movements in strabismus and amblyopia. PhD dissertation, Department of Physiological Optics, University of California, Berkeley, 1978.

Kenyon RV, Ciuffreda KJ, Stark L. Binocular eye movements during accommodative vergence. Vision Res 1978;18:545–55.

Kenyon RV, Ciuffreda KJ, Stark L. Dynamic vergence eye movements in strabismus and amblyopia: symmetric vergence. Invest Ophthalmol Visual Sci 1980a;19:60–74.

Kenyon RV, Ciuffreda KJ, Stark L. Unexpected role for normal accommodative vergence in strabismus and amblyopia. Am J Optom Physiol Opt 1980b;57:566–77.

Kenyon RV, Ciuffreda KJ, Stark L. Dynamic vergence eye movements in strabismus and amblyopia: asymmetric vergence. Br J Ophthalmol 1981;65:167–76.

Kirschen DK, Flom MC. Visual acuity at different retinal loci of eccentrically fixating functional amblyopes. Am J Optom Physiol Opt 1978;55:144–50.

Kirschen DG, Kendall JH, Riesen KS. An evaluation of the accommodative response in amblyopic eyes. Am J Optom Physiol Opt 1981;58:597–602.

Kretschemer S. La fausse correspondence retinienne. Doc Ophthalmol 1955;9:46.

Krishnan VV, Phillips S, Stark L. Frequency analysis of accommodation, accommodative vergence, and disparity vergence. Vision Res 1973;13:1545–54.

Krishnan VV, Shirachi D, Stark L. Dynamic measures of vergence accommodation. Am J Optom Physiol Opt 1977;54:470–73.

Liu JS. et al. Objective assessment of accommodation orthoptics. I. Dynamic insufficiency. Am J Optom Physiol Opt 1979;56:285–94.

Lyle K, Jackson S. Practical orthoptics. Philadelphia: Blakiston, 1941.

Mackensen G. Reaktionszeitmessungen bei Amblyopie. Albrecht Von Graefes Arch Klin Exp Ophthalmol 159:636–42.

Maddox E. Investigations on the relationship between convergence and accommodation of the eyes. J Anat 1886;20:475–505;565–84.

Manas L. The inconstancy of the ACA ratio. Am J Optom Arch Am Acad Optom 1955;32:304–15.

Manas L. The effect of visual training upon the ACA ratio. Am J Optom 1958;35:428–37.

Manas L, Shulman P. The variation in the accommodation-convergence accommodation (ACA) ratio upon periodic retesting. Am J Optom Arch Am Acad Optom 1954;31:385–95.

Mann SM. Amblyopia: accommodation as a causative factor. Optom Weekly 1975;67:177.

Mariani G, Pasino, L. Variations in the angle of anomaly and fusional movements in cases of small angle convergent strabismus with harmonious anomalous correspondence. Br J Ophthalmol 1974;48:439–43.

Martens TG, Ogle KN. Observations on accommodative convergence: especially its nonlinear relationships. Am J Ophthalmol 1959;47:455–62.

Morgan MW. Analysis of clinical data. Am J Optom Arch Am Acad Optom 1944a;21:477–91.

Morgan MW. Clinical measurements of accommodation and convergence. Am J Optom Arch Am Acad Optom 1944b;21:301–21.

Morgan MW. Accommodation and vergence. Am J Optom Arch Am Acad Optom 1968;45:417–54.

Morgan MW, Peters HB. Accommodative-convergence in presbyopia. Am J Optom Arch Am Acad Optom 1951;28:3–10.

Morris CW. Constancy of the ACA ratio. Am J Optom Arch Am Acad Optom 1957;34:117–27.

Mueller J. Elements of Physiology. Vol. 2. Baly W, trans. London: Taylor & Walton, 1826.

Ogle KN. Researches in binocular vision. New York: Hafner, 1950.

Ogle KN. The accommodative convergence accommodation ratio and its relation to the correction of refractive error. Trans Am Acad Ophthalmol Otolaryngol 1966;70:322–30.

Ogle KM, Dyer JA. Some observations on intermittent exotropia. Arch Ophthalmol 1965;73:58–73.

Ogle KN, Martens TG. On the accommodative convergence and the proximal convergence. Arch Ophthalmol 1957;57:702–15.

Ogle KN, Martens TG, Dyer JA. Oculomotor imbalance in binocular vision and fixation disparity. Philadelphia: Lea & Febiger, 1967.

Ogle KN, Mussey F, Prangen, AdeH. Fixation disparity and the fusional process in binocular single vision. Am J Ophthalmol 1949;32:1069–87.

Ono H. Accommodative-vergence and Hering's Law of equal innervation. Presented at the Association for Research in Vision and Ophthalmology, Sarasota, May 1981.

Otto J, Graemiger A. Uber Unzweckmabige Akkommodation Amblyoper Augenmit Exzentrischer Fixation. Albrecht Von Graefes Arch Klin Exp Ophthalmol 1967;173:125–40.

Otto J, Safra D. Uber das Akkommodation verhalten Hochradig Amblyoper Augen. Klin Monatsbl Augenheild 1974;165:175–79.

Otto J, Safra D. Methods and results of quantitive determination of accommodation in amblyopia and strabismus. In: Moore S, Mein J, Stockbridge L, eds. Orthoptics: past, present, future. New York: Stratton Intercontinental Medical Book Corp., 1976.

Owens DA. A comparison of accommodative responsiveness and contrast sensitivity for sinusoidal gratings. Vision Res 1980;20:159–67.

Parks MM. Abnormal accommodative convergence in squint. Arch Ophthalmol 1958;59:364–80.

Phillips SR. Ocular neurological control systems: accommodation and the near response triad. PhD dissertation, Department of Mechanical Engineering, University of California, Berkeley, 1974.

Phillips SR, Stark L. Blur: a sufficient accommodative stimulus. Doc Ophthalmol 1977;43:65–89.

Pickwell LD. Variations in ocular motor dominance. Br J Physiol Opt 1972;27:115–19.

Pickwell LD, Hampshire R. Jump-convergence test in strabismus. Ophthalmic Physiol Opt 1981;1:123–24.

Pratt-Johnson J, Wee HS. Suppression associated with exotropia. Can J Ophthalmol 1969;2:136–44.

Pratt-Johnson J, Wee HS, Ellis S. Suppression associated with esotropia. Can J Ophthalmol 1967;4:284–91.

Quere MA. Abnormal ocular movements in amblyopia. Trans Ophthalmol Soc UK 1979;99:401–6.

Quere MA, Pechereau A, Laveiant F. Etude electrooculographique des mouvements de vergence: I. La vergence symetrique. J Fr Ophtalmol 1981;4:25–32.

Rashbass C, Westheimer G. Disjunctive eye movements. J Physiol 1961;159:339–60.

Riggs LA, Niehl EW. Eye movements recorded during convergence and divergence. J Opt Soc Am 1960;50:913–20.

Robinson DA. The mechanisms of human vergence eye movement. J Pediatr Ophthalmol 1966;3:31–37.

Rosenberg R, Flax N, Brodsky B, Abelman L. Accommodative levels under conditions of asymmetric convergence. Am J Optom Arch Am Acad Optom 1953;30:244–54.

Saladin JJ, Stark L. Presbyopia: new evidence from impedance cyclography supporting the Hess-Gullstrand theory. Vision Res 1975;15:537–41.

Schapero M, Nadell M. Accommodation and convergence in beginning and absolute presbyopes. Am J Optom Arch Am Acad Optom 1957;34:606–22.

Schober HA, Dehler H, Kassel R. Accommodation during observations with optical instruments. J Opt Soc Am 1970;60:103–107.

Schoessler JP. Accommodative and fusional vergence in anomalous correspondence. Am J Optom Physiol Opt 1980;57:676–80.

Schlodtmann W. Studien uber anomale Sehrichtungsgemunschaft bei Schielenden. Albrecht Von Graefes Arch Klin Exp Ophthalmol 1900; 51:256.

Sears M, Guber D. The change in stimulus AC/A ratio after surgery. Am J Ophthalmol 1967;54:872–76.

Selenow A, Ciuffreda KJ. Vision function recovery during orthoptic therapy in an exotropic amblyope with high unilateral myopia. submitted.

Semmlow JL. Oculomotor response to near stimuli: the near triad. In: Zuber BL, ed. Models of oculomotor behavior and control. Miami: CRC Press, 1981.

Semmlow JL, Tinor T. Accommodative convergence response to off-foveal retinal images. J Opt Soc Am. 1978;68:1497–1501.

Semmlow JL, Venkiteswaran N. Dynamic accommodative vergence in binocular vision. Vision Res 1976;16:403–11.

Shirachi D, Liu J, Lee M, Jang J, Wong J, Stark L. Accommodation dynamics: range nonlinearities. Am J Optom Physiol Opt 1978;55:631–41.

Stark L. Neurological control systems. New York: Plenum Press, 1968.

Stark L, Takahashi Y, Zames G. Biological control mechanisms: human accommodation as an example of a neurological servomechanism. Theor Exp Biophys 1967;1:129–66.

Stark L, Vossius G, Young LR. Predictive control eye tracking movements. IRE Trans Hum Factor Electronics 1962;HFE-3:52–57.

Stoddard KB, Morgan MW. Monocular accommodation. Am J Optom Arch Am Acad Optom 1942;19:460–65.

Toates FM. Accommodation function of the human eye. Physiol Rev 1972;52:828–63.

Travers T. Suppression of vision in squint and its association with retinal correspondence and amblyopia. Br J Ophthalmol 1938;22:577–604.

Troelstra A, Zuber BL, Miller D, Stark L. Accommodative tracking: a trial-and-error function. Vision Res 1964;4:585–94.

Urist MJ. Primary and secondary deviation in comitant squint. Am J Ophthalmol 1950;48:647–56.

van der Wildt GJ, Bouman MA, van de Kraats J. The effect of anticipation on the transfer function of the human lens system. Optica Acta 1974;21:843–60.

von Noorden GK. Reaction time in normal and amblyopic eyes. Arch Ophthalmol 1961;66:694–701.

von Noorden GK. Divergence excess and simulated divergence excess: diagnosis and surgical management. Doc Ophthalmol 1969;26:719–28.

Westheimer G. The inconstancy of the ACA ratio. Am J Optom Arch Am Acad Optom 1955a;32:435–36.

Westheimer G. The relationship between accommodation and accommodative convergence. Am J Optom Arch Am Acad Optom 1955b;32:206–12.

Westheimer G. Amphetamine, barbiturates and accommodation convergence. Arch Ophthalmol 1963;70:830–36.

Westheimer G, McKee SP. Visual acuity in the presence of retinal-image motion. J Opt Soc Am 1975;65:847–50.

Westheimer G, Mitchell AM. Eye movement responses to convergent stimuli. Arch Ophthalmol 1956;55:848–56.

Westheimer G, Rashbass C. Barbiturates and eye vergence. Nature (Lond) 1961;191:833–34.

Whiteside TCD. The problems of vision in flight at high altitude. London: Butterworths, 1957.

Wilson D. A center for accommodative vergence motor control. Vision Res 1973a;13:2491–2503.

Wilson D. Noise coupling between accommodation and accommodative vergence. Vision Res 1973b;13:2505–13.

Windsor CE. Surgery, fusion, and accommodative convergence in exotropia. Int Ophthalmol Clin 1971;11:46–52.

Wood ICJ, Tomlinson A. The accommodative response in amblyopia. Am J Optom Physiol Opt 1974;52:243–47.

Yamamoto H. Studies on accommodative convergence. Jpn J Ophthalmol 1968;12:155–61.

Yamamoto H. Further studies on accommodative convergence. Jpn J Ophthalmol 1970;14:102–10.

Yoshida T, Watanabe A. Analysis of interaction between accommodation and vergence feedback control systems of human eyes. Bull NHK Broadcast Sci Res Labs 1969;3:72–80.

Zuber BL, Stark L. Dynamical characteristics of fusional vergence eye-movement system. IEEE Trans Syst Sci Cybernet 1968;SSC 4:72–79.

6

The Near Response: Theories of Control

John L. Semmlow
George K. Hung

Motility requirements imposed by binocular foveal vision are well met by the oculomotor system. Visual-motor research over the past few decades indicates that these demands are achieved largely through the lavish use of neural control processes. This strategy is implemented by dividing oculomotor responsibilities into a number of specific motor tasks: saccades, smooth pursuit, compensatory version movements, ocular vergence, and lens movements. Each task is mediated by a separate neural center responding to a different feature of the visual target or to vestibular information.

Even a single oculomotor task may be influenced by multiple control sources. For example, vergence eye movements assigned to follow changes in target depth are controlled by at least two neural centers. The disparity controller is driven by disparate retinal images formed in the two eyes. On the other hand, the accommodative controller, which senses target blur stimulation provided by the same change in target depth, also drives the vergence response.[1] Additionally, so-called higher level controls driven by an awareness or impression of distance or volition can influence the vergence response.

Our understanding of the oculomotor response to changes in target

[1] In keeping with the terminology suggested by Stark, Kenyon, Krishnan, and Ciuffreda (1980) we call the motor movement driven by disparate retinal images disparity vergence, and the movement driven by blur accommodative vergence.

depth, often termed the near response, is complicated by a richness of control processes and the multitasking of these processes. The motor movement involved holds interest for both visual-motor researchers and clinicians; therefore it is not surprising to find a long history associated with efforts to describe the controlling processes, their stimuli and, particularly, their interactions. This chapter sketches this history, presents current views along with associated experimental evidence, and defines the major unresolved issues in near triad control. The relevant physiological structures and behavioral features are only briefly discussed since a recent review covers them in some detail (Semmlow, 1981).

GENERAL ORGANIZATION OF THE NEAR TRIAD

Three distinct oculomotor activities involving separate neuromuscular structures are observed in response to changes in visual target distance: vergence, or disjunctive (oppositely directed) eye movements, changes in lens dioptic power, and changes in pupil diameter. Blur and retinal disparity provide the primary drive, although other factors may be involved. While the blur and disparity generated by a particular depth change are geometrically related, they can be isolated using optical techniques. Under such conditions each stimulus is capable of evoking all three motor responses.

The motor responses to a step change in target depth can directly modify the amount of stimulus: vergence movement decreases disparity while lens movement reduces blur. (Although changes in pupil diameter should theoretically modify blur by changing the optical depth of field, little effect is observed over normal pupil sizes) (Ripps et al., 1962). Thus for vergence and lens responses the notion of feedback control is applicable wherein lens and vergence movements continue until their respective errors are reduced to some acceptable level. Within this basic framework these controlled responses could be effectively mediated by independent feedback control systems, each responding to, and compensating for, one stimulus. Nonetheless, it is well known that the two systems interact, perhaps to provide redundancy or perhaps to achieve subtle control advantages. This interaction greatly complicates theoretical analysis of near triad control and is largely responsible for historical misunderstandings and currently unresolved issues.

EARLY THEORIES OF NEAR TRIAD CONTROL

Early theories were predominantly qualitative and centered on a presumed dominance of one stimulus and its associated control component.

As early as 1886 Maddox proposed that the near triad motor response was driven primarily by blur. He acknowledged the existence of a disparity-driven component, but ascribed to it a minor "supplemental" role (see Chapter 2). In his hierarchical theory, a vergence response is primarily evoked by blur, which in conjunction with a tonic component positions the eyes near the desired final position. Any remaining vergence error is then taken up by the feedback-controlled disparity-driven component, a process described by Toates (1974) as fine-tuning. The interactions among near triad processes predicted by the Maddox theory are shown in block diagram form in Figure 6.1. Many current clinical and research components such as fusional demand and fusional reserve are directly related to the Maddox structuring of vergence components.

His hierarchical theory was shaped by the experimental evidence available to him, which in turn was limited by instrumentation and related technology. Blur-driven vergence response (accommodative vergence) is relatively easy to expose and was quantitatively described as early as 1826 by Müller. Disparity-driven lens movements (vergence accommodation) are much more difficult to observe and were only vaguely described during Maddox's time. Thus the Maddox theory with its heavy emphasis on blur-driven components gained early popularity. The later discovery of a significant disparity-driven accommodation component did not much weaken the theory, since it was widely held that the role of disparity components, at least under normal circumstances, is "small and relatively unimportant for the basic process of near seeing" (Alpern, 1962).

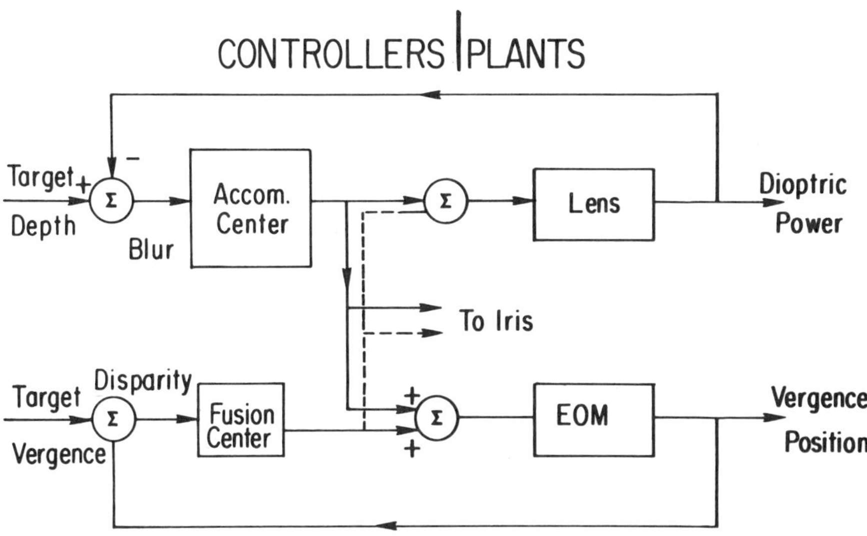

FIGURE 6.1. Block diagram presentation of near triad control components and their interrelationship as suggested by the Maddox theory.

Taking a nearly opposite view, Fincham and Walton (1957) readily acknowledged the strong vergence-accommodation interaction and proposed that it is disparity-driven components that dominate near triad responses. Their arguments are analogous to those presented by Maddox and Alpern, except disparity is used in place of blur, and accommodative vergence is replaced by vergence accommodation. Rather than dismiss the leftover interactive component (in this case, accommodative vergence) as functionally insignificant, Fincham and Walton suggest that it is not really a separate component after all. That is, only one neural "near center" exists, controlling both vergence position and lens dioptric power. As the feedback for either response is eliminated,[2] freeing that response from tight control, the single interactive process is exposed. Hence accommodative vergence is the movement produced by the near center in the vergence plant while vergence accommodation is the movement produced by that same center in the lens. While Fincham and Walton left the details of stimulus interaction somewhat vague, a probable arrangement satisfying their basic theoretical constraints is shown in block diagram form in Figure 6.2.

Evidence supporting or refuting these first two theories is detailed elsewhere (Semmlow, 1981), and is only summarized here. The Maddox-Alpern theory of near triad synkinesis involves two basic assumptions: (1) accommodative vergence adds algebraically to other vergence components to produce a binocular response and (2) the value of accommodative vergence during binocular fixation is the same as that observed monocularly for the same accommodative stimulus.

The most direct support for the first assumption is provided by the shape of the zone of clear single vision. In its usual representation, the horizontal boundaries of the zone depicting maximum and minimum vergence responses are assumed to be approximately parallel to the phoria line (Alpern, 1969; Balsam and Fry, 1959); that is, these vergence limits are related to the phoria position by a positive and negative constant. Assuming that the maximum and minimum attainable magnitude of the disparity component is constant, or at least independent of accommodative stimulation (Fry, 1939), the vergence limits are easily explained as the sum of this component (positive and negative) and the monocular accommodative vergence (Semmlow and Venkiteswaran, 1976).

Additional support for the first assumption of the Maddox theory is seen in fixation disparity experiments that suggest that the AC/A_s ratio under binocular viewing conditions is similar to that measured monocularly (Ogle and Martens, 1957). These results indicate that accommodative vergence is an active, additive vergence component during binoc-

[2] Using an optical pin-hole to remove blur feedback and monocular vision to eliminate disparity.

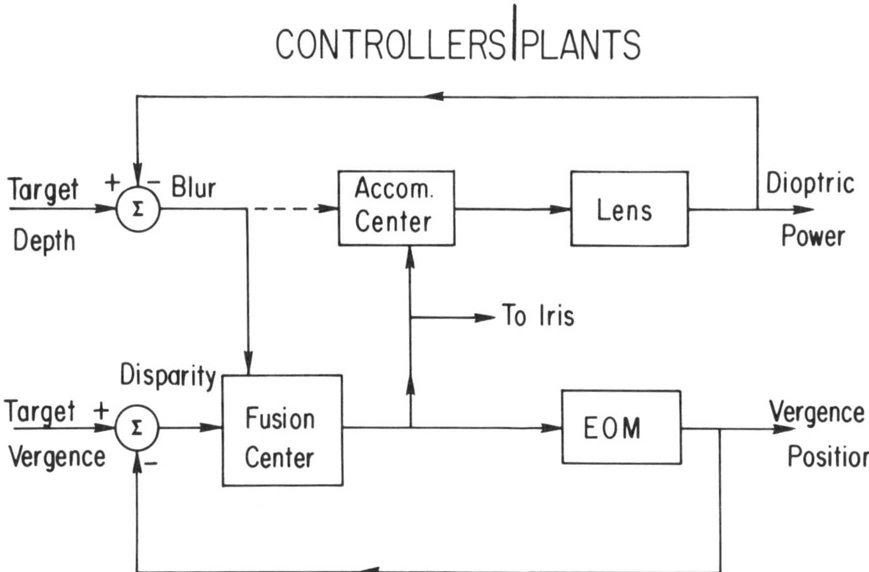

FIGURE 6.2. Block diagram presentation of near triad control components and their interrelationship as suggested by Fincham.

ular fixation. Finally, the summation of accommodative vergence with other components during a dynamic binocular response is shown in two recent experiments: binocular accommodative stimulation alone was shown to elicit a transient vergence response (Semmlow and Venkiteswaran, 1976); and vergence dynamics show a small, but consistent contribution due to added blur when compared to disparity-only dynamics (Semmlow and Wetzel, 1979).

While evidence exists that the first assumption is correct, there is little support for the second. In fact, evidence reflecting a difference in monocular and binocular accommodative vergence levels is indicated by a lack of strong correspondence between dissociated (monocular) phoria and associated phoria[3] (Ogle et al., 1967). These results coupled with their clinical experience led these investigators to conclude that monocular phoria measurements "often cannot be presumed to be a measure of the oculomotor imbalance when fusion is maintained."

Further evidence for a difference in monocular and binocular accommodative vergence is seen in recent experiments (Semmlow and Heerema, 1979) that examined the disparity component during binocular fixation of an orthophoric stimulus (that is, a binocular stimulus in which

[3] Associated phoria is defined by Ogle, Martens, and Dyer (1967) as the disparity stimulus required to produce zero fixation disparity.

the disparity stimulus was adjusted to equal the monocular response produced by accommodative vergence and tonic components). Under this stimulus condition the Maddox-Alpern theory predicts the disparity component will be zero since no "supplemental vergence" is necessary. Interruption of binocular fixation, however, produced a slow transient divergence movement with a time characteristic identical to a normal fusional decay movement (Semmlow and Heerema, 1979). This response was interpreted as evidence of a non-zero disparity-driven component in violation of an important prediction from the Maddox-Alpern theory.

Fincham's theory also implies two fundamental consequences: (1) disparity is the dominant stimulus in normal, binocular near response and (2) only a single interactive process exists.

Arguments supporting the concept that disparity-driven components dominate near triad motor responses have been summarized by Crone (1973). In addition to the fact that CA/C ratios generally exceed AC/A ratios when expressed in analogous units such as meter angles and diopters, the response latency of disparity-driven movements is less than blur-driven movements. Finally, the disparity stimulus is more accurate and without the direction ambiguity of blur.

While the evidence supporting the first prediction of Fincham's theory is largely circumstantial, the second prediction suggests behavioral characteristics that can be experimentally verified. Specifically, the AC/A_s and CA/C ratios should be reciprocally related in any given subject. Also, it should be impossible for accommodative vergence and vergence accommodation to maintain different values at the same time if they are manifestations of the same interactive process.

Most available data suggest that AC/C_s and CA/C ratios are not reciprocally related. Fincham himself reports CA/C ratios of around 1 D per meter angle for younger people (Fincham and Walton, 1957) as opposed to AC/A_s ratios around 0.7 meter angle per D (Morgan and Peters, 1951). Experimental errors in measuring the two ratios (particularly the CA/C) make such data an inconclusive test of Fincham's theory.

A direct test of the existence of two separate interactive components was the objective of a recent experiment (Semmlow and Hung, 1981; Semmlow, 1981). Using a technique described as time dissection, which is based on the difference in time characteristics of blur-driven and disparity-driven components, an approximate measure was obtained for the accommodative vergence component during strong overconvergence. If only a single interactive process exists, accommodative vergence must necessarily follow the increase in convergence accommodation associated with a strong disparity stimulus. Yet results showed accommodative vergence to be below the normal phoria level under these circumstances, suggesting accommodative vergence and vergence accommodation must be mediated by separate interactive processes and supported by separate and distinct neural mechanisms. Thus, as with the Maddox theory, a fundamental prediction of Fincham's theory has been experimentally disproved.

EARLY MODELS OF THE NEAR TRIAD

In the mid 1950s the high numbers of engineers entering the life sciences, since termed biomedical engineering, found an intriguing beachhead in oculomotor studies. Theory making became more quantitative, and the ability to evaluate a hypothesis rigorously using modeling and computer simulation was introduced. System analysis methods such as the use of block diagrams provided powerful organizational structures for widely scattered experimental evidence. This approach also made it possible to link conjectures to underlying physiological processes, the so-called homeomorphic model (Stark, 1968).

The new methods required that theories be stated more specifically, although not necessarily more transparently, to those not versed in the mathematics. To achieve more definitive statements, simplifications were usually necessary. By far the most common simplification was to model only one feedback control system, ignoring interactions with the other system. Since it is possible to isolate each system, at least under controlled laboratory conditions, experimental data could be obtained to evaluate such models. The fundamental assumption was that these systems behave more or less the same in isolation as they do when combined in normal binocular movement. Clearly, the absence of significant adaptive and interactive processes must be assumed.

Both accommodative and disparity feedback control systems have been modeled in isolation. Following the initial quantitative experiments of Campbell and Westheimer (1960), Stark, Takahashi, and Zames (1965) developed a complex model for accommodation, which included a nonlinear operator (saturation) and transport delay together with a second-order linear term and an integrator (Figure 6.3). No attempt was made to relate the mathematics to specific physiological processes, but the model was simulated and a comparison showed good representation of sinusoidal responses except for low-frequency phase angles, which the authors attributed to subject prediction.

A somewhat more homeomorphic feedback control model was proposed by Toates (1970). Particular emphasis was placed on the nonlinearities associated with depth of field, stimulus contrast, and physical saturation of the lens plant. Toates also argued for a proportional rather than integral controller based on sustained steady-state error in accom-

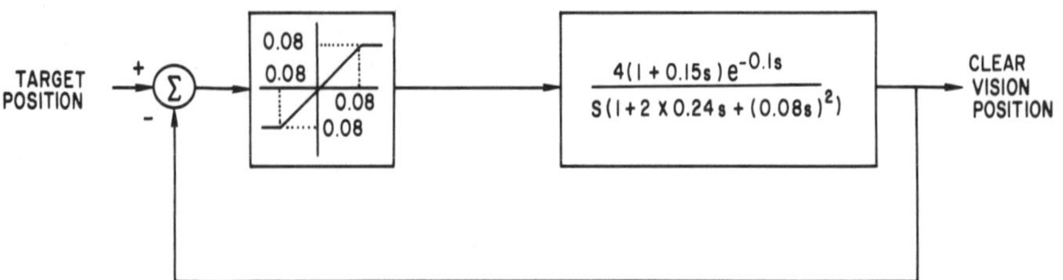

FIGURE 6.3. Early quantitative model of the isolated accommodative feedback control system. Reprinted by permission of the publisher, from Krishnan VV, Stark L. Integral control in accommodation. Comparative Proceedings in Biomedicine, 1975, Elsevier/North-Holland Biomedical Press.

modative response, the so-called lazy lag (Morgan and Olmstead, 1939). Unfortunately, the model was not simulated, perhaps because its function was to serve as an organizational structure for previous experimental findings.

The question of basic controller type was taken up by Krishnan and Stark (1975) in a series of no target experiments. Results suggested a "leaky" integrator (a first-order lag term, i.e., $1/(s + a)$), which they incorporated into a model together with a parallel derivative controller[4] to improve transient stability (Figure 6.4). As was later shown by Hung and Semmlow (1980), a leaky integrator has the same static characteristics as a proportional controller, a fact anticipated by Toates (1970) who included such an element in his proportional model.

A particularly useful application of system analysis methods is to facilitate transfer of information across boundaries defined by a given experiment, a specific subject, or even a specific species. The knowledge gained through one experimental paradigm can be translated into a model that could be applied in total, or as a submodel in analyzing quite different experiments. As an example, Thompson (1975) used data gathered during ciliary nerve stimulation of monkey to construct a model of the lens neuromuscular apparatus. The model consisted of a second-order, overdamped dynamic process with appropriate time constants, a transport delay, and saturating nonlinearity. Thompson was able to use this plant model to represent the lens in a larger model of the human accommodative control system.

A model of the isolated vergence system was first described, although not explicitly shown, by Zuber and Stark (1968). An analysis of their experimental data implied a unity feedback control system containing asymmetry and amplitude dependent nonlinearity followed by linear dynamic terms. Toates (1974) also developed a feedback model of dis-

[4] Actually a lead-lag term, $s/(s + a)$, was used.

parity vergence, principally to serve as an organizational tool for an extensive review. It included an integral controller and showed the points at which interaction with the accommodative control system occurred, although the consequences of this interaction were avoided.

In another example of information transfer between experimental paradigms, Krishnan and Stark (1977) used a plant model derived from saccadic eye movement data (Cook and Stark, 1967) within a larger model of the disparity vergence system. To the plant model they added a time delay and a controller made up of a leaky integrator and parallel derivative (lead-lag) element (Figure 6.5). The model was simulated, and results closely matched experimental responses for both sinusoids and steps; however, an analysis of the static, or fixation response of their model shows large errors when compared to actual data (Hung and Semmlow, 1980).

A model principally directed at representing static and long-term adaptive behavior has recently been developed by Schor (1979, 1980) (see Chapter 14). Using a configuration similar to the model in Figure 6.5, Schor added to the controller a parallel element consisting of a leaky integrator with a very long time constant. This added element functions essentially as an adaptive offset, or bias signal, reducing over the long term the maintenance signal level required from the transient, fast-response controller. Simulation results suggest this model adequately represents the slow modification of fixation disparity that occurs during sustained disparity stimulation.

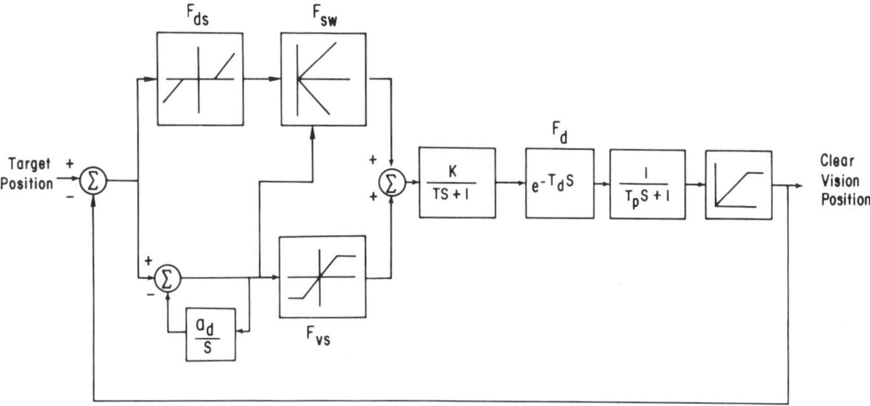

FIGURE 6.4. Quantitative model of the isolated accommodative feedback control system emphasizing dynamic properties of the neural controller. Reprinted by permission of the publisher, from Krishnan VV, Stark L. Integral control in accommodation. Comparative Proceedings in Biomedicine, 1975, Elsevier/North-Holland Biomedical Press.

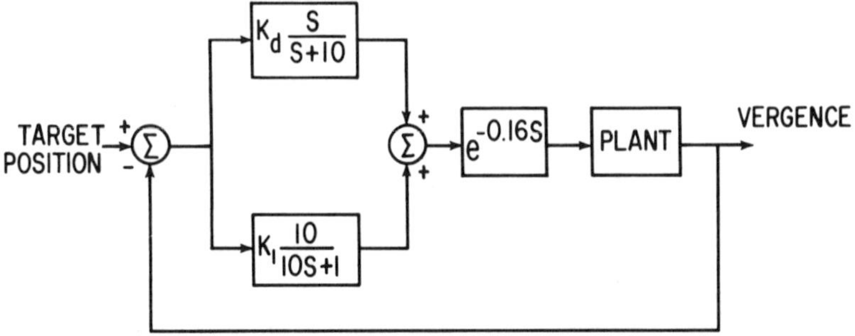

FIGURE 6.5. Quantitative model of the isolated disparity vergence feedback control system. Reprinted by permission of the publisher, from Krishnan VV, Stark L. A heuristic model of the human vergence eye movement system. Institute of Electrical and Electronics Engineers Transactions in Biomedical Engineering, © 1977 IEEE.

COMPLETE MODELS OF THE NEAR TRIAD

Westheimer (1963) proposed the first descriptive block diagram model to include both accommodative and disparity feedback control systems. Although very general, the description did feature distinct accommodation and vergence neural control centers each linked to the other through separate neural channels. Westheimer found this organizational structure helpful in explaining the effects of amphetamines and barbiturates on accommodative vergence. A similar model with a more specifically defined controller and cross-link structure was subsequently proposed by Toates (1968).

The first interactive model to be quantitatively specified and tested through computer simulation was developed by Semmlow and Jaeger (1972) as shown in Figure 6.6. The major feature of the model was that accommodation and vergence controllers were considered to be separate, and interaction of the two systems occurs by way of feed-forward "cross-links" from the controller outputs. This configuration is consistent with the experimental evidence mentioned earlier (Semmlow and Hung, 1981). The controllers themselves were simple integrators. It was found that while the static open-loop behavior of the model was consistent with human data for a wide variety of model values, the range for acceptable closed-loop behavior was quite limited. A model having a similar structure was recently proposed by Krishnan, Phillips, and Stark (1977); however, except for transport delays, the model was not quantitative.

The most recent comprehensive near triad model, Figure 6.7, has been developed by Hung and Semmlow (1980) as an extension of the earlier model by Semmlow and Jaeger (1972). It is concerned only with

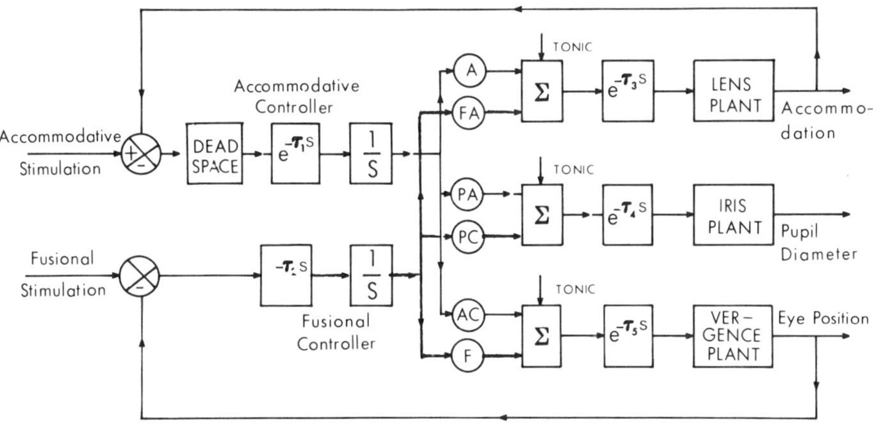

FIGURE 6.6. Early quantitative model of the complete near response showing separate but interacting disparity-driven and blur-driven controllers. Reprinted by permission of the publisher, from Semmlow JL, Jaeger R. Modelling the visual motor triad: an example of a multiple input-output biocontrol system. Proceedings 25th Alliance for Engineering in Medicine and Biology, 1972.

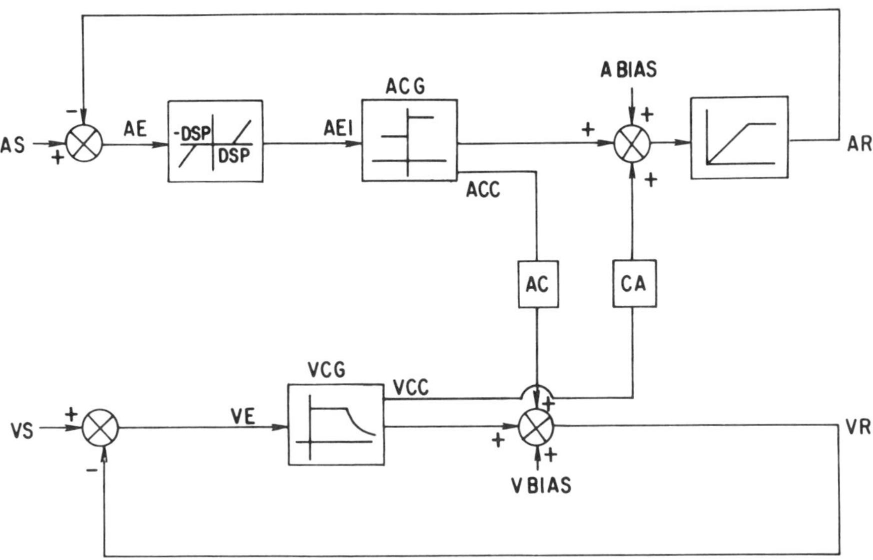

FIGURE 6.7. Recent quantitative model of the complete near response. Reprinted by permission of the publisher, from Hung G, Semmlow J. Static behavior of accommodation and vergence. Institute of Electrical and Electronics Engineers Transactions in Biomedical Engineering, © 1980 IEEE.

short-term static responses. Adaptive processes such as those described by Schor (1979, 1980) have not yet been incorporated. The model does include major accommodative and disparity nonlinearities and has been subjected to rigorous evaluation using computer simulation.

One of the main difficulties with the modeling of the combined system has been lack of multiple input/output experimental data performed on the same subject. Krishnan and associates (1973) analyzed the frequency response of accommodation, accommodative vergence, and disparity vergence; however, their results provide no information on static behavior. Hence Hung and Semmlow (1980) collected a consistent set of data on all static stimulus-response combinations from four subjects.

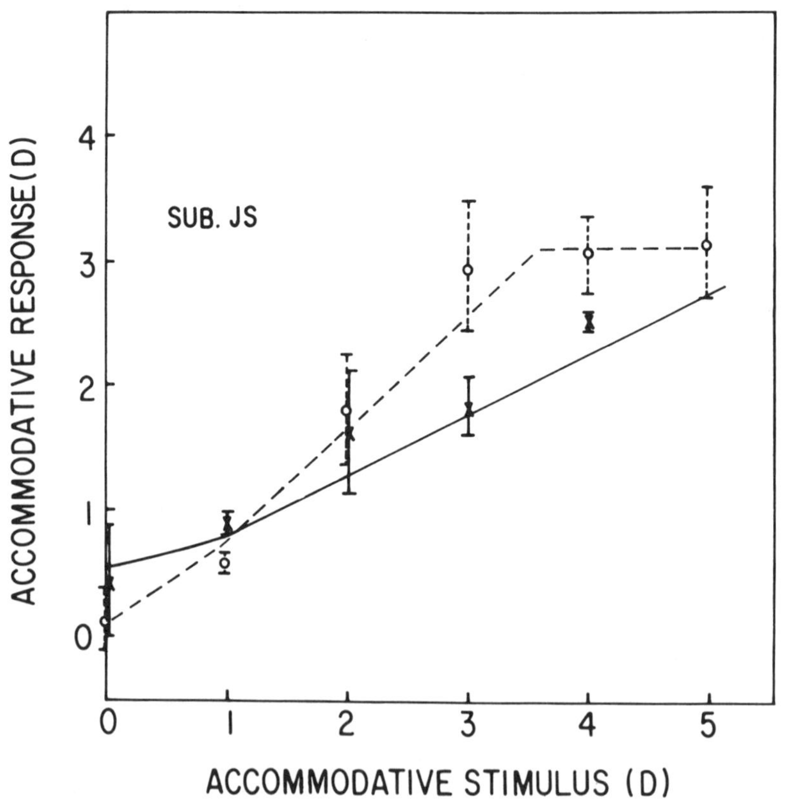

FIGURE 6.8. Comparison of static human experimental data and model simulations for seven of the eight possible stimulus-response combinations in this system. Reprinted by permission of the publisher, from Hung G, Semmlow J. Static behavior of accommodation and vergence. Institute of Electrical and Electronics Engineers Transactions in Biomedical Engineering, © 1980 IEEE.

Since there are two feedback-controlled motor responses,[5] two primary stimuli, and each feedback system can be either open-loop or closed-loop, eight experiments in all are possible. Data were collected from seven of the eight possible stimulus conditions using a paradigm that reduced long-term adaptive processes (Hung and Semmlow, 1980). Results were then compared with model simulations, and after appropriate parameter adjustment (see Hung and Semmlow, 1980 for details) good correlations were obtained for all seven (Figure 6.8). Furthermore, allowing for the adjustment of only six basic values (Table 6.1), the results from all four subjects could be replicated.

The success of the model under rather stringent evaluation provides support for its basic configuration, and hence its theoretical foundation. Unlike the qualitative theories of Maddox and Fincham, the model suggests that both stimuli contribute to near triad responses, at least in the short-term static response, and that both interactive pathways are active.

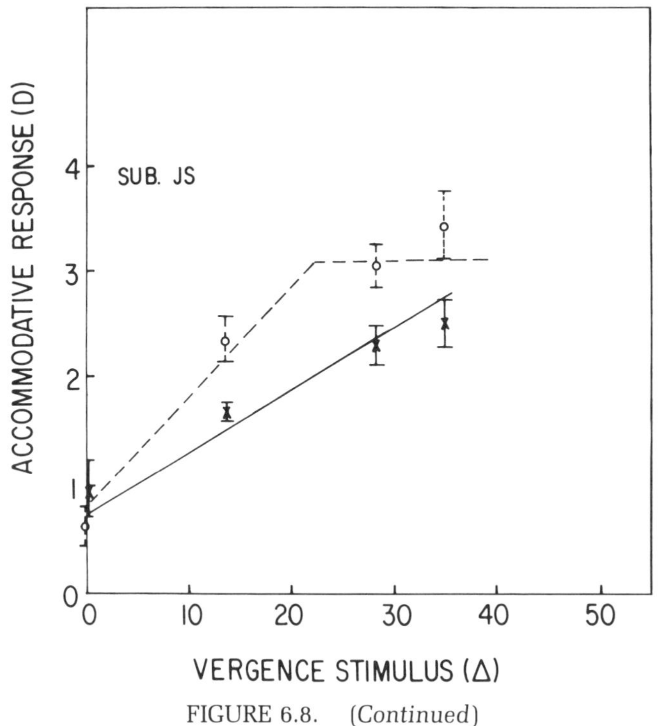

FIGURE 6.8. *(Continued)*

[5] Iris response was ignored since its feedback effects on the two stimuli are quite small (Ripps et al., 1962).

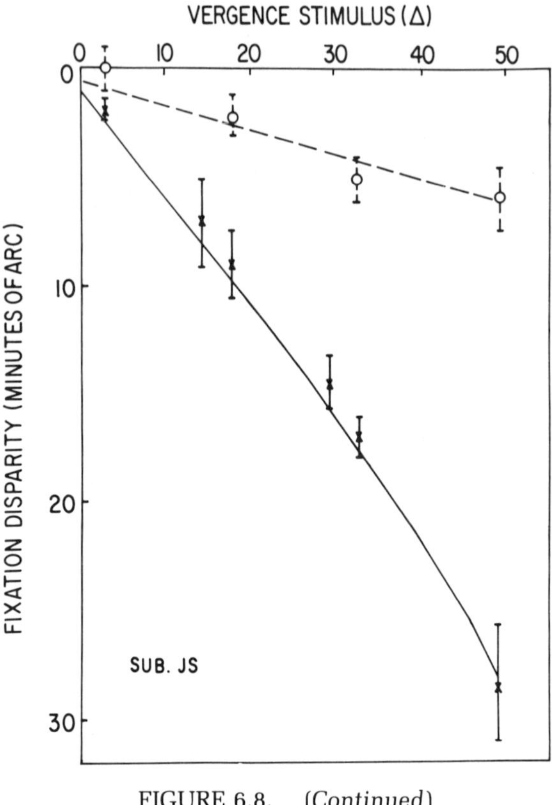

FIGURE 6.8. *(Continued)*

TABLE 6.1. Linear model parameters for four subjects

	Values for Subject			
Parameter	*JS* (Age 37)	*GH* (Age 32)	*FR* (Age 21)	*JM* (Age 18)
ABIAS(D)	0.42	1.70	0.75	2.20
VBIAS(MA)	−0.62	1.00	0.19	0.93
VCG	293.0	141.0	126.0	166.0
ACGP	8.53	2.60	10.7	2.32
CA(D/MA)	0.66	0.50	0.85	0.47
AC(MA/D)	1.15	1.76	0.49	0.63

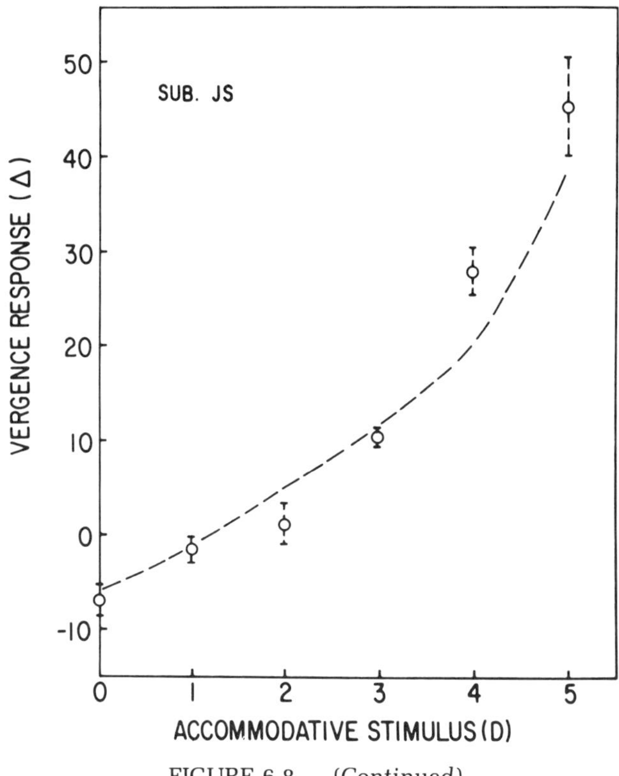

FIGURE 6.8. *(Continued)*

MODEL APPLICATIONS

One advantage of a comprehensive model of the oculomotor near response is that it provides, through simulation, very detailed predictions concerning both internal and external behavior. An example of model usage in "dissecting" the internal structure is shown in a recent parameter sensitivity study (Hung and Semmlow 1981). The influence of the magnitudes of the interactive cross-links (pathways CA and AC in Figure 6.7)[6] on internal control patterns was documented. Specifically, the relative control exerted by the two major controllers on near triad responses was analyzed under varying values of cross-link effectiveness.[7] Results are

[6] For large stimulus values, it can be shown that $CA/C \cong CA^* \dfrac{VCG}{1 + VCG}$ and $AC/A_s \cong AC^* \dfrac{ACG}{1 + ACG}$. Since VCG is large (VCG = 293 for subject JS), for all practical purposes CA/C = CA; however, ACG is relatively small (ACG = 8.47 for subject JS). Hence AC/A_s is proportional to, but slightly smaller, than AC.

[7] Cross-link effectiveness was adjusted by modifying the gain of the CA and AC pathways. This is analogous to varying the AC/A_s and CA/C ratios.

displayed in Figure 5.9 as the percentage of a near triad motor response associated with a given controller under varying combinations of AC/A_s and CA/C values. From the data in Figure 6.9 we note that when the CA/C ratio equals 1 D per meter angle, a value not uncommon in young subjects (Fincham and Walton, 1957), the disparity controller completely dominates the near triad motor responses (100% of both lens and vergence responses). This dominance can be attributed to the tight control (high loop gain) associated with this feedback control system; in other words, the same control features that produce such small vergence fixation errors (fixation disparity) result in control dominance given a reasonably strong CA/C ratio. As the CA/C ratio diminishes the influence of the disparity controller declines, particularly as the AC/A_s ratio is increased. Even with a CA/C ratio of 0.5 D per meter angle and a AC/A_s ratio of 1 meter angle per D, the model predicts that the disparity controller still exercises approximately 20% of the total control.

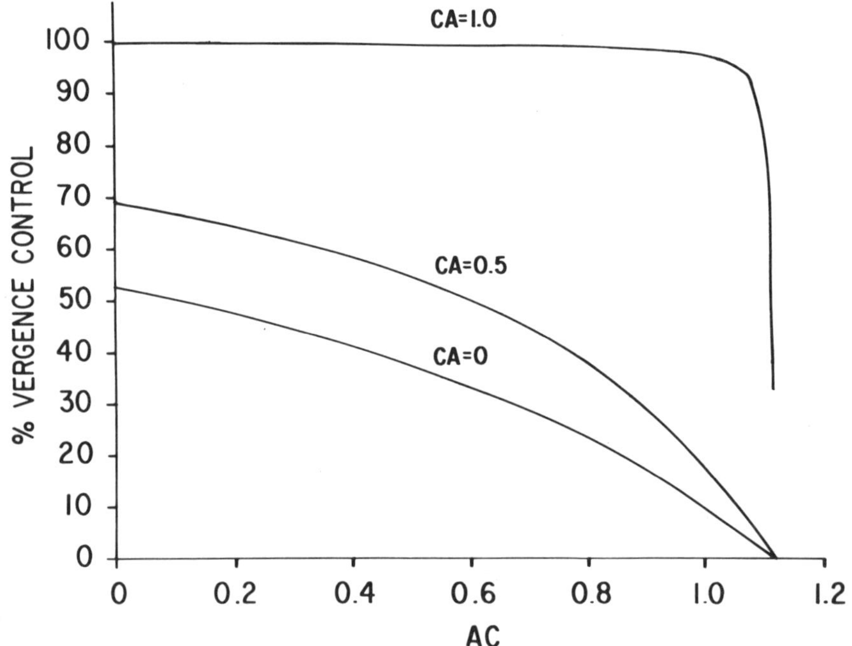

FIGURE 6.9. Results of model simulations on the relative influence of major near response controllers. A Percentage of vergence response controlled by the disparity controller for various values of cross-link effectiveness. The percent control exercised by the accommodative controller would be the complement of the curve shown. B Percentage of lens response controlled by the accommodative controller for various values of cross-link effectiveness. The percent control exercised by the disparity controller would be the complement of the curve shown.

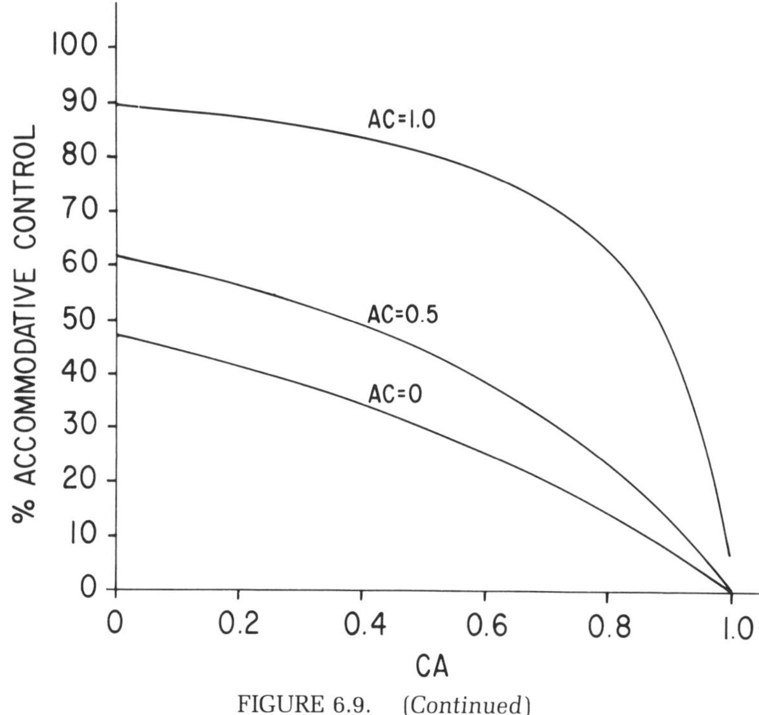

FIGURE 6.9. *(Continued)*

The results of Figure 6.9 are simply highly specific predictions extracted from a well-defined theory. As both controller outputs are strictly internal variables, these predictions cannot be experimentally verified directly; however, the model demonstration of a well-defined shift of controller dominance with CA/C and AC/A ratios suggests a number of confirmatory experiments. As these experiments are currently in the planning phase in the authors' laboratory, details are left to the imagination of the reader.

Another application of the model is quantative description of clinical abnormalities. As an example, amblyopia is a reduction in monocular acuity that is not correctable by refraction or attributable to obvious structural or pathological abnormalities (Schapero et al., 1968). The afflicted eye shows a reduced accommodative response (Wood and Tomlinson, 1975), and as this is a monocular condition only the accommodative control system is involved (disparity-driven components are absent).

Referring to the model of Figure 6.7, one possible explanation for decreased accommodative response is a reduction in accommodative controller gain (ACG).[8] Simulations of accommodative response for normal

[8] The controllers in Figure 6.7 are taken to include sensory processes, the probable origin of this abnormality.

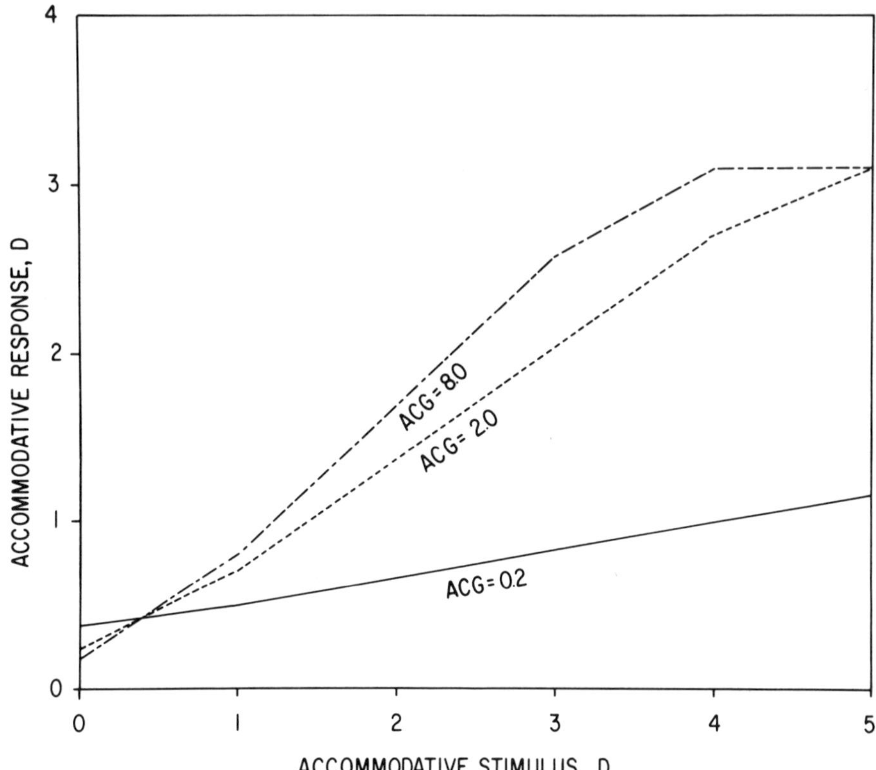

FIGURE 6.10. Computer simulation of an amblyopic response showing the effect of decreased accommodative controller gain (ACG = 0.2, 2) on accommodative response. Response of a normal eye (ACG = 8) is shown for comparison. Reprinted with permission from the Proceedings of the 9th Annual Northeast Bioengineering Conference, Hung G, Ciuffreda KJ, Semmlow JL, Modelling of human response disorder, 1981, Pergamon Press, Ltd.

and low values of controller gain are shown in Figure 6.10 plotted as a function of stimulus (Hung et al., 1981). A marked reduction in response is noted as accommodation controller gain is reduced. All other parameters used in this simulation were those of a normal (although somewhat presbyopic) subject.

CONCLUSIONS

Theories of neural control of near triad motor responses represent a line of scientific inquiry extending over 100 years. Recent approaches have brought powerful analytical techniques to bear on both experimental design and theoretical analysis. Yet the significant questions remain largely unresolved. Specifically, the exact nature of the stimulus to near triad motor responses, primarily blur, primarily disparity, or a specific combination of the two, is just now being systematically studied.

In a head-to-head comparison of binocular vergence to disparity-only responses (with the accommodation system open-loop) an overall similarity in dynamics was noted (Semmlow and Wetzel, 1979). The addition of blur stimulation over disparity alone brought only a slight increase in response velocity and only toward the end of the response. From these experiments it can be concluded that blur information contributes little to the dynamic vergence response, but what of the steady-state response or the lens movement? The influence of blur on fixation disparity convincingly demonstrates the potential of this stimulus to influence the steady-state vergence response, and presumably the steady-state lens response as well, but the same could be said for the marked influence of disparity on steady-state lens dioptric power (see Figure 6.8).

Theoretically, pupil responses could also be used to resolve the question of stimulus dominance; that is, by comparing pupil response to disparity, blur, and combined stimuli the relative importance and timing of each control component could be determined. Unfortunately, pupil dynamics are heavily influenced by the plant—the iris musculature—and control dynamics would likely be overshadowed by this sluggish plant.

The most recent comprehensive model of the near response predicts stimulus dominance depends in part on the combination of AC/A_s and CA/C ratios. Taking the nominal range of these ratios into consideration, the model predicts that in most subjects, most of both the lens and vergence response to a near target is controlled by disparity-driven components. The model further suggests that this dominance is the result of a more tightly controlled (higher gain) disparity feedback system.

The experimental evidence to date also indicates disparity driven signals, with their unambiguous sign information and shorter latency (the process required for neural decoding of disparity appears more straightforward than that required for blur) dominate near triad motor behavior, but this evidence is largely circumstantial. Experimental verification could be achieved by comparing lens responses to disparity-only, blur-only, and combined binocular stimulation. As in earlier times, critical experiments are restricted by available instrumentation; eye movement associated with normal disparity or binocular stimulation generates substantial artifacts in current dynamic optometers. Advances in optometer design to permit artifact-free recording of lens power on a moving eye are crucial to the continued growth of our knowledge of near triad control.

REFERENCES

Alpern M. Accommodation: evaluation of theories of preobyopia. In: Davson H, ed. The eye. Vol. 3. 1st ed. New York: Academic Press, 1962.

Alpern M. Types of movement. In: Davson H, ed. The eye. Vol. 3. 2nd ed. New York: Academic Press, 1969;65–174.

Balsam MH, Fry GA. Convergence accommodation. Am J Optom Arch Am Acad Optom 1959;36:567–15.

Campbell FW, Westheimer G. Dynamics of accommodation responses of the human eye. J Physiol (Lond) 1960;151:285–95.

Cook G, Stark L. Deviation of a model for the human eye-positioning mechanism. Bull Math Biophys 1967;29:153–75.

Crone RA. The control of eye movements. In: Diplopia. New York: American Elsevier, 1973.

Fincham EF, Walton J. The reciprocal actions of accommodation and convergence. J. Physiol (Lond) 1957;137:488–508.

Fry G. Further experiments of the accommodative convergence relationship. Am J Optom Arch Am Acad Optom 1939;16:325–34.

Hung G, Semmlow JL. Static behavior of accommodation and vergence: computer simulation of an interactive dual-feedback. IEEE Trans Biomed Eng 1980;BME-27:439–47.

Hung G, Ciuffreda KJ, Semmlow JL. Modeling of human near response disorder. Proceedings of the 9th Annual Northeast Bioengineering Conference, March 1981, Piscataway, N.J.

Krishnan VV, Stark L. Integral control in accommodation. Comput Programs Biomed 1975;4:237–45.

Krishnan VV, Stark L. A heuristic model for the human vergence eye movement system. IEEE Trans Biomed Eng 1977;BME-24:44–49.

Krishnan VV, Phillips S, Stark L. Frequency analysis of accommodation, accommodative vergence and disparity vergence. Vision Res 1973;13:1545–54.

Maddox E. Investigations on the relationship between convergence and accommodation of the eyes. J Anat 1886;20:475–505, 565–84.

Morgan MW, Olmstead JHD. Quantative measurements of relative accommodation and relative convergence. Proc Soc Exp Biol Méd 1939;41:303–307.

Morgan MW, Peters H. Accommodative convergence in presbyopia. Am J Optom Arch Am Acad Optom 1951;28:3–10.

Müller J. Elements of physiology. Vol. 2. Taylor W, Walton J, trans. London: 1842, pp. 207–17.

Ogle KN, Martens TG. On the accommodative convergence and the proximal vergence. Arch Ophthamol 1957;51:702–15.

Ogle KN, Martens TG, Dyer JA. Oculomotor imbalance. In: Binocular vision and fixation disparity. Philadelphia: Lea & Febiger, 1967.

Ripps H, Chin NB, Siegel IM, Breinen GM. Effect of pupil size on accommodation convergence and the AC/A ratio. Invest Ophthalmol 1962;1:127–35.

Schapero M, Cline D, Hofstetter H. Dictionary of visual science. Philadelphia: Chilton Book Co., 1968.

Schor CM. The influence of rapid prism adaptation upon fixation disparity. Vision Res 1979;19:757–65.

Schor CM. Fixation disparity: a steady state error of disparity-induced vergence. Am J Optom Physiol Opt 1980;57:618–31.

Semmlow, JL. The oculomotor near response. In: Zuber B, ed. Models of oculomotor behavior. Chemical Rubber, New York, 1981.

Semmlow JL, Hung G. Experimental evidence for the independence of accommodative convergence and convergence accommodation. Doc Ophthalmol 1981;51:209–224.

Semmlow JL, Heerema D. The synkinetic interaction of convergence accommodation and accommodative convergence. Vision Res 1979;19:1237–42.

Semmlow JL, Jaeger R. Modelling the visual motor triad: an example of a multiple input-output biocontrol system. Proceedings of the 25th Association Engineering in Biology & Medicine, January 1972, Bal Harbor, Fla.

Semmlow, JL, Venkiteswaran N. Dynamic accommodative vergence in binocular vision. Vision Res 1976;16:403–11.

Semmlow, JL, Wetzel P. Dynamic contributions of binocular vergence components. J Optom Soc Am 1979;69:639–45.

Stark L. Neurological control systems: studies in bioengineering. New York: Plenum Press, 1968.

Stark L, Takahashi Y, Zames G. Nonlinear servoanalysis of human lens accommodation. IEEE Trans Systems Sci Cybernet 1965;SSC-1:78–83.

Stark L, Kenyon RV, Krishnan VV, Ciuffreda KJ. Disparity vergence: a proposed name for a dominant component of binocular vergence eye movements. Am J Optom Physiol Opt 1980;57:606–9.

Thompson H. The dynamics of accommodation in primates. PhD thesis, University of Illinois at the Medical Center, Chicago, Ill., 1975.

Toates FM. Control of the eye intrinsic muscles. Trans Inst Meas Contr 1968;1:T129–T132.

Toates FM. A model of accommodation. Vision Res 1970;10:1069–76.

Toates FM. Vergence eye movements. Doc Ophthalmol 1974;37:153–214.

Westheimer G. Amphetamine, barbiturates and accommodative convergence. Arch Ophthalmol 1963;70:830–36.

Wood I, Tomlinson A. The accommodative response in amblyopia, Am J Optom Physiol Opt 1975;52:243–47.

Zuber BL, Stark L. Dynamical characteristics of the fusional vergence eye-movement system. IEEE Trans System Sci Cybernet 1968;SSC-4:72–79.

IV
DISPARITY VERGENCE

7

Sensory Processing of Binocular Disparity

Christopher W. Tyler

HISTORY

One principle in the progression of science is that major phenomena can emerge from the investigation of second-order effects. What was once a wrinkle on a primary effect becomes a field of study in its own right. Binocular disparity is a prime example. As early as the eleventh century, Arabic ophthalmologists such as Alhazen knew that similar images are projected onto the two retinas (Winter, 1954). (This idea of projection onto the retinas is itself remarkable, since the prevailing doctrine from Euclid onward was that the world was sensed by rays emitted outward from the eye.) In the seventeenth century, Aguilonius (1613) appreciated that these two projected images were slightly different, and defined the positions in space that would project to corresponding points in the two eyes. It was not until the nineteenth century that an expansion of interest in vision led to the recognition of the unique role of binocular disparity in depth perception.

In 1833 Wheatstone made the discovery of a new sensory dimension, stereopsis (Meyer, 1833; Wheatstone, 1838). As a result, the second-order phenomenon of slight differences between the retinal images became the field of study of vision in the third dimension. Since that time there have

Supported by NIH grants EY-03622 and EY-01186 and the Smith-Kettlewell Eye Research Foundation.

been two major phases of growth in the field, in the mid-nineteenth century and the mid-twentieth centuries. This chapter concentrates on the early contributions to geometric analysis of visual space that have been largely ignored in this century, and on recent advances in stereopsis, which will be cast into a new framework for understanding this aspect of neural processing.

Sensory Consequences of Binocular Disparity

The presence of binocular disparity between the images has a number of distinct sensory consequences, depending on the precise configuration of the stimuli and the sensory dimension of interest.

Binocular Visual Direction

Visual direction is the perceived frontal plane position of a stimulus in relation to the observer: up, down, left, or right. When specified with the eyes in their primary positions (i.e., with no eye movements), visual direction provides the basic metric of the visual position sense. It can be specified either for the binocular perception of the stimulus, or for the perceived monocular images if there is sufficient binocular disparity between the two monocular images for them to be perceived separately (see below). Monocular points that project at the same perceived visual direction in the two eyes are called corresponding points, defining zero binocular disparity, and are considered to project to the same region of visual cortex. There is a limited set of physical points in space that project to corresponding retinal points and define the horopter for a given fixation position.

Sensory Fusion and Diplopia

If the images in the two eyes are similar but one is moved slightly to produce a small binocular disparity, the binocular stimuli will still be perceived as fused into a single image. The range of binocular disparities over which the image remains fused and single has been classically known as Panum's (1858) fusional region. Beyond this region the stimuli to each eye are perceived separately. This perception of the stimulus as doubled is known as diplopia.

Dichoptic Stimulation

If the images arriving at corresponding regions of the two retinas are very different, the perception will not be diplopia, in which both monocular images are seen simultaneously, but binocular rivalry, in which the monocular images are perceived alternately with a random rate of alternation in any given retinal region.

Under certain circumstances the transient suppression of the non-perceived image may turn into continuous interocular suppression in a given retinal region. This can occur if either the stimulus characteristics or organismic factors operate to give one retinal input dominance over the corresponding input from the other retina.

Stereopsis

If the binocular disparity between similar images in the eyes is small and horizontal, the image will be seen in vivid depth nearer or farther than the point of fixation, but the impression of depth is degraded by the presence of vertical disparities. Depth perception is experienced under conditions of binocular fusion and also where the disparity is large enough to cause diplopia. In other words, stereopsis is independent of the state of fusion.

Vergence

A final aspect of binocular physiology that relates to space perception is the direction in which the two eyes are pointing. If we define the visual axis of an eye as the line passing through the fovea and the optical nodal point of the eye, the angle between the two visual axes is the vergence angle. This angle is convergent if the visual axes cross closer than infinity, otherwise it is divergent. The vergence angle affects many aspects of binocular vision.

These five aspects of binocular perception form the major subdivisions of sensory binocular processing.

BINOCULAR VISUAL DIRECTION AND THE HOROPTER

Binocular Visual Direction

The study of the perceived visual direction of a binocular image has a long history dating back to Hering (1864). Consider a situation in which point light sources are projected to corresponding points on the two retinas, for example, to the fovea of each eye. By definition, the points have zero binocular disparity and will be perceived as a single fused point of light. If the point in the right eye is moved rightward to the limit of Panum's fusional region (assuming no eye movements), a single fused point will still be perceived (Figure 7.1), but the monocular visual direction of the point in the right eye has been changed by perhaps 10 arcminutes. The question is, how will the binocular fused image change its visual direction? The answer proposed by Hering was that the binocular visual direction lies approximately halfway between the directions of the monocular images.

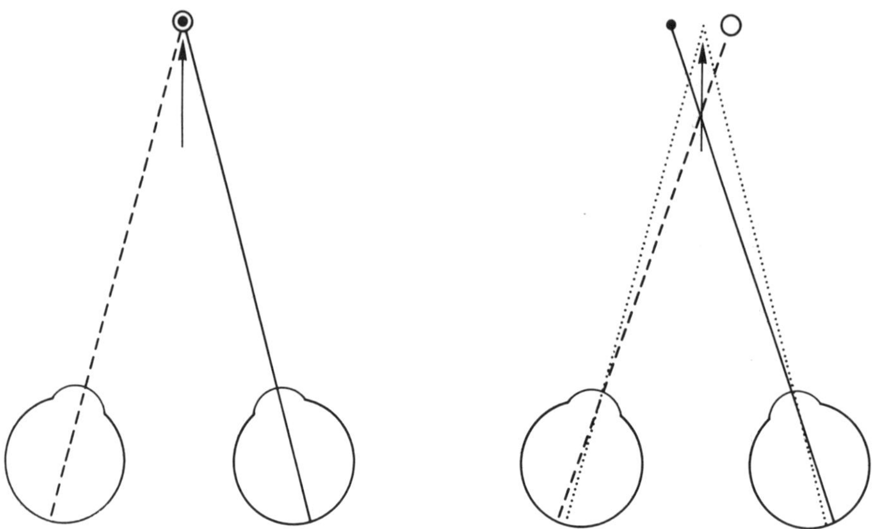

FIGURE 7.1. Visual direction. When the right (.) and left (o) eye images are in correspondence (*left panel*) visual direction (*arrow*) is unambiguous, but when the two images fall on disparate points (*right panel*) the perceived visual direction lies part way between them (*arrow*) depending on eye dominance. Reprinted by permission of the publisher, from Tyler CW and Scott AB. Binocular Vision. In: Records R, ed. *Physiology of the Human Eye and Visual System*. Hagerstown: Harper and Row, 1979.

Subsequently, investigators such as Verhoeff (1902), Fry (1950), and Ogle (1958) generally upheld this conclusion but reported a good deal of variability in the percepts both for a given observer and between observers. This may have been partly due to a lack of control of vergence eye movements. The definitive study on this topic is that of Sheedy and Fry (1979), who used a stimulus with a complex binocular surround, which effectively held vergence at a fixed value. They also used a stimulus line with a vertical disparity, to study the fusion system without contamination from the stereoscopic system. Under these conditions, variability in each estimate of the position of the binocular image was low and was close to that of the monocular images for their eight observers. Across observers the mean position of the binocular image was almost exactly halfway between the two monocular positions, although each observer tended to see it closer to one monocular position than the other.

Corresponding Retinal Points

In the analysis of binocular space perception, the perceived relative distances of objects from the observer are determined in general by the binocular disparity between the images falling on the retinas of the two eyes (in conjunction with the convergence of the eyes).

It is necessary to define more precisely the concept of corresponding points, that is, points have zero binocular disparity on the two retinas. The simplest definition is based on ocular geometry (Figure 7.2), in which corresponding points on the two retinas are defined as being at the same horizontal and vertical distance (as measured by the monocular visual directions) from the center of the fovea of each eye. (The rotation of the eyes must be taken into account but may be considered identical when the eyes are in the primary, or straight ahead, position.)

For every position of binocular fixation there must be a set of points in space for which the binocular disparity is zero. The locus of these points is known as the *horopter* (the horizon of vision), a term introduced

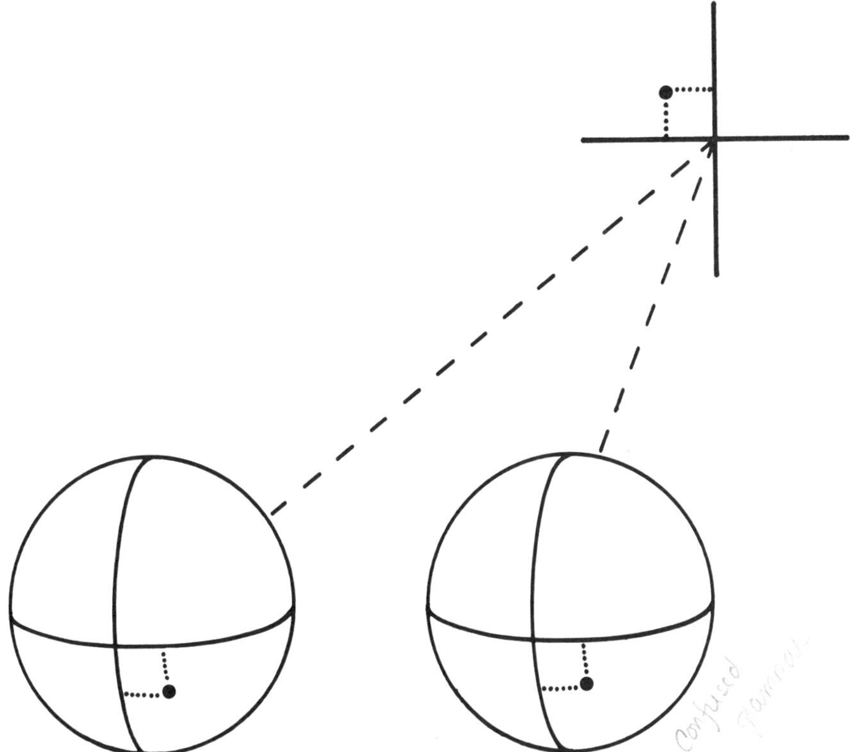

FIGURE 7.2. Geometric retinal correspondence. When the eyes are aligned and viewing a point at infinity at a given vertical and horizontal distance away from the fixation point projects equivalent distances horizontally and vertically away from the fovea in each eye. These two projections are then in geometric correspondence. Reprinted by permission of the publisher, from Tyler CW and Scott AB. Binocular Vision. In: Records R, ed. *Physiology of the Human Eye and Visual System*. Hagerstown: Harper and Row, 1979.

by Aguilonius (1613). The *point horopter* is the locus of zero disparities for point stimuli (i.e., where both horizontal and vertical disparities are zero). Ideally, the point horopter is a horizontal circle and a vertical line intersecting at the point of fixation, although in certain restricted circumstances it may become a two-dimensional surface. Under no circumstances is the point horopter ever a sphere or a torus.

Types of Horopters

There has been a considerable amount of confusion in the literature caused by laxity in defining horopter. Walls (1952), for example, maintained that there is only one, with many ways of measuring it. This is incorrect. The form of horopter depends in principle on its definition, which can be based on zero binocular disparity, zero horizontal disparity, zero deviation from equal perceived distance from the observer, and so on. In each case the horopter is different.

The definition used thus far has been purely geometric and based on the concept of binocular retinal correspondence with zero binocular disparity. This geometric horopter must be distinguished from the empirical horopter measured on a given observer, which may be found to deviate from the geometric construction. Such empirical deviation may occur either if physiological correspondence departs from the geometric definition of corresponding points or if there are optical distortions of the images.

Furthermore, in extending the horopter concept to perception of objects in space, it is possible to base the definition on distance from the observer rather than on binocular disparity per se. The perception of distance from the self involves activity at a higher level of the perceptual apparatus, which may add compensations or distortions to the form of the binocular correspondence horopter. The distance horopter is therefore not as fundamental a concept as the binocular correspondence horopter. Two procedures have been used to measure the distance horopter. In one, stimuli in different directions are set to appear equidistant. This establishes the equidistance horopter. In the other, stimuli are set to form an apparent fronto-parallel plane. This defines the fronto-parallel horopter. A fuller description of these types of distance horopter is beyond the scope of this chapter.

The horopter based solely on horizontal disparities is especially interesting because it is these disparities that are involved in depth perception. This is equivalent to a horopter measured with long vertical lines, and is therefore known as the longitudinal horopter by analogy with the vertical lines of longitude on the globe of the earth. This is the one most commonly specified in texts and most often measured empirically. It is important to note that whereas the point horopter is an intersecting curve and line (except for fixation at infinity), the longitudinal horopter is a two-dimensional surface.

A final type of empirical horopter is the locus of points in space that appear binocularly fused to the observer. The fusion horopter is a three-dimensional volume in space extending around the point horopter. The fusion horopter is the one preferred in ophthalmologic practice, and is described in the section on binocular fusion.

Significance of the Point Horopter

Much of the literature since the time of Helmholtz and Hering has concentrated on the longitudinal horopter, which ignores the influence of vertical disparities. While it is true that vertical disparity does not give rise to depth perception directly (Hering, 1864; Ogle, 1955), the presence of vertical disparity at a point will degrade the perception of depth from horizontal disparities at that point. Ogle (1955), studying stereoacuity at 0.5° above the fovea, found the degradation to be a continuous function of the vertical disparity, and that it began to be detectable at a vertical disparity of about 10 arc-minutes. A similar conclusion was reached by Friedman et al. (1978). Mitchell (1970) found that horizontal vergence eye movements were attenuated by the presence of vertical disparities of up to 1°, depending on the stimulus configuration. Thus for both depth perception and vergence eye movements the presence of vertical disparities has a substantial (if negative) effect on disparity processing.

Vertical disparities are also of direct relevance to the fusion system, since their presence can cause diplopia even more readily than do horizontal disparities. Schor and Tyler (1981), for example, showed that vertical disparities as small as 1 arc-minute may be out of the fusional range for some types of stimuli.

It follows that a description of the metric of binocular space in terms of horizontal disparities alone is incomplete, and that the longitudinal criterion for the definition of the horopter is insufficient. For this reason an extensive description of the neglected point horopter, which takes vertical disparity fully into account, follows.

THE POINT HOROPTER AND EFFECTS OF CONVERGENCE

Fixation at Infinity and Shear of "Vertical" Meridians

The simplest case of all for the point horopter is when fixation is at optical infinity. Here rays from each point in the frontal "plane" at infinity are parallel and this is therefore the only case where the geometric point horopter can be considered a plane; however, there is already a complication. Volkmann (1859) and Helmholtz (1866) found that corresponding meridians in the vertical direction are each tilted outward about 1° from the true vertical where the eyes are in the primary position of gaze. No such tilt of corresponding meridians appears in the horizontal direction. Since this tilt is anisometropic to the vertical direction, it is best described as a shear of retinal correspondence.

The Helmholtz shear completely alters the plane of the point horopter for parallel fixation. Figure 7.3 shows the projection through the

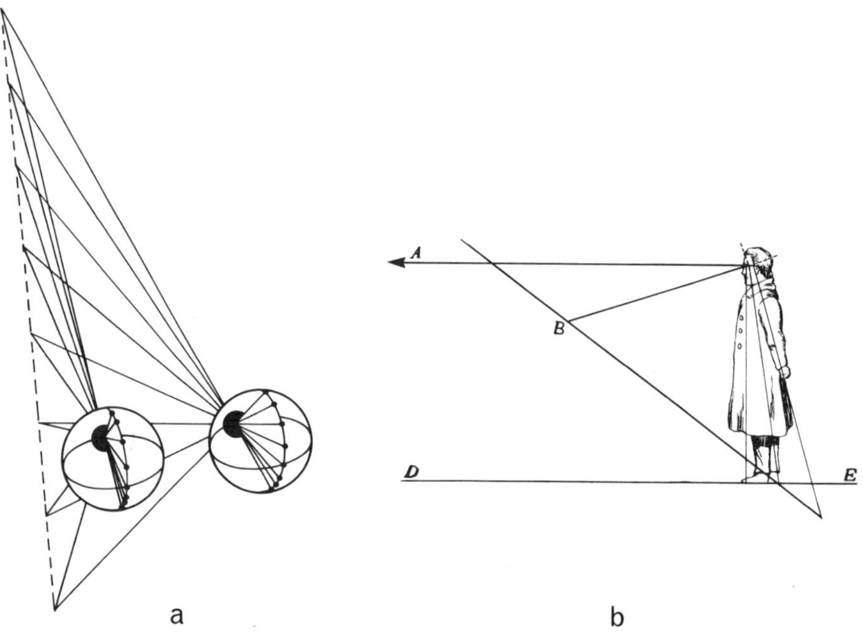

FIGURE 7.3. A Projection of vertical meridians, showing that if the meridians are straight (i.e., great circles) they must project in two planes that meet in a straight line, rather than any kind of circle. In addition, if the vertical meridians are tilted relative to each other, the line in which they meet will be inclined in the third dimension relative to the observer. B The angle of inclination of the midline horopter line depends jointly on the tilt of the vertical meridians and the fixation distance. The average midline tilt is 2°, which means the midline horopter will pass approximately through the feet (shown here for fixation at B). With fixation at infinity (A), the midline horopter (D, E) will become horizontal, lying in the ground plane. (After Helmholtz, 1866) At this point the horopter itself becomes a plane. Reprinted by permission of the publisher, from Tyler CW and Scott AB. Binocular Vision. In: Records R, ed. *Physiology of the Human Eye and Visual System*. Hagerstown: Harper and Row, 1979.

pupil of the corresponding "vertical" meridian of each eye, when convergence is parallel and symmetric. Each projection forms a plane in space, and the intersection of these two planes defines the horopter in the vertical midline plane, which is inclined backward in space. If the relative tilt or shear of the corresponding "vertical" meridians is fixed, it follows that the inclination of the vertical horopter varies with fixation distance. For fixation at infinity, the projected planes meet in a horizontal line running below the eyes, roughly in the plane of the ground when the observer is standing. For parallel fixation on the horizon the projections of all other meridians' corresponding points will also intersect in the ground plane extending to the horizon. Helmholtz therefore suggested that the 2° shear has an adaptive function of bringing the horopter into the plane of the ground, on which are located most of the objects of survival value to the human organism.

Point Horopter with Symmetric Fixation in the Visual Plane

To introduce the basic form of the point horopter, a simplified case will be considered with only symmetric fixation in the visual plane. In this position eye torsion may be considered to be zero. Retinal correspondence will be defined geometrically and optical aberrations will be assumed to be absent.

Allowing symmetric convergence at points closer to the observer than infinity has another consequence of significance concerning points away from the horizontal or vertical axes. It will be analyzed on the assumption that no cyclorotatory eye movements occur. As shown in Figure 7.4, it is generally the case that off-axis points in space project to the two retinas with both horizontal and vertical disparities. With convergence, the only exceptions are when a point is at the distance corresponding to the horopter, which would nullify the horizontal disparity. Note that nothing can be done to nullify the vertical disparity produced by off-axis points being necessarily closer to one eye than the other, with a resulting difference in the projection angle in the two eyes. Thus all off-axis points in a frontal plane through the fixation point (except at infinity) project with some vertical disparity to the two eyes, and are therefore not included in the horopter.

The only points in space that will project in correspondence in this case are those in the vertical midline as described above, and those along the horizontal midline through the fovea. The latter form a component of the symmetric point horopter designated as the Vieth-Müller circle (although it was first specified by Aguilonius, 1613). The Vieth-Müller circle passes horizontally through the point of fixation and the nodal points of the two eyes, since in this circle all points on the circumference

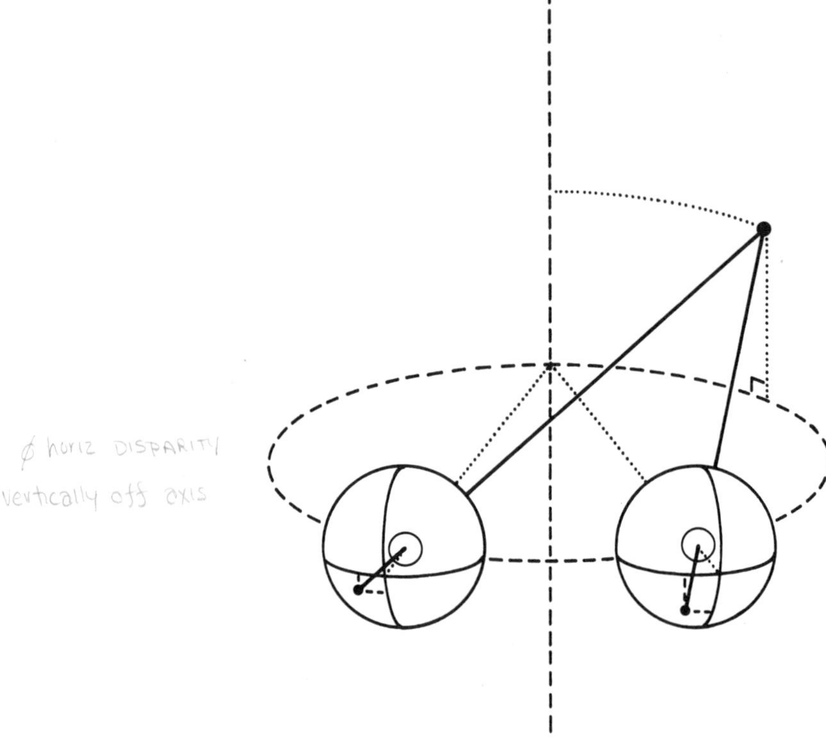

FIGURE 7.4. For convergence at any distance other than infinity, all points that do not lie on the Vieth-Muller circle or the midline horopter project to the retina with either a vertical disparity or both a vertical and horizontal disparity. Dashed lines show geometric horopter for symmetric fixation. Construction lines are dotted. Solid lines represent relevant light rays. The vertical disparity arises from the differential magnification occurring when the point is closer to one eye than the other, as must occur with all points off the vertical axis. The three-dimensional point horopter is therefore not a surface but a line and a circle in space. Reprinted by permission of the Mayo Foundation, from Ogle KN. *Researches in Binocular Vision*. Philadelphia: W.B. Saunders Company, 1950.

have the same disparity between the two nodal points. It should be emphasized that all other points in space project with some horizontal or vertical disparity to the two eyes, and are therefore not part of the point horopter. The geometric point horopter for symmetric fixation in the horizontal visual plane, therefore, consists solely of an inclined vertical line and a horizontal circle (see Figure 7.4).

Point Horopter with Asymmetric Convergence in the Visual Plane

In asymmetric convergence the point of convergence lies outside the median plane of the head. This is an important case to consider, not only because it occurs in normal viewing, but also because in many respects it is equivalent to symmetric fixation with a unilateral image magnification (aniseikonia), such as occurs in unilateral aphakia (lens removal). The simplest type of asymmetric convergence is where the point of convergence lies in the visual plane of the eyes. Here the same logic that generated the Vieth-Müller circle implies that as the eyes fixate at different points around a given Vieth-Müller circle, the horizontal horopter always falls on the same circle.

The vertical line component of the horopter also remains essentially fixed in space directly in front of the observer as the eyes are moved around the Vieth-Müller circle, rather than following the position of the fixation (Figure 7.5A). This occurs because the difference in image mag-

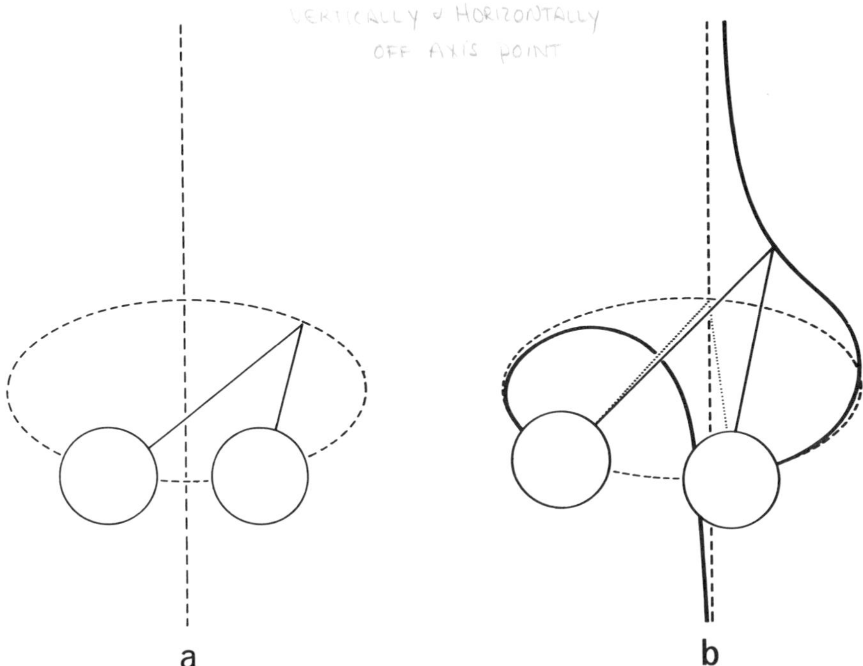

FIGURE 7.5. A Geometric horopter with asymmetric fixation (*dashed lines*). Note that both the Vieth-Müller circle and the vertical horopter lines remain fixed in space as fixation moves around Vieth-Müller circle. B Geometric horopter with asymmetric fixation away from both horopter lines. Horopter (*solid line*) becomes a one-turn helix winding around the symmetric horopter (*dashed line*).

nification away from the "vertical" meridian is a function of the distance of the image from each eye, which is essentially unaffected by ocular rotation (except that the center of rotation differs slightly from the nodal point of the eye). Thus in eccentric fixation to the left, the foveal image in the left eye is magnified relative to that in the right eye. The magnification is equal only for the stimuli lying in the median plane of the head, which project onto peripheral lines on the retinas. The direct consequence of this geometry is that in eccentric fixation, regions projecting immediately above and below the fovea have an inherent vertical disparity that must affect both stereopsis and fusion.

Generalized Point Horopter in Asymmetric Convergence

Finally, the most general case is to allow fixation at any point, involving asymmetric convergence away from both the median and horizontal planes. This case was developed in detail by Helmholtz (1866) and is a curve of the third degree that forms a single-loop spiral (Figure 7.5B) within an abstract cylinder projected up and down from the Vieth-Müller circle. For any point of asymmetric fixation, the point horopter consists solely of this single-loop spiral line.

Helmholtz's curve may be construed as the geometric result of stretching the line and circle horopter so as to pass through the point of asymmetric fixation. Thus the generalized helix of the point horopter is constrained to pass through the point of fixation and the nodal points of the two eyes, and to become asymptotic to the vertical line at infinity.

Effects of Eye Torsion on the Form of Horopter

The occurrence of eye torsion with different positions of gaze and degrees of convergence is discussed in Chapter 16. The main point of interest here is that with both convergence and gaze elevation the eyes rotate in opposite directions about the visual axes (cyclovergence), producing either intorsion or extorsion according to whether the tops of the eyeballs move toward or away from each other. This section is concerned with the effects of such cyclovergence on the form of the horopter.

One point to emphasize is that the effects of cyclovergence differ substantially from the effects of the shear of the vertical meridians shown in Figure 7.3. Consider, for example, the situation of parallel vergence. If there were neither shear of the vertical meridians nor relative ocular torsion, a frontal "plane" at infinity would project in correspondence at every point, forming a horopter surface. As described above, a purely horizontal shear in the correspondence tilts the entire horopter surface into the horizontal plane at some distance above or below the observer's eyes, depending on the sign and degree of the shear. Ocular cyclovergence, on the other hand, reduces the parallel vergence horopter to a single line in the median plane, inclined according to the degree of torsion. The reason for this constriction of the horopter from a surface to a line is that cyclovergence introduces vertical disparities at all points away from the vertical meridian, which are maximal in the horizontal meridian. Wherever there is a vertical disparity there is no point horopter. The only region where such disparities are zero is an inclined line in the median plane. Note, however, that this example is given merely to illustrate the difference between shear and cyclovergence. In the normal eye, there is no ocular torsion with fixation in the primary position, and hence the shear of correspondence is the only effect that need be taken into account.

In normal individuals, cyclovergence occurs under two conditions—when the eyes are converged and when the gaze is directed downward. The extent is detailed in Chapter 16, but in each case reaches a maximal value of about 3°. The effects of the two conditions are additive. Figure 7.6A shows the effect of convergent extorsion on the point horopter with fixation at eye level before (dashed curve) and after (solid curve) cyclovergence is taken into account. The vertical horopter becomes inclined with the top further away from the observer, while still passing through the fixation point. The Vieth-Müller circle becomes inclined down out

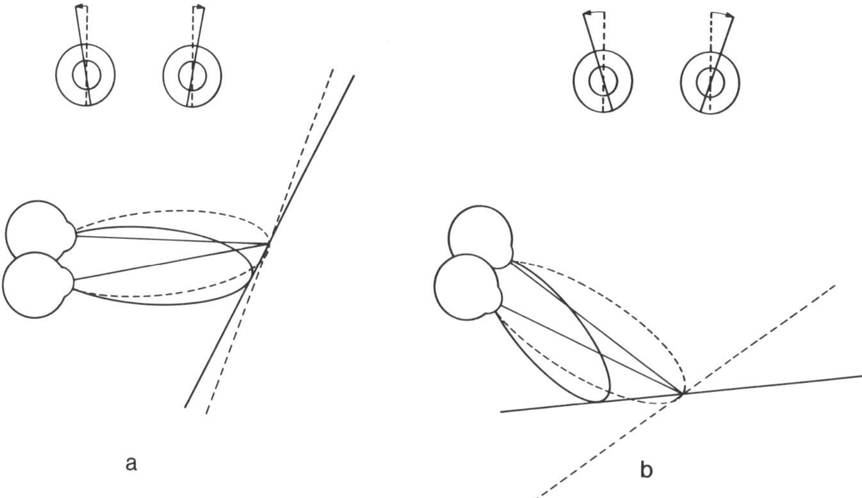

FIGURE 7.6. A Additional tilt of horopter produced by cyclovergence occurring with convergence (*solid lines*). Inset shows frontal view of ocular torsion. Dashed lines show horopter without cyclovergence, for the same fixation position. B Further tilt of horopter (*solid line*) from geometric position in down gaze (*dashed line*) caused by convergent plus down gaze extorsion.

of the visual plane. As before, no other points in visual space are in both horizontal and vertical correspondence.

Directing the gaze up or down without altering convergence also induces cyclovergence, generally extorsion. The most consistent effect is in down gaze, which is the only case discussed here. Two conditions are considered: down gaze with fixation at infinity and down gaze with convergence.

Parallel down gaze, which is unlikely for a standing observer, might occur if the observer were lying on the ground with the head raised at 45° to look at the horizon. In this situation, the eyes would extort by about 3°, conveniently causing the horopter to become horizontal in the manner described above. It will be below but parallel to the ground plane, although as already pointed out, the fact that it is being produced by cyclovergence will constrain it to a single line rather than a plane.

Finally, extorsion accompanying down gaze will add to that induced by convergence if fixation is brought to a near point (Figure 7.6B). This is a common occurrence; it occurs, for example, when a person reads a book. It will further incline the vertical horopter in relation to its position in down gaze if no cyclovergence were to occur. This case is illustrated in Figure 7.6B, with the dashed lines showing the position of the horopter without cyclovergence, and the full lines indicating its position after cyclovergence is taken into account.

EMPIRICAL EVIDENCE FOR THE FORM OF THE HOROPTER

Vieth-Müller Circle in the Visual Plane

As mentioned previously, the measurements of the empirical longitudinal horopter by Hering (1864) and Hillebrand (1893) and Ogle (1932) showed consistent deviations from the geometric Vieth-Müller circle, with somewhat different forms if the horopter was measured in terms of equal visual direction or by the more perceptual criteria of the range of fusion or equal perceived distance.

Ogle (1932, 1950) showed that the empirical horopter in the visual plane is well described by a curve from the mathematical class of conic sections, which would imply that it is a circle, ellipse, straight line, or hyperbola, depending on the radius of curvature at the point of fixation. If the Hering-Hillebrand deviation from the Vieth-Müller circle is equivalent to a fixed amount of angular disparity at each angle of eccentricity, the form of the horopter will change with fixation distance. (It is only when there is no deviation from the Vieth-Müller circle that the horopter will remain a circle as fixation distance varies.) A family of curves for different fixation distances is shown in Figure 7.7, illustrating how the

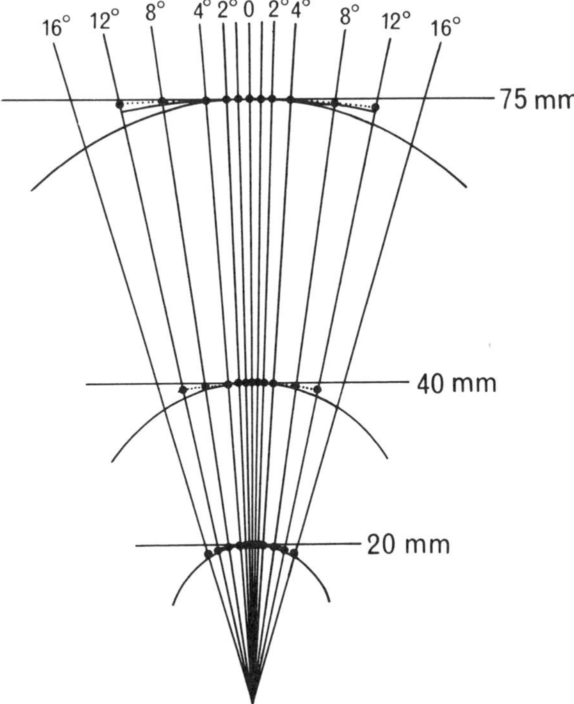

FIGURE 7.7. Hering-Hillebrand deviation (*dashed lines*) from the geometric horopter circle (*solid line arcs*). Note the change in form of the deviation with fixation distance, although the retinal disparity maintains a fixed deviation from geometric correspondence. Reprinted by permission of the Mayo Foundation, from Ogle KN. *Researchers in Binocular Vision*. Philadelphia: W.B. Saunders Company, 1950.

empirical horopter progressively curves away from the observer as fixation distance increases. In fact, these data are for the criterion of a frontoparallel plane, but the nonius horopter undergoes similar changes (Ogle, 1932).

Some form of the Hering-Hillebrand deviation would be expected if nasal eccentricity were larger than temporal eccentricity for every pair of corresponding points, and this difference increases with eccentricity. A point in the left visual field must project at a greater angle from the fovea on the nasal retina of the left eye than on the temporal retina of the right eye to hit corresponding receptors. Hence the point must lie behind the geometric Vieth-Müller circle. If the noncongruence of corresponding retinal points is fixed, it would be equivalent to a constant angular deviation of the empirical horopter from the Vieth-Müller circle, as the empirical horopter varies its curvature with fixation distance. In fact, the angular deviation of the nonius horopter changes with the viewing distance, but it is not clear whether this change represents a plasticity of correspondence or perhaps the stretching of the retina during accommodation (Hollins, 1974).

Empirical Vertical Horopter

The discussion of the inclined line that constitutes the vertical horopter was based on Helmholtz's (1866) analysis of the tilt of "vertical" meridians measured monocularly. It is only very recently that any direct measurements of binocular correspondence in the vertical meridian have been attempted. Direct measurements over a 60° range using a method of minimal interocular apparent movement were reported by Nakayama, Tyler, and Appelman (1977) and Nakayama (1977) in both horizontal and vertical meridians. The data for four observers are shown in Figure 7.8.

The first requirement is to establish whether there is any cyclovergence between the two eyes. This was achieved by measuring vertical disparities for stimuli within the horizontal meridians (lower graphs in Figure 7.8). It can be seen that there is very little systematic deviation in this meridian, so that cyclovergence is less than 1° for any observer. For horizontal disparities with stimuli in the vertical meridian, a substantial deviation from the geometric zero line is evident (upper graphs in Figure 7.8). This corresponds to an interocular tilt between the corresponding "vertical" meridians of between 2° and 5°.

These data essentially confirm Helmholtz's analysis in three interesting particulars:

1. There is a relative extorsion of the corresponding "vertical" meridians of the two retinas, which has substantial implications for the form of the horopter away from the median plane.
2. This extorsion is not due to cyclorotation or optical factors, but must be attributed to a shear in the cortical representation of the retinal projections from the two eyes.
3. The data are a good fit to a straight line, confirming that the empirical vertical horopter is a straight (inclined) line in space, and does not form a toroid or any other curved surface, as has sometimes been supposed.

The tilt of the vertical horopter can explain some results of Breitmeyer, Julesz, and Kropfl (1976), who set out to do stereoperimetry in the foveal region using dynamic random-dot stereograms with a six-minute (6′) stereoscopic test field. They found an up-down anisotropy such that in the upper field best detection was behind the point of fixation, while

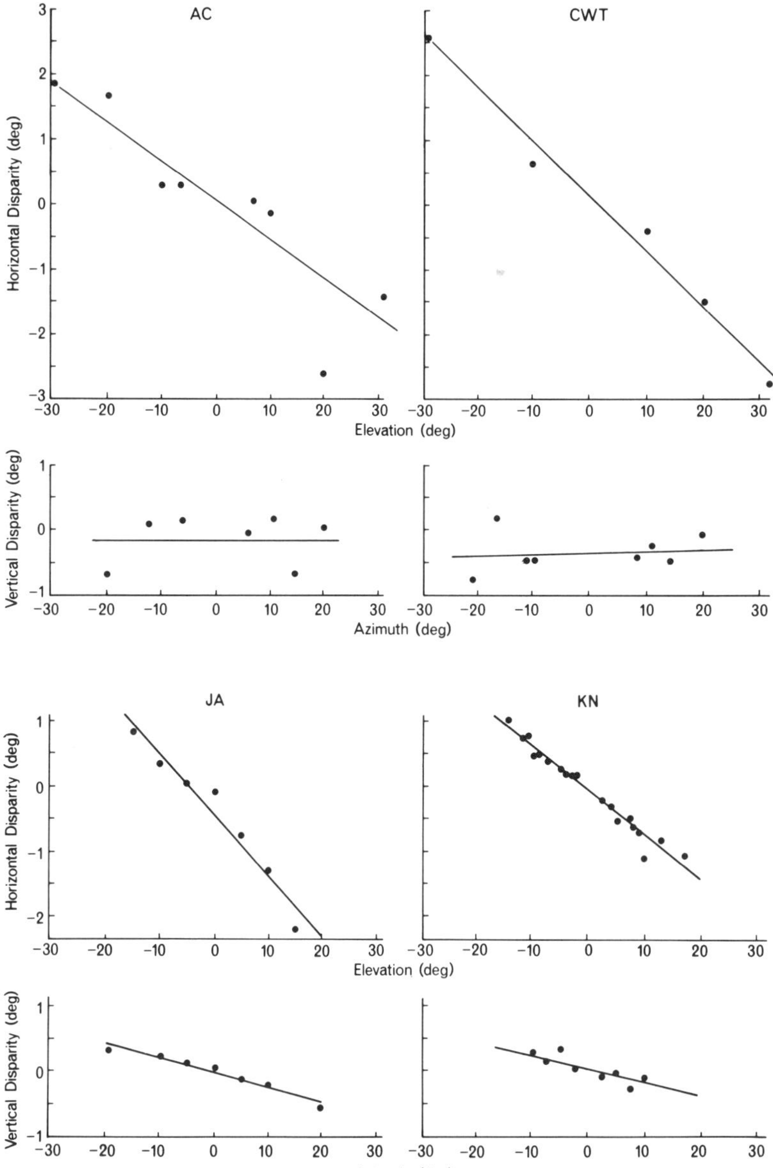

FIGURE 7.8. Measurements of the tilt of the vertical horopter by nulling the visual direction of interocular apparent motion for four observers. Upper graphs of each pair show horizontal disparities as a function of distance up and down the vertical meridian. Lower graphs are control data for ocular cyclovergence, showing vertical disparities along the horizontal meridian.

in the lower field it was in front of the point of fixation. The regions of best detection correspond well with the points at which the stereoscopic plane formed by the random dots projects onto the inclined vertical horopter, although the authors were unaware of Helmholtz's analysis at the time.

The next question that might be asked is, how does the shear of the vertical horopter affect the perception of vertical planes in front of an observer? This was addressed by Cogan (1979), who made a direct comparison between horopter inclination and perceived inclination in depth. He first confirmed in a dichoptic task that the observers showed a relative shear of the "vertical" meridians (between 1.5° and 3.2° for his eight observers). At the viewing distance of 1 m these tilts corresponded to a mean inclination in space of 31° (top of line tilting backward). He then asked observers to set a binocularly viewed line to appear vertical. On average, they inclined the line only 3° backward. Thus the perception of vertical was almost veridical, and perceptual compensation for the shear of the "vertical" meridians was almost complete.

Another phenomenon that can be explained by the inclination of the vertical horopter is the appearance of binocular moiré fringes observed in vertical gratings (Piggins, 1978). Such fringes are best observed in counterphase gratings, and seem to occur because the grating breaks up into horizontal strips along the angle of the vertical horopter (Tyler, 1980). This and the above result exemplify the way in which the rather abstract construct of the vertical horopter can influence perception of diverse stimuli.

BINOCULAR FUSION

Classical Theories of Fusion

There have been four classic approaches to the binocular fusion of stimuli in the two eyes into a single percept: the synergy, local sign, eye movement, and the suppression hypotheses. Each is subject to serious misgivings and all four have been rendered essentially obsolete by neurophysiological data on binocular responses of cortical neurons, which give rise to a fifth, physiological hypothesis. Since elements of several of the classic hypotheses are incorporated into the physiological hypothesis, they will be briefly described.

In the synergy hypothesis, Panum (1858) originated the suggestion that binocular fusion is due to the "binocular synergy of single vision by corresponding circles of sensation." By this he appeared to mean that the stimulus in one retina could be physiologically fused with a range of similar stimuli around the point of precise correspondence in the other retina. This range is now known as Panum's area. Nevertheless, information as to which point within the "corresponding circle of sensation" is stimulated is not lost, but remains available in the visual system for perception of depth. This last stipulation is necessary because while the range of binocular disparities allowing fusion is typically in the region of 10 to 20 arc minutes, stereoscopic depth may be perceived from a disparity 100 times smaller.

The problem with the synergy hypothesis is that it seems contradictory that the positional information within the region of the corresponding circle of sensation is simultaneously lost for fusion and available for stereopsis. Thus Panum's hypothesis progresses little beyond a description of the data.

The local sign hypothesis was first applied to stereopsis and binocular fusion by Hering (1864). Essentially, when any point on the retina is stimulated, its position is coded as a "local sign" (or what computer users call an address) as to where the stimulation occurred. As in the synergy hypothesis, there is a small range of binocular disparities for which the local sign is identical, and therefore the image is seen as single. The finer resolution of stereoscopic depth is treated by positing a further "depth sign" that codes the precise binocular disparity information separately from the lateral sign information.

The difficulty with the local sign hypothesis is that it does not explain rivalry between dissimilar forms projected to corresponding points in the two eyes (Helmholtz, 1866). For example, a dot to one eye may fall in precise correspondence with one part of a line to the other eye. Fusion is not obtained, rather there is rivalry and suppression between the dot and line in the region of correspondence. This is contradictory to the local sign hypothesis since each stimulus should have the same local sign at this point and therefore be perceived as fused.

As an alternative, Helmholtz (1866) proposed an eye movement hypothesis of fusion based on the idea that small eye movements make the image so unstable that precise specification of stimulus position is impossible. It was suggested that the range of imprecision corresponds to the region of fusion. The eye movement hypothesis of fusion is immediately invalidated by the fact of the extremely fine resolution of stereoscopic depth (as described above), which should imply a similar resolution of fixed images.

Developed in an early form in the eighteenth century by du Tour, the suppression hypothesis was more recently revived by Verhoeff (1935). It builds on observations that dissimilar stimuli in corresponding regions of the two retinas rival for attention. It is assumed that the rivalry is due to reciprocal suppression of signals in the visual cortex and that this suppression occurs between similar as well as dissimilar stimuli, although it is not consciously observed when the stimuli are similar. What is ignored by the suppression hypothesis is that alternation between disparate but similar images would produce a perception of apparent motion or displacement of a single stimulus from one position to another. No such displacement is observed in fused disparate images. Thus while interocular suppression undoubtedly occurs in many situations, it cannot provide an explanation for fusion.

The low variability of estimates of binocular visual direction argues strongly for a true binocular fusion mechanism involving a shift in visual direction, as opposed to the other three hypotheses. Similar conclusions were reached by Kertesz (1972) on the basis of a cyclodisparity stimulus. The tendency for observers to see the binocular image closer to one of the two monocular images indicates that some kind of ocular dominance is giving preferential weighting of one eye over the other in the fusion situation. This dominance represents a partial expression of the suppression hypothesis, but complete dominance/suppression was seen in only one of Sheedy and Fry's (1979) eight observers, and then only for smaller disparities.

The conclusion to be reached is that although each hypothesis may have some degree of validity in special circumstances, none provides a complete explanation of sensory fusion, one of the most compelling phenomena of binocular vision.

Physiological Basis of Fusion and Diplopia

An appropriate resolution of the controversy over fusion arises from consideration of the physiological basis of binocularity in the visual cortex, as suggested by Roenne (1956). An initial version of the hypothesis was based on the distribution of disparities of the binocular receptive fields (Joshua and Bishop, 1970). In its current form this hypothesis would rely on neurophysiological data on different types of binocular neurons in the visual cortex. Hubel and Wiesel (1962) showed that some neurons in cat cortex could be driven by stimulation of an appropriate region of either eye (binocular neurons), whereas others responded only to stimulation of one eye (monocular neurons). In addition, several groups of investigators (Barlow et al., 1967, Hubel and Wiesel, 1970) have found that while some binocular neurons had receptive fields at exactly corresponding points on the two retinas, others had receptive fields with various degrees of binocular disparity in one of any of the retinal meridians. Their interpretation of these disparite neurons detectors as the basis for stereoscopic depth perception is open to question, but the relevance for the theory of binocular fusion is hard to dispute.

Thus neurophysiologically we may define four classes of neurons having binocular corresponding, binocular disparate, monocular right, and monocular left receptive fields (Figure 7.9). Presumably, each neuron is labeled for a specific visual direction. The visual direction is unam-

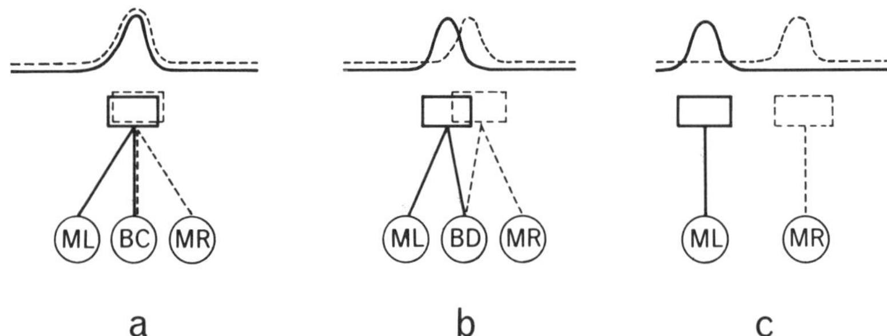

FIGURE 7.9. Model of binocular fusion and diplopia, considered from the point of view of four classes of cortical neuronal receptive field with similar visual directions: monocular, left eye (ML); monocular, right eye (MR); binocular corresonding (BC); and binocular disparate (BD). Monocular stimulus inputs to these receptive fields are shown as solid (L) and dashed (R) lines; A = zero; B = small; and C = large binocular disparities. Reprinted by permission of the publisher, from Tyler CW and Scott AB. Binocular Vision. In: Records R, ed. *Physiology of the Human Eye and Visual System*. Hagerstown: Harper and Row, 1979.

biguous for all classes except the binocular disparate, where we shall assume that it falls midway between the visual directions of the two monocular receptive fields for that neuron.

When sets of stimuli are presented to each of the two eyes so that they project to corresponding points, the binocular corresponding neurons and monocular right and left neurons with the same local sign are stimulated. Since all three types have the same visual direction label, there is no conflict and the stimulus, encoded as the sum of all neurons responding, is seen as single.

When a small disparity is introduced between the sets of points, some binocular disparate neurons are stimulated and the binocular corresponding neurons should cease responding. Now, however, the monocular right and monocular left neurons that receive equivalent images have local signs slightly to either side of the mean visual direction signaled by the binocular disparate neurons (Figure 7.9). It is assumed that the two monocular visual directions (which would be discriminably different if presented singly) are integrated with that signaled by the binocular disparate neurons. There should therefore be a range of small disparities that gives a unitary perception of a fused stimulus.

Finally, if the disparity between the sets of points is increased beyond the range in which binocular response can be integrated with the two monocular responses, each monocular response is associated with a different visual direction and two diplopic sets of stimuli are perceived.

Thus the neurophysiology results can explain many perceptual states arising from binocular stimulation. Note, however, that the basic disparity in binocular receptive fields has been considered as a basis for fusion and departures from it, rather than for stereopsis.

CHARACTERISTICS OF FUSION

Retinal Eccentricity, Fusion, and Cyclofusion

The limiting disparity at which binocular fusion breaks down varies as a function of retinal eccentricity (Figure 7.10) (an average of the three observers fully measured) by (Ogle, 1950). Thus Panum's area is not a fixed size, but increases roughly in proportion to distance from the fovea.

This increase in fusion limit is adaptive from three standpoints. One is that the size of retinal receptive fields and hence visual acuity both show a proportional change with eccentricity. It is appropriate for the size of Panum's area to be matched to the monocular grain of the retina at each point.

The increase in Panum's area is also adaptive in terms of the bi-

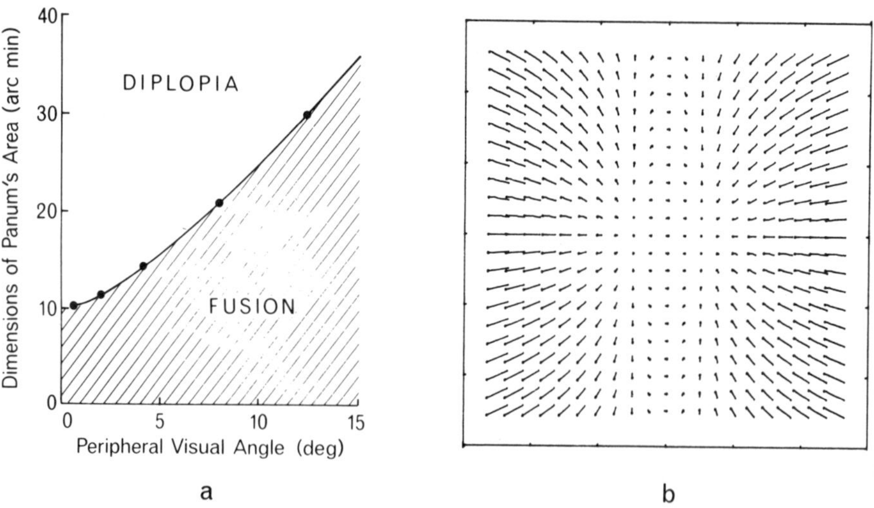

FIGURE 7.10. A Variation in the horizontal disparity of Panum's area of binocular fusion with retinal eccentricity (the average of three observers measured by Ogle, 1950). B The field of geometric disparities of a flat plane viewed at 20 cm and slightly in front of the fixation point. Field size is ±38° in each direction. Relatively large disparities can occur in peripheral regions under conditions that might occur while reading or writing. Reprinted by permission of the publisher, from Nakayama K. Geometrical and physiological aspects of depth perception. In: *Image Processing*, S. Benton, Ed. Proceedings of the Society of Photo-Optical Instrumentation Engineers, 1977.

nocular environment. Figure 7.10 shows the disparities produced by binocular viewing of a plane inclined at the angle of the vertical horopter at a distance of 50 cm. This situation might occur when a person reads a book or other flat material at a comfortable reading distance. The disparities of points lying in the plane at large distances from the foveas are substantial, and increase roughly in proportion to degree of eccentricity. A corresponding increase in Panum's area therefore allows a much larger region of such a plane to appear fused than would otherwise be the case.

The third reason why it is helpful to have fusion increasing with eccentricity is that it allows a degree of sensory cyclofusion. If Panum's area remained constant at all eccentricities, the maximum cyclodisparity between two line images extending across the retinas would remain fused for only about 4′. As it is, the increase in Panum's area with eccentricity theoretically allows fusion for up to about 2° of cyclodisparity (Ogle, 1950). In practice, the extent of cyclofusion depends on the size and configuration of the stimulus (Kertesz, 1972), as does the extent of Panum's area itself (Tyler, 1973).

The Fusion Horopter

One can measure the total region of space around a given point of convergence for which point stimuli appear fused. This empirical fusion horopter is depicted in Figure 7.11 for the special case of symmetric convergence in the visual plane A and for the general case of asymmetric convergence off the visual plane B (from Tyler and Scott, 1979). Note that the fusion horopter runs wide of the geometric Vieth-Müller circle due to the Hering-Hillebrand deviation. The narrowing of Panum's area near fixation produces thinning of the asymmetric fusion horopter B in this region. The case for asymmetric fixation is based on the Helmholtz one-turn helix described in a previous section. The rather strange forms in Figure 7.11 represent the only regions of space that produce fused visual images of point sources of light under the selected conditions of fixation. Linksz (1954) has suggested that the fusion horopter has the form of a torus, but his analysis is based on an incorrect assumption and is not empirically validated (as has been pointed out).

Spatial Limits

It is a common experience that larger objects in the field remain fused over a greater range of disparities than smaller objects. To this extent, fusion depends on the spatial extent of the stimulus. It is also evident that blurred images will show a greater fusional range than sharply focussed images.

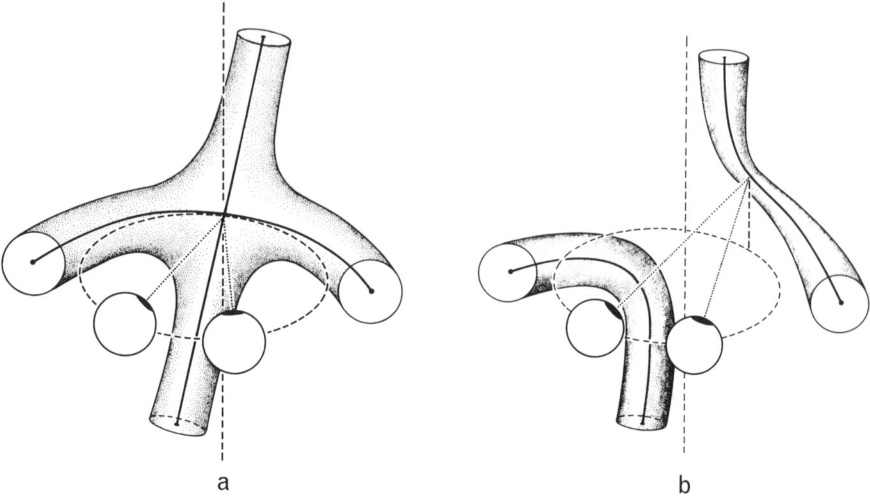

Figure 7.11. A The empirical fusion horopter for symmetric fixation in the visual plane. Note the spread away from the geometric horopter (*dashed line*) due to the Hering-Hillebrand deviation, and the vertical inclination due to the Helmholtz shear of the vertical meridians. B The generalized empirical fusion horopter for any other fixation point. Note that asymmetric fixation produces a dramatic reduction of the fused region near the fixation point. Reprinted by permission of the publisher, from Tyler CW and Scott AB. Binocular Vision. In: Records R, ed. *Physiology of the Human Eye and Visual System*. Hagerstown: Harper and Row, 1979.

More systematically, fusion has been studied as a function of size of the waves in a sinusoidal line stimulus (Tyler, 1973). A sinusoidal wavy line was presented to one eye to be fused with a straight line in the other. When the lines were horizontal, the threshold for fusion of vertical disparities remained reasonably constant (Figure 7.12), but when they were vertical, Panum's area for horizontal disparities varied dramatically with the size of the waves. The maximum horizontal disparity could be as much as 1° when the waves had a period of 30° per cycle, and became as small as 2′ when the period was reduced to 20′ per cycle. This all occurred with the stimulus passing through the fovea.

Thus the traditional concept of Panum's area as a fixed property of a given retinal region must be abandoned. Instead, the fusional extent is strongly dependent on the stimulus used to measure it. Hence the fusional horopter presented above is not a fixed range around the point horopter, and the depictions of Figure 7.11 must be taken only as an indication of the fusional range in the real world, which will expand and contract according to the objects present in the field and the optical characteristics of the eyes viewing them.

Temporal Aspects

One interesting aspect of the fusion is that it is established in a very short time. Helmholtz (1866) had experimented with fusion in stereograms illuminated by a (microsecond) electric spark. Woo (1974) examined the effect of duration systematically and found that fusion appeared to be complete by about 30 msec. This is probably the same as the luminance integration time under his conditions, so the speed of fusion for flashed targets seems to be limited mainly by the rate of integration of luminance.

However, the extent of Panum's area is affected substantially by the temporal characteristics of the stimulus presentation. Fender and Julesz (1967), using a binocular retinal image stabilizer to control eye move-

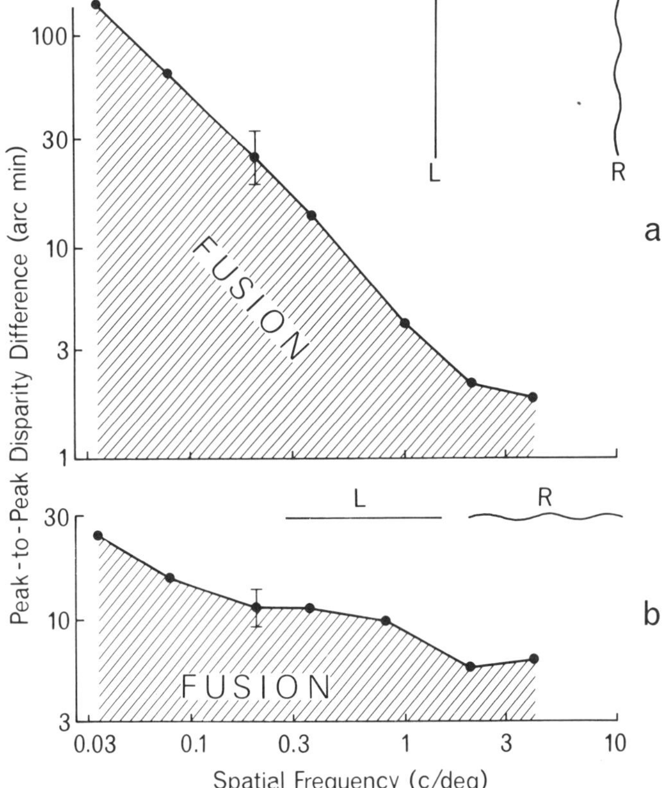

FIGURE 7.12. Fusion limit as a function of stimulus pattern. For horizontal disparities (A) fusion limit increases for stimuli with large cycles and decreases for stimuli with very small cycles. For vertical disparities (B) the fusion limit remains much more constant. Insets show left (L) and right (R) eye views of the stimulus.

ments, increased horizontal disparity from zero at various fixed rates. They found that for line stimuli Panum's area could be increased from the classical value of 14 arc-minutes to 65 arc-minutes of uncrossed disparity by continuously increasing disparity at a rate of 2 arc-minutes per second. (Note that the larger range found for random-dot stimuli was not in a fusion task but a depth perception task, and thus has nothing to do with the fusion mechanism.) In a follow-up study, Diner (1978) found that much of this increase could be attributed not to an extension of Panum's area, but to a shift in the mean disparity about which fusion occurred. The maximum rate for which this shift could be obtained was 8 arc-minutes per second.

Another approach to the temporal characteristics of fusion is to use sinusoidal temporal modulation of the disparity. Schor and Tyler (1981) applied this approach using vertical lines 0.5° on either side of the fovea, which were disparity-modulated in counterphase. This display effectively controlled the effects of eye movements since vergent tracking of one stimulus to reduce its disparity would increase the disparity of the other. For eight observers the horizontal extent of Panum's area reached about 18 arc-minutes for low temporal frequencies up to 0.25 Hz, and then gradually declined with increasing frequency to about 3 arc-minutes by about 5 Hz (Figure 7.13, open circles). Thus high temporal frequencies of horizontal disparity modulation appear to constrict Panum's area in a fashion similar to flashed presentations.

Vertical disparities showed a different pattern of behavior. When the whole display was rotated by 90° the lines were horizontal above and below the fovea and the disparities were vertical. The filled circles in Figure 7.13 show that with the same kind of disparity modulation the vertical range of Panum's area reached only about 6 arc-minutes at low temporal frequencies, and fell to about the same value as the horizontal range at high temporal frequencies (3 arc-minutes). Thus it appears that the horizontal range of fusion is extended by low rates of modulation (stimulus velocities), while the vertical range is approximately constant.

Spatiotemporal Interactions

The foregoing sections review evidence for profound interactions between size of the fusion area and both spatial and temporal characteristics of the stimulus. This raises the question of interactions between the effects of these two domains, that is, spatiotemporal effects on the fusional area. This question was also addressed by Schor and Tyler (1981) for both the horizontal and vertical extents of Panum's area. A line stimulus similar to that described above was used, but with both spatial and temporal modulation of disparity. Thus each line in each eye had a sinusoidal

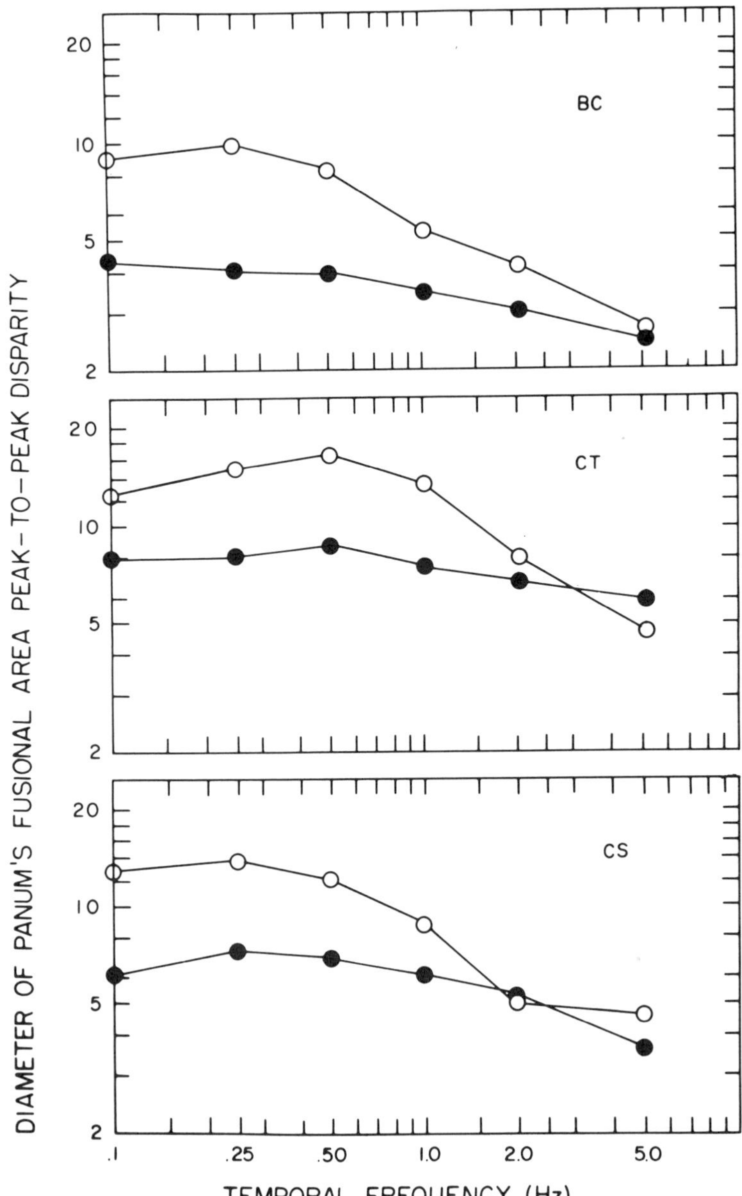

FIGURE 7.13. Open and filled circles depict the size of Panum's area for temporal variations of horizontal and vertical disparities respectively. The vertical disparity of Panum's area is relatively unaffected by temporal frequency for three observers.

spatial modulation that was amplitude-modulated sinusoidally in time (Figure 7.14).

The data are summarized in Figure 7.14 for a full range of stimulus conditions. Each ellipse represents the disparity ranges of Panum's area under given conditions of spatial and temporal modulation of disparity. This figure emphasizes the large variation in size and shape of Panum's area with stimulus conditions. The main effect of spatial frequency of

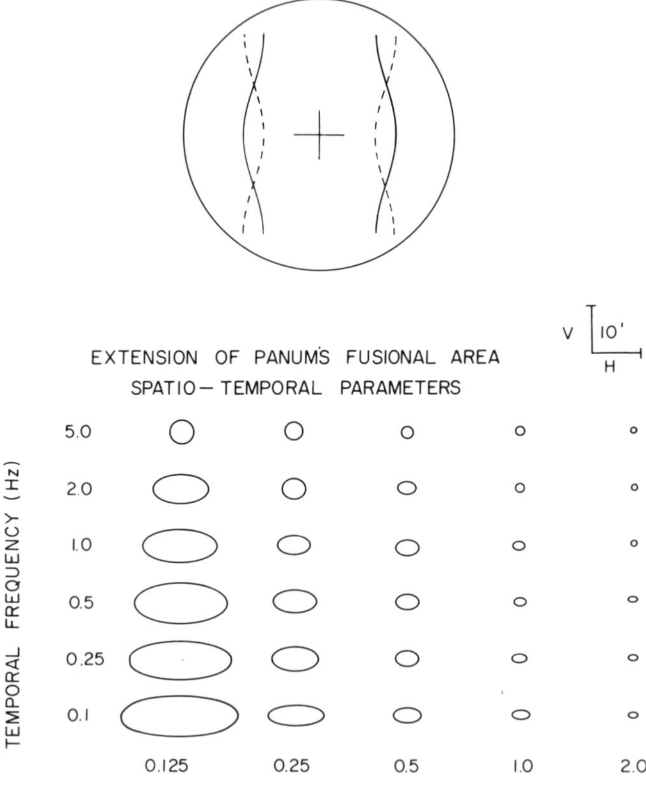

FIGURE 7.14. The size and shape of Panum's area varies with both temporal and spatial characteristics of disparity modulation. The horizontal but not the vertical diameter of the area varies from a maximum of 20 to a minimum of 1.5 arc-minutes. At low temporal and spatial frequencies, the area is elliptical with a ratio of 2.5:1 between the horizontal and vertical extents. At high temporal frequencies the horizontal extent is reduced to equal the fixed vertical extent and the shape becomes circular. Both the horizontal and vertical extents are reduced to 1.5 arc-minutes by increasing spatial modulation frequency to an upper limit of 2 cycles per degree.

disparity modulation occurs at low temporal frequencies, and affects both the horizontal and vertical fusion range. Conversely, the main effect of temporal frequency occurs at low spatial frequencies, but temporal frequency affects the horizontal fusion range much more than the vertical fusion range. Thus the largest extent of Panum's area (25′ by 10′) occurs for slowly changing stimuli with a large spatial extent, while the smallest range (1.5′ by 0.6′) is obtained for fine spatial variations of disparity almost regardless of the rate of temporal change.

In summary, these data radically revise our conception of Panum's area (in unstabilized vision with normal eye movements). Instead of a fixed fusional region there is a strong dependence of fusion on the local stimulus characteristics. Panum's area is a dynamic entity that is continually being adapted to the prevailing features of the stimulus environment.

Evoked Potentials

Many types of binocular interaction are reflected in the cortical visual evoked potential (VEP) recorded from the human scalp. These fall into the categories of binocular summation, binocular rivalry and suppression, and stereopsis, which will be considered separately in the appropriate sections.

Evoked potential amplitude shows partial binocular summation under most conditions, whether the stimulus is a uniform or patterned flickering field (Gouras et al., 1964; Perry et al., 1968; Harter et al., 1973) or an alternating pattern of some kind (Campbell and Maffei, 1970). Complete summation would occur if binocular response were the algebraic sum of the two monocular responses, or when the stimulus contrast required to produce a given response was half as great for binocular stimulation as for a monocular stimulation. In fact, most of the studies cited report only partial binocular summation, in which the binocular response was about 1.4 times greater than the mean monocular response, both near and well above threshold.

These studies all involved transient evoked potentials measured at a single peak. In an earlier study by Spekreijse (1966) the stimulus was a sinusoidally flickering uniform field. This revealed that in many circumstances high-amplitude stimulation produced saturation of the VEP, which could eliminate any appearance of binocular summation. Conversely, an appropriate choice of contrast and field size would reveal full (2.0) summation. Full summation in the evoked potential is compatible with what is known of the neurophysiology. A monocular stimulus should stimulate monocular neurons strongly and binocular neurons partially, whereas a congruent stimulus in the other eye should stimulate the monocular neurons for the other eye, and enhance the response of the binocular neurons. (Note that on this model a response to binocular stimulation is nevertheless partially attributable to monocular neurons). When partial summation is seen in the evoked potential it is indicative of some more complex process at work, such as saturation, inhibition, or other undetermined factor. If a certain stimulus produced a strong response in exclusively binocular neurons but only a weak response in monocular neurons, the summation characteristics would be described as facilitation beyond the level of full summation.

All of these types of summation occur under different stimulus con-

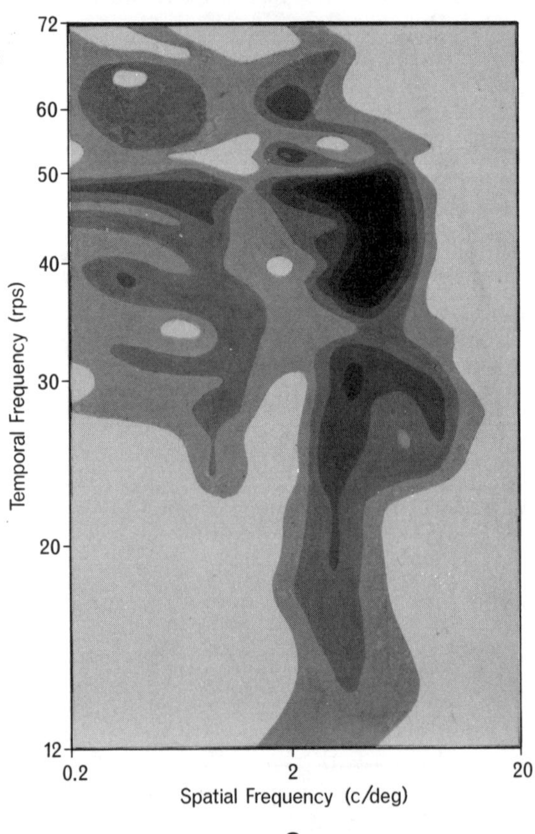

FIGURE 7.15. A Spatiotemporal frequency response plots for the amplitude of the synchronous pattern VEP under monocular conditions. B Degree of binocular facilitation (*hatched areas*) of binocular response relative to monocular response is taken to indicate the responses of purely binocular neurons. Reprinted by permission of the publisher, from Apkarian PA, Nakayama K, Tyler CW. Binocularity in the visual evoked potential: facilitation summation and suppression. Electroencephalography and Clinical Neurophysiology, Elsevier/North-Holland Scientific Publishers Ltd., 1981.

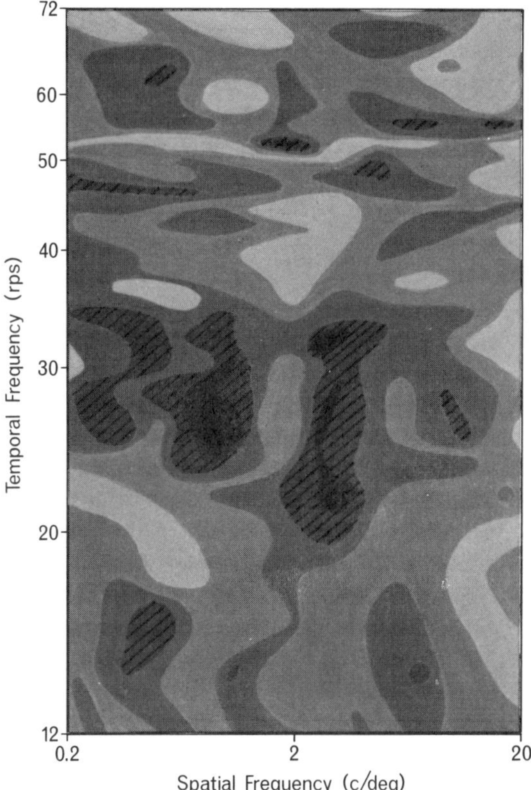

FIGURE 7.15. (*Continued*)

ditions in the normal evoked potential. In fact, the degree of binocular summation is highly specific to the precise spatiotemporal properties of the stimulus. Apkarian, Nakayama, and Tyler (1981) have systematically explored the effects of spatial frequency and temporal frequency (Figure 7.15), and also of contrast and orientation on the amplitude of the synchronous evoked potential induced by alternating sinusoidal gratings. Binocular facilitation up to a ratio of five relative to the monocular responses was seen, but only for narrowly defined spatiotemporal frequency conditions (Figure 7.15). Varying the spatial frequency by 50% or the temporal frequency by 20% could alter the response from maximum facilitation to simple summation, as could rotating the orientation from vertical to horizontal or varying the contrast by 20%. The particular response conditions varied markedly for different observers and different electrode configurations.

These results suggest that the scalp VEP contains components from many highly specific neural populations, and that the stimulus conditions can be used to separate out the responses from these populations. The binocular facilitation responses, for example, probably arise largely from specifically binocular neurons, whose properties can then be studied in the human. In the study by Apkarian and colleagues (1981), facilitation was seen only for spatial frequencies below 5 cycles per degree and temporal frequencies below 30 reversals per second (i.e., 15 Hz). This suggests that the binocular neural population has low spatiotemporal resolution, in contrast to the monocularly driven population, which gives pattern responses up to 30 cycles per degree and as high as 90 reversals per second (Tyler et al., 1978).

DICHOPTIC STIMULATION

Stimulation will be defined as dichoptic when different stimuli fall at the corresponding points in the two eyes. There are six classes of percept that may be obtained by dichoptic stimulation, depending on the degree of noncorrespondence between the stimuli:

1. Depth with fusion.
2. Depth with diplopia.
3. Diplopia without depth.
4. Binocular mixture.
5. Binocular rivalry and suppression.
6. Binocular luster.

The first two classes are dealt with in the section on stereoscopic vision. They are not generally referred to as dichoptic, since the two retinal patterns are sufficiently similar as to be combined into a unified impression (particularly for fused stereopsis). The last four classes are clearly dichoptic. There is little to be said about diplopia except as an indicator of the failure of fusion. This section on dichoptic stimulation is therefore restricted to three topics; binocular mixture, binocular rivalry and suppression, and binocular luster.

Binocular Mixture

Under certain circumstances, different images in the two eyes can be mixed to form a combined visual impression. The earliest known instance of this phenomenon occurs in the description of a telescopic device invented by Galileo in 1613 (Drake and Kowal, 1980). Because Galileo's telescope produced a virtual image, he was unable to superimpose a measuring grid directly on the celestial field for the estimation of planetary and star positions. He circumvented this problem by using an external grid attached to the telescope, which could be viewed with the eye not looking through the instrument. Although the two images were very different, he found that they could be visually superimposed and it was in this way that he made the first observations of the planet Neptune (which he thought was a fixed star). His visual measurements were so accurate that the current computations of Neptune's orbit have been called into question (Drake and Kowal, 1980).

The key to the binocular mixture occurring in this example is that the visual stimuli were bright elements on a dark field so that at each retinal location there was usually an object in only one eye, which would predominate over the dark corresponding region in the other eye. Hence the two images could be mixed binocularly with little or no rivalry occurring between them.

Reports of binocular color mixture of uniform fields of different colors in the two eyes were collated by Helmholtz (1866), although he was unable to obtain the effect himself. Similarly, this author perceives only a grading of contrast during the rivalry of dichoptic colors, without the production of the expected intermediate hues.

Binocular Rivalry

Binocular Rivalry and Suppression

If the images in the two eyes are so different that they fail to fuse when falling on roughly corresponding areas, the resulting conflict is resolved not by binocular summation, but by a temporal alternation between one image and the other. In a given region of retina, the image in one eye predominates while the other is suppressed, and suddenly the suppressed image emerges into perception and dominates the region (Figure 7.16).

Binocular rivalry fluctuations are similar in many respects to fluctuations of attention, and are widely supposed to be under voluntary control. Actually, several studies have found that there is very little voluntary control over which eye dominates at any given time (Blake et al., 1971). The change of dominance is not affected by eye blinks (Barany and Hallden, 1947) or by variations in accommodation or pupil size (Lack, 1971). In fact, the fluctuations in rivalry are well described by a sequentially independent random variable with no periodicities, as though the arrival of each change in dominance had no effect on the occurrence of subsequent changes (Levelt, 1965).

Recently, a series of studies by Fox and co-workers into the characteristics of binocular rivalry have made some headway in determining its location in the visual pathway. Even though this was inferred from psychophysical evidence, the results revealed significant facts about the

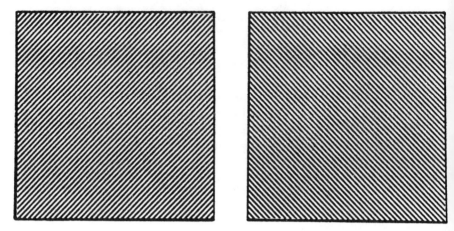

FIGURE 7.16. Stimulus demonstrating strong binocular rivalry when left panel is viewed by left eye and right panel is viewed by right eye in the same retinal location. (After Levelt, 1965) Reprinted by permission of the publisher, from Tyler CW and Scott AB. Binocular Vision. In: Records R, ed. *Physiology of the Human Eye and Visual System*. Hagerstown: Harper and Row, 1979.

processes of binocular cooperation and their breakdown in pathological conditions. With the use of a monocular detection probe stimulus, Fox and Check (1966a) found that suppression has a number of interesting characteristics.

1. The suppression state is inhibitory. Sensitivity was reduced in the suppressed eye for a variety of test probes and testing procedures, including forced-choice detection of incremental light flashes, forced-choice recognition of letter forms, and reaction time for detection of targets set into motion during suppression (Fox and Check, 1966a, 1966b, 1968; Collyer and Bevan, 1970; Wales and Fox, 1970).
2. The magnitude of the inhibitory effect varies among subjects and with stimulus conditions, but is generally on the order of 0.5 log units, a value frequently observed in studies of saccadic suppression and visual masking.
3. The inhibitory effect of suppression endures throughout the duration of the suppression phase, and the magnitude of the inhibition remains constant (Fox and Check, 1972).
4. The inhibitory suppression state acts nonselectively on all classes of test stimuli regardless of their similarity to the rivalry stimulus. Evidence of nonselectivity is the attenuation of several different kinds of test probe stimuli. More systematic evidence of nonselectivity is provided by the use of a spatial frequency grating as a rivalry stimulus while changing either frequency or orientation of the grating during suppression, keeping

mean luminance and contrast constant. Changes in orientation of 45° and of an octave or more in frequency remain undetected (Blake and Fox, 1974a).

These studies suggest that rivalry is a process that is rather independent of monocular pattern recognition, but is triggered by a binocular mismatch and then continues with its own characteristics independently of most stimulus parameters. One factor that is very important, however, is the stimulus effectiveness in each eye. The higher the stimulus strength (in terms of luminance, contrast, or movement) in one eye, the greater the suppression of the other. If the stimulus strength is increased in both eyes equally, the rate of alternation between the two increases (Levelt, 1965; Breese, 1899; Kakizaki, 1960; Fox and Rasche, 1969).

Finally, two interesting experiments have explored the relationship between aftereffects of visual adaptation and rivalry suppression. For the motion aftereffect (Lehmkuhle and Fox, 1975), threshold elevation, and spatial frequency shift after adaptation to a grating (Blake and Fox, 1974b), perceptual occlusion of the stimulus during binocular rivalry did not affect the strength of the aftereffect, whereas equivalent physical occlusion of the stimulus reduced the aftereffect dramatically. In effect, the brain was adapting to an invisible stimulus. Since these aftereffects are almost certainly cortical, binocular rivalry must be occurring at a higher level in the cortex.

Evoked Potentials

A pattern reversal VEP can be recorded during binocular rivalry conditions. Cobb, Morton, and Ettlinger (1967) presented vertical bars to the left eye and horizontal bars to the right eye, with contrast reversals at 12 Hz that were 180° out of phase for the two eyes. The phase changes of the pattern VEP response were well correlated with the subjective responses, indicating changes in perceptual dominance at any given moment. No correlation was found between rivalry suppression and the amplitude of potentials evoked solely by luminance changes.

Similarly, van der Tweel, Spekreijse, and Regan (1970) found that perceptual suppression of a flickering pattern presented to one eye by a static pattern presented to the other eye was accompanied by almost complete suppression of the VEP from the stimulated eye.

How do the VEP rivalry data accord with neurophysiology? The two are in conflict, for the known neurophysiology would suggest that during rivalry the monocular neurons for both eyes are stimulated, whereas the VEP reflects the subjective suppression of one eye at a time. It therefore appears that the site at which the pattern VEP is generated (at least for low frequencies of alternation) is beyond the level of binocular rivalry in the cortex. The rivalry process must then inhibit the response of one set of monocular neurons at a time, producing the reduction in VEP amplitude.

Binocular Luster

Binocular luster is the final class of perception that can occur with non-corresponding stimuli. It occurs in areas of uniform illumination in which the luminance or color is different for the two eyes. It was described by early authors in visual science, such as Panum (1858) and Helmholtz (1866), as a kind of lustrous or shimmering surface of indeterminate depth.

In fact, it may be said that the lustrous appearance of surfaces such as a waxed tabletop or a car body is essentially due to binocular luster. It results from the different position of partially reflected objects in the surface by virtue of the different positions of the two eyes. It is distinct from both the shininess of a surface as seen monocularly by reflected highlights, and from the clear depth image seen in a mirror. The lustrous surface has a translucent quality of depth due to diffusion from the surface, providing a fixation plane at which the large disparities of the partial reflections produce areas of binocular luminance difference.

That the phenomenon of binocular luster has been largely ignored, except as an incidental observation, is surprising in view of the fact that it is qualitatively different from depth, diplopia, or rivalry. The lustrous region cannot be localized in depth, but seems unitary and does not fluctuate in the manner of binocular rivalry.

Recent work (Julesz, 1960; Julesz and Tyler, 1976; Tyler and Julesz, 1976) has demonstrated that binocular luster may also be observed in static and dynamic random-dot stereograms in which all the elements have opposite contrast in the two eyes. When the dots are identical in the two eyes they are perceived as fused, while when they are complemented in contrast in the two eyes the perception is of a lustrous surface. For the identical dot condition fusion will persist even though the dots are rapidly changing in position, providing they always occupy corresponding positions in the two eyes. Such a stimulus provides an opportunity to examine the speed of fusion and defusion in complex stimuli. A change from matching luminance to complementary contrast between the eyes is not visible to either eye alone when the random dots are dynamically changing.

Julesz and Tyler (1976) used this paradigm to show that the average time required for perception of a binocularly identical field interposed between two periods of lustrous stimuli (complemented fields) was 30 msec. The mean time required for detection of the complemented (lustrous) array between two periods of fusion was only 4 msec. This kind of temporal anisotropy was found to be a particular property of the fusion/luster mechanism and no equivalent effect was found for a comparable stereoscopic task. The remarkable performance in luster detection is the most rapid so far demonstrated for any exclusively binocular task, and suggests that binocular luster is a phenomenon worth further study.

STEREOSCOPIC VISION

Binocular Disparity

Stereoscopic vision may be defined as the ability to perceive distances of objects on the basis of visual information available only to a two-eyed observer. Because the two eyes are separated horizontally they receive slightly disparate views of objects at different distances. The field of horizontal retinal disparities combined with information about the directions of the gaze of the two eyes (convergence) provides precise, quantitative information about the distances of the objects from the observer.

Consider the situation close to the line of sight in the normal observer. If both eyes fixate a point object at a given distance (bifoveal fixation), an image of it will fall on the fovea in each eye and there will be no binocular disparity between the images. If the point object is moved closer to the observer, the change in depth may be signalled in two ways: (1) by the resulting binocular disparity and (2) by change in convergence.

1. If an object is placed at a distance other than the fixation distance, there will be a binocular disparity between the images on the retinas (Figure 7.17). This can be interpreted by the observer as separation in depth of the object from the point of convergence. When the object is in front of this point, the lines of sight of the monocular images intersect in front of the point of convergence giving rise to a crossed disparity. If the object is moved away from the observer, the lines of sight cross beyond the convergence distance, and the disparity is described as uncrossed (Ogle, 1952a).

The mistake has sometimes been made of regarding the nasal or temporal halves of the *retinas* as being associated with specific depth information. A nasal shift in crossed disparity and a temporal shift for uncrossed disparity do *not* mean that the images fall on the nasal and the temporal halves of the retinas, respectively, unless the images are at or close to the foveas. Thus if the near object is viewed at 5° eccentricity in the right field (see Figure 7.17), the images will always fall on the temporal retina in the left eye and the nasal retina in the right eye for all disparities (up to 5°), whether crossed, zero, or uncrossed.

2. A second result of moving a point object closer is that the eyes

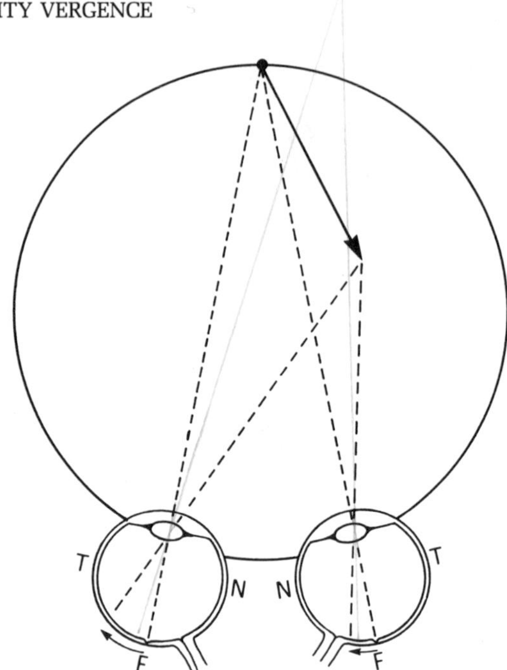

FIGURE 7.17. Objects at different distances (e.g., head and tail of arrow) give rise to horizontal disparities between the images on the two retinas. Such disparities produce stereoscopic depth impressions. Reprinted by permission of the publisher, from Tyler CW and Scott AB. Binocular Vision. In: Records R, ed. *Physiology of the Human Eye and Visual System*. Hagerstown: Harper and Row, 1979.

may converge to the new vergence angle so as to reacquire bifoveal fixation. The difference in convergence angle provides the only cue to the new distance of the point, since the binocular disparity is again zero.

Processing Binocular Disparity

In discussing a field of study it is useful to provide a basic mnemonic of the nature of the domain in question. In the case of binocular disparity, the most relevant feature is the depth (or distance along the line of sight) produced by a given binocular disparity. Figure 7.18 shows schematically how the perceived depth varies as a function of binocular disparity, either crossed or uncrossed. It is derived from experiments in which the perceived depth of briefly flashed disparate images were matched to full-cue depth stimuli (Richards, 1971) or determined by magnitude estimation (Richards and Kaye, 1974).

The aspect of concern here is not so much the magnitudes of disparity or perceived depth, but the form of the function. Near zero disparity there is the stereoacuity threshold below which depth appears to be zero, or indiscriminably different from a flat stimulus. Then there is a region where perceived depth matches the actual depth implied by a given disparity. If all the data were veridical in this way they would fall on the dashed line in Figure 7.18. Beyond a certain point the perceived depth falls away from this line and is less than veridical. Disparity is not being fully processed, but it still gives rise to a large depth sensation. In fact the perceived depth continues to increase up to a maximum, then decreases as the disparity is further enlarged, up to some point (the upper disparity limit) where the disparity is so great that the perceived depth falls to zero (up to 10° of disparity, depending on the stimulus) (Richards and Kaye, 1974).

Figure 7.18 also depicts Panum's limit of binocular fusion. For disparities smaller than the fusion limit the images in the two eyes are perceived as a single, fused object in space. Beyond this limit, the image in each eye is seen separately, causing double vision or diplopia. It is important to note that the largest amount of depth is perceived in this region of diplopia, even though the depth is not veridical. Many students of stereopsis have assumed that depth is weaker or less effective in the region of diplopia, but in fact the reverse is the case. A large range of

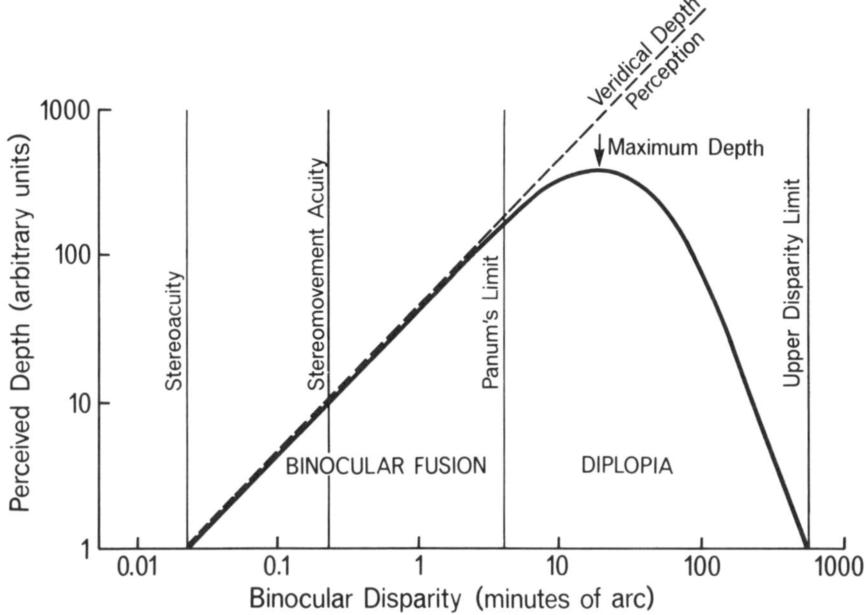

FIGURE 7.18. Schematic of some stereoscopic limits of perceived depth and fusion as a function of binocular disparity (see text for details).

disparities gives rise to depth sensations, and the maximum perceivable depth occurs under diplopic conditions.

This account of stereoscopic limits is at variance with the rubric suggested by Ogle (1950), who maintained that stereopsis up to the point of maximum depth was obligatory (or patent), while beyond this point it was qualitative and variable. Richards (1971) has shown that depth magnitude may be quantified throughout the range of perceived depth, so that there is no region of purely qualitative stereopsis. Instead one might wish to divide depth percepts into a region of veridical depth perception (which is smaller than Ogle's region of patent stereopsis) and the remaining region of nonveridical depth perception. "Veridical" is used here to imply that if the distance of an object at zero disparity is perceived at its true distance, then the change in distance for a given disparity is also correctly perceived.

In Richards' (1971) data for normal observers, the region of fusion coincides with the region of veridical depth perception. It is not known whether this observation applies to other situations in which the stimulus conditions change either the perceived depth or the range of fusion.

Precision of Stereoscopic Localization

Under normal conditions, most observers with no ocular abnormalities can discriminate a depth difference that produces a relative disparity of only about 10 arc-seconds (0.0028°). The best values reported in the literature have been obtained by the method of constant stimuli, in which the observer is asked to report whether a vertical test rod is nearer or further than similar comparison rods for each of several separations in depth between the rods (Howard, 1919). Whether monocular information is present or eliminated (Woodburne, 1934), the best observers achieve a 75% discrimination level close to 2 arc-seconds (0.00056°).

This appears to be one of the finest discriminations of which the human visual system is capable. It represents a truly amazing accomplishment, particularly considering that the resolution limit for dark lines is more than 10 times larger at the intensities used in stereoscopic discrimination tasks (Hecht and Mintz, 1939), and also that the discrimination requires the observer to compare images in continuous motion on the two retinas due to eye movements. To illustrate the refinement of this discrimination, it can be converted into real distances for the near and far limits of vision. For the closest fixation distance of 10 inches, the best stereoscopic threshold corresponds to the appreciation of a depth of one-thousandth of an inch (25 μ). For comparison, this is finer than the size of a typical human ovum (100 μ) or the cell body of a typical neuron (50 μ). Conversely, when fixation is on the horizon, it enables stereoscopic discrimination that objects two miles away are nearer than the horizon.

This allows, for example, stereoscopic discrimination of depth in the nearer types of clouds. These limits provide useful stereopsis over an extensive range of environmental conditions.

The Three-Dimensional "Fovea" for Stereoacuity

Although stereoacuity is excellent at the fovea, it deteriorates with an accelerating function as the stimulus is moved into the periphery (Ogle, 1952b), so that stereopsis rapidly becomes very poor outside the circle passing through the two blind spots in the binocular visual fields. Stereoacuity decreases exponentially with eccentricity. Although there are few relevant measurements away from the horizontal meridian, a similar reduction of stereoacuity presumably occurs along any retinal meridian. (Such measurements require that the backward inclination of the vertical horopter be taken into account.) The result is a two-dimensional distribution of stereoacuity that has its own maximum coinciding approximately with the anatomic foveas of the two eyes, although there may be some small discrepancy in the precise alignment (Hirsch and Weymouth, 1948).

Since stereopsis is a three-dimensional sense, one can ask about the distribution of stereoacuity in the third dimension of space. Is it degraded as the test display is moved away from the horopter without changing the mean visual direction? This operation corresponds to an experimental fixation disparity, and was the subject of a careful study by Blakemore (1970a). He simulated changes in distance by varying the disparity between dichoptic stimuli in a stereoscope and found that indeed, stereoacuity was rapidly degraded with increasing disparity from the horopter in the direction of both crossed and uncrossed disparities. He was able to show that the degradation was exponentially proportional to the disparity from the horopter over a range of horizontal eccentricities. This simple relationship together with the exponential decrease in stereoacuity with eccentricity should allow specification of stereoacuity anywhere in visual space by a simple analytic function. Such a function is shown as the solid lines for the horizontal (x) and disparity (z) dimensions in Figure 7.19. This may be regarded as the three-dimensional equivalent of a fovea for stereopsis (the y dimension is not shown, but is probably similar to the x dimension). Although schematic, this figure provides a useful conceptualization of the range of stereoacuity in visual space, for which the empirical details have still to be gathered.

Cyclopean Stereopsis

An important advance in both experimental analysis and controlled clinical testing of stereopsis was the development of random-dot stereograms

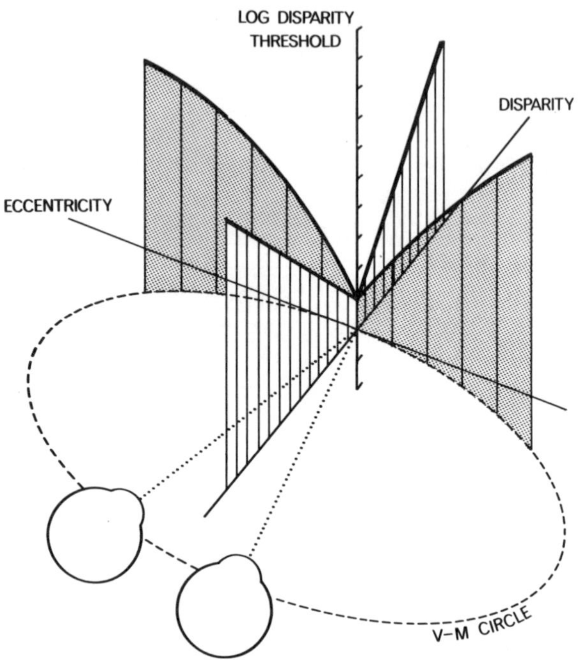

FIGURE 7.19. Depiction of the spatial function of stereoacuity around the point of fixation. Note that stereoacuity falls off approximately linearly in log coordinates with distance from the fovea in both lateral and depth directions.

(RDS) by Julesz (1960). The basic idea is to present to each eye a field of random dots containing a camouflaged stereoscopic figure. An early version of this approach was conceived by Ames in the form of a "leaf room" (Ogle, 1950). All sides of the room were covered with leaves to obscure the monocular perspective information of its shape. The room appeared almost flat when viewed with one eye, but appeared to spring into vivid depth on opening the other eye. The perceived shape of the room was predictably altered by placing different types of magnifying lens before one eye and altering the disparity relationships on the two retinas.

Julesz (1960) demonstrated with computer-generated random-dot patterns that it is logically possible to produce complete dissociation between the monocular and binocular patterns. If the dot pattern in one eye is completely random, then selected elements may be shifted and rearranged, but the result is another random pattern with no hint of the local rearrangement that has occurred. If the two patterns are presented dichoptically, the visual system may use the correlation between the two to perceive relative pattern shifts. If the shifts are horizontal, they constitute a binocular disparity and give rise to a stereoscopic depth figure that is literally invisible with either eye alone. (Other types of shift give rise to various kinds of binocular rivalry and luster percept.)

An example of an RDS with a complex stereofigure (a stereoscopic checkerboard) is shown in Figure 7.20, in a new type of "autostereogram" designed for free fusion without the need for a stereoscope or anaglyph glasses. Only a single random-dot field is required, and there is no limit to its size. An entire wall may be covered if desired, giving cyclopean vision over the full visual field. The basis for an autostereogram is the repetition of a random pattern (Tyler and Chang, 1977). If the eyes are converged by one repetition width, each random strip will be dichoptically superimposed on its neighbor, giving the percept of a new plane at a disparity corresponding to the repetition width in the original plane. It is now possible to control this disparity by varying the repetition width at each point in the field. Any stereoscopic surface with variations in both the horizontal and vertical directions may be generated by this means. Complex cyclopean figures may be appreciated, as illustrated by the two autostereograms shown in Figure 7.21, which depict respectively

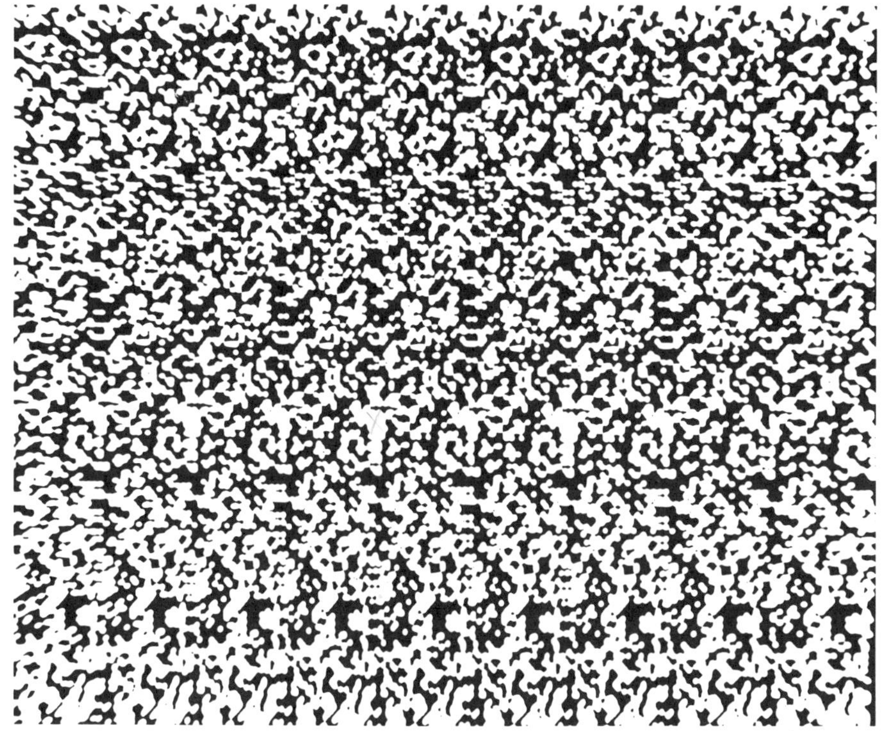

FIGURE 7.20. Random-dot stereogram of a checkerboard generated by a new autostereogram technique. At 40 cm viewing distance hold a finger about 10 cm above page and fixate finger continuously. The stereoscopic percept will gradually emerge in the plane of the finger, which can then be removed for free viewing within the stereospace.

an eyeball and a vortex figure inspired by Leonardo da Vinci. The main constraint is that the disparity may be varied only in discrete values corresponding to the dot size. This gives rise to the steps visible in the autostereogram of Figure 7.21.

To facilitate the viewing of the autostereogram, one can fixate on a finger held in front of the page. When vergence is maintained in this fashion, a stereoscopic percept will gradually emerge by virtue of the disparities between adjacent repetitive strips of the autostereogram. A good deal of patience may be required on the first attempt, since one must dissociate convergence and accommodation. Once stereopsis is achieved,

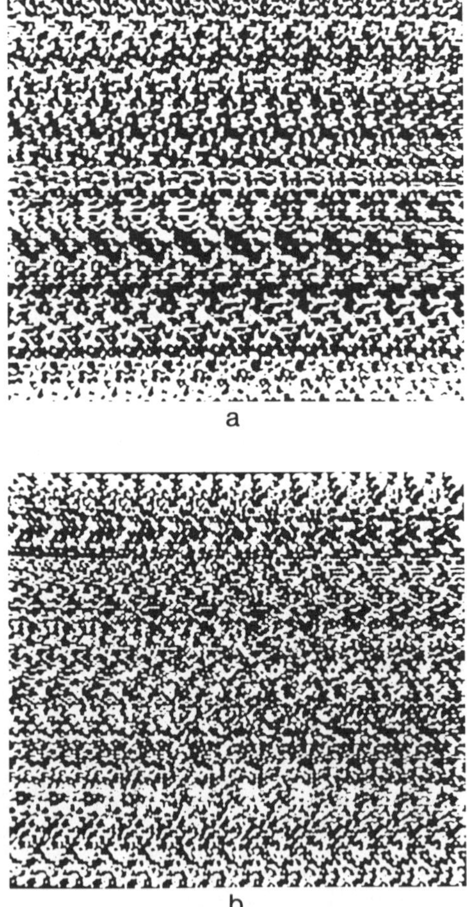

FIGURE 7.21. Autostereograms of A an eyeball and B a spiral figure inspired by da Vinci's Star of Bethlehem drawing (c. 1513) from the vortex series. (Royal Library of Windsor Castle Collection)

the observer is free to inspect the entire field of the autostereogram without losing the depth percept.

The importance of random-dot stereograms is that they demonstrate that a monocular form is not necessary for the perception of a stereoscopic form. The stereoscopic form is first present at a binocular level in the cortex, which Julesz designated as cyclopean. (This term should be distinguished from the cyclopian eye of Hering, which refers to the imaginary position in the head from which binocular visual direction is perceived.)

The cyclopean level of neural processing provides a bench-mark for determining the relative locus in the nervous system of different functions. For example, Julesz (1971) has found that a large number of visual illusions persist when presented so as to be visible only at the cyclopean level. The processes responsible for the residual illusion must therefore be located in the cortex rather than the eye.

Random-dot stereograms are useful in the clinical diagnosis of defects in stereopsis because it is impossible to fake the response by looking first with one eye and then the other, since neither contains the stereoscopic figure. Perception of the form may be possible by binocular luster alone, however. To demonstrate depth perception unambiguously one must ask the observer whether the cyclopean figure appears in front of or behind the surround, rather than merely what form is visible.

Physiological Basis of Stereopsis by Spatial Disparity

The first requirement for neural processing of the stereoscopic depth information is some means of assessing minute differences in the relative positions of similar images in the eyes. In the visual cortex the comparison can be made by neurons with binocular receptive fields. Accordingly, the first attempt at an explanation of the physiological basis of stereopsis was in terms of binocular neurons with disparities between the positions of the receptive field in each eye (Barlow et al., 1967; Hubel and Wiesel, 1970). This now seems more likely to be the basis for binocular fusion only, since the minimum size of receptive fields in monkey cortex (Hubel and Wiesel, 1962) is about 15′. This would give a range of disparities of about half a degree—a far cry from the disparities of a few arc-seconds that can be discriminated behaviorally.

A much more sensitive mechanism of tuning cells for binocular disparity is revealed by looking at binocular interactions with simultaneous stimulation of the two retinal receptive fields (Barlow et al., 1967; Pettigrew et al., 1968; Joshua and Bishop, 1970; Poggio and Fischer, 1977; von der Heydt et al., 1978). Many cells show facilitatory and inhibitory interactions as binocular disparity is varied within the range of the receptive fields (as defined by stimulation of each eye separately). The region of disparity over which binocular facilitation occurs may be an order of magnitude narrower than the size of the receptive fields. Furthermore, stimulation of flanking regions often shows binocular inhibition of the response, providing further tuning of the disparity range of the cell. The region of facilitation is so fine that it is difficult to compare its peak disparity from cell to cell because of drift in the physiological preparation. Pettigrew and Konishi (1976) were the first investigators to establish the presence of different peak disparities of the facilitation range by recording from more than one cell simultaneously. Thus the substrate for cell coding of disparity may be by means of binocular facilitation in an array of neurons. Such interactions are probably the first stage of the mechanism by which the cortex processes the hairsbreadth disparities present between the retinal images.

Some support for this view is provided by the human evoked potential evidence of Apkarian, Nakayama, and Tyler (1981). It was argued that the binocular facilitation which occurred with vertical gratings (see Figure 7.16), represented the activity of binocular facilitatory neurons. Such facilitation was reduced to binocular summation when the gratings were rotated to horizontal, in which position they were presumably invisible to neurons selective for horizontal disparity (von der Heydt et al., 1978). Thus facilitation appears to be limited to the system encoding depth from retinal disparity.

A THEORETICAL FRAMEWORK FOR STEREOPSIS

Overview

The conceptual framework proposed here is based largely on neurophysiological results (both in stereopsis and in other sensory domains) and on psychophysical studies. It is concerned with a series of simple interactions between local cortical elements sensitive to the disparity field, and similar processing at higher levels, as opposed to the inherently global models of such authors as Julesz (1971). The region of space to be processed by this system is optimized by means of both versional and vergent eye movements.

The point of departure is Nelson's (1975) simple model of a parallel array of cortical disparity "detectors," each responding to the presence of a stimulus with a particular location in x, y, z, coordinates (represented by the first rectangle in Figure 7.22, with the y axis omitted for clarity). There may be neural interactions in both the lateral (spatial) domain and the disparity domain. These inhibitory interactions introduce an element of "globality" into the model, in the sense that the processing of disparity at one point depends on the disparity relationships in other regions of

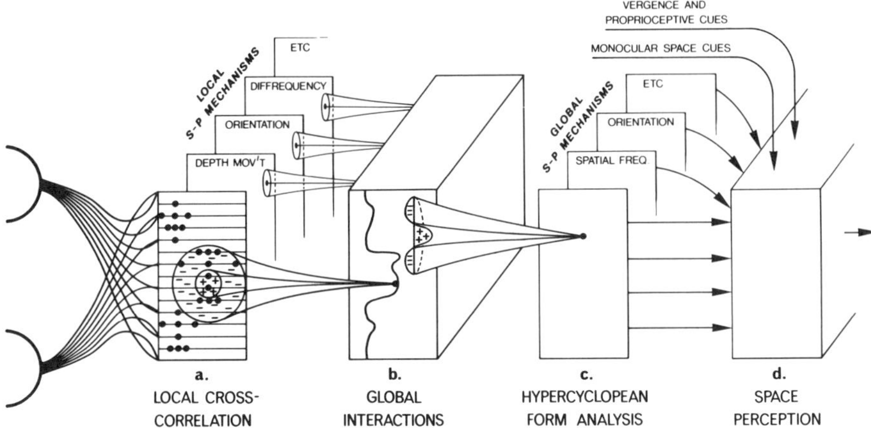

FIGURE 7.22. The four stages (A-D) of the proposed model of stereoscopic space perception. Note that each stage is a two-dimensional representation of a three-dimensional array, and many possible interconnections are unknown. The parallel planes represent arrays of special-purpose (S-P) mechanisms (details in text).

the image. Nevertheless, they are processes with great physiological plausibility, and since they operate with a few simple neural connections, they are appropriate to account for the rapidity of stereoscopic detection (Tyler, 1977a). These two criteria of physiological plausibility and explanatory range are predominant in the analysis of stereopsis presented below.

The second feature of the analysis is reliance on arrays of special-purpose mechanisms to account for certain attributes of the stereoscopic process. Such mechanisms are not properties of Nelson's model, and are represented by the sketched rectangles extending behind the first one in Figure 7.22. Examples of such attributes that will be discussed are the direction selectivity for motion in depth and selectivity for orientation of the stereoscopic figure in random-dot stereograms. Such selectivities are not predicted by inhibition or facilitation between simple disparity-selective neurons. Each special-purpose array is assumed to operate in parallel with other such arrays at the same processing level, with the overall output being determined either by a combination of the processes or by the most sensitive process under particular stimulus conditions.

The third characteristic is to break down the global nature of stereopsis (Julesz, 1978) into a sequence of serial processes (Figure 7.22) that are empirically separable. Within this serial structure is a further parallel organization for analyzing specialized global features of the stereoscopic image.

The final aspect of the analysis is its treatment of eye movements. While many theories of stereopsis have assumed that vergence eye movements play a major role in building up the components of the stereoscopic image, recent data suggest a modification of this view. Vergence may operate merely to optimize the region of best stereopsis in relation to the objects of interest in the three-dimensional field. Rather than acting to build up a percept of the field piece by piece, large regions of the stereoscopic image may be processed rapidly in parallel over much of the range of interest. It is mainly when fine stereoscopic discrimination is required that vergence is necessary to bring the stimuli close to the horopter region, which then acts as a disparity analogue of the fovea in being the region of finest discrimination. Vergence is also of value in processing particularly large disparities (Foley and Richards, 1972) for which the degree of convergence provides a further depth cue that can be used in addition to the retinal disparity information.

Special-Purpose Mechanisms

Before the analysis is described in detail, some justification will be provided for including special-purpose mechanisms, the most radical aspect of the analysis. There are numerous indications that specialized arrays of mechanisms exist to process specific attributes to the disparity field, in contrast to the general-purpose system that is often proposed. Proposal of these mechanisms forms a major departure from previous types of model, which have all assumed a unitary array of serial processes operating on the disparity field, with interactions occurring within the array. Each special-purpose mechanism is assumed to operate in parallel with the others, in a manner analogous to the "feature-specific" conception of neurons in striate cortex proposed by Hubel and Wiesel (1962). Note that here it is the processing *arrays* of neurons that are in parallel, since even in unitary models the processing array operates on parallel inputs from the retinas. Inclusion of these mechanisms is justified by four considerations.

1. There are several types of specialized neural response within the disparity domain that have been reported in neurophysiological experiments. They establish that special-purpose mechanisms are a significant facet of stereoscopic processing.

2. There is substantial psychophysical evidence for the existence of these mechanisms, with features in common with those suggested by the neurophysiological evidence (see following sections).

3. Special-purpose mechanisms are an efficient method of network operation, allowing rapid processing under a wide range of operating conditions. Presumably such mechanisms have developed to meet specific environmental conditions for which a general-purpose physiological mechanism would be too unwieldy. A similar path is being taken in the

current design of computer architecture, now that the inherent constraints of electronic components are becoming clear.

4. Current models of nonstereoscopic cortical function also strongly favor the existence of special-purpose processing as opposed to a more general, linear matrix representation. Examples are provided by neurons (or neural circuits) selectively sensitive to direction and velocity of retinal motion, color-opponent neurons, and neurons with orientation-specific excitation and inhibition.

Special-purpose mechanisms may themselves exist in two classes according to whether specialization occurs at the local level (retinal-receptive-field characteristics) or global level (cortical interactions). Examples of local mechanisms that are discussed are those specialized for the detection of stimuli with specific sizes and orientations, orientational disparities, motion in depth, and spatial frequency differences between the eyes. Mechanisms in the second class (global mechanisms) use conventional spatial disparity information from the two retinas, but respond to a specialized aspect of the disparity information at the global level of stereopsis. Examples are global lateral inhibition, specificity for cyclopean size and orientation, and processes specialized for sinusoidal stereograting detection.

Structure of the Model

Stereoscopic space perception seems to involve at least four levels of processing beyond the retinal level (see Figure 7.22). At each level there may be parallel arrays of neurons processing specialized aspects of the previous level (although such arrays are needed at only the first and third levels to account for the evidence to be presented).

As depicted in Figure 7.22, the initial stage of binocular combination is a disparity detection that might be achieved by the various types of neuron with facilitatory responses to different disparities, recorded in the visual cortex of cat and monkey. This may be considered as a local cross-correlation process, performed by neurons tuned to different disparities, occurring at each location in the binocular visual field. As the eyes vary their vergence, cortical "images" of the visual scene slide over one another to obtain the shift (or disparity) that produces the best match or correlation in each local region of the visual field. The images matched in this way are said to be in register. In practice there are, of course, two dimensions of field location, and there is no reason to suppose that the array is as regular as depicted here.

All disparities in the cortical image should give rise to a response somewhere in the neural disparity field, but they will not all necessarily produce veridical depth images, since in complex stereograms there may be many disparities arising from spurious correlations between adjacent points (Julesz, 1960). In dynamic RDS any degree of decorrelation, such as produced by images well out of register, will tend to be visible as depth noise, a dynamic cloud of depth (Julesz and Tyler, 1976). For static departures from register, such depth noise is not visible except with very short duration exposures and hence the depth image must involve further processing beyond local disparity detection, as has been amply demonstrated by Julesz (1962, 1971). The further processing for depth is identified with the second, global processing level (Figure 7.22), although it may not be physiologically distinct from the first level.

The result of the first two processing levels is a three-dimensional representation of the visual scene. Although some neural processing has been involved, this representation has advanced little beyond the form of a direct projection of the stimulus field into the brain. It is reasonable to suppose that there is a further stage of pattern processing that extracts specific features of this image to be extracted for perceptual analysis. This has been called the hypercyclopean level (Tyler, 1975a) as shown in Figure 7.22. The studies described show that there are hypercyclopean processes operating on the stereoscopic depth images that are similar to some of the cortical processes operating on the two-dimensional retinal image. For example, there seems to be specific representation of the size and orientation of features of the stereoscopic image.

Even beyond the hypercyclopean level there may be a further level of abstract spatial representation in which stereoscopic information is integrated with other spatial representations, such as those from the motion vector field (Gibson, 1950; Nakayama and Loomis, 1974), the texture gradient field (Gibson, 1950), and accommodation, vergence, vestibular, and other nonstereoscopic cues. This level of integration is indicated by the fourth element of Figure 7.22. For the present purposes only the relationship to the vergence system is considered in detail.

Outline

The consideration of the various levels of stereoscopic processing from Figure 7.22 is broken into a number of subsections.

Local processes
1. Local/global separation.
2. Local cleaning operations to remove ghost images.
3. Specialized local stereoscopic processes.

Global processes
1. Global lateral inhibition.
2. Global processing limitations.

3. Specialized global stereoscopic processes.
4. Hypercyclopean perception.

LOCAL PROCESSES

Local/Global Separation

Definitions

Before the topic of local/global separation is discussed, several related dichotomies must be distinguished: local/global, cyclopean/noncyclopean, fine/coarse, and fused/diplopic disparity. Much of what follows requires clear specification of these concepts.

1. Local/global. In this context, local mechanisms are defined as those that involve no interactions at or beyond the initial disparity processing level, whereas global mechanisms are those that do have such interactions. Thus local disparity mechanisms are those that process disparity in one region on the visual field without reference to the disparities present in other regions. They must also be local with respect to other disparities present in the same region of the field.

2. Cyclopean/noncyclopean. Although Julesz (1971) has tended to regard cyclopean as equivalent to global, this identification blurs an important distinction between stimulus and mechanism. Cyclopean is defined here as applicable to any stimulus feature that is invisible monocularly but visible by means of the disparity-processing mechanisms. These mechanisms may be local or global in terms of the definition above, whether the stimulus is cyclopean or not.

Note that on the one hand this does not limit cyclopean stimuli to random element stereograms, while on the other hand stimuli that are cyclopean in one mode of presentation may become noncyclopean in another. An example of the latter is that when two (cyclopean) static RDS with different disparities are presented in succession, there can be a monocularly visible differentiation of the central square. To render the change invisible monocularly, dynamic RDS must be used.

3. Fine/coarse disparity. Another concept reviewed below is the existence of separate mechanisms for processing fine (small) and coarse (large) disparity stimuli. It should be stressed that in principle each of these mechanisms might operate by either local or global processes, and also that each might operate on either cyclopean or noncyclopean stimuli. Thus the three dichotomies are logically independent, although there may be empirical correspondence among them.

4. Fusion/diplopia. One myth that should be dispelled is that the transition between fine and coarse disparity processing (or for either of the other dichotomies) is connected with Panum's fusional limit. While

stereopsis operates on horizontal disparities, Panum's limit is a property of the fusion mechanism for either horizontal or vertical disparities, and does not exist for cyclopean RDS. No matter how large the disparity, an RDS will not appear diplopic, although the static type will eventually go into rivalry.

Thus the limits of global, cyclopean, and fine disparity processing are each logically independent of the fusion limit and of each other. That there may be empirical coincidences for a particular stimulus configuration does not detract from the functional independence of these limits over the range of potential stimuli.

Analysis of Local/Global Distinction

A local disparity process is one in which the disparity at one location in the field is processed without reference to the disparities present at other locations, or to other disparities present at the same location. Local disparity processes may well be affected by retinal stimulus features, however, such as the size and orientation of the retinal images carrying the disparity signal. Local processes may also be affected by retinal image features at other locations on the retina, such as retinal lateral inhibition. This may be regarded as a retinal globality (as opposed to the cortical globality in which interactions occur between local disparity detectors in the cortex). A final feature of local processing is that it is not necessarily limited to small disparities. In fact, the evidence to be reviewed suggests that it is the larger disparities that are processed by local mechanisms.

Global, interactive processing does seem to be limited to the small-disparity range. Many different types of global processing have been proposed, from lateral interactions between disparity detectors to iterative computation of the best stereoscopic figure in the disparity array. A definition that encompasses them all is that it involves interactions between local disparity-detection mechanisms.

Previous Theories

The separation of stereoscopic processing into two types, fine and coarse disparity processes, has been a feature of many recent theories (Julesz, 1978). Each theory has a slightly different concept of the fine/coarse division.

Something of this dichotomy was embodied in Ogle's (1950) distinction between patent and qualitative stereopsis. He suggested that for small disparities, depth perception was linearly proportional to the magnitude of the disparity (patent), while for larger disparities there was a (qualitative) region of crude depth perception related only to the sign of the disparity. He did not specifically suggest that these were processed by two separate systems.

Julesz (1962) developed in algorithmic form the concept of a global system that searched for dense planes in the local array of disparity detectors that were stimulated by the stereoscopic image. This global system was supposed to operate only on fine disparities. He also recognized the existence of a separate local system that would account for the perception of large disparities in the range of qualitative stereopsis. Thus he not only postulated separate fine and coarse disparity mechanisms, but associated the fine mechanism with both global and cyclopean processing, while the coarse mechanism was considered to be local and noncyclopean.

Several other theorists have made fine, global processing of some sort a feature of their models (Sperling, 1970; Nelson, 1975; Marr and Poggio, 1976, 1979; Mayhew and Frisby, 1980). They have also introduced coarse local disparity processes as a means of signaling the vergence eye movement system to bring the image into the range of small disparities for sensory processing by the fine system. Most of these theorists have specifically repudiated the idea of perception of large disparities despite psychophysical evidence for its occurrence. Therefore they cannot be regarded as suggesting a fine/coarse distinction in the sensory processing of disparity for perception.

Richards and Kaye (1974) obtained data showing that the range of depth perception increased continuously with the width of the stimulus elements, which they took to indicate that the apparent dichotomy between fine and coarse disparity processes was in fact a continuum. Their smallest disparity (15 arc-minutes) was larger than the range proposed by Julesz (1971) for fine global stereopsis. Thus in his terms they were studying only the local (coarse) disparity system.

In summary, although the idea of a separation between fine and coarse processes for depth perception has been mooted in various forms, it has not been a central concern of previous theorists, who have usually concentrated on either fine or coarse mechanisms without considering the relative roles of the two.

Psychophysical Separation of Fine and Coarse Mechanisms

Psychophysical evidence for a distinction between mechanisms processing fine and coarse disparities exists in the form of different perceptual phenomena in the two disparity ranges. One of the more direct examples is in the appearance of multiple depth planes. When one views an RDS containing two overlaid disparity planes with a small disparity separation, they are fused to form the perception of a single dense plane (called pykno-stereopsis, from the Greek for dense), whereas in the range of larger disparity separations between the two depth stimuli two transparent depth surfaces may be seen (called dia-stereopsis, from the Greek for separate or transparent). Within the pykno-stereoscopic range there is averaging of the depths of the component planes (Figure 7.23), while the dia-stereoscopic range gives the three-dimensional equivalent of lateral diplopia (or even polyopia) beyond the range of binocular fusion.

Schumer (1979) was the first to study depth averaging in the pykno-stereoscopic range using dynamic RDS stimuli. He found that the averaging was approximately linear for a variety of stereofigures and flat planes up to disparities of about 20 arc-minutes. Beyond this value the two stereofigures were perceived separately and no averaging of separate depth surfaces occurred.

There are other differences that seem to be related to the same distinction. With a psychophysical technique, Mitchell and Baker (1973) found that the depth aftereffect produced by prolonged inspection of a disparate line target was optimal for a 5-arc-minute adapting stimulus, but could not be obtained for disparities greater than 15 to 20 arc-minutes. Felton, Richards, and Smith (1972), however, have shown that the optimal disparity for the production of this aftereffect depends on the size of the bars used, with larger bars producing optimal aftereffects at larger disparities. Blakemore and Julesz (1971) reported that their best disparity aftereffect occurred rather narrowly around 10 arc-minutes for a static RDS. Depth aftereffects produced by the inspection of disparate stimuli thus seem to be characteristic of fine rather than coarse disparities.

Another effect that occurs only for fine disparities is induced movement in the disparity domain (Norcia and Tyler, unpublished observations). A dynamic RDS contained a set of stereoscopic bars alternating

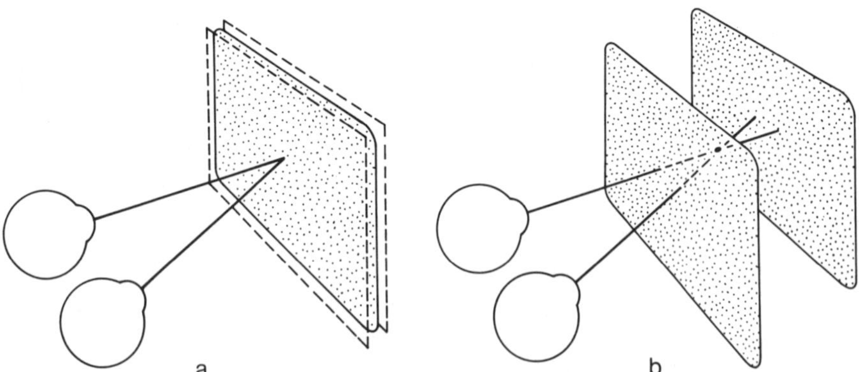

FIGURE 7.23. A Pykno-stereopsis: depth averaging of two RDS planes at a small disparity into the percept of a single dense surface. B Dia-stereopsis: the separation of two RDS planes at a large disparity into a percept of two transparent surfaces in depth.

between two positions in depth while the intervening regions remained fixed in depth. At small disparities the alternating bars induced counterphase motion in their stationary neighbors. At larger disparities, induction was not seen. Here again, the different perceptual properties of the fine and coarse disparity regions support the existence of a separate fine process.

Jones (1977) has shown that persons with normal stereoacuity (fine stereopsis) may have vergence eye movement and perceptual anomalies associated with large disparities. He also suggested that the temporal properties of coarse and fine stereopsis may be different. Similarly, Langlands (1926) and Ogle and Weil (1958) have reported that fine stereopsis was improved with long exposure durations, such that maximum stereoacuity was obtained for about three-second exposure. Conversely, coarse disparity judgments are optimal with short exposures (Ogle, 1962b).

Another case in which eye movements are differentially involved is in the initial learning behavior for depth perception in RDS (Saye and Frisby, 1975). Monocular contours were used to guide the eye movements of naive observers in viewing RDS. A marked improvement was found for large-disparity stereograms, but no effect was seen when using small (5′) disparities.

Neurophysiological Studies

Until recently, neurophysiological studies concentrated on showing neural selectivity to specific disparities. A new approach was taken by Poggio and Fischer (1977), who suggested that binocular interactions of neurons in the behaving monkey cortex may be grouped into four classes (Figure 7.24). Neurons that are predominantly binocular (in the classical sense of having identifiable receptive fields for monocular stimulation of each eye) tend to show a region of either binocular facilitation (A) or binocular occlusion (B). More surprisingly, they found that cells with classically monocular receptive fields showed binocular facilitation for either crossed (C) or uncrossed (D) disparities only. Whereas the type A cells showed facilitation in a narrow range around zero disparity, types C and D tended to give facilitation over a large range of either crossed or uncrossed disparities.

These results are exciting as they suggest a neural basis for fine and coarse stereopsis based on different types of receptive field wiring rather than different ranges of the same type of receptive field. Receptive field type A would correspond to fine stereopsis, while types C and D would provide the basis for coarse stereopsis. The inhibitory type B might well be involved in the mechanism of binocular rivalry. It could interact with the stereoscopic system by activating suppression of stereopsis when stim-

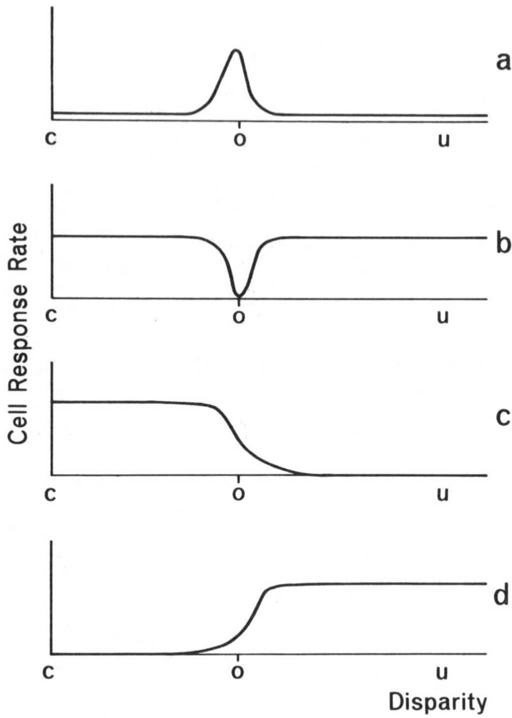

FIGURE 7.24. Four classes of binocular disparity sensitivity in monkey cortex: A binocular facilitation; B binocular occlusion; C "monocular" crossed; D "monocular" uncrossed sensitivities. Reprinted by permission of the publisher, from Tyler CW and Scott AB. Binocular Vision. In: Records R, ed. *Physiology of the Human Eye and Visual System*. Hagerstown: Harper and Row, 1979.

uli occur beyond a certain range of disparities or beyond a certain proportion of binocular mismatches.

Evoked Potential Studies

Further support for the local/global mechanisms in human stereopsis comes from an evoked potential study by Norcia and Tyler (1980). They used a dynamic RDS in which a depth plane alternated between equal crossed and uncrossed disparity positions. The entire display area was occupied by this plane, not merely a central square. A fixation marker with nonius lines was provided to control vergence eye movements. The evoked potential was recorded from bipolar electrodes near the inion and synchronized to each stimulus event (reversal of the disparity plane from crossed to uncrossed, or vice versa). Three types of datum can be obtained from this kind of recording: response amplitude, phase of the response relative to the input stimulus, and delay of the response with respect to the stimulus. Response delay is computed from the rate of change in response phase as a function of the temporal frequency (Regan, 1972), and is therefore logically independent of the phase at a given temporal frequency.

Differentiation between fine and coarse disparity mechanisms was evident in the data of Norcia and Tyler (1980) for all three measures. As indicated in Figure 7.25, the response amplitude showed a peak at about 15 arc-minutes with a pronounced dip followed by a second peak as disparity was increased. The phases of the responses were different for the small and large disparities, and were separated by nearly 180° between the two peaks (15 and 40 arc-minutes). The delay computed at these peak amplitudes was about 50 msec shorter for the coarse disparity mechanism than for the fine disparity mechanism. It was concluded that the two ranges of disparity are processed by discrete, separable mechanisms that may correspond to Poggio and Fischer's (1977) binocular neural classes (A) for fine disparities and (C) and (D) for coarse disparities, respectively (see Figure 7.24).

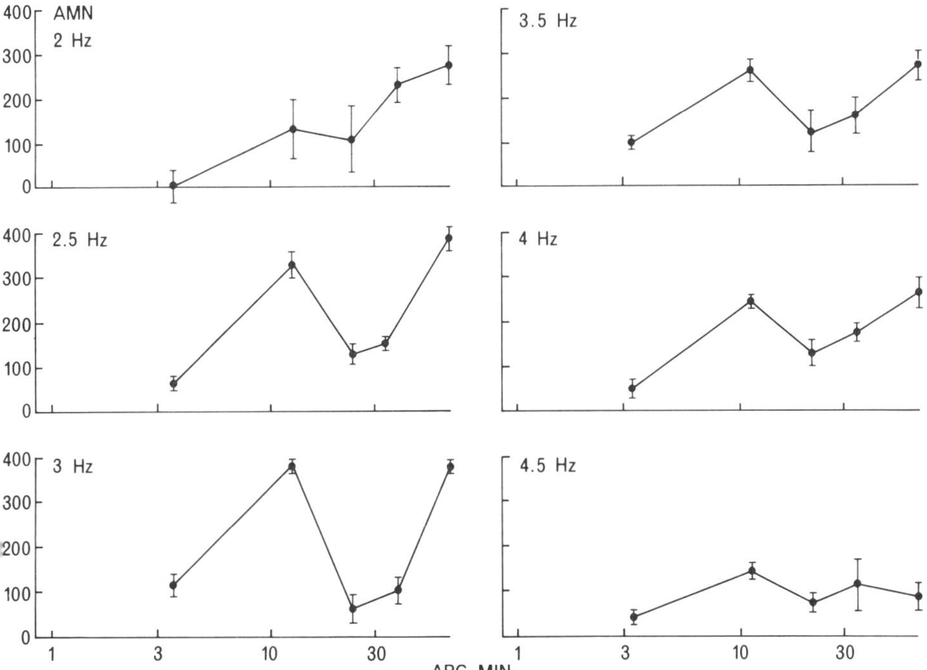

FIGURE 7.25. Synchronous evoked potential amplitudes to RDS disparity stimulation as a function of disparity at six temporal frequencies (recording frequency was at the stimulus reversal rate, i.e., twice the fundamental frequency).

Local Cleaning Operations

The neural problem of establishing corresponding details in disparate images in the two eyes was highlighted by the invention of random-dot stereograms. Julesz (1962) pointed out that the ambiguity of which elements should be paired between the eyes to give the appropriate depth image increases with the square of the number of points in each horizontal line, and felt that the solution of this problem required a cooperative process in the cortex. In fact, correspondences between dots with some vertical displacement must also be considered, so that the ambiguity problem actually increases with the fourth power of the number of dots, up to the correspondence limits. Given that there may be as many as ten thousand positions within the correspondence limits for the foveal region, the potential number of spurious dot correspondences, at 50% density, is 10^8 for a 10×10 stimulus array and 10^{16} for the limiting 100×100 array. Thus the processes by which the brain might reduce the ambiguity problem are of considerable interest.

Local Stereoscopic Bandwidth Limitation

For a perceptual system that can detect stimulus modulations down to zero frequency, the spatial bandwidth of that system is defined as the maximum number of cycles of modulation that can be resolved per unit visual angle of the relevant stimulus variable. For the monocular acuity system for luminance contrast the bandwidth is therefore about 50 cycles per degree.

There appears to be a limitation of stereoscopic bandwidth that is partly precyclopean and partly at the cyclopean level of the cortex. That is, there is a limitation on the spatial bandwidth of (precyclopean) retinal signals that can be accepted for input into the stereoscopic system, and a further limitation on the (cyclopean) spatial disparity profile that can be generated from the retinal information. Evidence for some precyclopean bandwidth limitation is provided from three sources.

1. Limitation in spatial pattern bandwidth. The bandwidth of spatial patterns that can produce stereopsis is lower by a factor of two than monocular resolution (Blakemore, 1970b).
2. Binocular frequency reduction in visual noise. For binocular viewing the appearance of both dynamic visual noise (MacKay, 1961) and static visual noise (Tyler, 1975c) is lower in spatial frequency by about a factor of two than for with monocular viewing.
3. Cortical receptive field size. In monkey visual cortex the predominantly binocular complex and cells have receptive fields from 1.5 to 2 times the size of the predominantly monocular simple cells (Hubel and Wiesel, 1968).

These three lines of evidence all concur in suggesting a precyclopean binocular limitation of spatial bandwidth of about a factor of two.

A physiological basis for the bandwidth limitation is suggested by the functional architecture of monkey visual cortex (Hubel and Wiesel, 1968) as opposed to the sizes of receptive fields. There are different arrangements of orientation and disparity preferences of cells in area 18 of monkey cortex. Columns or strips of cells responding to similar orientations were found to be very narrow compared to those responding to binocular disparity. This was also indicated in autoradiographic studies of the anatomy of 2-deoxyglucose uptake during stimulation with an oriented stripe pattern (Hubel et al., 1978). One might therefore expect the spatial integration across the cortex to be coarser for depth than for form processing, providing a possible basis for the poor cyclopean spatial resolution of stereoscopic information.

Depth Averaging

Kaufman (1964) with RDS, and Foley (1976) using classical stimuli, have demonstrated the occurrence of depth averaging for images with different disparities lying in the same or similar retinal locations. In RDS, many spurious disparities associated with unintended dot comparisons occur, and may lie in the same retinal location as the intended image. In particular, as Tyler (1977a) has pointed out, for every spurious disparity in a flat plane of dots, there is a conjugate disparity in the same visual direction symmetrically in front of or behind the plane. The depth impression should therefore average out to zero. Thus depth averaging or cancellation can eliminate many spurious correlations even in complex RDS images. For a flat plane, all spurious correlations would be eliminated in this way, even in the limiting case of close to 10^{16} of them.

Specialized Local Stereoscopic Processes

Size Specificity

The first type of specialization is for the size of the retinal image, with different sizes being processed by different mechanisms. If such mechanisms all had equivalent disparity ranges, the separation of size specificity would have little to do with the stereoscopic system. There is evidence, however, that the disparity range over which such mechanisms operate is proportional to the size of their receptive fields.

The only authors to provide systematic evidence of the relation of size and disparity of neuronal receptive fields were Pettigrew, Nikara, and Bishop (1968). Their method for determining selectivity was to measure the disparity of the monocular receptive fields in the two eyes. As was argued previously, this may have more to do with the fusion mechanism than the stereoscopic mechanism, but it does provide some indication of the binocular organization of receptive fields. The correlation between disparity and receptive field size was 0.81 for their data (Tyler, 1973).

Further evidence for a size/disparity relationship is available from psychophysics. Richards and Kaye (1974) found that both the maximum perceived depth and the maximum range of disparity that would evoke any depth sensation increased progressively with the width of the stimulus. The increase was proportional to the square root of stimulus width rather than linear, as pointed out by Tyler and Julesz (1980a), but this still provides the basis for a marked economy in disparity processing.

Julesz and Miller (1975) showed that the stereoscopic information carried by channels tuned to different retinal sizes could be processed independently. They filtered RDS so that low and high spatial-frequency components of the pattern each contained either stereoscopic or rivalrous information. Observers could simultaneously see the stereoscopic form and experience rivalry in the other spatial frequency band. Although this experiment does not address the question of a size/disparity correlation, it shows that the binocular system contains parallel channels for different sizes of retinal input.

Size-specific mechanisms in stereopsis and other specialized local processes could help to disambiguate complex stereograms such as RDS (Marr and Poggio, 1979). The ambiguity is substantially reduced by the retinal specificity of the local processes outlined in this section, so that Marr and Poggio (1979) were able to extract the stereoscopic image from a RDS with a noncooperative algorithm that incorporated only the size specificity. Specialized local processes could therefore be of great importance in simplifying the task of the cortex in extracting depth information.

Orientation Specificity

It is also possible that the orientation of the stimulus on the retina provides a basis for a specialization in the local disparity-processing system. Although the neurophysiological evidence for orientation specificity in binocular receptive fields is too well known to require a review (Hubel and Wiesel, 1968), one psychophysical experiment does not support its role in human stereopsis. Mayhew and Frisby (1979) found that filtering an RDS at one orientation tended to destroy the stereoscopic information, while combining the monocularly filtered stereograms for two orthogonal orientations restored the stereoscopic impression. It must be concluded that if oriented filters are involved, they are combined in a nonlinear (facilitatory) fashion such that the information from a set of detectors tuned to only one orientation is not available to perception.

Orientational Disparity

Blakemore, Fiorentini, and Maffei (1972) have pointed out that the oriented receptive fields of cortical cells suggest that there may be orientational disparities between the receptive fields of the eyes, in addition to a spatial binocular disparity. They found such orientational disparities present for cat neurons, and hypothesized that they might be involved in the processing of inclination (depth tilt). Detection of an inclination in this manner has the advantage that the orientational cues are independent of the distance (and hence the spatial disparity of the object).

Psychophysical support for this suggestion comes from an experiment by von der Heydt, Adorjani, and Hanny (1977) using one-dimensional random visual noise with different orientations in the two eyes. The visual noise stimuli, which looked like bundles of straight sticks, were made uncorrelated between the eyes with the intention of precluding normal disparity relationships. Although uncorrelated stimuli can give rise to random depth relationships (Tyler 1974b, 1977a; Julesz and Tyler, 1976), this does not seem to apply to static stimuli, when the uncorrelated images give rise to rivalry but not stereopsis (Julesz, 1971). If von der Heydt and associates (1977) thus succeeded in controlling the conventional disparity cues, the introduction of a difference in orientation between the eyes should have no further effect. In fact, they observed a dramatic inclination in the median plane (Figure 7.26), providing a perceptual example of the use of orientational disparity cues when conventional disparity cues are inoperative.

The possibility of a separate orientational disparity system is particularly interesting in light of the mathematical demonstration by Koenderink and van Doorn (1976) that orientational disparity can provide robust depth information. By mathematically analyzing the disparity vector field they found that the orientation disparity cue is less disturbed by various transformations, such as convergence, than are other cues. Thus from the point of view of ecological optics orientational disparity provides a relatively invariant perceptual depth cue.

Binocular Spatial-Frequency Difference

Corresponding to stereopsis from orientation differences, which produces an appearance of inclination, there is also the possibility of stereopsis from spatial frequency differences between the images in the eyes, producing an impression of lateral depth tilt. The term "binocular spatial frequency difference" is so unwieldy that it will be replaced by the term "diffrequency," by analogy with "disparity" for positional differences between the eyes.

The first suggestion that diffrequency might be a specialized cue for stereopsis was made by Blakemore (1970b). He used vertical sinusoidal

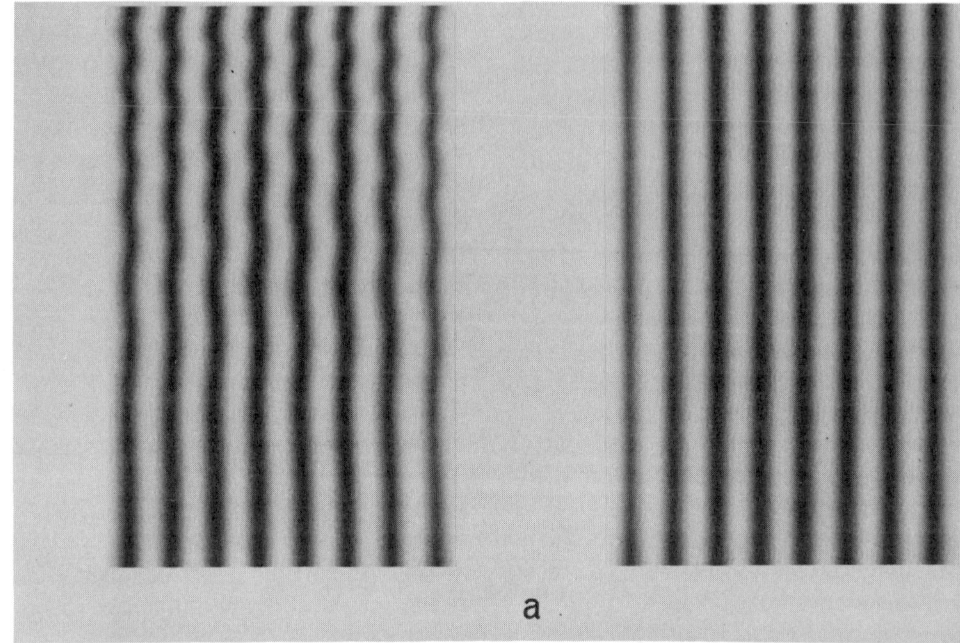

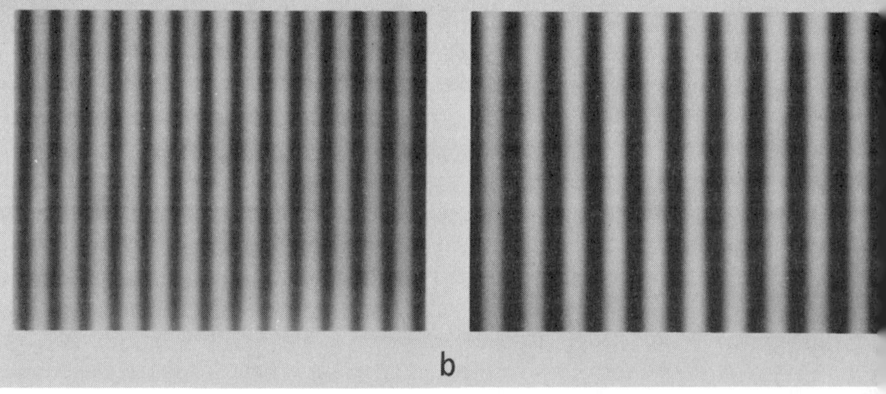

FIGURE 7.26. A Stereogram of the stimulus as used by von der Heydt et al (1977) to demonstrate the existence of a special-purpose mechanism for orientational disparity. B Stereogram showing diffrequency in grating stimuli as used by Blakemore (1970).

gratings in the frontal plane as stimuli (Figure 7.26), and found that binocular diffrequencies gave rise to a horizontal depth tilt up to a ratio of 1.4:1 between the frequencies in the eyes. The suggestion was taken up by Tyler and Sutter (1979), who designed several stimulus paradigms to ensure that conventional disparity cues were not involved. The simplest of these consisted of sinusoidal grating stimuli moving in opposite directions in the two eyes. When the velocity was slow, conventional disparity cues gave the perception of a flat plane moving toward the observer. Each time the gratings had moved the distance of a complete cycle, the plane flipped back and continued to move toward the observer. As the velocity was increased a point was reached at which the depth movement failed and was replaced by a perception of rivalry between the two monocularly moving images. At this point (a velocity of 4° per second), conventional disparity cues had been eliminated.

If the spatial frequency in one eye was now changed by a small amount, the observers reported that the plane was simultaneously rivalrous *and* tilted into depth. Thus the rivalry within the conventional disparity system was maintained, superimposed on the depth attributable to the diffrequency between the eyes, clearly demonstrating that diffrequency is a separate depth cue from disparity. Depth was detectable up to diffrequency ratios of 2:1.

A second experiment by Tyler and Sutter (1979) used dynamic, one-dimensional visual noise, which was uncorrelated between the two eyes to avoid conventional disparity cues. As in the orientational experiment of von der Heydt and co-workers (1977), horizontal depth tilt was visible when the noise was uncorrelated between the eyes, but only for diffrequency ratios between 1.2:1 and 2:1. For ratios less than 1.2:1, depth tilt was visible only when the stimuli were correlated between the eyes, and thus presumably needed only conventional disparity cues.

Disparity-Specific Lateral Motion

A further stimulus that appears to be processed by specialized stereoscopic mechanisms is lateral motion at non-zero disparities, for example, motion to the right in a stimulus with a crossed disparity. Neurophysiologically, most disparity-specific neurons have directional selectivity, and the directions are distributed fairly evenly around the clock, including all combinations of horizontal and vertical directions. Psychophysical support for the role of such neuronal direction specificity in depth perception has been provided by Regan and Beverley (1973a). They adapted observers to rotatory motion in depth (Figure 7.27) and found that the sensitivity reduction was strongly specific to the direction of rotation. Rotation in depth is made up of two components: motion in depth toward and away from the observer, and lateral motion at crossed and uncrossed disparities. Under the RDS conditions used by Regan and Beverley, the extent of movement was small compared with the size of the moving stimulus. Thus the motion-in-depth component covered approximately the same retinal region for both directions of depth movement, and there should have been no resultant direction-specific adap-

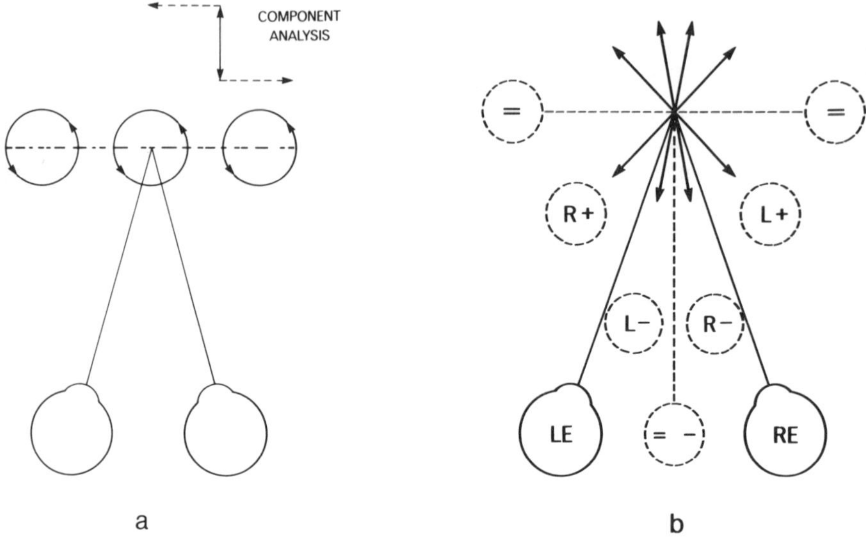

FIGURE 7.27. A Rotary motion in depth, as used by Regan and Beverley (1973a). Motions of three points are shown. Component analysis indicates the interpretation of direction specific adaptation of lateral motion at two disparities (*dashed arrows*), while depth motion (*solid arrow*) is not stimulated in a directionally specific manner. B The four classes of depth motion in the Beverley and Regan (1973) experiment. The eye in which the motion is greater is indicated by L or R (or = when they are equal) and in phase or counterphase motion is indicated by + or −.

tation (except in a thin strip at the edges of the moving stimulus). The component of lateral movement occurred, for example, at a crossed disparity when moving leftward and an uncrossed disparity when moving rightward, for clockwise motion in depth. The opposite association would occur for counterclockwise motion in depth. Each direction of rotation was associated with a single direction of lateral motion at each disparity. The rotation-specific adaptation is therefore most simply explained as a disparity-specific adaptation of direction of lateral motion.

Regan and Beverley (1974) have also provided evoked potential evidence for this using a similar adaptation paradigm and comparing the evoked potential amplitude before and after directional adaptation at specific disparities.

Motion in Depth

Just as cortical receptive fields may exhibit a preferential response for one direction of lateral motion, so may they show directional specificity for motion in depth. Pettigrew (1973) has reported cells in the two eyes with opposite preferred directions. Such cells would be well suited to detect motion in depth toward or away from the observer. Cynader and Regan (1978) have shown that many cells, particularly those showing binocular occlusion, have a binocular interaction specific for motion in depth, that is, motion in opposite directions on the two retinas.

In a series of papers, Beverley and Regan (1973, 1975, 1979) studied the psychophysical characteristics of the mechanisms involved. Using an adaptation paradigm, they showed that there are four separately adaptable classes for different directions of motion in depth according to whether the motion passes outside the line of sight of the right eye, between the right line of sight and the midline, between the midline and the line of sight of the left eye, or outside the left line of sight.

An alternative representation is to consider these directions in terms of the relations between the retinal motions of the two eyes (Figure 7.27). This is an important framework for the discussion that follows. The retinal motion may be categorized in terms of a 2 × 2 matrix according to whether it is in the same or opposite directions in the two eyes, and also whether it is of greater amplitude in the left eye or the right eye. These categories are denoted by the convention L+, L−, R−, and R+, where L+ means that motion in the left retina is greater than right retinal motion and is in the same direction, L− means left retinal motion greater than right retinal motion in the opposite direction, and so on. The way in which retinal motion is related to direction of motion in space is indicated in Figure 7.27. (The precise directions for which L = R and L = −R are indicated by = and = − respectively.)

Beverley and Regan (1973) found that prolonged stimulation with sinusoidal motion in a given direction in space produced adaptation throughout one or more of these ranges of direction. For exposure to stimuli in the extreme ranges (L+ and R+), adaptation occurred only for the stimulated range. Within the range, adaptation was identical for a given test stimulus regardless of the adapting stimulus direction.

For the intermediate directional ranges (L− and R−) the results were more complex. For example, exposure to a stimulus within the L− range produced adaptation for all test stimuli oriented on that side of the midline (i.e., both the L+ and L− ranges). The converse was true for exposure within the R− range. The only exposure stimulus that did not adapt the extreme ranges (L+ and R+) was motion directly along the midline (L= −R). This equal counterphase stimulus adapted both the L− and R− ranges. Thus a shift in the amplitude ratio between the two eyes of only 20% could produce a radical change in the adaptation range of stimuli close to the midline. The authors did not test to see whether a similar situation occurs for stimuli near the L = R point.

In summary, these results provide strong evidence for neural channels specific to the direction of motion in space. These channels have some curious properties in that their adaptation characteristics are not independently determined, despite the authors' attempt to depict their isolated characteristics. There is an asymmetry, in that exposure to counterphase movement adapts for in-phase movement (except for equal retinal amplitudes), while exposure to in-phase movement does not adapt for counterphase movement. This suggests a one-way interaction between these two types of motion processing.

Further evidence for the existence of separate processes for in-phase (lateral) and counterphase (depth) motion comes in the form of a substantial difference in psychophysical threshold for the two types of motion. It was originally found that the detection threshold for sinusoidal motion in depth was about three times higher than that for detection of each monocular component of the motion (Tyler, 1971, 1975d). Thus the depth motion system was not only less sensitive than the lateral motion system, indicating that the two systems have different motion-processing characteristics, but also less sensitive than each monocular motion system. This suggests that activation of the stereomovement system causes suppression of some information that is otherwise available to the monocular and binocular lateral movement systems.

This stereomovement suppression effect is not only operative to the same extent over a large range of temporal frequencies, but also occurs for pulsed changes in depth (Tyler and Foley, 1975). Under certain stimulus conditions stereomovement suppression does not occur, and there can even be an enhancement of depth movement over lateral movement detection (Regan and Beverley, 1973a; Tyler, 1975d), but for many classes of stimuli it is a general phenomenon (Regan and Beverley, 1973c; Tyler, 1974c) operating for both horizontal and vertical changes in disparity (Tyler, 1975d). This latter fact implies that the suppression is occurring in the binocular fusion system, since vertical disparities have no input to the stereoscopic depth system. In this way, stereomovement suppression reveals much about the interactions between the three systems involved in binocular movement processing (binocular lateral movement, binocular depth movement, and binocular fusion).

GLOBAL PROCESSES IN STEREOPSIS

Global Lateral Inhibition

Methods

The main tool for the study of global processes in stereopsis is the random-dot stereogram (RDS) developed by Julesz (1960). He has applied this technique to a vast array of problems in both the local and global domains, which are fully reviewed in a recent publication (Julesz, 1978). There is space only to touch on a few of the complex aspects of this work. Instead emphasis will be placed on a modification of the method—the sinusoidal stereograting—that can be used for studies of the basic questions of the global domain.

A stereograting is produced by spatial modulation of the disparity across the field of view (Tyler, 1974a; Tyler and Raibert, 1975). Such disparity modulation can be added to any two-dimensional image (e.g., a line image), a contrast grating, or an RDS. Thus the term stereograting refers solely to the disparity profile, not to the monocular image. If the monocular image is an RDS the result is a cyclopean stereograting, in which the monocular image contains no information about the modulation. An example is shown as an autostereogram in Figure 7.28. The disparity modulation can be square wave, sine wave, or any other repetitive waveform, and can be oriented in any direction (although it is difficult to produce sinusoidal stereogratings that are cyclopean except with vertical modulation, i.e., horizontal bars in depth).

Having developed the concept of disparity modulation, the tools of the contrast modulation paradigms can be applied to the disparity domain to study such questions as the existence of global lateral inhibition.

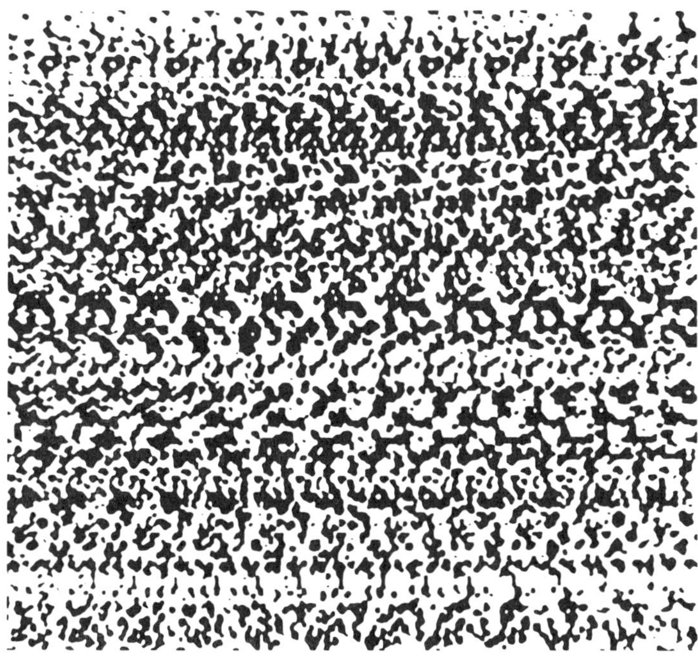

FIGURE 7.28. Autostereogram of a sinusoidal stereograting with horizontal bars, to be viewed as for Figure 6.20.

Edge Effects

Lateral inhibition in the global stereoscopic representation (as opposed to inhibition across disparity at the same visual direction locus) was first evinced by Anstis, Howard, and Rogers (1978). Following the logic of the Craik-O'Brien-Cornsweet illusion, they generated an RDS in which the disparity profile was that of a differentiated edge between two planes of equal disparity. The perceived depth of the planes differed, such that the depth on either side of the edge was assimilated to some extent into the perceived depth of the plane into which it merged.

While this is an interesting illusion, its interpretation in terms of lateral inhibitory processes is indirect. The assumption is that lateral inhibition would tend to differentiate a depth edge and that the differentiated edge would then be restored to its undifferentiated form by higher processes. This restoration process is what gives rise to the illusion when the system is presented with a physically differentiated depth edge. Apart from the implied nonlinearity, it is rather a long chain of reasoning to infer the presence of lateral inhibition from a demonstration of the restoration process.

Periodic Disparity Modulation

A more direct demonstration of global lateral inhibition is obtained from another technique derived from contrast modulation experiments. Lateral inhibition should reduce the sensitivity to stereogratings of low spatial frequency, because they consist mainly of shallow ramps in which the strength of the depth signal at any point is approximately equal to the sum of the signals some distance on either side of that point. Thus the lateral inhibitory network is fully stimulated and produces the maximal reduction in sensitivity at low spatial frequencies. High spatial-frequency stereogratings escape the inhibitory effect because the lateral inhibitory network cannot resolve the disparity modulation, while the excitatory process still can, up to some spatial frequency. (Obviously, if the excitatory and inhibitory processes had the same spatial resolution, no purpose would be served other than to reduce the response equally for all stimuli.)

The disparity amplitude threshold for detection of the presence of sinusoidal stereogratings over a range of spatial frequencies is shown in Figure 7.29. The data were obtained by a forced-choice technique using a dynamic random-dot stereograting generator with a 20° field. There is a linear increase in threshold with reduction in spatial frequency over the low range from 0.4 to 0.05 c/degree, as would be predicted from the lateral inhibition model. This reduction is unlikely to be caused by probability summation effects resulting from the decreasing number of bars in the stimulus, since such effects are known to predict a much more

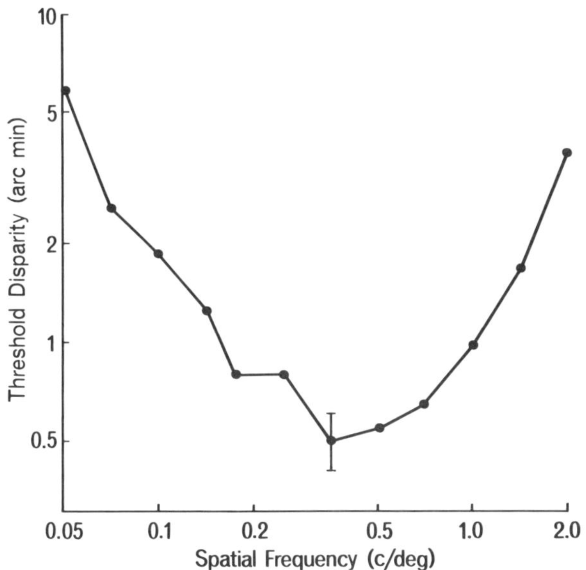

FIGURE 7.29. Threshold stereoacuity function for sinusoidal stereogratings. Note similarity to contrast MTF, except that all features occur at 10 times lower spatial frequency. Increase in threshold at very low frequency suggests operation of cyclopean lateral inhibition.

limited change in threshold (Graham et al., 1978). Note that the lateral inhibition implied by these data is cyclopean.

In comparison with the contrast threshold for luminance gratings, the whole disparity threshold function is shifted down in spatial frequency by about one log unit. The peak sensitivity occurs at about 0.4 cycles per degree, which corresponds approximately to the resolution limit of the global inhibitory process (depending on the exact model of the interactions between inhibition and excitation). The limited frequency resolution in this domain is discussed in the next section.

The existence of cyclopean lateral inhibition is in contradiction to the conclusion drawn from earlier, noncyclopean experiments using wavy line stimuli (Tyler, 1973, 1975b). A straight vertical line was presented to one eye and a line consisting of vertical segments displaced alternately to the left and right to the other eye (Tyler, 1973). On fusion, the segments are seen alternately forward and back from the fixation distance. Although the disparity-modulated stimuli showed a reduction in sensitivity at low spatial frequencies, a similar reduction in sensitivity was seen for monocular wavy lines. It was therefore concluded that no additional stereoscopic lateral inhibition was implied.

The evidence for cyclopean lateral inhibition casts a new light on the situation and requires the conclusion either that monocular stimuli are processed independently of the stereoscopic stimuli, or that noncyclopean stimuli are processed independently of the cyclopean stimuli. Since an independence between monocular and stereoscopic stimuli has recently been demonstrated by other techniques (Wolfe and Held, 1981), the first explanation seems preferable. This would imply that the stereoscopic system has a veridical input of the monocular components that is not directly available to (monocular) perception, but that a cyclopean lateral inhibition is added so that the two curves match as a result of similar but parallel processes in the monocular and stereoscopic domains.

Since the data of Figure 7.29 are threshold measurements, the cyclopean lateral inhibition operating to reduce low spatial-frequency sensitivity must be occurring between detectors at very similar disparities near threshold. It remains a question whether there is also lateral inhibition between detectors separated by larger disparities. This was addressed in a noncyclopean study by Tyler (1975b) in which the dependent variable was not the threshold but the maximum disparity for which any depth could be perceived. This upper disparity limit (UDL) was compared for sinusoidal and square wave spatial modulation of the disparity. If lateral inhibition were operative across large changes in disparity then it should tend to reduce the effective amplitude of a sinusoidal disparity modulation, as it does near threshold, while having no effect on the apparent amplitude of square wave disparity modulation, which contains no gradual slopes of disparity. Hence the sinusoidal modulation should have a larger physical value than the square wave modulation before the UDL is reached. This result was obtained in the Tyler (1975b) study, in which the sinusoidal UDL exceeded the square wave UDL by about a factor of three at all spatial frequencies of disparity modulation up to 1 cycle per degree. This suggests that lateral inhibition has a substantial effect on adjacent disparities, and is not limited in operation to detectors at the same disparity.

Global Processing Limitations

Apart from the effects of cyclopean lateral inhibition on stereograting threshold, there are two other major limitations on the processing of cyclopean images. The first is the maximum spatial frequency of disparity modulation that can be resolved (corresponding to the grating acuity limit in the contrast domain). This is the global bandwidth limitation mentioned earlier. The second is the limitation of the maximum disparity that can give rise to depth perception (upper disparity limit), and its variation with the structure of the disparity profile.

Global Bandwidth Limitation

Stereograting resolution is limited to between 3 and 5 cycles per degree for disparity modulation of both line stimuli (Tyler, 1973, 1975b) and cyclopean RDS (Tyler, 1974a; Schumer and Ganz, 1979; Tyler and Julesz, 1980a). This therefore seems to be a fundamental limitation in stereoscopic processing. It has been computed (Tyler, 1977b) that this limitation, which constitutes a reduction in bandwidth of about a factor of 10 in relation to the contrast bandwidth of the monocular channels, reduces by a factor of 10,000 the number of interocular point comparisons required to process the mean disparity of each point in a 10° × 10° image. This cuts the total number of comparisons required, or neurons needed, to process a 200-msec dynamic RDS from perhaps 10 million to about one thousand, which is clearly an enormous saving in brain processing capacity for the extraction of stereoscopic images.

Cyclopean Size/Disparity Scaling

The second type of limitation is that of the maximum disparity that can give rise to depth perception. Although it is well known that disparities greater than about 10° cannot be processed for depth, it was only recently that the dependence of this limit on the form of the disparity image was determined (Tyler, 1973, 1974a, 1975b). In fact, for repetitive modulation of disparity in both line and random-dot stereograms, the upper disparity limit (UDL) increases in direct proportion to the spacing of the disparate segments (i.e., inversely with the spatial frequency of disparity modulation). The maximum disparities for which depth was perceived was inversely proportional to vertical length of the segments over more than a 2-log unit range from 3 arc-minutes to 10° (upper portion of Figure 7.30), for both multiple and single cycles of disparity modulation. This relationship was termed disparity scaling of the upper disparity limit with stimulus size, since the form of the stimulus remains constant but is scaled uniformly to reach the UDL. Disparity scaling provides a further massive saving in the processing capacity required for fine detail in the disparity domain. At the same time it allows very large variations in disparity to be processed if they occur over a sufficiently large spatial extent.

Interestingly enough, the existence of disparity scaling in cyclopean RDS does not provide conclusive evidence that the scaling is a global phenomenon. If there is a correlation between the size of a receptive field and the disparity it processes, then low spatial frequencies of disparity modulation could be processed by large receptive fields with large dis-

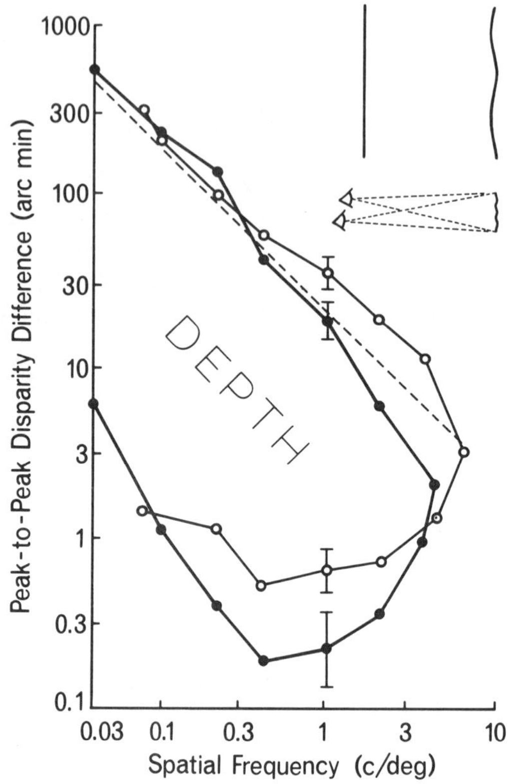

FIGURE 7.30. Complete region of depth perception as a function of spatial frequency of disparity modulation. Inset shows the left and right eye views of the stimulus together with a depiction of the binocular impression. Region marked DEPTH contains all stimuli in which depth modulation is visible. Filled circles = fixed aperture of 20°. Open circles = variable aperture such that one cycle was visible at each frequency. Dashed line has slope of −1.

parity preference, while high-modulation frequencies could be processed only by small receptive fields with fine disparity tuning. This would result in the kind of disparity scaling of the UDL observed on the basis of a local, rather than a global mechanism.

The global nature of disparity scaling can be established, paradoxically, by recourse to noncyclopean stimuli. Such an approach was taken by Pulliam (1982). Instead of presenting disparity modulation in an RDS format, he produced it in conventional sinusoidal contrast gratings. An example of this kind of stereograting is shown in Figure 7.31, in which the sinusoidal disparity modulation itself varies in frequency downward. Such gratings constrain the input to the cortex to essentially a single size of receptive field, with strong attenuation of the activation of those receptive fields that do not match the grating bar width (Albrecht et al., 1980). Nevertheless, the UDL showed the same kind of dependence on disparity modulation frequency as occurred in the line and RDS stereograms. Since only one size of receptive field is activated, this disparity scaling cannot be explained by the local size/disparity correlation. Given that disparity scaling occurs in line, grating, and RDS stimuli, it is presumably a truly global limitation of the processing of disparity modulation.

Figure 7.30 therefore depicts the complete range of disparity processing as a function of the spatial organization of the disparity stimulus, in terms of the spatial frequency of vertical modulation of horizontal disparity. The lower part of the figure shows the stereograting threshold with a peak sensitivity at about 0.4 cycle per degree. The right-hand portion of the curve represents the frequency resolution limit at about 4 cycles per degree, and the disparity scaling in the upper portion has been described.

No disparity modulation can produce sensations of depth variations outside these limits, which therefore constitute an important rubric for the construction of stereograms. This principle is frequently ignored in the presentation of stereograms in such fields as biochemistry, where stereograms are used for the depiction of large organic molecules. An example is shown in Figure 7.32, which may be seen stereoscopically by free-fusion if the reader is practised at this ability. Note that large ranges of depth are visible throughout the image, but in the complex segment near the arrow stereopsis fails because the spatial changes in disparity

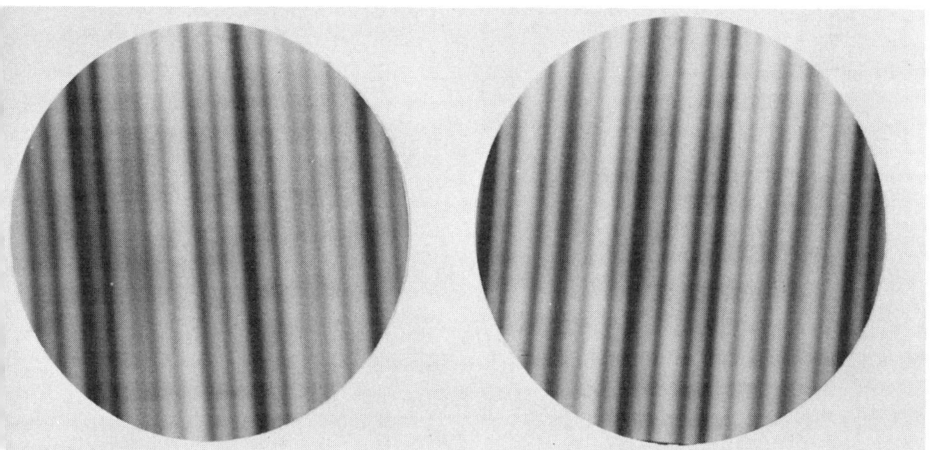

FIGURE 7.31. Disparity-modulated luminance grating. If the two halves of the stereogram are dichoptically fused, a percent of a sinusoidal surface in depth is obtained. The spatial frequency of disparity modulation increases toward the bottom of the image where the depth wrinkles become invisible because modulation has exceeded the upper depth limit due to disparity scaling.

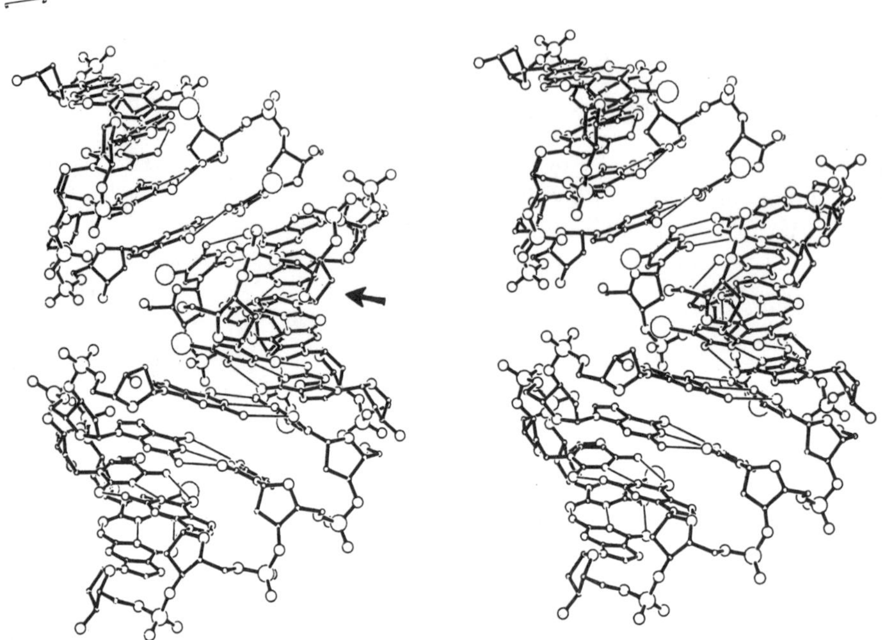

FIGURE 7.32. Stereogram of a DNA molecule showing region in which depth cannot be resolved because it exceeds the disparity scaling limit (*arrow*). Reprinted by permission of the publisher, from Dickerson RE, Drew HR, Conner BN, Wing RM, Fratini AV, Kopka ML. The anatomy of A-, B-, and Z- DNA. Science 1982, 216:475–485, American Association for the Advancement of Science.

are too rapid for cortex to process. This region of the molecular stereogram corresponds to the upper right-hand region of the disparity modulation space of Figure 7.30.

Specialized Global Stereoscopic Processes

In addition to global processing limitations, there are numerous specialized processes that occur within the cortical representation of the three-dimensional matrix of stereoscopic space (actually four-dimensional, since temporal phenomena are also of significance). One is the distinction between the pykno-stereoscopic and dia-stereoscopic ranges of fused depth surfaces and the range in which surfaces may be seen at different depths in the same visual direction. The others are a series of global stereoscopic phenomena such as hysteresis, which are described in detail by Julesz (1978) and therefore mentioned only briefly.

Pykno-Stereopsis and Dia-Stereopsis

The distinction between the fused depth range of pykno-stereopsis and the transparent surfaces of dia-stereopsis is emphasized here because it has important theoretical implications. For example, all models of stereopsis that rely on the determination of a single optimum surface within the disparity matrix presented to the eyes fail to account for the perception of coexistent diaphanous surfaces in RDS. Such surfaces are visible in the ambiguous stereograms generated by Julesz and Johnson (1968), who nonetheless suggest that only one surface is seen at a time.

Of course, it may be possible to modify the models to take the dia-stereoscopic range into account, but in their present form they apply only to the pykno-stereoscopic range, which has been measured at ±20 arc-minutes by Schumer (1979). Within this range there is depth averaging of the depths of the component images. This also appears to be the range of the stereoscopic depth aftereffects referred to previously. Since depth can be perceived up to several degrees in RDS (Tyler and Julesz, 1980a), the ±20-arc-minute range of pykno-stereopsis is only a small fraction of the range of global stereopsis. Furthermore, perception of multiple depth planes is not possible in local stereopsis (Foley, 1976), so it must be regarded as a global stereoscopic phenomenon.

Global Hysteresis

Hysteresis in global stereopsis was first described by Fender and Julesz (1967). Using a binocularly stabilized eye-movement system they found that the mean disparity in RDS could be increased to about 2° before the stereoscopic percept was destroyed, but that the disparity then had to be reduced to less than 10 arc-minutes for stereopsis to be reactivated. It is important to note that this was specifically a stereoscopic depth hysteresis and should not be considered relevant to the binocular fusion system, since it is difficult to tell whether or not an RDS is binocularly fused. A much smaller range of hysteresis was found for the binocular fusion of line stereograms. One problem in interpreting the Fender and Julesz result as a true hysteresis is that the RDS contained a central square with a disparity of 1° in relation to the surround, so it may be that differential attention to these two disparity planes could have produced part of the result.

A possible explanation for the hysteresis effect comes from the rivalry system, discussed earlier in the chapter. Once stereopsis has been destroyed, the rivalry mechanism could operate to interdict stereoscopic processing until the disparity was small enough to fall within the fusion range. The advantage of such an explanation is that it enlists the known switching behavior of the rivalry system to explain the hysteresis, and does not require additional hysteresis within the global stereoscopic process itself.

A second type of specialized global mechanism has been described by Julesz and Chang (1976). Using ambiguous dynamic RDS in which two planes were potentially visible at equal disparities in front of and behind fixation, these investigators "seeded" one of the planes by introducing a small percentage (4% to 25%) of unambiguous points. For presentation times as short as 50 msec the seeding introduced a strong dominance in the direction of the seeded disparity, which persisted at a reduced strength even when the seeding points were at a different disparity than the ambiguous planes. This seeding effect argues for a rapid parallel processing of the disparity image, with pooling between detectors at different disparities within the cyclopean image.

Summary of Cyclopean Limits

At this point it is worth summarizing some of the domains that have been discussed in a cyclopean equivalent (Figure 7.33) of the noncyclopean limits shown in Figure 7.18. Many of these limits have been studied only recently, so some of the details of the diagram are still sketchy. The outer curve of depth perception and the upper and lower disparity limits for noncyclopean perception are included from Figure 7.18 for comparison with the cyclopean limits.

Cyclopean stereoacuity is probably similar to noncyclopean stereoacuity, as both are typically measured at between 10 and 20 arc-seconds.

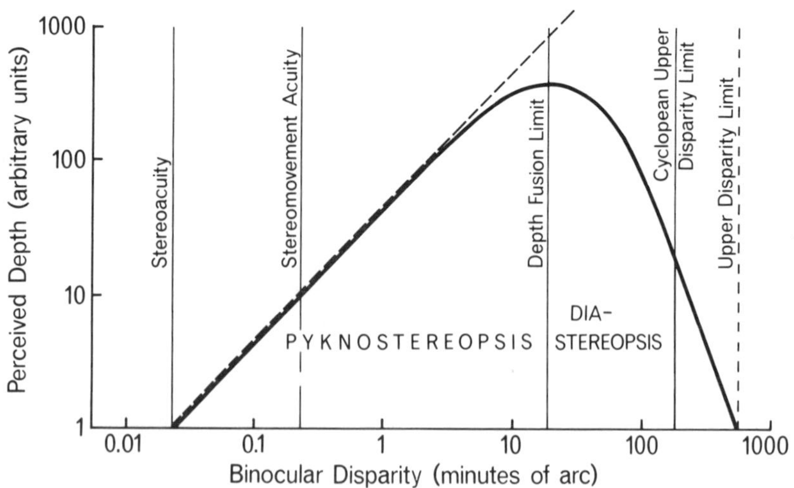

FIGURE 7.33. Schematic of some cyclopean disparity limits (see text for explanation).

The highly practised, forced-choice paradigms that give stereoacuity values of less than 5 arc-seconds have not yet been applied in a cyclopean paradigm, so that a real difference remains to be established.

A cyclopean stereomovement limit of about 30 arc-seconds was reported by Norcia (1980), who also determined the depth fusion limit between the ranges of pykno-stereopsis and dia-stereopsis. Since this limit varies with stimulus parameters, its position in the diagram is indicated only qualitatively.

As described, Tyler and Julesz (1980a) found that the cyclopean upper disparity limit (CUDL) was lower than its noncyclopean equivalent. Both limits depended in a similar fashion on the stimulus characteristics. It should be noted, however, that cyclopean stereopsis occurs across much of the noncyclopean range, and that the CUDL is not reached until well beyond Panum's fusional limit (compare Figures 7.18 and 7.33).

Thus the main point of this diagram is to emphasize that there is a series of limits in cyclopean stereopsis that are distinct from the noncyclopean limits, but may or may not take the same numerical values in cases where the two types are similarly defined.

Hypercyclopean Perception

The concept of hypercyclopean analysis refers to the third level of processing of stereoscopic images described in Figure 7.22. Just as images processed by the retina are then viewed by cortical neurons having retinal receptive fields with specific characteristics, so there is the possibility of a higher level of neurons in cortex having "receptive fields" at the level of the "cleaned" cyclopean depth image. These hypercyclopean receptive fields would have characteristics defined in terms of the *form* of the cyclopean image but independent of its specific disparity characteristics, that is, which particular disparity is stimulated at any given retinal location.

The existence of such a hypercyclopean level of processing can be demonstrated by means of an adaptation paradigm (Tyler, 1975a). The analogy is with the demonstration of cortical involvement in processing luminance gratings by adaptation to drifting gratings on the retina (Blakemore and Campbell, 1969; Kelly and Burbeck, 1980). Since the grating is drifting, there can be no retinal afterimage, and hence the threshold elevation, which is specific to both spatial frequency and orientation of the adapting grating, must be occurring at a higher, presumably cortical level of processing. In just the same way, if adaptation is found for a stereograting that is moving across the retina, it represents the activity of a level of form processing beyond that of the cyclopean processing for depth per se. Although there is no particular reason to expect a neural specificity for this type of stimulus, there are nevertheless several lines of evidence that suggest the existence of channels selective for the spatial frequency of the disparity modulation (as opposed to spatial frequency selectivity for the monocular contrast distribution).

Hypercyclopean Spatial Frequency Specificity

The first demonstration of a hypercyclopean aftereffect (Tyler, 1975a) was based on the Blakemore and Sutton (1969) experiment showing a perceived spatial frequency shift in a luminance grating after adaptation to one of a slightly different spatial frequency. In the hypercyclopean experiment, adaptation to a random-dot stereograting of one spatial frequency produced the perception of an increased spatial frequency of disparity modulation in another stereograting of slightly higher spatial frequency, and a corresponding decrease when testing with a slightly lower spatial frequency. The use of scanning eye movements during adaptation ensured that this result was not due to local disparity adaptation, but was a hypercyclopean effect. The result is suggestive of the existence of channels selective to the spatial frequency of disparity modulation.

Schumer and Ganz (1979) used an adaptation paradigm to investigate stereograting specificity. They adapted for eight minutes to one spatial frequency of disparity modulation and measured the threshold elevation for stereogratings across a range of spatial frequencies. Adaptation was maximal at the spatial frequency of the adapting stereograting, and showed a rather broad function with a bandwidth of about ±1 octave around each adapting frequency.

Although the adaptation approach has been widely used in psychophysics to establish the existence of selective neural channels, it may be criticized on the grounds that only those channels that are adaptable may be revealed by this technique. Other channels may exist that are not adaptable by the stimulus exposure used. Furthermore, the adaptation might not have a linear characteristic, and thus might distort the apparent shape of the channels when measured by this method. For example, if adaptation were very rapid in the case of stereogratings, the eight-minute adaptation period used by Schumer and Ganz (1979) might have saturated the system and given the appearance of artifactually broad channels.

The reason for this detailed analysis of the adaptation paradigm is that an alternative approach has suggested that the stereograting channel bandwidth is much narrower. This approach is based on the narrow-band masking paradigm introduced by Stromeyer and Julesz (1972) for contrast gratings. By masking the test grating with a one-octave band of noise at various center frequencies, they showed that frequency-selective channels in the contrast domain extended throughout the suprathreshold range, with bandwidths similar to those found by the threshold adaptation paradigm. Using a comparable technique, Tyler and Julesz (1980b) found that frequency selectivity for stereogratings was much narrower than found with the adaptation paradigm.

Figure 7.34 illustrates the paradigm used by Tyler and Julesz (1980b). The test stimulus was a sinusoidal stereograting of fixed spatial frequency. Masking noise in the form of the sum of six sinusoids across a one-octave band was added to the test stimulus with various separations between the noise and test. Each presentation had a 200-msec duration and thresholds were determined by a temporal two-alternative forced-choice paradigm. Figure 7.34 shows data for threshold elevation at three stereograting spatial frequencies as a function of the spatial frequency separation from a

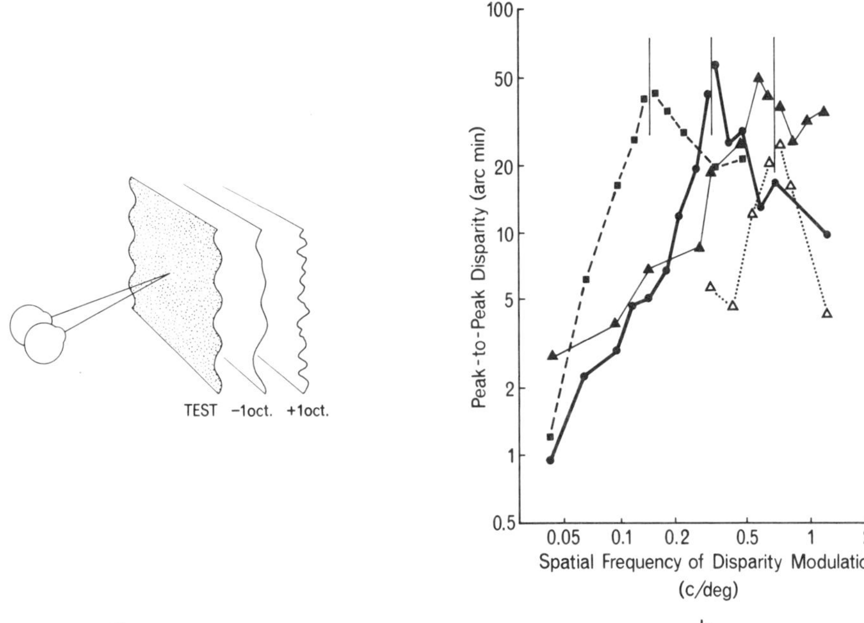

FIGURE 7.34. A Paradigm for hypercyclopean masking of stereograting perception in dynamic RDS. The detection stimulus is a stereograting masked by a one-octave band of disparity-modulation noise, which is added to the stimulus. Noise fields extending one octave below and one octave above the test frequency are depicted separately from the stimulus for clarity. B Threshold masking functions for stereogratings of three spatial frequencies (0.15, 0.3, and 0.6 cycles per degree) as a function of separation from the masking noise. (Masking is constant at the maximum value when the stereograting frequency is within the noise band, so these values are collapsed at the test frequency, as indicated by the vertical lines.) Dotted curve shows effect of reducing noise amplitude by a factor of three for the 0.6-cycle-per-degree condition. Note narrow tuning for disparity modulation revealed by masking technique.

one-octave band of masking noise. In each case the threshold elevation function has a bandwidth of about one-quarter octave on the low side and one-half octave on the high side.

The stereograting channel bandwidths implied by the masking data are very narrow in comparison to those found with the adaptation paradigm, indicating the presence of narrowly tuned mechanisms that were not adaptable by the technique used by Schumer and Ganz (1979). These data seem to imply the existence of specialized mechanisms for processing repetitive patterns of disparity modulation on the cyclopean retina.

Further evidence of such specialization is indicated by the difference in slopes of the cyclopean upper disparity limit (CUDL) for a single square in depth versus a stereograting. In RDS the CUDL for a single square increases with the square root of area, whereas the CUDL for a stereograting increases in direct proportion to the size of each cycle. A similar difference in slope is apparent for a single-cycle versus periodic modulation of the disparity in line stereograms (Tyler, 1973). These differences imply that specialized processing is involved in the perception of periodic disparity stimuli, in accord with the concept of channels selective for periodic disparity modulation.

Hypercyclopean Frontal Orientation Specificity

An argument similar to that adduced for spatial frequency can be developed for the existence of orientation specificity in the hypercyclopean domain. An experiment in support of this idea (Tyler, 1975a) was based on the well known tilt aftereffect paradigm (Gibson and Radner, 1937; Campbell and Maffei, 1971). Adaptation to a stereograting with an orientation at some angle away from horizontal produced a perceived tilt in a horizontal test stereograting. The magnitude of tilt aftereffect is plotted as a function of orientation difference between test and adapting stereogratings in Figure 7.35. This has a conventional form but peaks at about 25° in comparison to the 12° peak obtained for contrast gratings (Campbell and Maffei, 1971).

One can ask whether the hypercyclopean tilt aftereffect is independent of the contrast tilt aftereffect, or whether there is any cross-adaptation between them. The relative degree of cross-adaptation indicates the extent to which the two systems share a common pathway. Cross-adaptation was tested by adapting to a contrast grating of the same spatial frequency and measuring the tilt aftereffect obtained in a stereograting (which, it should be emphasized, had no orientation specificity in the contrast domain, i.e., the random-dot matrix). A cross-adaptation tilt aftereffect was obtained, but with about half the magnitude of the pure hypercyclopean effect (or, indeed, a pure contrast effect). It was therefore concluded that there are some oriented elements common to the two systems. Since the stimulus specification essentially precludes a common basis at the early stages of

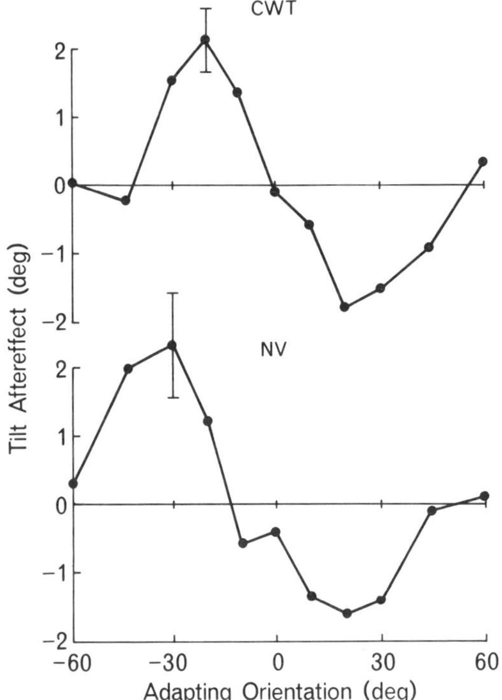

FIGURE 7.35. Hypercyclopean aftereffect of adaptation to orientation of stereograting. Angle of perceived horizontal of test stereograting is shown as a function of adapting orientation.

visual processing, it seems most likely that this common orientation specificity occurs even beyond the hypercyclopean level. Perhaps there is a high-level oriented "map" of the visual world that draws together the orientation information from previous levels, and is slightly rotated by adaptation to either contrast or cyclopean form information (see next sections).

Depth Orientation Specificity

The previous section addressed the question of cyclopean orientation specificity only for the two frontal dimensions of orientation. The three-dimensional nature of stereoscopic space also permits representation of orientation in the third (depth) dimension. Is there a specialized processing of such inclination in depth? One way to examine this is to look for visual illusions that are specific to inclination.

In his studies of cyclopean visual illusions, Julesz (1971) coded all his visual illusions in two-dimensional frontal planes using disparity only as a code to replace the brightness levels of the classical illusions. One can also ask whether there are (cyclopean) illusions in the third dimension of space. Figure 7.36 shows an original example based on the Hering illusion of line curvature induced by small, tilted line segments. This autostereogram, which should be viewed by the free-fusion technique, shows two sets of strips of opposite inclination. The overall planes in which they are embedded are not tilted and yet the tilted strips induce tilts in these planes.

Thus it appears that there are orientation interactions in the third dimension of visual space. Since the cyclopean presentation contains no

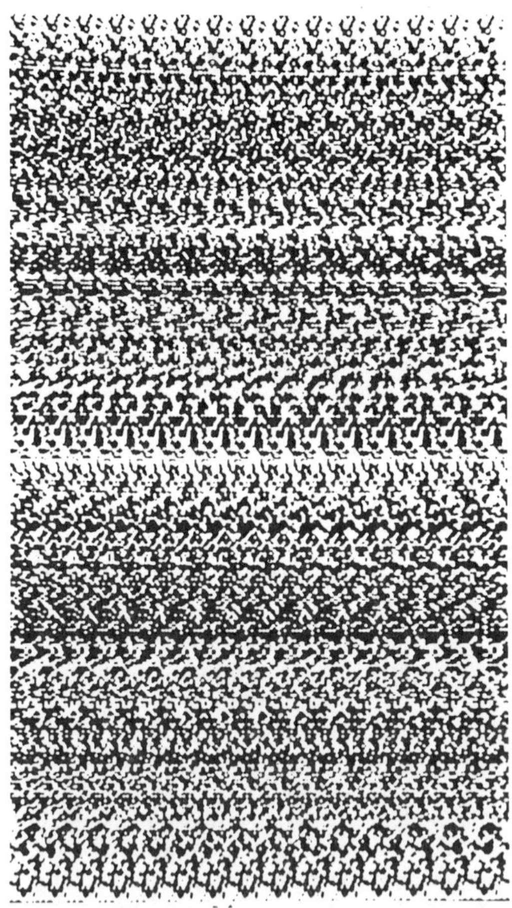

FIGURE 7.36. Autostereogram showing simultaneous depth tilt induction. Stereogram depicts "venetian blind" of tilted horizontal segments (in opposite directions in upper and lower halves of the image), inducing a perceived overall tilt of the two halves. Autostereogram should be viewed as described for Figure 7.20.

associated cues to monocular tilt, the mechanism must be different from those involved in the classical illusions of orientation. Mechanisms at the global cyclopean level are equally unable to account for the effect, since the processes should be the same in each bar, and therefore cause no perceived inclination of the overall planes. Only interactions specific to the inclination of the cyclopean plane constitute a sufficient explanation, and therefore represent a hypercyclopean selectivity for inclination in depth.

Hypercyclopean Object Constancy

Pushing further into the realms of complex space perception, one can approach the question of object constancy from the point of view of stereoscopic processing. Object constancy is the ability to perceive an object as having a rigid three-dimensional structure even while the retinal image is distorted by motion of the object in space. Although the contours of the object are undergoing continuous transformation, the brain often has the capability to reduce the motions to a single projective transformation within which the object retains its rigid form.

This concept can be applied to transformations of stereoscopic images. When an RDS is rotated or the observer moves around with respect to the stereogram, the cyclopean form is perceived as undergoing shape distortions in the form of relative motion between the different disparity planes (Julesz, 1971). This percept occurs even though the monocular half-images consist of flat planes in which there is no objective relative motion. This induced stereomovement has been attributed to the operation of object constancy (Tyler, 1974c) since it occurs at depth edges where the planes at different depths would move past each other, if the stereoscopic form were a rigid object undergoing rotation. When the object does not behave as expected, the stereoscopic object seems to become distorted in a nonrigid fashion, inducing relative perceived movements of the stereoscopic planes.

The dynamic characteristics of the object constancy system were measured by determining the sensitivity limits for induced stereomovement as a function of temporal frequency of rotation (Tyler, 1974c). At low frequencies the object constancy mechanism, as evinced from the induced stereomovement effect, operated down to about twice the amplitude of stereomovement threshold itself. As frequency was increased the object constancy mechanism progressively failed, and no induced stereomovement was seen above about 5 Hz, which was still close to the peak sensitivity for binocular movement perception. A remarkable observation was that in the region in which induced stereomovement was absent, substantial stereoscopic rotation could be perceived, and the stereoscopic form actually appeared to be a rotating rigid object. Thus there seems to be a clear perceptual dissociation of the stereomovement and object constancy systems.

It is perhaps premature to speculate on the relationship between the object constancy system and the cross-adaptable spatial rotation system described in the previous section. Nevertheless, if they are associated with perceptual processing beyond the hypercyclopean level, these paradigms may open the door to systematic investigation of the hierarchy of processes involved in human space perception.

VERGENCE

Role of Vergence in Stereopsis

Vergence eye movements have been invoked in a number of theories of stereoscopic processing (Sperling, 1970; Julesz, 1971; Marr and Poggio, 1979). If the range of disparities covered by the cortical disparity detectors were small, vergence eye movements would allow the processing of each part of a stereoscopic scene to be entered piece by piece into some higher perceptual representation of the full range of three-dimensional space. Such a process is taken to account for the ability to improve perception of RDS with continued exposure. After the initial presentation of a stereogram, the vergence system is already primed as to the appropriate fixation procedure, and depth could thus be achieved more rapidly than on the initial exposure.

Although vergence movements are undoubtedly important for binocular alignment, there are several problems with assigning them a major role in stereoscopic perception. The first of these is the large range of stereopsis without eye movements.

Stereopsis without Eye Movements

The original demonstration that stereopsis could occur without eye movements was provided by Dove (1841). He showed that depth could be seen with an electric spark of very brief duration, but did not measure the range of stereopsis obtainable. Extensive evidence for stereoscopic performance in the absence of vergence movements has been reviewed throughout this chapter, as typified by Richards and Kaye's (1974) finding of depth discrimination up to about 10° of disparity, which is similar to the range for which vergence movements can be initiated (Westheimer and Tanzman, 1956). If $\pm 10°$ represents the maximum range of neural disparity processing, it is sufficient to cover most of visual space, that is, from optical infinity down to 17 cm away from the observer's eyes. The range of $\pm 2°$ that is possible in cyclopean stereopsis allows depth perception from infinity down to 86 cm from the observer. For noncyclopean stereopsis, veridical depth perception is obtained up to about 2° of disparity for large stimuli (although it fails earlier if the stimuli are small). Thus there is little need to build up a higher cortical representation piecemeal, since such a large range is captured by the parallel disparity processing. Of course, best discrimination occurs near the fixation position, so that vergence eye movements can improve stereoscopic performance within this range, but they are not necessary for overall perception of stereoscopic space.

The stereoscopic situation is analogous to perception of two-dimensional space with a high-acuity fovea controlled by lateral eye movements. It is clear that the general layout of objects in two-dimensional space is readily perceived across the 180° field without lateral eye movements, as fixation on any scene will demonstrate. What the eye movements accomplish is detailed perception of a chosen part of the perceived scene. It seems reasonable to suppose that vergence movements serve the same role for the third dimension, bringing regions of interest into the range of best disparity discrimination.

Having reviewed the evidence for stereopsis without eye movements, it should be clear that vergence is not necessary for the operation of much of stereoscopic perception. The question remains whether vergence plays a role in building up stereoscopic images under some circumstances, or whether it merely serves to optimize the region of best stereopsis. This question has been approached in three ways: the role of vergence in immediate stereoscopic perception, the role of vergence in stereoscopic learning tasks, and the integration of vergence information into the perception of distance.

Immediate Stereoscopic Perception

The first question is whether voluntary eye movements are necessary for optimal stereoacuity. In general, it seems that the presence of vergence eye movements does not improve stereoacuity (Wright, 1951; Rady and Ishak, 1955; Ogle, 1956). Furthermore, it is unaffected by lateral movement of the stimuli across the retina at velocities up to 2° per second (Lit, 1964; Westheimer and McKee, 1978). Thus it appears that stereoacuity is not dependent on eye movements of either the vergence or versional type, but is in fact rather well insulated from such disturbances.

The next question is whether eye movements play a role in suprathreshold stereopsis, as opposed to the extraction of depth information from convergence per se, which will be considered later, as will the scaling of depth with mean convergence angle. The specific question here is whether differential depth appreciation is aided by vergence movements within a given stereoscopic image. Marr and Poggio (1979), for example, have argued that the depth image close to each convergence angle is processed directly and added serially to a higher cortical representation of visual space with each new vergence position.

Experiments purporting to demonstrate that eye movements increase the range of perceived depth (Foley and Richards, 1972) have been confounded by the influence of nonstereoscopic cues to depth from the vergence angle itself, which is a difficult factor to dissociate. Other experiments suggest that the use of convergence does not enhance depth perception in complex random-dot stereograms (Frisby and Clatworthy, 1975). On balance, therefore, it appears that suprathreshold stereopsis is not enhanced by vergence eye movements.

Stereoscopic Learning and Vergence

If, as Julesz (1971) and others have suggested, improved vergence performance is the explanation for stereoscopic learning in RDS, then preceding exposure of the RDS by a stimulus that covers the relevant vergence range should also improve perception time for stereopsis. Frisby and Clatworthy (1975) conducted such an experiment for an RDS of a complex spiral, using as a preceding stimulus a physical model of the spiral, which was also covered with random dots. They further included test conditions in which noncyclopean contours outlined the stereofigure, and the observers were required to fixate on a fixation point. None of these conditions had a significant effect on the perception time for the test stereogram compared with the control condition without a preceding stimulus, either on first presentation or during the subsequent learning phase. Other conditions in which verbal descriptions of the stimulus preceded the presentation actually showed retardation of perception time.

Thus not only did the contours, designed as a guide for eye movements, not improve the stereoscopic performance, but prohibition of eye movements by requiring fixation did not degrade stereoscopic performance. Apparently, vergence movements play no role in the perception of complex RDS containing disparities up to 1°. Furthermore, such learning as did occur was essentially complete by the third trial, so that the phenomenon of stereoscopic learning was largely confined to naive observers and perhaps difficult types of stereogram. This observation again tends to minimize the role of vergence in mature stereopsis.

Curiously, Frisby (1979) seems to disregard these findings and favors the vergence hypothesis of stereoscopic learning, although his own evidence (Saye and Frisby, 1975) shows that it applies only under extreme disparity conditions with a single square stereofigure. Under these conditions the vergence information may have provided a nonstereoscopic cue to depth. Clearly, disparity distributions in the real world are generally more like a complex stereogram with multiple, graded surfaces than a single square standing at a disparity of 1°. The Frisby and Clatworthy

(1975) study shows that vergence eye movements provide no advantage for depth perception in such complex stimuli.

An experiment by Ramachandran and Braddick (1973) suggests that the key to stereoscopic learning may lie in the monocular structure of the noise of which the stereogram is composed. They exposed observers to a random-line stereogram constructed from oblique line segments at $+45°$ orientation. On repeated exposure the perception time was progressively reduced. When these observers were shown a stereogram containing the same cyclopean depth image but made from segments at $-45°$ orientation, there was little transfer of the stereoscopic learning except on the first trial, and the stereogram had essentially to be learned all over again.

In a second experiment Ramachandran (1976) altered the micropatterns of the (nonoriented) noise in an RDS after it had been learned, keeping the stereofigure unchanged. No decrement of performance was produced by this alteration. Taken together these experiments showed that the learning had not occurred with respect to stereoscopic form or to specific micropatterns but largely with respect to structural constraints of the monocular patterns, and therefore had little relation to any vergence learning that may have occurred during observation of the original stereogram.

Role of Vergence in Space Perception

Although the case has been made that vergence is not necessary for stereoscopic processing of binocular disparity, it nevertheless plays a substantial role in the calibration of depth into perceived distance and the perception of three-dimensional space. The effects of vergence and conjunctive eye position on the form of the horopter have been considered in detail at the beginning of this chapter.

Depth Perception by Means of Vergence Alone

The question of how much depth is perceived by means of vergence has been addressed in a landmark paper by Foley (1978), in which a large body of data from a century of experimentation is integrated into a formal model of binocular distance perception. Without reviewing this work in detail, the main conclusions can be summarized succinctly. Perceived depth increases linearly with vergence angle to a good approximation for most observers, but the relation is not veridical because the vergence signal is underestimated. (In many tasks vergence is not controlled directly, but the stimuli are set at different distances and the observers permitted free eye movements, so that vergence generally corresponded to the absolute binocular disparity at each distance.)

The degree to which vergence information is underestimated depends on the depth estimation task, and is expressed in terms of the slope of the linear relation between vergence angle and perceived depth. Three types of task have been used: stereoscopic distance estimation, manual pointing, and verbal estimation of depth magnitude. In each case, the relation between perceived depth and absolute disparity (i.e., vergence angle) is reasonably linear, but each has a characteristic slope.

For tasks estimating stereoscopic distance, which involve some method of setting the relative perceived distances of stereoscopic stimuli, the slope is typically about 0.5. This implies that the convergence signal controls stereoscopic depth perception at about half-strength, such that distances closer than the resting vergence position (Gogel, 1961) are perceived as not so close and those farther than the resting vergence position as not so far away.

For manual pointing tasks, in which the observer has to point to the perceived distance of the stereoscopic object while the hand is not visible, the depth/disparity functions have a shallow slope of about 0.25 (Foley, 1977). Thus the convergence signal seems to be less available to the motor output system than to the visual system directly. When the task is a verbal estimation of the amount of perceived depth, slopes of about 0.8 are found (Foley, 1977), so that by the time the depth is processed by higher perceptual mechanisms it approaches the veridical value of 1.0. In order to understand the basis of these differences it is important to bear in mind the precise nature of each task. One factor that may be significant is the time taken to make each type of judgment. If the vergence signal for depth had a rapid decay time, it is possible that the task differences in slope could be attributed to differences in the time taken to form each type of judgment. This factor cannot be estimated in experiments using free eye movements, but would require more controlled experiments. The fact that the verbal estimation had the highest slope is suggestive, however, since it was based on the observers' immediate impression, and did not require the time for a visual or manual matching procedure.

Vergence Calibration of Relative Stereoscopic Depth Perception

The depth perceived between objects with a relative disparity depends on the convergence angle with which the objects are viewed (see Foley, 1978 for review). A well-known example of this effect can be seen in random-dot stereograms. For example, if the autostereograms of Figures 7.20, 7.21, and 7.28 are viewed from one distance and then moved away, it will be seen that the absolute amount of perceived depth (in cm) appears to increase with viewing distance.

A similar experiment can be done on perceived stereoscopic depth with all distance cues eliminated except for vergence angle. If the effect of convergence angle were veridical there should be a linear relationship (depth constancy), such that halving the viewing distance should halve the perceived depth. In fact, perceived depth varies less than this veridical prediction. Foley (1978), however, has demonstrated that for a wide variety of stimuli, perceived depth varies linearly with perceived viewing distance, after taking the reduced gain of the vergence system (0.5) into account. It is as though the stereoscopic system makes a perfect calibration of the perceived depth according to the distance information received, but the vergence system is unable to supply it with a veridical estimate of the distance. Thus the fault lies not in our stereopsis but in our proprioception.

From a teleological point of view it is puzzling that in distance perception, as for much other proprioceptive input, the brain appears to have all the apparatus available to achieve a veridical representation of the spatial world yet falls short for want of an adequate gain factor. Surely, if the information is sufficiently accurate to provide a linear distance signal from the convergence angle, it should be simple enough to give the appropriate gain.

One possibility is that the experimenters are asking the wrong question in determining depth constancy for the convergence signal when it is the only cue to depth. It presumably evolved to operate in conjunction with all the other depth cues, which combine to provide a veridical distance estimate (Holway and Boring, 1941). If Foley (1978) is correct that imperfections of stereoscopic depth constancy are entirely attributable to weak convergent input, then veridical depth constancy should be expected when there are full cues. The rules of combination of the various cues to depth (which are not known at present) may require that the gain of each alone be less than unity.

CONCLUSION

This chapter describes an attempt to take a representative portion of the data of binocular vision and develop a coherent framework of binocular processing and its relation to vergence eye movements. This is in contrast to many previous models that limit their description to a narrow subset of the available data. As in many branches of science, the story has to become more complicated before it gets simpler. It seems that the series/parallel concept of Figure 7.22 provides a place for most of the puzzling findings in the current literature, many of which are at odds with previous theoretical treatments. It is hoped that it will continue to serve the same function for some time into the future.

Naturally, what has been gained in inclusiveness has tended to detract from predictive rigor. At this stage, the model contains little that can define specific outcomes for future experiments, which is why it has been discussed as a theoretical framework rather than a theory as such. By their nature, parallel systems are more difficult to analyze from their response characteristics than serial systems. This may be regarded as one of the central dilemmas of the brain sciences, and it is not made easier by failing to recognize it.

In fact, most neurophysiological and anatomic techniques are oriented toward analysis of parallel systems. Many single neurons process different information from the same retinal location, and each different type can be considered to belong to an array across the retina for each type of stimulus feature. Then there is increasing evidence for multiple representation of the retinal input in a series of cortical regions. To date very little of such neurophysiological structure is known to apply to stereoscopic processing, due to difficulty of controlling with sufficient accuracy the minute disparities in animal preparations.

In the psychophysical domain, the main technique for the study of parallel systems is by selective adaptation (e.g., Blakemore and Campbell, 1969). Again, this has yet to be applied to stereopsis in the kind of detail that would provide a test of the proposed model. Finally, the third pathway into the human brain, the evoked potential, is beginning to show a surprising degree of selectivity to a wide variety of stimulus parameters. As implied by the organization of this chapter, a cooperative program using a combination of all these approaches may be the best way to untangle the complexities of human stereopsis and other sensory processing.

REFERENCES

Aguilonius F. Opticorum libri sex. Antwerp: Plantin, 1613.

Albrecht DG, DeValois RL, Thorell LG. Visual cortical neurons: are bars or gratings the optimal stimuli? Science 1980;207:88–90.

Anstis SM, Howard IP, Rogers B. A Craik-O'Brien-Cornsweet illusion for visual depth. Vision Res 1978;18:213–18.

Apkarian PA, Nakayama K, Tyler CW. Binocularity in the visual evoked potential: facilitation, summation and suppression. Electroenceph Clin Neurophysiol 1981;51:32–48.

Barany EH, Hallden U. The influence of some central nervous system depressants on the reciprocal inhibition between the two retinas as manifested in retinal rivalry. Acta Psychol Scand 1947;14:296–316.

Barlow HB, Blakemore C, Pettigrew JD. The neural mechanism of binocular depth discrimination. J Physiol 1967;193:327–42.

Beverley KI, Regan D. Evidence for the existence of neural mechanisms selectively sensitive to the direction of movement in space. J Physiol 1973;235:17–29.

Beverley KI, Regan D. The relation between sensitivity and discrimination in the perception of motion-in-depth. J Physiol 1975;249:387–98.

Beverley KI, Regan D. Separable aftereffects of changing-size and motion-in-depth: different neural mechanisms? Vision Res 1979;19:727–32.
Blake R, Fox R. Binocular rivalry suppression: insensitive to spatial frequency and orientation change. Vision Res 1974a;14:687–92.
Blake R, Fox R. Adaptation to invisible gratings and the site of binocular rivalry suppression. Nature 1974b;249:488–90.
Blake R, Fox R, McIntyre C. Stochastic properties of stabilized-image binocular rivalry alternations. J Exp Psychol 1971;88:327–32.
Blakemore C. The range and scope of binocular depth discrimination in man. J Physiol 1970a;211:599–622.
Blakemore C. A new kind of stereoscopic vision. Vision Res 1970b;10:1181–1200.
Blakemore C, Campbell FW. On the existence of neurones in the human visual system selectively sensitive to the orientation and size of retinal images. J Physiol 1969;203:237–60.
Blakemore C, Julesz B. Stereoscopic depth aftereffect produced without monocular cues. Science 1971;171:286–88.
Blakemore C, Sutton P. Size adaptation: a new aftereffect. Science 1969;166:245–47.
Blakemore C, Fiorentini A, Maffei L. A second neural mechanism of binocular depth discrimination. J Physiol 1972;226:725–49.
Breese BB. On inhibition. Psychol Monogr 1899;3:1–65.
Breitmeyer B, Julesz B, Kropfl W. Dynamic random-dot stereograms reveal up-down anisotropy and left-right isotropy between cortical hemifields. Science 1976;187:269–70.
Campbell FW, Maffei L. Electrophysiological evidence for the existence of orientation and size detectors in the human visual system. J Physiol 1970;207:635–52.
Campbell FW, Maffei L. The tilt aftereffect: a fresh look. Vision Res 1971;11:833–40.
Cobb WA, Morton HB, Ettlinger G. Cerebral potentials evoked by pattern reversal and their suppression in visual rivalry. Nature 1967;216:1123–26.
Cogan AI. The relationship between the apparent vertical and the vertical horopter. Vision Res 1979;19:655–65.
Collyer SC, Bevan W. Objective measurement of dominance control in binocular rivalry. Percept Psychophysics 1970;8:437–39.
Cynader M, Regan D. Neurons in cat parastriate cortex sensitive to the direction of motion in three-dimensional space. J Physiol 1978;274:549–69.
Dickerson, RE, Drew HR, Conner BN, Wing RM, Fratini AV, Kopka ML. The anatomy of A-, B-, and Z-DNA. Science 1982;216:475–85 [Fig. 1].
Diner D. Hysteresis in binocular fusion: a second look. Ph.D. dissertation, California Institute Technology, 1978.
Dove HW. Uber Stereoskopie. Ann Phys 1841;2,110:494–98.
Drake S, Kowal CT. Galileo's sighting of Neptune. Sci Am 1980;243:74–81.
Felton TB, Richards W, Smith RA. Disparity processing of spatial frequencies in man. J Physiol (Lond) 1972;225:349.
Fender D, Julesz B. Extension of Panum's fusional area in binocularly stabilized vision. J Opt Soc Am 1967;57:819–30.
Foley JM. Binocular depth mixture. Vision Res 1976;16:1263–68.
Foley JM. Effect of distance information and range on two indices of perceived distance. Perception 1977;6:449–60.

Foley JM. Primary distance perception. In: Held R, Leibowitz HW, Teuber H-L, eds. Handbook of sensory physiology. Vol. VII. Perception. Berlin: Springer-Verlag, 1978.

Foley JM, Richards W. Effects of voluntary eye movement and convergence on the binocular appreciation of depth. Percept Psychophysics 1972;11:423–27.

Fox R, Check R. Binocular fusion: a test of the suppression theory. Percept Psychophysics 1966a;1:331–34.

Fox R, Check R. Forced choice recognition of form during binocular rivalry. Psychonom Sci 1966b;6:471–72.

Fox R, Check R. Detection of motion during binocular rivalry suppression. J Exp Psychol 1968;78:388–95.

Fox R, Check R. Detection of motion during binocular rivalry suppression. J Exp Psychol 1972;78:388–95.

Fox R, Rasche F. Binocular rivalry and reciprocal inhibition. Jpn Psychol Res 1969;2:94–105.

Friedman RB, Kaye MG, Richards W. Effect of vertical disparity upon stereoscopic depth. Vision Res 1978;18:351–52.

Frisby JP. Seeing: illusion, brain and mind. Oxford: Oxford University Press, 1979.

Frisby JP, Clatworthy JL. Learning to see complex random-dot stereograms. Perception 1975;4:173–78.

Fry GA. Visual perception of space. Am J Optom 1950;27:531–53.

Gibson JJ. The perception of the visual world. Boston: Houghton Mifflin, 1950.

Gibson JJ, Radner M. Adaptation, aftereffect and contrast in the perception of tilted lines. I. Quantitative studies. J Exp Psychol 1937;20:453.

Gogel WC. Convergence as a cue to absolute distance. J Psychol 1961;52:287–301.

Gouras P, Armington JC, Kropfl W, Gunkel RD. Electronic computation of human retinal and brain responses to light stimulation. IV. Neurophysiology 1964;115:763–75.

Graham N, Robson JG, Nachmias J. Grating summation in fovea and periphery. Vision Res 1978;18:815–26.

Harter MR, Seiple WH, Salmon L. Binocular summation of visually evoked responses to pattern stimuli in humans. Vision Res 1973;13:1433–46.

Hecht S, Mintz EU. The visibility of single lines at various illuminations and the retinal basis of visual resolution. J Gen Physiol 1939;22:593–612.

Helmholtz HL. Handbuch der physiologische Optik. Hamburg: Voss, 1866.

Hering E. Beitrage zu Physiologie. Leipzig: W Engelman, 1864.

Hering E. The theory of binocular vision (1868). Bridgeman B, Stark L, eds, trans. New York: Plenum Press, 1977.

Hillebrand F. Die Stabilitat der Raumwerte auf der Netzhaut. Z Psychol 1893; 5:1–59.

Hirsch MJ, Weymouth FW. Distance discrimination. II. Effect on threshold of lateral separation of the test objects. Arch Ophthalmol 1948;39:224–31.

Hollins M. Does the central human retina stretch during accommodation? Nature 1974;251:729–30.

Holway AH, Boring EG. Determinants of apparent visual size with distance variant. Am J Psychol 1941;54:21–37.

Howard HJ. A test for the judgment of distance. Am J Ophthalmol 1919;2:656–75.

Hubel DH, Wiesel TN. Receptive fields, binocular interaction and functional architecture in the cat's visual cortex. J Physiol 1962;160:106–54.

Hubel DH, Wiesel TN. Receptive fields and functional architecture of monkey striate cortex. J Physiol 1968;195:215–43.

Hubel DH, Wiesel TN. Stereoscopic vision in macaque monkey. Nature 1970;225:41–42.

Hubel DH, Wiesel TN, Stryker MP. Anatomical demonstration of orientation columns in macaque monkey. J Comp Neurol 1978;177(3):361–80.

ones R. Anomalies of disparity detection in the human visual system. J Physiol (Lond) 1977;264:621–40.

oshua DE, Bishop PO. Binocular single vision and depth discrimination. Exp Brain Res 1970;10:389–416.

Julesz B. Binocular depth perception of computer-generated patterns. Bell Syst Tech J 1960;39:1125–62.

Julesz B. Towards the automation of binocular depth perception (AUTOMAP-I). In: Popplewell CM, ed. Proc. IFIPC Amsterdam: Elsevier North-Holland, 1962.

Julesz B. Foundations of cyclopean perception. Chicago: University of Chicago Press, 1971.

Julesz B. Global stereopsis: cooperative phenomena in stereoscopic depth perception. In: Held R, Leibowitz HW, Teuber H-L, eds. Handbook of sensory physiology. Vol. VII. Perception. Berlin: Springer-Verlag, 1978.

Julesz B, Chang JJ. Interaction between pools of binocular disparity detectors tuned to different disparities. Biol Cybernet 1976;22:107–19.

Julesz B, Johnson SC. Mental holography: stereograms portraying ambiguously perceivable surfaces. Bell Syst Tech J 1968;49:2075–83.

Julesz B, Miller J. Independent spatial-frequency-tuned channels in binocular fusion and rivalry. Perception 1975;4:125–43.

Julesz B, Tyler CW. Neurontropy, an entropy-like measure of neural correlation, in binocular fusion and rivalry. Biol Cybernet 1976;22:107–19.

Kakizaki S. Binocular rivalry and stimulus intensity. Jpn Psychol Res 1960;2:94–105.

Kaufman L. On the nature of binocular disparity. Am J Psychol 1964;77:393–402.

Kelly DH, Burbeck CA. Motion and vision. III. Stabilized pattern adaptation. J Opt Soc Am 1980;70:1283–89.

Kertesz AE. The effect of stimulus complexity on human cyclofusional response. Vision Res 1972;12:699–704.

Koenderink JJ, van Doorn AJ. Geometry of binocular vision and a model for stereopsis. Biol Cybernet 1946;21:29–35.

Lack LC. The role of accommodation in the control of binocular rivalry. Percept Psychophysics 1971;10:38–42.

Langlands, NMS. Experiments on binocular vision. Trans Opt Soc 1926;28:230–38.

Lehmkuhle S, Fox R. The effect of binocular rivalry suppression on the motion aftereffect. Vision Res 1975;15:855–60.

Levelt WJM. On binocular rivalry. Ph.D. thesis, Institute for Perception, RVO-TNO, Soesterberg, The Netherlands 1965.

Linksz A. The horopter: an analysis. Trans Am Ophthalmol Soc 1954;52:877–946.

Lit A. Equidistance settings (photopic) and target velocity. J Opt Soc Am 1964;54:83–88.

MacKay DM. Visual effects of non-redundant stimulation. Nature 1961;192:739–40.

Marr D, Poggio T. Cooperative computation of stereo disparity. Science 1976;194:283–87.

Marr D, Poggio T. A theory of human stereopsis. Proc R Soc B 1979;204:301–28.

Mayhew JEW, Frisby JP. Surfaces with steep disparity variations in depth pose difficulties for orientationally tuned disparity filters. Perception 1949;8:691–98.

Mayhew JEW, Frisby JP. The computation of binocular edges. Perception 1980;9:69–86.

Meyer H. Handbuch der Physiologie. Berlin: MH Romberg, 1833.

Mitchell DE. Properties of stimuli eliciting vergence eye movements and stereopsis. Vision Res 1970;10:145–62.

Mitchell DE, Baker AG. Stereoscopic aftereffects: evidence for disparity specific neurones in the human visual system. Vision Res 1973;13:2273–88.

Nakayama K. Geometrical and physiological aspects of depth perception. In: Benton S, ed. Image processing. Proc Soc Photo-Opt Instr Eng. 1977;120:1–8.

Nakayama K, Loomis JM. Optical velocity patterns, velocity sensitive neurons and space perception: a hypothesis. Perception 1974;3:63–80.

Nakayama K, Tyler CW, Appelman J. A new angle on the vertical horopter. Invest Ophthalmol (Suppl) 1977;16:82.

Nelson JI. Globality and stereoscopic fusion in binocular vision. J Theoretical Biol 1975;49:1–88.

Norcia AM. Frequency domain analysis of human stereopsis. Ph.D. thesis, Stanford University, Palo Alto, California, 1980.

Norcia AM, Tyler CW. Frequency domain analysis of human stereopsis. Soc Neurosci Abs 1980;6:483.

Ogle KN. Analytical treatment of the longitudinal horopter. J Opt Soc Am 1932;22:665–728.

Ogle KN. Researches in binocular vision. Philadelphia: WB Saunders, 1950.

Ogle KN. Disparity limits of stereopsis. Arch Ophthalmol 1952a;48:50–60.

Ogle KN. On the limits of stereoscopic vision. J Exp Psychol 1952b;44:253–59.

Ogle KN. Stereopsis and vertical disparity. Arch Ophthalmol 1955;53:495–504.

Ogle KN. Stereoscopic acuity and the role of convergence. J Opt Soc Am 1956;46:269–73.

Ogle KN. Fixation disparity and oculomotor imbalance. Am Orthopt J 1958;8:21–36.

Ogle KN. Spatial localization through binocular vision. In: Davson H, ed. The eye. Vol. 4. Visual optics and the optical space sense. New York: Academic Press, 1962a.

Ogle KN. The problem of the horopter. In: Davson H, ed. The eye. Vol. 4. Visual optics and the optical space sense. New York: Academic Press, 1962b.

Ogle KN, Ellerbrock VJ. Cyclofusional movements. Arch Ophthalmol 1946;36:700–36.

Ogle KN, Weil MP. Stereoscopic vision and the duration of the stimulus. Arch Ophthalmol 1958;59:4–17.

Panum PL. Physiologische Untersuchungen uber das Sehen mit zwei Augen. Kiel: Schwering, 1858.

Perry NW, Childers DG, McCoy JG. Binocular addition of the visual evoked responses at different cortical locations. Vision Res 1968;8:567–73.

Pettigrew JD. Binocular neurones which signal change of disparity in area 18 of cat visual cortex. Nature New Biol 1973;241:123–24.

Pettigrew JD, Konishi M. Neurons selective for orientation and binocular disparity in the visual Wulst of the barn owl (*Tyto alba*). Science 1976;193:675–78.

Pettigrew JD, Nikara T, Bishop PO. Binocular interaction on single units in cat striate cortex: simultaneous stimulation by single moving slits with receptive fields in correspondence. Exp Brain Res 1968;6:391–410.

Piggins D. Moirés maintained internally by binocular vision. Perception 1978;7:679–81.

Poggio GF, Fischer B. Binocular interaction and depth sensitivity of striate and prestriate cortical neurons of behaving rhesus monkeys. J Neurophysiol 1977;40:1392–1405.

Pulliam K. Spatial frequency analysis of three-dimensional vision. Proc Soc Photo-Opt Instr Eng 1982;303:17–23.

Rady AA, Ishak IGH. Relative contributions of disparity and convergence to stereoscopic acuity. J Opt Soc Am 1955;45:530–34.

Ramachandran VS. Learning-like phenomena in stereopsis. Nature 1976;262:382–84.

Ramachandran VS, Braddick OL. Orientation-specific learning in stereopsis. Perception 1973;2:371–76.

Regan D. Evoked potentials in psychology, sensory physiology and medicine. London: Chapman & Hall, 1972.

Regan D, Beverley KI. Disparity detectors in human depth perception: evidence for directional selectivity. Science 1973a;181:877–79.

Regan D, Beverley KI. Some dynamic features of depth perception. Vision Res 1973b;13:2369–79.

Regan D, Beverley KI. The dissociation of sideways movements from movements in depth: psychophysics. Vision Res 1973c;13:2403–15.

Regan D, Beverley KI. Electrophysiological evidence for the existence of neurones sensitive to the direction of movement in depth. Nature 1974;246:504–6.

Richards W. Anomalous stereoscopic depth perception. J Opt Soc Am 1971;61:410–14.

Richards W, Kaye MG. Local versus global stereopsis: two mechanisms? Vision Res 1974;14:1345–47.

Roenne G. The physiological basis of sensory fusion. Acta Ophthalmol 1956;344:1–28.

Saye A, Frisby JP. The role of monocularly conspicuous features in facilitating stereopsis from random-dot stereograms. Perception 1975;4:159–71.

Schor CM, Tyler CW. Spatio-temporal properties of Panum's fusional area. Vision Res 1981;21:683–92.

Schumer RA. Mechanisms in human stereopsis. Ph.D. thesis, Stanford University, Palo Alto, California, 1979.

Schumer RA, Ganz L. Independent stereoscopic channels for different extents of spatial pooling. Vision Res 1979;19:1303–14.

Sheedy JE, Fry GA. The perceived direction of the binocular image. Vision Res 1979;19:201–11.

Spekreijse H. Analysis of EEG responses to diffuse and patterned light in human. The Hague: DW Junk, 1966.

Sperling G. Binocular vision: a physical and neural theory. J Am Psychol 1970;83:461–534.

Stromeyer CF III, Julesz B. Spatial frequency in vision: critical bands and spread of masking. J Opt Soc Am 1972;62:1221–32.

Tyler CW. Stereoscopic depth movement: two eyes less sensitive than one. Science 1971;174:958–61.

Tyler CW. Stereoscopic vision: cortical limitations a disparity scaling effect. Science 1973;181:276–78.
Tyler CW. Depth perception in disparity gratings. Nature 1974a;251:140–42.
Tyler CW. Stereopsis in dynamic visual noise. Nature 1974b;250:781–82.
Tyler CW. Induced stereomovement. Vision Res 1974c;14:609–13.
Tyler CW. Stereoscopic tilt and size aftereffects. Perception 1975a;4:187–92.
Tyler CW. Spatial organization of binocular disparity sensitivity. Vision Res 1975b;15:583–90.
Tyler CW. Observations on binocular frequency reduction in random noise. Perception 1975c;4:305–9.
Tyler CW. Characteristics of stereomovement suppression. Percept Psychophysics 1975d;17:225–30.
Tyler CW. Spatial limitations in stereopsis. Proc Soc Photo-Opt Instr Eng 1977a;120:36–42.
Tyler CW. Stereomovement from interocular delay in dynamic visual noise: a random spatial disparity hypothesis. Am J Optom 1977b;54:374–86.
Tyler CW. Binocular moiré fringes and the vertical horopter. Perception 1980;9:475–78.
Tyler CW, Chang JJ. Visual echoes: the perception of repetition in quasi-random patterns. Vision Res 1977;17:109–16.
Tyler CW, Foley J. Stereomovement suppression for transient disparity changes. Perception 1975;3:287–96.
Tyler CW, Julesz B. The neural transfer characteristic (neurontropy) for binocular stochastic stimulation. Bio Cybernet 1976;23:33–37.
Tyler CW, Julesz B. On the depth of the cyclopean retina. Exp Brain Res 1980a;40:196–202.
Tyler CW, Julesz B. Narrowband spatial frequency tuning for disparity gratings in the cyclopean retina. J Opt Soc Am 1980b;70.
Tyler CW, Raibert M. Generation of random-dot stereogratings. Behav Res Methods Inst 1976;7:37–41.
Tyler CW, Scott AB. Binocular vision. In: Records R, ed. Physiology of the human eye and visual system. Hagerstown, Md.: Harper & Row, 1979;643–71.
Tyler CW, Sutter EE. Depth from spatial frequency difference: an old kind of stereopsis? Vision Res 1979;19:859–65.
Tyler CW, Apkarian PA, Nakayama K. Multiple spatial frequency tuning of electrical responses from human visual cortex. Exp Brain Res 1978;33:535–50.
van der Tweel LH, Spekreijse H, Regan D. A correlation between evoked potentials and point-to-point interocular suppression. Electroenceph Clin Neurophysiol 1970;28:209–12.
Verhoeff FH. A theory of binocular perspective. Am Ophthalmol 1902;11:201.
Verhoeff FH. A new theory of binocular vision. Arch Ophthalmol 1935;13:151–75.
Volkmann AW. Die Stereoskopischen Erscheinungen in ihrer Beziehung zu der Lehre von den identischen Netzhautpunkten. Albrecht Von Graefes Arch Klin Exp Ophthalmol 1859;2:1–100.
von der Heydt R, Adorjani C, Hanny P. Neural mechanisms of stereopsis: sensitivity to orientational disparity. Experientia 1977;33:786.
von der Heydt R, Adorjani C, Hanny P, Baumgartner G. Disparity sensitivity and receptive field incongruity of units in the cat striate cortex. Exp Brain Res 1978;31:523–45.

Wales R, Fox R. Increment detection thresholds during binocular rivalry suppression. Percept Psychophysics 1970;8:90–94.

Walls GL. The common-sense horopter. Am J Optom (Monogr 133) 1952.

Westheimer G, McKee SP. Stereoscopic acuity for moving retinal images. J Opt Soc Am 1978;68:450.

Westheimer G, Tanzman IJ. Qualitative depth localization with diplopia images. J Opt Soc Am 1956;46:116–17.

Wheatstone C. Some remarkable phenomena of binocular vision. Phil Trans R Soc 1838;128:371–94.

Winter HJJ. The optical researches of Ibn Al-Haitham. Centaurus 1954;3:190–210.

Wolfe J, Held R. Binocular adaptation that cannot be measured monocularly. Invest Ophthalmol Visual Sci (Suppl) 1981;21:223.

Woo GCS. The effect of exposure time on the foveal size of Panum's area. Vision Res 1974;14:473–80.

Woodburne LS. The effect of a constant visual angle upon the binocular discrimination of depth differences. Am J Psychol 1934;46:273–86.

Wright WD. The role of convergence in stereoscopic vision. Proc Phys Soc Lond 1951;B64:289–97.

8

Horizontal Disparity Vergence

Ronald Jones

The neuroanatomic organization of the human visual system brings into association discrete regions of the retinas of the two eyes. These small areas are referred to as corresponding points and have the perceptual characteristic of giving rise to identical visual directions. The distribution of these pairs of points is nearly identical in the two eyes and it is for this reason that Hering (1868) referred to corresponding points as "cover points." The term was conceived from the notion that if the two retinas could be placed one on top of the other so that the foveas align, corresponding points would be juxtaposed.

An object in space normally will be seen singly if its images in the two eyes fall on corresponding retinal points. It is the role of disjunctive eye movement to eliminate noncorresponding stimulation, a condition referred to by Fechner (1860) as retinal disparity. The precision of disjunctive eye movement is normally such that the tolerance for disparity at the point of regard is less than about 6 arc-minutes. Although all comprehensive theories of fusion recognize that disjunctive eye movements provide the substrate for sensory unification, this realization does not "explain" sensory fusion. Rather, it begs the following important question: what is the nature of the sensory process that recognizes retinal disparity and directs the eyes to eliminate it?

This chapter was supported by a grant from the National Eye Institute, grant R01 EY0-2532.

Maddox (1886) classified vergence eye movements into distinct or independent categories that are now generally referred to as tonic, accommodative, proximal, and fusional. The major vergence component that occurs independently of accommodation is termed fusional according to this classification. Retinal disparity is the adequate stimulus to fusional vergence (Westheimer and Mitchell, 1956), but two different means of disparity introduction are commonly used to elicit it. Disparity may be introduced slowly using ramp stimulation, or suddenly using step or pulse disparity waveforms. Clinically, the former paradigm is the mode and in this case the ocular response time is such that disparity is immediately nullified. The result is that manifest disparity is kept small enough to sustain sensory fusion. This chapter is concerned primarily with the results of using retinal disparities of sufficient magnitude to produce diplopia. The distinction is not arbitrary as there is experimental evidence to suggest that these two aspects of fusional vergence are physiologically distinct (Jones, 1980). The term disparity vergence, after the suggestion of Stark and associates (1980), is used to describe those eye movements obtained using manifest disparities.

PSYCHOPHYSICAL DISPARITY

In anomalous retinal correspondence, cover points obtained with foveal alignment do not define retinal corresponding points. Rather, it is as if the two retinas are slipped with respect to each other. This problem is not discussed here, but psychophysical evaluation of the nature of correspondence in normals must be described to define the stimulus to disparity vergence. Disparity may be defined psychophysically as the angular difference in visual direction (measured at the entrance pupils) between the two images of a common object. The two images associated one with each eye are properly termed half-images or haplopic images.

Specification of disparity is a classical problem in physiological optics and involves determination of the horopter. This chapter is limited to discussion of lateral eye movements, thus the relevant horopter surface is called the longitudinal horopter. This is the object surface with image points of zero disparity, and is very nearly a circle passing through the two entrance pupils and the fixation point (the Vieth-Müller circle). The psychophysical description of corresponding points is very much simplified by assuming that the horopter corresponds exactly to the Vieth-Müller circle. This is equivalent to Hering's assumption that corresponding points are bilaterally symmetric and hence cover points.

A further assumption facilitates calculation of retinal disparity, namely, that the visual directions associated with retinal points (local signs) are uniformly distributed over the retinas. This is a more demanding

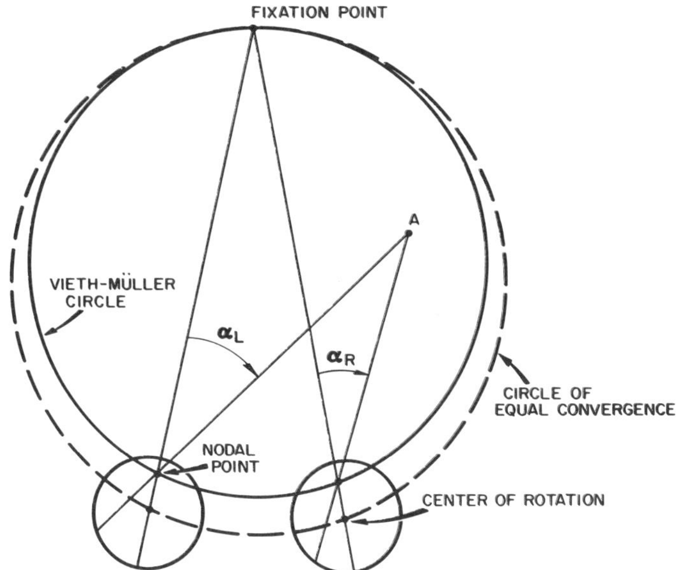

FIGURE 8.1. The retinal disparity of A is equal to the difference in the longitudinal angles ($\alpha_L - \alpha_R$) and is approximately equal to the amount of disparity vergence required to fixate the point.

assumption as it requires more than just ocular bilateral symmetry. Monocular partition experiments have shown that small, systematic asymmetries are in reality present (Ogle, 1950). Nevertheless, it is commonly assumed that corresponding points are both symmetric and uniformly distributed across the retinas. The error associated with these assumptions is probably less than our present precision of eye movement recording. Disparity at position A (Figure 8.1) may thus be easily computed from:

$$\text{disparity} = \alpha_L - \alpha_R \qquad (a)$$

where α_L and α_R are defined as the longitudinal angles.

To the extent that the above assumptions are correct, equation (*a*) accurately describes the perceived separation of the visual images. Moreover, since the distance between the entrance pupil of the eye and the center of ocular rotation is small, equation (*a*) approximates the amount of relative convergence required to fixate a target of given disparity.

In the example in Figure 8.1, A is not on the midline and thus its fixation requires a conjugate eye movement in addition to convergence in going from the fixation point to A. The amount of conjugate eye movement is:

$$\text{conjugate amplitude} = \alpha_L + \alpha_R. \qquad (b)$$

The conjugate and disjunctive components of eye movement that are specified in equations (*a*) and (*b*) are derived from Hering's law of equal innervation (Jones and Kerr, 1971).

MEASUREMENT OF OCULAR VERGENCE

Disjunctive eye movements can be measured by determining the ocular rotation of each eye and subtracting right from left. Similarly, the conjugate component corresponds to the addition of the two ocular rotations. It must be noted, however, that only if Hering's law of equal innervation is obeyed rigidly by the vergence control system will there be an absence of a conjugate ocular response component to a disparate stimulus. To avoid ambiguities and to allow for cases in which Hering's law is not obeyed, it would seem appropriate to make a formal distinction between the terms used to specify the magnitude and direction of eye movement and the names for the individual movements. The terms disjunctive and conjugate are used as independent descriptors of eye position, and the terms vergence and version refer to the physiological responses. Using this terminology a vergence response (e.g., accommodative vergence) will be strictly disjunctive and a version (e.g., cycloversion) strictly conjugate only if Hering's law is upheld.

BASIC CHARACTERISTICS OF DISPARITY VERGENCE

As has been noted, the adequate stimulus to disparity vergence is disparity. This fact was best demonstrated by Westheimer and Mitchell (1956) who showed that vergence responses could be elicited by stereoscopically produced disparate stimuli in the absence of any actual changes in target distance. The responses shown in Figure 8.2 are the results of a replication of this experiment. The disparate stimuli consisted of vertical line targets (0.1° by 3°) that abruptly replaced a fixation cross. The line presented to the right eye was 0.5° to the left of the former fixation point whereas the line seen by the left eye was presented 0.5° to the right of the former fixation point. This represents a +1° lateral step disparity (equation *a*) calling for relative convergence of the eyes. The response begins after a latency period of from 130 to 250 msec (Krishnan et al., 1973) but usually near 160 msec. There is an initial period of more or less uniform velocity that lasts for a time equal to the latency period. Subsequently the response decelerates, taking approximately 1 second to be completed in this case. If the duration of the disparate stimulus is less than the time required for response completion the vergence responses are attenuated in amplitude. Rashbass and Westheimer (1961a) pointed out that these

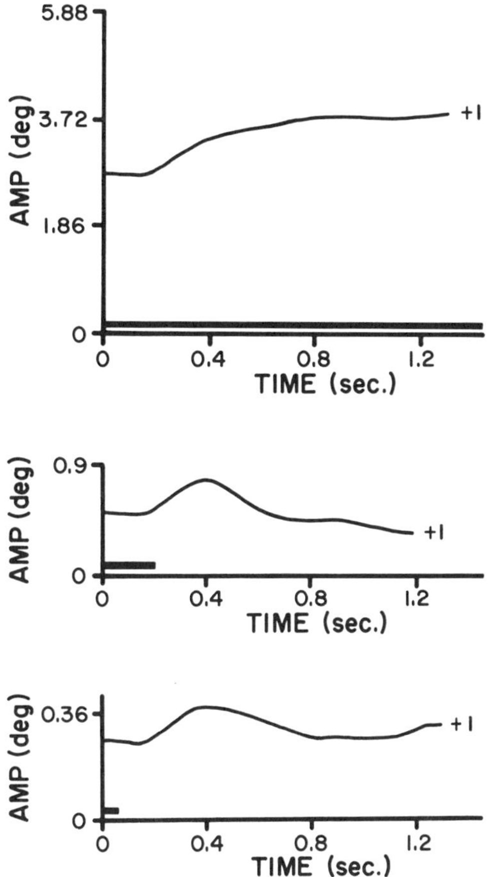

FIGURE 8.2. Disparity vergence responses for a 1-degree convergent (crossed) disparity for a step presentation (*upper*), a 200-msec pulse (*middle*), and a 50-msec pulse (*lower*). The 50-msec response is the computer average of five individual responses.

attributes indicate that disparity vergence is continuously controlled. This distinguishes vergence eye movements from saccadic movements, which have a discontinuous control system and thus exhibit all-or-none responses.

Although it has been appreciated that continuous control predicts attenuated vergence responses for briefly exposed disparities, such control also requires that disparity vergence exhibit a minimum response duration. For explanatory purposes the response to a disparity pulse exposed for a period less than the response latency (160 msec) may be analyzed into three components. The initial component should be a uniform vergence response having a velocity proportional to the stimulating disparity and a duration equal to that of the stimulus. This should be followed immediately by a period of zero velocity. The period of zero velocity is predicted by the fact that a zero disparity stimulus is present during the period from the end of the stimulus to the beginning of the initial response. The period of zero velocity response, therefore, should last for a time equal to the latency period minus the stimulus duration. Finally, there will be an opposite vergence eye movement in response to the disparity generated by feedback from the initial vergence response. The final response should be slower than the initial response because the disparity generated by the response is less than the initial stimulus. The entire vergence response to a disparity pulse, therefore, should have a duration longer than one latency period.

Actual responses for short exposure pulse disparities differ from the predictions of this simple continuous model. Data for short exposures (Figure 8.3) obtained by Zuber and Stark (1968) fail to reveal the predicted period of zero velocity (for 100 msec pulses the trace should be horizontal between about 260 msec to 320 msec). Additionally, the return velocity is more rapid than expected. These characteristics have been confirmed in our laboratory using even shorter pulses to extend the predicted period

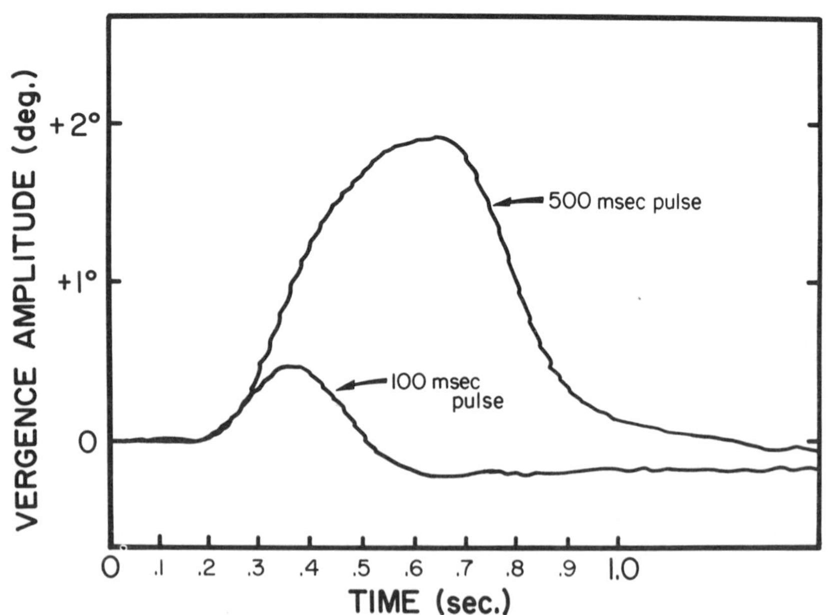

FIGURE 8.3. Averaged disparity vergence responses obtained for 2-degree convergent disparity pulses of 100 msec and 500 msec. Adapted from Zuber BL, Stark L. Dynamical characteristics of the fusional vergence eye movements system. Institute of Electrical and Electronics Engineers Transactions in Systems, Science, and Cybernetics, © 1968 IEEE. Reprinted by permission of the publisher.

of zero velocity response. A computer average of 5 convergence responses to +1.0 disparity exposed for 50 msec is shown in Figure 8.2. Also shown for comparison in Figure 8.2 is a response to a 200 msec stimulus for which no period of zero velocity is predicted. The 50 msec and 200 msec responses are unexpectedly similar as they appear to differ only in their amplitude. (The presentation sequence from which these responses were obtained were random so that individual stimuli were unpredictable in terms of their magnitude and direction.)

The differences between actual responses and the predictions of an ideal continuous controller might be considered reflective generally of the sluggishness of disparity vergence. Small amplitude sinusoidal disparate stimuli have been employed to analyze the frequency response characteristics of fusional vergence (Rashbass and Westheimer, 1961a; Zuber and Stark, 1968). But this technique is not directly applicable to disparity vergence because of the different range of disparities utilized. Theoretically, the frequency response of a linear system can be determined by taking the Fourier transform of an impulse response. The Fourier transform of the responses of Figure 8.2 yields a transfer function that is characteristic of integration beyond a corner frequency of about ⅓ Hz, however, the validity of this quantitative approach remains to be demonstrated.

The frequency response limitation on disparity vergence is not imposed by ocular inertia or muscle dynamics because other types of eye movement do not have similar limitations. Nor does the suggestion (Alpern and Wolter, 1956) that the sluggishness is due to the utilization of small, nonmedullated nerve efferents appear to be justified (Keller and Robinson, 1972). Thus it seems reasonable to place the source of the frequency response limitations in the central nervous system controller of vergence and conclude that significant temporal integration of disparity is involved.

RELATIONSHIP BETWEEN DISPARITY AND VERGENCE AMPLITUDE

The gain characteristics of disparity vergence were first extensively investigated by Rashbass and Westheimer (1961a). On a small number of subjects they determined the velocity of vergence as a function of disparity under closed-loop and open-loop circumstances. Since the initial velocity of vergence response to a step disparity is unmodified by response feedback, its measurement unveils the response amplitude of disparity vergence to the full magnitude of the disparate stimulus. A form of stabilized retinal imagery also was employed by Rashbass and Westheimer (1961a) to measure the open-loop response of disparity vergence directly. The relationships between vergence velocity and disparity that were revealed using these two approaches were in close agreement. Vergence velocity was found to be approximately linear over the range of $+-5°$ being 7° to 10° per second per degree of disparity.

The gain of disparity vergence alternately may be determined from measurement of the peak amplitude of vergence response to brief duration pulses. The peak amplitude will be proportional to the vergence velocity provided the pulse durations do not exceed the latency period. This method overcomes the uncertainty in measuring the initial response velocity that is posed by the presence of some initial acceleration (rounding) in response. This approach has been applied extensively to the study of disparity vergence (Westheimer and Mitchell, 1969; Mitchell, 1970; Jones and Kerr, 1971, 1972; Jones, 1977, 1980).

The relationship of vergence velocity to disparity magnitude is subject to large individual differences. Convergence and divergence are often unequal but either may be more responsive (Mitchell, 1970; Jones and Kerr, 1971, 1972; Jones, 1977). The disparity-amplitude relationship is nonlinear and influenced by target luminance (Mitchell, 1970), fixation distance (Jones, 1980), and other variables to be discussed. This makes application of control systems analysis especially difficult. An approach used to investigate individual differences (Jones, 1977), is the disparity vergence profile illustrated in Figure 8.4. This is a plot of the peak amplitude of vergence against disparity size for 200-msec disparity pulses. The targets in this case were narrow vertical lines (1.7° by 0.05°). The amplitude, linearity, and relative efficacy of convergence relative to divergence are readily visualized in this form of presentation. A non-monotonic relationship is typical; the vergence response is normally maximum for disparities between 2° and 3°. In about 20% of the sample investigated (Jones, 1977) a marked (greater than 3 : 1) asymmetry between the convergence and divergence amplitudes was present. In several cases convergence or divergence was absent, or almost so, under these conditions (Figure 8.4). A notable feature of all cases in which asymmetries were found was the presence of low-amplitude vergence responses to zero disparity. Zero disparity stimuli were actually monocular targets consisting of two fine vertical lines separated by a distance equal to a disparity used in a binocular trial. This target has the same appearance as a disparate stimulus if an individual is unable to use disparity as a distance cue.[1]

As the duration of the pulse is lengthened, the vergence asymmetries present for brief exposures are modified. Figure 8.5 shows the responses of a vergence-anomalous subject as the duration is increased. For the

[1] Subsequent experiments have shown that true zero disparities produced by substitution of a binocular vertical line target for the binocular fixation point give similar responses to the monocularly created zero disparities.

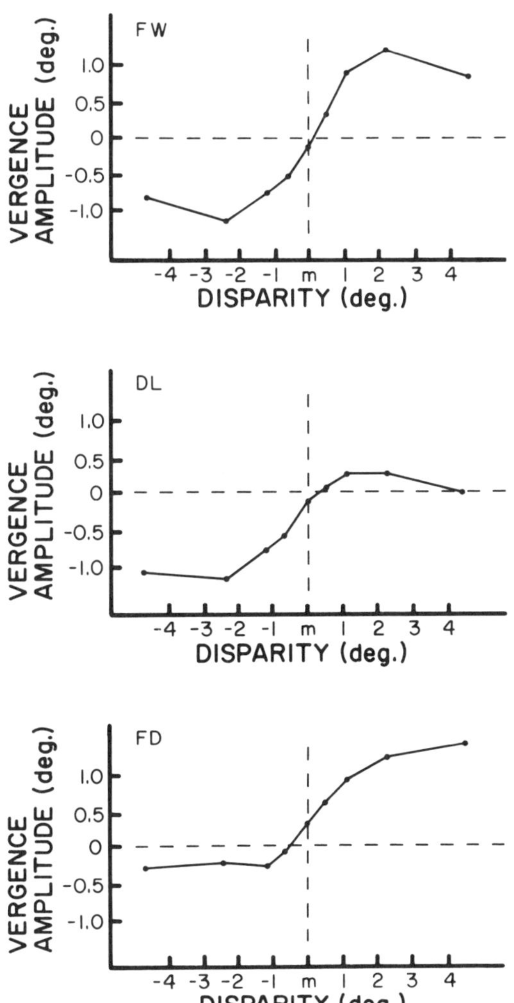

FIGURE 8.4. Disparity vergence profiles for three subjects. Each data point is the average peak amplitude of 5 to 6 responses to 200-msec pulse stimuli at the indicated disparity.

longest pulse duration (1 second) the asymmetry reveals itself only as a slightly increased latency period and a slower velocity of response. The clinical significance of these anomalies of vergence is not apparent, as this subject had normal binocular vision as determined by standard clinical tests (Jones, 1972).

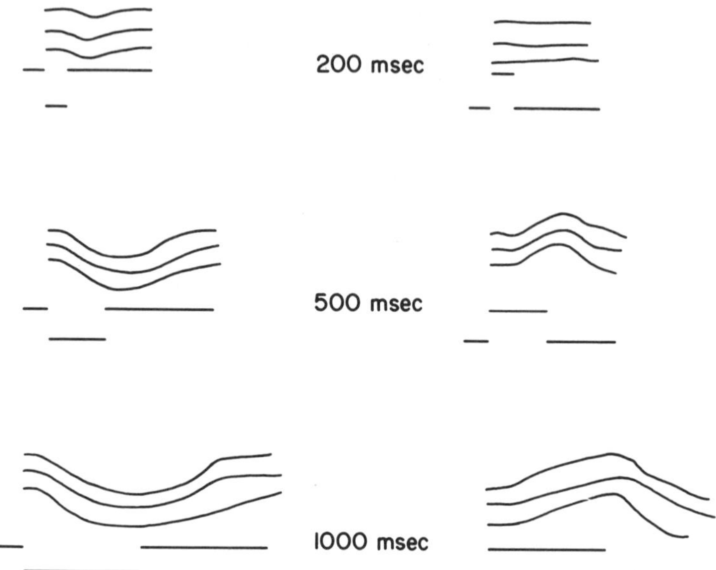

FIGURE 8.5. Disparity vergence responses obtained to convergent (+) and divergent (−) 4 prism-diopter (2.3 degree) pulse disparities of 200, 500, and 1,000 msec. Three responses are shown for each stimulus condition. The stimulus trace is indicated below the responses; divergence is downward, convergence is upward. The height of the stimulus traces corresponds to the 4-pd stimulus amplitude, the pulse width specifies the time scale.

TARGET INFLUENCES ON DISPARITY VERGENCE

Thin vertical lines or small spot targets have been the targets of choice in the investigations of disparity vergence reported above. The effect of changes in the binocular target used in creating the disparity has received little attention. Mitchell (1970) reported that the amplitude of disparity vergence decreases when the luminance of the disparate stimulus is decreased but there remains the need for parametric investigation of this effect. Luminance effects denote a kind of luminance-disparity reciprocity and are consistent with the notion that disparities are pooled prior to the site of vergence initiation (Jones, 1977).

Preliminary results of our experiments on the effect of target size on disparity vergence are given in Figure 8.6. Targets consisted of vertical bars having widths ranging between 0.1° and 3° and were presented using pulse exposures of 200 msec on a dark surround. The fixation point was a diagonal cross at 4 m that was extinguished during stimulus presentation to promote reflex eye movement. For wide bars a long latency (greater than 300 msec) convergence response was superimposed on the re-

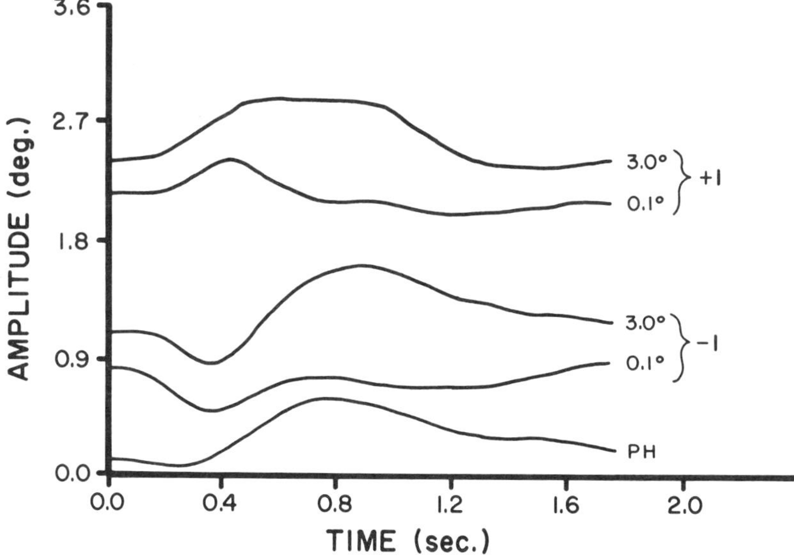

FIGURE 8.6. Disparity vergence responses to 1-degree convergent (+) and divergent (−) disparities showing the effect of pupillary response artifacts for 3-degree wide targets. The response labeled PH was obtained under monocular conditions (see text).

sponses. Wide bars calling for divergence often produced an initial correct response but this was followed by a longer latency convergence response. This bias was not present in all subjects but is typical and was observed in both experienced and naive observers.

Intermixed with the stimulus presentation sequence from which the data of Figure 8.6 were taken were trials in which the target to one eye was extinguished during the 200-msec exposure period. A long latency response, identical to that obtained for a zero-disparity stimulus, is obtained to such stimuli (labeled PH). This finding indicates that the long latency response cannot be disparity vergence. The weight of present evidence leads us to conclude that this is a response artifact due to pupillary constriction. Pupillary light reflexes recorded during these trials were much larger for large bars than for small. Also, retesting after the introduction of a pupillary dilator (phenylephrine hydrochloride) eliminated these long latency components. Eye movements were recorded using a modulated infrared limbal tracker (Biometrics, model SGHV-2). At the high sensitivity required to record the small vergence responses no adjustment could be maintained that would eliminate these artifacts reliably. Their presence poses a caveat in the investigation of disparity vergence.

Interactions between disparity vergence and other oculomotor ad-

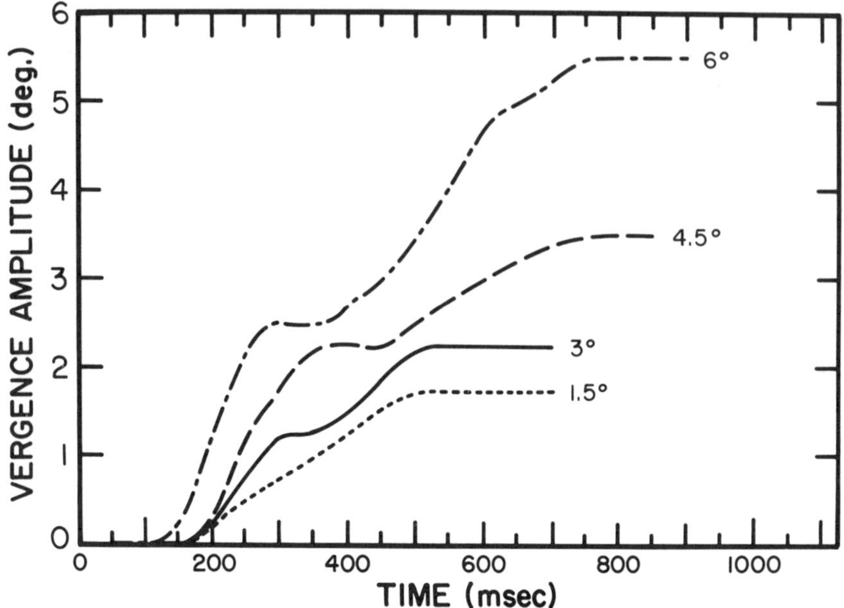

FIGURE 8.7. Disparity convergence responses to step disparities of the indicated magnitudes. Adapted from Westheimer G, Mitchell AM. Eye movement responses to convergent stimuli. American Medical Association Archives of Opthalmology, 55: 848–856. Copyright 1956, American Medical Association. Reprinted by permission of the publisher.

justments have been reported in the literature. The intrusion of accommodative convergence on convergence elicited by ramp introduction of disparity, such as is employed in clinical vergence testing, is well documented (Alpern, 1969). Moreover, accommodative changes to introduction of step disparities have been measured using simultaneous accommodative and eye movement recording (Krishnan et al., 1977) and have been inferred in earlier investigations.[2] Westheimer and Mitchell (1956) found that disparity vergence obtained for large step disparities is diphasic. Their data are reproduced in Figure 8.7. It can be seen that a second longer latency component follows the initial vergence response; this they suggested was accommodative convergence. Accommodative convergence appears to replace disparity vergence in certain

[2] Changes in accommodation have been found for step disparity (Krishnan et al., 1977) and were called vergence accommodation. There remains controversy as to whether convergence accommodation and accommodative convergence are distinct entities. A detailed discussion is given by Alpern (1962). The perceived need for the distinction rests in large part on the effect of age on the relationship of accommodation and convergence. The results of Fry (1959) seriously question the need for this distinction.

patients having binocular deficiencies (Kenyon et al., 1980). Since these responses may be voluntary (Eskridge, 1971), the possibility of contamination by accommodative convergence is always present in research on disparity vergence.

DISPARITY VERGENCE AND FIXATION DISTANCE

It is to be expected that factors known to influence neural disparity detection would be reflected by the response characteristics of disparity vergence. Fixation distance has been shown to modify psychophysical responses to disparity as revealed in measurements of stereopsis and sensory fusion. Suprathreshold disparity has been shown to become more effective as fixation distance is decreased, but crossed and uncrossed disparities are influenced differently (Richards, 1971; Richards and Foley, 1971; Woo and Sillanpaa, 1979). Although stereothreshold does not appear to change consistently with fixation distance (Ogle, 1958; Jameson and Hurvich, 1959; Woo and Sillanpaa, 1979), the stereoscopic depth interval for a given (suprathreshold) disparity increases substantially with increased convergence (Foley, 1967). Convergence results in an increase in sensitivity to suprathreshold disparity (Richards and Foley, 1971) and an expansion of Panum's limits of single vision (Richards, 1971). The effects on crossed and uncrossed disparity detection are probably independent since distance related effects occur primarily for uncrossed disparity (Jones, 1974).

The influence of convergence on the amplitude of disparity vergence has been investigated and is found to be generally consistent with the known suprathreshold sensory changes (Jones, 1980). Measurements of the peak amplitude of disparity vergence for 500 msec presentations of crossed and uncrossed disparities are shown in Figure 8.8. The results were obtained at seven different convergence positions of the eyes with the stimulus to accommodation set at zero diopters. A large amplitude change is observed with increasing convergence but only for uncrossed disparities. It cannot be concluded that this convergence effect is independent of accommodation since reflex accommodation cannot be avoided in this stimulus situation (Alpern, 1969).

SENSORY STIMULUS TO DISPARITY VERGENCE

How does the visual system extract disparity information? This question is central to our understanding of the control of disparity vergence. Barlow, Blakemore, and Pettigrew (1967) formulated a model of disparity detection based on the neurophysiological findings of single cell record-

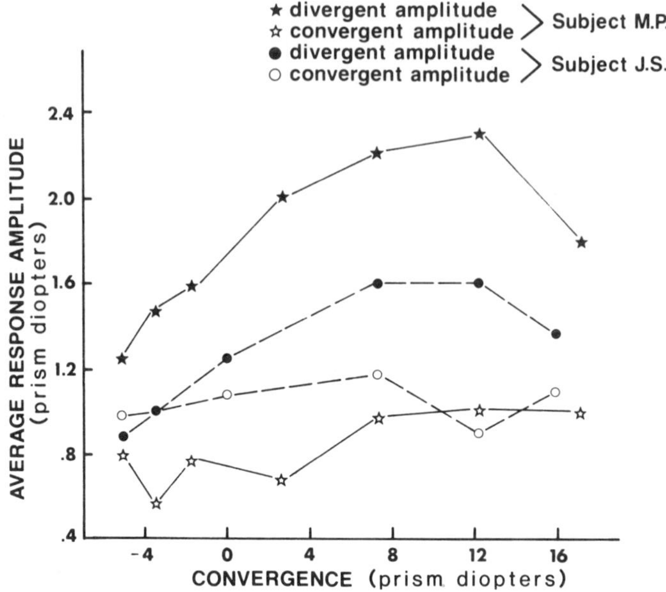

FIGURE 8.8. Disparity vergence responses obtained for various amounts of sustained convergence of the fixation point.

ings in cat visual cortex. The receptive field properties of disparity-detector units in the visual cortex of cat require a high degree of similarity of the haplopic images to extract the disparity information. This result suggested a filter mechanism whereby disparity is automatically extracted for similar images in the two eyes. The model would seem to predict that for disparity vergence to occur the haplopic images would need to be relatively similar. The proposal was in agreement with the known facts at the time. Ogle (1950) held that disparity vergence required that the images be similar enough to permit them to be fused, that is, differences must be less than the extent of Panum's areas. The results of Westheimer and Mitchell (1969), Mitchell (1970), and Jones and Kerr (1971, 1972) subsequently revealed that similarity of the haplopic images is not important to the initiation of disparity vergence. A new model is needed to explain these results.

A quantitative investigation of the limits within which haplopic images could differ in form and vertical offset while still initiating disparity vergence was first reported by Mitchell (1970). A haploscope was employed to allow pulse presentations (200 msec) of disparate targets consisting of letters or fine lines while objectively recording vergence eye movement. Between stimulus presentations only a fixation point was visible. Mitchell found that vergence responses elicited by similar targets (e.g., fusable vertical lines) were identical to those obtained for dichoptic targets having grossly different shapes (e.g., vertical line to one eye, horizontal line to the other). Moreover, vertical offsets between targets sufficient to prevent fusion did not deter disparity vergence. For large offsets, however, the probability of a disparity vergence response was reduced, as was the velocity of the obtained response. A 50% probability of response was present for a 2° vertical offset and response cessation occurred at between 3° to 4° of vertical offset.

Mitchell concluded that if cortical disparity detector units are responsible for the initiation of human disparity vergence the receptive field properties must be much less selective to shape than those known to exist in cats and lower primates. It might be argued that despite the gross dissimilarity of the targets used, Mitchell's experiments do not offer a decisive test of the question of whether contour selective mechanisms are operative in the control of disparity vergence because they are the only targets in the binocular field. This criticism was specifically addressed in later investigations (Jones and Kerr, 1971, 1972), the results of which confirmed and extended Mitchell's conclusion.

Figure 8.9 illustrates the haploscopic target configuration that was used in our laboratory to test the contour-selective properties of disparity vergence. Two opposite disparities, simultaneously exposed for 500 msec, replaced the fixation point at 3-second intervals. This target configuration is similar to Panum's limiting case: the single target to the right eye may be combined with either of the two targets in the left eye. Using this target

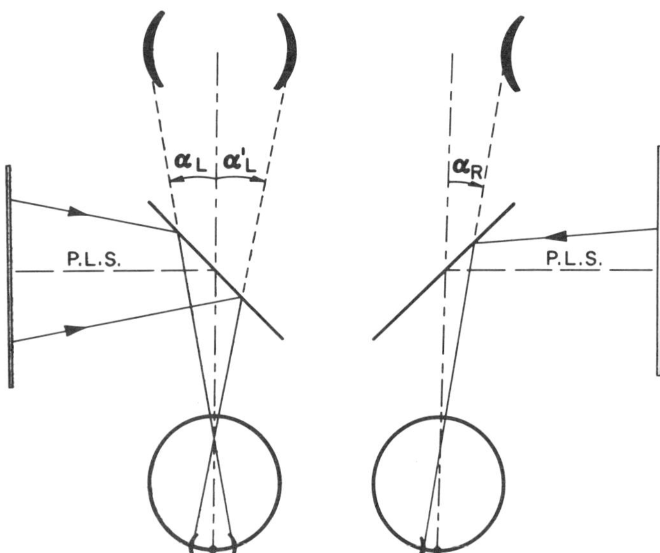

FIGURE 8.9. Haploscopic target presentation used to test the shape-selectivity of disparity vergence.

as an example, if the right eye target combines with the target in the left eye having the same form, there is an uncrossed disparity equal to

$$disparity = \alpha_L - \alpha_R. \qquad (c)$$

Alternatively, if the right eye target combines with the left eye target of dissimilar form, the crossed disparity is equal to

$$disparity = \alpha_L' - \alpha_R. \qquad (d)$$

Two opposite stimuli to conjugate eye movements are also present. From equation (*b*) the similar pairings require a leftward saccade equal to

$$conjugate = \alpha_L + \alpha_R. \qquad (e)$$

The dissimilar pair requires a rightward saccade equal to

$$conjugate = \alpha_L' + \alpha_R. \qquad (f)$$

Using this principle a large number of different targets were designed having a range of disparities. The double target separation was held constant at 6 degrees; this constrained the stimulus presentations such that the sum of the crossed and uncrossed disparities always equaled 6 degrees. The magnitude of the similar and dissimilar pairings was randomized to produce all possible combinations of conjugate and disjunctive stimuli in a balanced block design. Vergence and version responses were recorded objectively and the determination of preferred pairings was based on the direction of the recorded response. Ambiguity in interpreting the response direction was avoided since the brief exposures used always elicited unidirectional responses.

The results were unequivocal in those subjects who had nearly equal response velocities of convergence and divergence. Disparity vergence was always in the direction of the smaller of the two opposing disparities regardless of target shape considerations. If the magnitude of the opposing disparities was equal, a random response distribution was obtained. Thus no shape selectivity was exhibited by disparity vergence under any of the conditions (Jones and Kerr, 1971).

Preference for the smaller of the two opposing disparities is consistent with the response characteristics of disparity vergence revealed by the disparity vergence profiles. The smaller of the two stimuli is closer to the response peak of the profile (Figure 8.4) and thus is the more effective stimulus. It appears that the disparity vergence response is the result of simple algebraic addition of the potential responses to the individual component disparities. These responses may be explained entirely by a binocular disparity-detection process that is devoid of shape identification properties.

Some subjects had significant differences between the velocities of their convergence and divergence movements when exposed to single disparities. When tested in the similar-dissimilar paired-target paradigm these individuals also failed to show any response preference for the similar pair. Rather than responding to the smaller disparity, they always selected the disparity corresponding to the more proficient of their disparity vergence responses. This is consistent with a vergence profile that is asymmetric, such as those shown in Figure 8.4.

Further evidence was obtained using the similar-dissimilar experimental paradigm in support of the view of Rashbass and Westheimer (1961b) that vergence and version eye movements have independent physiological control mechanisms. Subjects could be instructed to look voluntarily to the right or left target during the stimulus presentation in order to force the version response to a particular target pairing (either similar or dissimilar). When this was done the direction of the disparity vergence response (either convergence or divergence) was found not to be affected.[3]

A SCENARIO FOR DISPARITY VERGENCE CONTROL

The existence of large asymmetries within the normal population between the amplitudes of disparity convergence and disparity divergence has been interpreted as evidence that each is controlled by independent physiological control mechanisms (Jones, 1972, 1977). It has been noted above that crossed and uncrossed disparity detection in stereopsis and sensory fusion also appear to involve independent physiological processes; however, evidence that the sensory and motor modalities share the same neural mechanisms of disparity detection is as yet circumstantial (Jones, 1977). Another major characteristic of disparity vergence control is that it integrates across disparity. These facts suggest that disparity is pooled over two broad overlapping domains that feed to separate operators responsible for the initiation of convergence and divergence. Disparity detection within each pool must be very coarse to account for the lack of feature-selectivity and for the reciprocity of disparity and luminance. According to this model, the net amplitude and direction of vergence response corresponds to the difference in the activity in these two disparity pools. If the two types of anomalous vergence responses shown in Figure 8.4 may be attributed to the absence of one or the other of these pools, then the sensitivities of each pool can be derived from these disparity vergence profiles. This origin of vergence anomaly is analogous to the reduction hypothesis proposed for many color vision defects. The

[3] Reflex saccadic fixation was normally in the direction of the targets that were closer together, i.e., had the smaller disparity, except a preference for haplopic images that projected to the same hemisphere of the brain was also exhibited. Disparity vergence did not show a significant hemispheric preference.

predicted relationship for the velocity of disparity vergence obtained using this assumption is illustrated in Figure 8.10.

This model predicts several characteristics of disparity vergence that cannot be easily reconciled with models of disparity detection that presume that local disparity detectors encode specific vergence responses. The small amplitude disparity vergence responses, which occur for brief exposures of zero disparity, are easily explained on the basis of the commonly observed imbalance between the convergence and divergence pools. The major advantage of this model, however, is its freedom from false disparity detection when presented with multiple targets. False detections can arise because geometry allows us to calculate four disparities given only two objects at different distances from the eyes. Two can be determined from combining the appropriate haplopic images and another pair from combinations of images in the eyes that do not belong to the same object. Elimination of such false or "ghost" combinations is a central problem for most models disparity detection. It can be shown, however, that the sum of the disparities for the correct pair equals the sum of the ghost pair. Ghost combinations therefore are irrelevant if disparities are summed (pooled) to provide the sensory stimulus to disparity vergence.

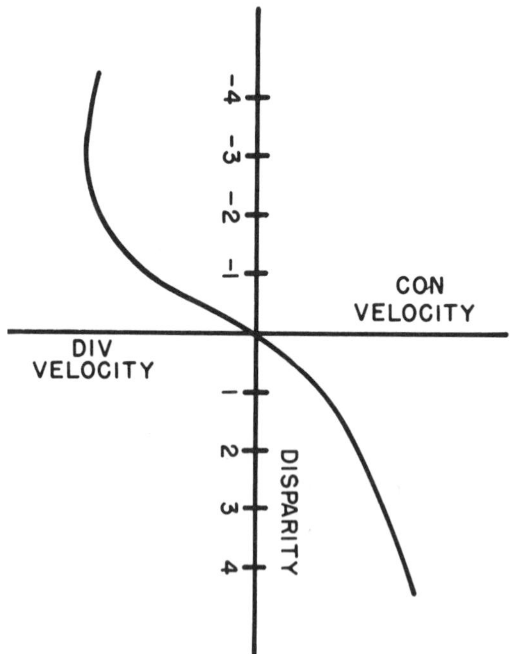

FIGURE 8.10. Hypothetical velocity versus disparity characteristics of disparity vergence. Derived by taking the difference between the disparity vergence profiles (Figure 7.4) of a convergence-anomalous and a divergence-anomalous individual.

Most of the characteristics of disparity vergence reviewed in this chapter do not appear consistent with the demands of sensory fusion. Principally, it is known that to sustain fusional vergence with the great precision required, similarly shaped images in the two eyes are required. This dichotomy suggests that fusional vergence is a two-stage process having separate initiation and sustaining phases each with distinct physiological characteristics (Jones, 1972, 1977). Evidence for this proposal has been recently reviewed (Jones, 1980) and is analogous to the hypothesis of Bishop and Henry (1971) that stereopsis is a dual process consisting of fine and coarse neural mechanisms of disparity detection. The spatial and temporal properties of disparity vergence and sustained fusional vergence suggest that this dichotomy reflects the respective activity of transient and sustained classes of visual neurons.

There is a distinct advantage to such a two-stage transient-sustained control process. Since the visual system is sensitive to a very broad range of disparity (Richards and Foley, 1971), an exorbitant amount of visual processing would be necessary to seek out similar haplopic images over this entire region. The proposed zone model reduces processing demands through the use of a broadly sensitive but nonselective initiation stage. This permits the second fusion-sustaining stage to have a narrow range of sensitivity. The search for similar contours is thereby simplified by the expedient of limiting the search area to a relatively narrow region—perhaps the size of the region of binocular single vision.

REFERENCES

Alpern M, Wolter JR. The relation of horizontal saccadic and vergence movements. AMA Arch Ophthal 1956;56:685–90.

Alpern M. Types of eye movements. In: Davson H. ed. The eye, Vol 3. New York: Academic Press, 1962.

Alpern M. Physiological characteristics of the extraocular muscles. In: Davson H, ed. The eye. Vol 3. 2nd ed. New York: Academic Press, 1969.

Barlow HB, Blakemore C, Pettigrew JD. The neural mechanism of binocular depth discrimination. J Physiol 1967;193:327–42.

Bishop PO, Henry GH. Spatial vision. Rev Psychol 1971;22:119–61.

Eskridge B. An investigation of voluntary vergence. Am J Optom 1971;48:741–46.

Fechner GT. Elemente der Psychophysik I. Aufl. Leipzig, Breitkopf and Härtel, 1860.

Foley JM. Disparity increase with convergence for constant perceptual criteria. Percept Psychophysics 1967;2:605–608.

Fry GA. The effect of age on the AC/A ratio. Am J Optom 1959;36:299–303.

Hering, E. The theory of binocular vision, English translation by Bridgeman B. and Stark L. New York: Plenum Press, 1977.

Jameson D, Hurvich L. Note on factors influencing the relationship between stereoacuity and absolute distance. J Opt Soc Am 1959;49:639.

Jones R. Psychophysical and oculomotor responses of normal and stereoanomalous observers to disparate retinal stimulation. Ph.D dissertation, Ohio State University, Columbus, Ohio, 1972.

Jones R. On the origin of changes in the horopter deviation. Vision Res 1974;14:1047–49.

Jones R. Anomalies of disparity detection in the human visual system. J Physiol 1977;264:621–40.

Jones R. Fusional vergence: sustained and transient components. Am J Optom 1980;57:640–44.

Jones R, Kerr KE. Motor responses to conflicting asymmetrical vergence stimulus information. Am J Optom 1971;48:989–1000.

Jones R, Kerr KE. Vergence eye movements to pairs of disparity stimuli with shape selection cues. Vision Res 1972;12:1425–30.

Keller EL, Robinson DA. Abducens unit behavior in the monkey during vergence movements. Vision Res 1972;12:369–82.

Kenyon RV, Ciuffreda KJ, Stark L. An unexpected role for normal accommodative vergence in strabismus and amblyopia. Am J Optom 1980;57:566–77.

Krishnan VV, Farazian F, Stark L. An analysis of latencies in the fusional vergence system. Am J Optom 1973;50:933–39.

Krishnan VV, Shirachi D, Stark L. Dynamic measures of vergence accommodation. Am J Optom 1977;54:470–73.

Maddox EE. Investigations on the relation between convergence and accommodation of the eyes. J Anat 1886;20:475–508.

Mitchell DE. Properties of stimuli eliciting vergence eye movements and stereopsis. Vision Res 1970;10:145–62.

Ogle KN. Researches in binocular vision. Philadelphia: WB Saunders, 1950.

Ogle KN. Note on stereoscopic acuity and observation distance. J Opt Soc Am 1958;48:794–95.

Rashbass C, Westheimer G. Disjunctive eye movements. J Physiol 1961a;159:149–70.

Rashbass C, Westheimer G. Independence of conjugate and disjunctive eye movements. J Physiol 1961b;159:361–64.

Richards W. Independence of Panum's near and far limits. Am J Optom 1971;48:103–9.

Richards W, Foley JM. Interhemispheric processing of binocular disparity. J Opt Soc Am 1971;61:419–21.

Stark L, Kenyon RV, Krishnan VV, Ciuffreda KJ. Disparity vergence: a proposed name for a dominant component of binocular vergence eye movements. Am J Optom 1980;57:606–9.

Woo G, Sillanpaa V. Absolute stereoscopic theresholds as measured by crossed and uncrossed disparities. Am J Optom 1979;56:350–55.

Westheimer G, Mitchell AM. Eye movement responses to convergent stimuli. Arch Ophthalmol 1956;55:848–56.

Westheimer G, Mitchell DE. The sensory stimulus to disjunctive eye movements. Vision Res 1969;9:749–55.

Zuber BL, Stark L. Dynamical characteristics of the fusional vergence eye-movement system. IEEE Trans Systems Sci Cybernet 1968;SSC-4:72–79.

9

Vertical and Cyclofusional Disparity Vergence

Andrew E. Kertesz

Human fusional response to retinal image disparity contains two components: (1) a motor component in the form of compensatory vergence eye movements and (2) a sensory or nonmotor component whose magnitude is limited to the extent of Panum's fusional areas. Traditionally, the fusional response has been studied in terms of the three orthogonal directions along which disparities are presented: horizontal, vertical, and torsional. Thus we speak of horizontal, vertical, and cyclofusional responses. There was no a priori reason to suspect that there would be substantial differences among these three components; however, recent experimental results revealed many. The horizontal fusional response is reviewed in the previous chapter. This chapter reviews the vertical and cyclofusional responses and points out differences and similarities among the responses according to three somewhat arbitrary criteria: (1) speed of response, (2) conformance to Hering's law of equal innervation, and (3) the effect of stimulus size on the magnitude of response.

VERTICAL FUSIONAL RESPONSE

Definitions

At this point, it may be useful to state clearly the meaning of each term associated with the vertical fusional response. If the disparity contained

This chapter was supported in part by research grant EY-1055 from the National Eye Institute.

in a stimulus is fused by the subject, the magnitude of fusional response is equal to the stimulus disparity. The fusional response has a motor or vergence component and a sensory or nonmotor component. Thus the term vergence is used to describe motor response, while the word fusion is used to describe the subject's percept and response, which depends on both motor (vergence) and sensory components.

A left hyper, or positive, vertical disparity is said to exist between the monocular stimulus images if the stimulus presented to the left eye is displaced in an upward direction with respect to the stimulus seen by the right eye. A right hyper, or negative, vertical disparity is said to exist between the monocular stimulus images if the stimulus presented to the right eye is displaced in an upward direction with respect to the stimulus seen by the left eye. The vertical fusional amplitude corresponding to a particular stimulus configuration is determined by finding the largest vertical disparity (maximum fusible) in a given direction that can be presented to an observer without destroying the fused percept of the stimulus. Presentation of disparities greater than the maximum fusible would destroy the fused percept and would bring about diplopia or suppression.

Background

The vertical fusional response was initially studied by subjective means (Burian, 1939; Ellerbrock, 1949, 1952). Subjects were asked to fixate a horizontal line visible to one eye only, while the position of a second horizontal line, visible to the other eye, was adjusted until the two lines were aligned horizontally. Thus the subjective measure of vertical phoria was used to estimate fusional amplitudes. Ellerbrock found that disparities up to 4° could be fused, but the fusional amplitude was a function of stimulus size, brightness, and the rate of introduction of stimulus disparity. In obtaining the 4° fusional amplitude, Ellerbrock introduced the disparity in quarter-degree increments at two-minute intervals. Fender and Julesz (1967) were first to use an objective binocular eye movement monitoring device to measure vertical fusional amplitudes under normal and stabilized retinal image viewing conditions. Their subjects were able to fuse vertical disparities up to 22 minutes of arc when the effect of fusional eye movements was negated, which provided clear evidence of the existence of a sensory component in vertical fusional response. Fender and Julesz did not study vertical fusional eye movements, but demonstrated that the magnitude of both sensory and motor components are a function of stimulus complexity and of the recent history of stimulation. The plasticity of these two components was demonstrated by slow introduction of disparity until the diplopia threshold was reached, at which point disparity was decreased until fusion was once again established. The breakpoint was found to be significantly larger than the refusion or recovery point under both conditions. The significant difference between break and recovery points during normal viewing conditions is a common clinical observation. The surprising result of the Fender and Julesz experiments is that this difference is preserved even under stabilized retinal image viewing conditions, which requires a certain plasticity within Panum's fusional areas.

Symmetric Disparity Presentations

Perlmutter and Kertesz (1978) examined the vertical fusional response to symmetric disparity presentations, that is, the monocular stimulus images were displaced by an equal amount but in opposite directions, using an objective binocular eye-movement measuring device. They examined the responses to step and ramp disparity presentations. Stimuli subtending 8.5° were displayed dichoptically on oscilloscopes and consisted of single horizontal lines whose intensified centers served as fixation points. At the beginning of each experimental run, the subject fixated the center of a zero-disparity stimulus for 15 seconds, which was followed by the presentation of a positive or negative disparity. Typical responses are shown in Figures 9.1 and 9.2.

Figure 9.1 shows averaged responses to positive and negative step disparity presentations. The movement of each eye was unequal both in magnitude and in time course. The slower moving left eye (part A) compensated for 51.2% of the stimulus disparity (or equivalently, followed 102.4% of its monocular stimulus movement), while the faster-moving right eye compensated for 32.5% of the disparity (or followed 65% of its stimulus movement), resulting in an overall motor compensation of 83.7%. Part B of the figure shows that when the direction of the step disparity was reversed, so were the relative motor contributions of the two eyes. In this case, the left eye was moving faster and compensated for only 30.5% of the stimulus disparity, while the slower-moving right eye compensated for 48.5%, as if the asymmetry between motor components were sensitive to the direction of disparity changes. The magnitude and time course of these eye movements did not conform to Hering's law of equal innervation.

Figure 9.2 shows an average of 18 responses to a vertical ramp disparity presentation. Once again, the two monocular contributions were unequal. The left eye compensated for 61.5% of the stimulus disparity, while the right eye only compensated for 20.5%, resulting in overall motor compensation of 82%.

Perlmutter and Kertesz (1978) also compared the responses to hor-

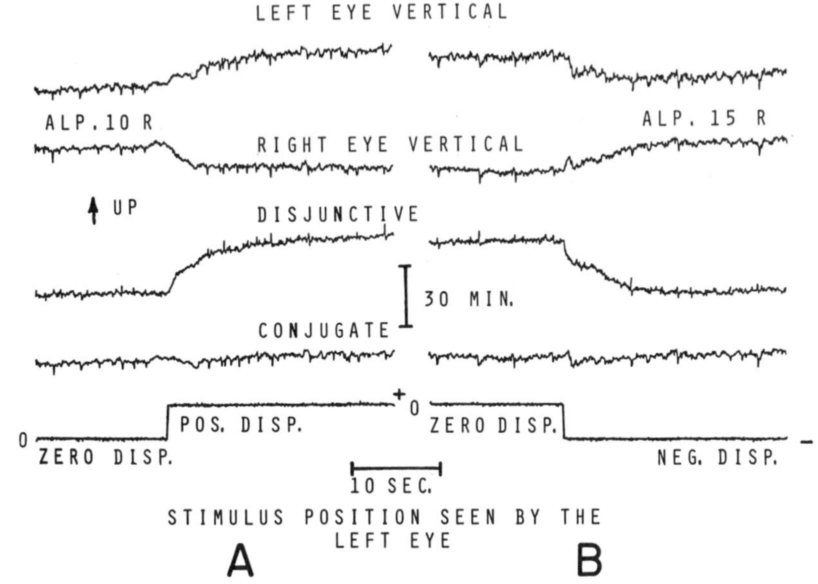

FIGURE 9.1. Eye movement responses to presentations of a vertical step disparity. The top two traces depict the vertical position of the left and right eyes, respectively. The disjunctive component represents the difference between left and right vertical eye position (D = L-R). The conjugate component was calculated by using C = ½(L-R). The bottom trace indicates the position of the stimulus seen by the left eye. (A) An average of 10 responses to the presentation of a 33.6-minute positive step disparity. (B) An average of 15 responses to the presentation of a 33.6-minute step disparity. Reprinted with permission from Vision Research, 18, Perlmutter AL, Kertesz AE, Measurement of human vertical fusional response, 1978, Pergamon Press, Ltd.

izontal and vertical disparity presentations and found basic differences between fusional responses. While horizontal disparities of 1.5° were readily fused by their subjects, the maximum fusible vertical disparity was less than 1°. The magnitude and time course of the horizontal vergence movements were symmetric and in accordance with Hering's law; the vertical fusional movements were often asymmetric both in time course and final contribution to the overall motor response. Horizontal fusional stimulation evoked a purely disjunctive motor response, whereas the vertical fusional response sometimes contained a direction-specific conjugate component as well. Vertical vergence movements were roughly eight times slower than horizontal ones, requiring approximately eight seconds for completion of motor response to a vertical step disparity change.

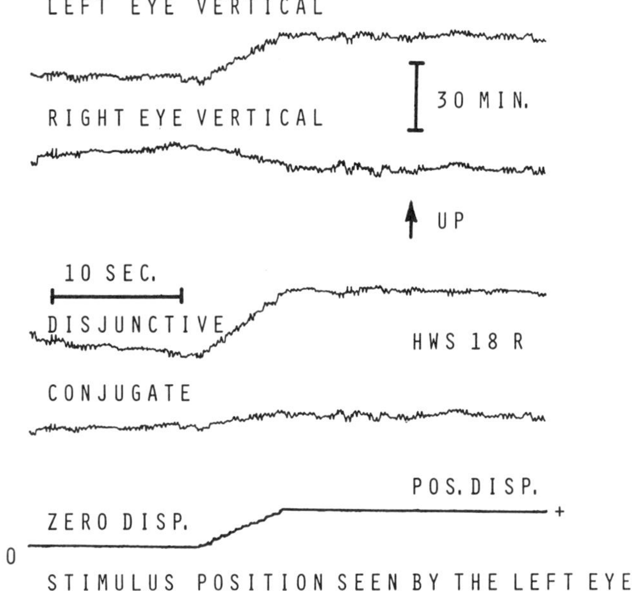

FIGURE 9.2. Eye movement responses to the presentation of a vertical positive ramp disparity of 33.6 minute maximum disparity. Reprinted with permission from Vision Research, 18, Perlmutter AL, Kertesz AE, Measurement of human vertical fusional response, 1978, Pergamon Press, Ltd.

These results emphasize the importance of objective and simultaneous monitoring of the movements of each eye during vertical fusional response. The motor compensation was always found to be incomplete so that the response contained a significant sensory component as well, and in addition, asymmetries were often observed in the time course and final contribution of the two eyes to the overall motor compensation. Therefore it is not enough to use a binocular eye-movement measuring technique and only evaluate the disjunctive component of the response. The monocular eye-movement records must also be examined to provide a complete characterization of the response.

Asymmetric Disparity Presentations

Perlmutter and Kertesz (1979) studied the vertical fusional response to asymmetric disparity presentations. Step or ramp disparities were introduced during dichoptic stimulus presentations by movement of only one of the monocular stimulus images, while horizontal and vertical movements of each eye were monitored with a resolution of 1′ of arc.

Figure 9.3 shows a typical motor response to a step disparity of 2° resulting from movement of the right stimulus only. After a reaction time of approximately 300 msec, the two eyes responded with conjugate saccades. The amplitudes of the two saccades were approximately equal, but each was greater than half of the disparity. Vergence movements followed the fast saccadic movements. The right eye compensated 90% of the stimulus disparity while the left eye failed to return to its original position. Thus the overall motor component only compensated 80% of disparity. Motor compensation averaged over 48 responses and 3 subjects was found to be 84.4%, with the range of 75% to 105%. Thus the response contained both motor and sensory components of varying amplitudes. When the step disparity was introduced, the subject experienced diplopia that was followed by a slow drift of the two stimulus images toward each other until they coalesced. It had taken 5.4 seconds to reestablish fusion subsequent to introduction of the step disparity. Response completion time was much longer than that observed during horizontal disparity presentations (Perlmutter and Kertesz, 1978).

No saccades were observed in the responses to presentations of vertical ramp disparities. The eye whose monocular image moved followed

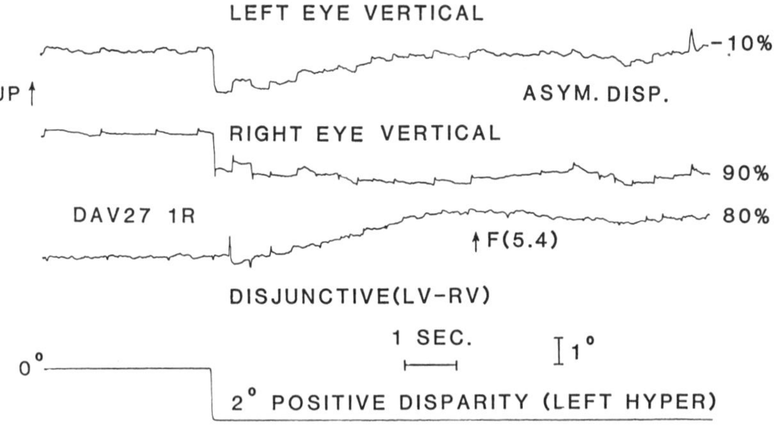

FIGURE 9.3. Eye movement responses to presentation of a 2° asymmetric vertical step disparity. The top two traces depict the vertical positions of the eyes. The disjunctive component represents the difference between left and right vertical eye positions (D = LV-RV). The bottom trace depicts the disparity contained in the stimulus. The small arrow indicates the time at which the subject fused the stimulus subsequent to the introduction of the disparity. The numbers on the right-hand side denote the portion of stimulus disparity that was compensated by each eye. The stimulus plot depicts stimulus position seen by the right eye. (From Perlmutter and Kertesz, 1979)

the stimulus closely, while the other eye did not move or moved only by a small amount. Thus the ramp disparity presumably elicited conjugate smooth pursuit and disjunctive vergence innervations, or movements of similar time course. The suggestion that vergence and smooth pursuit movements are additive for vertical ramp stimulation reinforces similar observations made by Miller, Ono, and Steinbach (1980) for the horizontal fusional response. The average motor compensation was found to be 87%, with a range of 60% to 105% of stimulus disparity.

In asymmetric disparity presentation, slower time course characterized the vertical vergence movements that were otherwise similar to the horizontal motor response.

Normal and Stabilized Disparity Viewing Conditions

It is standard engineering practice to study a feedback control system under open-loop and closed-loop conditions to obtain a description of the dynamic behavior of the system. Perlmutter and Kertesz (1980, 1981) studied the vertical fusional response under normal viewing conditions (closed-loop mode) and under stabilized disparity viewing conditions (open-loop mode) to symmetric disparity presentations. Disparity stabilization in the open-loop mode was achieved using vertical eye movement signals to move the appropriate monocular stimulus images so as to negate the effect of the movements on the retinal position of the stimulus. This was accomplished by feeding the vertical eye position signals directly to the oscilloscopes on which the stimuli were displayed and by adjusting the amplitude of these signals until a change in eye position resulted in an equal change in stimulus position.

Normal Viewing Conditions (Closed-Loop)

The step and ramp responses have already been discussed. Perlmutter and Kertesz (1980, 1981) also obtained the frequency response (steady state gain and phase curves) to predictable and unpredictable disparity presentations. A predictable disparity consisted of a single-frequency sinusoid, while an unpredictable one was composed of a mixture of 13 nonharmonically related sinusoids of different frequencies. As the circular symbols in Figure 9.4 show, 2 Hz was the maximum frequency at which the subject was able to fuse a sinusoidal disparity of 9.3′ peak-to-peak amplitude (these sinusoidal disparities were symmetric about zero disparity and were alternating between positive and negative values). The gain of the system (the ratio of disjunctive eye movement to stimulus disparity) was greater than 1 for frequencies up to 0.9 Hz. For frequencies higher than 0.9 Hz the vergence eye movements were attenuated, and beyond 2 Hz fusion began to break up. The difference between the meas-

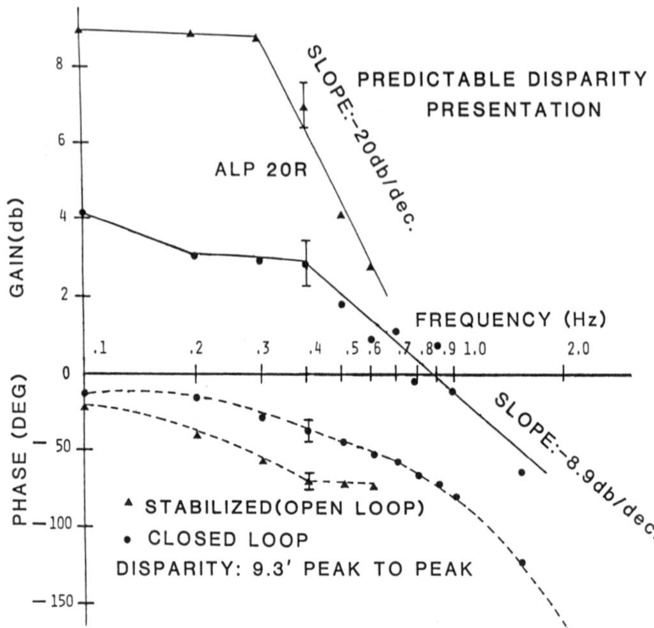

FIGURE 9.4. Steady-state gain and phase response of the vertical fusional vergence mechanism to stimuli containing sinusoidal disparities of 9.3′ peak to peak. The ● symbols denote normal viewing conditions (closed-loop), and the ▲ symbols denote stabilized disparity viewing conditions (open-loop). (From Perlmutter and Kertesz, 1981)

ured phase lag and that calculated from the gain curve can be represented by a simple time delay of 135 msec. No significant differences in phase lags were observed between the responses to predictable and unpredictable disparity presentations, indicating the lack of prediction in the response. The maximum frequency of 2 Hz at which subjects were able to fuse is only one-half of the corresponding frequency observed by Zuber and Stark (1968) for horizontal vergence response. Both horizontal and vertical vergence responses contained amplitude-dependent nonlinearities.

Stabilized Disparity Viewing Conditions (Open-Loop)

It was mentioned in the previous paragraph that the gain of the system was greater than 1 for frequencies up to 0.9 Hz under normal viewing conditions. This means that the magnitude of the disjunctive eye movements exceeded that of the disparity, and therefore a contribution from the sensory component of fusional response was required to assure fusion. Under normal viewing, the sensory component is only needed when the gain of the system is different from 1. Under open-loop conditions, however, it is only the sensory component that can bring about fusion since eye movements can no longer alter the magnitude of stimulus disparity because their compensatory effect is negated.

Rashbass and Westheimer (1961) reported that when a small horizontal step disparity is presented under open-loop conditions, the vergence response begins after a reaction time of 170 msec and it almost immediately attains a constant velocity that is maintained throughout the movement until either the stimulus is swept off the oscilloscope or an extreme value of vergence is attained. The velocity of the movement is proportional to the disparity and a constant of proportionality was derived for each subject. Based on these results, the presence of an integrator was stipulated in the forward branch of the horizontal disparity vergence mechanism.

Figure 9.5 shows the open-loop response to a 14.85′ vertical step disparity as measured by Perlmutter and Kertesz (1981). After a reaction

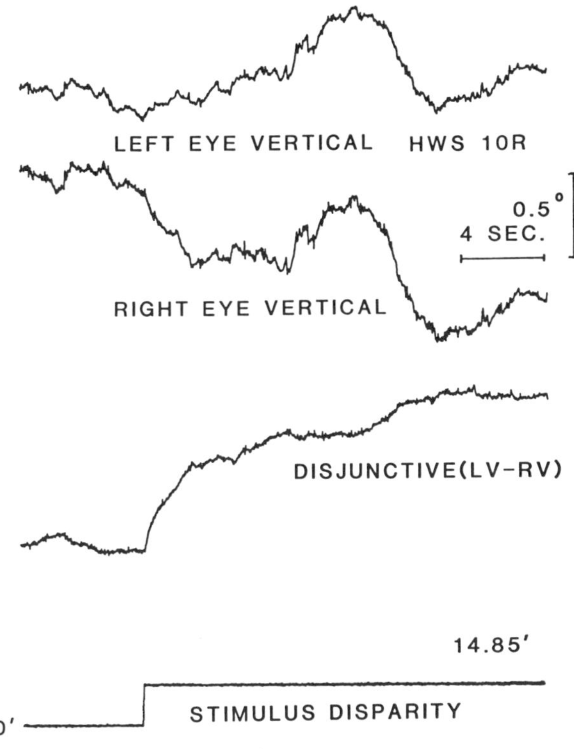

FIGURE 9.5. Vertical fusional vergence response to the introduction of a 14.85′ symmetric vertical step disparity under stabilized disparity viewing conditions. (From Perlmutter and Kertesz, 1981)

time of 180 msec, the initial velocity of the disjunctive component is 39.6′ per second, but this velocity is only maintained for 250 msec, after which the response begins to level off to a final positional value of 54′ of arc within 15 seconds. Therefore in the case of the vertical response to an open-loop step disparity, the maximum motor contribution is limited to less than 1°, and the initial velocity is only maintained for the relatively short time of 250 msec. The initial velocity, however, is proportional to the magnitude of the disparity, thus reinforcing the notion of the presence of an integrator in the forward loop. The effect of this integrator is not as strongly felt as in the horizontal case. Furthermore, as the individual eye movement records reveal, the response contains both version and vergence components. The initial velocities of the eyes also differ: the initial velocity of the right eye is 21.6′ per second and the left eye's velocity is 14.4′ per second. In general, the figure illustrates the need for recording individual eye movements as well as disjunctive components for a complete description of the fusional response.

Perlmutter and Kertesz (1981) also measured the frequency response under open-loop conditions for predictable and unpredictable stimuli. Figure 9.4 shows that for predictable stimuli the open-loop gain was always greater than 1 and was also higher than the closed-loop gain (a common characteristic of negative feedback systems). The highest frequency at which this subject was able to fuse under open-loop conditions was 0.6 Hz, which is significantly smaller than the corresponding 2 Hz observed for closed-loop conditions.

A comparison of frequency response to predictable and unpredictable stimuli under open-loop conditions shows no significant difference in phase lags and thus rules out the presence of a predictor in the system.

Effect of Stimulus Size and Complexity

The fusional response to stimulation within foveal and near foveal regions has received considerable attention, but only relatively recently have objective measurements been made to explore the role of more peripheral retinal regions. Ellerbrock (1949) observed that increasing the visual angle subtended by the stimulus from 0.25° to 8.25° brought about a significant increase in vertical fusional amplitudes. Fender and Julesz (1967) observed that increasing stimulus complexity also results in a significant increase in vertical fusional amplitudes.

Kertesz (1981) used an objective eye movement measuring technique to determine the effect of stimulus size and complexity on vertical fusional amplitudes and on the partitioning of the response between its motor and sensory components. The stimuli subtended from 5° to 57.6° and were composed of either a single horizontal line or 50 randomly segmented horizontal lines (Figure 9.6). The more complex segmented-line stimulus was more fusionally compelling because it evoked significantly larger fusional amplitudes than did the single-line stimulus.

Figure 9.7 shows that the increase in size of the single-line stimulus from 5° to 57.6° was accompanied by a significant increase in fusional amplitudes; however, this increase was overshadowed by the much larger—over twofold—increase in fusional amplitudes in response to the corresponding change in size of the complex stimulus. Thus inclusion of peripheral retinal regions in fusional stimulation has a significant effect on the fusional amplitudes. Identification of stimuli that evoke large fusional amplitudes is of special interest for the clinical treatment of vergence insufficiency where enlargement of vergence amplitudes is of primary importance.

Objective measurement of eye movements indicate that the increase in fusional amplitudes evoked by increasing stimulus size was brought about by proportionate increases in both motor and sensory components. The percentage of motor contribution varied from subject to subject but was typically in the range of 60% to 74%, allowing for a significant sensory component as part of the response. The amplitude of the sensory component was in some cases as large as 2.25°.

The existence of a small sensory fusional component limited to the extent of Panum's fusional areas is commonly accepted. It is also known

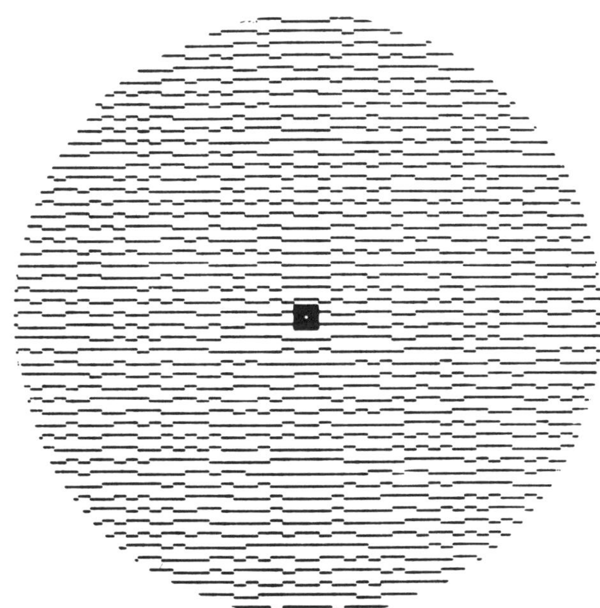

FIGURE 9.6. Stimulus consisting of randomly segmented lines.

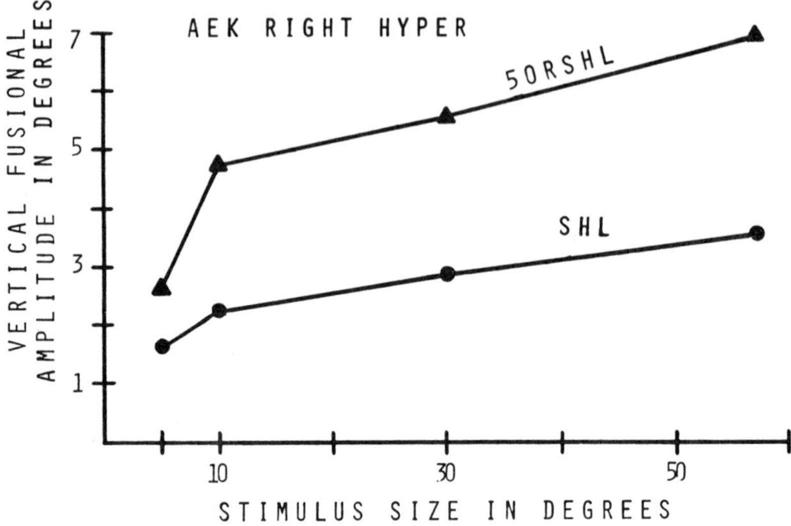

FIGURE 9.7. Vertical fusional amplitude vs stimulus size for either single horizontal line (●) or 50 randomly segmented horizontal lines (■). Data points represent an average of 10 observations with ±1 standard deviation contained within symbols. Reprinted by permission of the publisher, from Kertesz AE. The effect of stimulus size on fusion and vergence. Journal of the Optical Society of America, 1981.

that the magnitude of Panum's areas increases at increasingly peripheral retinal locations (Ogle, 1964). Since the sensory component is limited to the extent of Panum's fusional areas by definition (Ogle, 1964), Kertesz's results show that the extent of these areas is not always small; they can be quite substantial and are a function of stimulus size and complexity. The dependence of Panum's fusional areas on stimulus complexity and on the recent history of stimulation was first reported by Fender and Julesz (1967) and was later confirmed by others (Kertesz, 1972; Crone and Everhard-Halm, 1975). Kertesz's (1981) results add yet another stimulus parameter, size, that has a significant effect on the overall extent of Panum's areas. This is not equivalent to saying that Panum's areas increase at increasingly peripheral locations. During Kertesz's experiments the disparity contained in the stimulus was the same for the entire retinal region covered by that stimulus. Therefore a larger Panum's area at a peripheral location would not help to bring the disparity within the correspondingly smaller extent of the area at a more central retinal location unless some form of interaction occurred among neighboring retinal regions during fusional stimulation. The increase in sensory contribution corresponding to increased stimulus size is interpreted as evidence for interaction among adjacent retinal regions whereby inclusion of peripheral regions in the fusional stimulation increases the extent of Panum's areas in the more central retinal regions as well. Interactions between adjacent retinal regions was also observed during cyclofusional response and is discussed below.

Extrafoveal Stimulation

Burian (1939) was first to investigate the particular role of a strictly peripheral retinal disparity in binocular fusion. Using a subjective measure of vertical phoria, he found that strictly peripheral stimuli could elicit a fusional response. The most peripheral of his fusional stimuli was located 12° above each fovea, at which distance Burian's observer could not state whether or not they were actually fused, due to their "indistinct" appearance. Nevertheless, Burian estimated the fusional response magnitude by measuring the displacement of centrally located nonius lines that were shifted by the response to the peripheral stimuli. One of the surprising results was that peripheral fusion could actually disrupt central fusion, causing the subject to experience diplopia in the percept of a small fusional stimulus within the central visual field. Since Burian did not monitor eye positions during his experiments, he could not distinguish the relative contributions of the motor and sensory components to the overall fusional response.

Kertesz and Hampton (1980) examined the way in which vertical fusional amplitudes are apportioned between the motor and sensory components during extrafoveal stimulation. They used dichoptically presented circular disc stimuli that subtended 57°. One of the monocular stimuli contained a fixation point while the central 10° portion of the other monocular stimulus pattern was electronically blanked. This blanked region formed an artificial scotoma, whose position was electronically controlled and stabilized with respect to horizontal and vertical movements of the eye whose monocular image contained it. By using horizontal and vertical eye movement signals to negate the effect of eye movements, Kertesz and Hampton were able to stabilize the retinal position of the scotoma. The response to a 0.4° symmetric vertical step disparity was examined. The extrafoveal fusional stimulus elicited a disjunctive motor response that compensated for 75% of the stimulus disparity. The individual eye movement responses were asymmetric, however, with the nonscotomatic eye doing most of the disparity compensation. A comparison of full-field versus extrafoveal fusional stimulation indicates that the presence of the monocular scotoma exacerbated the asymmetry between the two monocular motor responses without appreciably affecting the magnitude of the overall disparity-compensating motor response.

The fact that disparities positioned extrafoveally are sufficient to evoke a fusional response should not surprise clinicians, as there are many examples of patients with macular degeneration, often bilateral, who are able to maintain ocular alignment. Clearly, in these cases it is the peripheral fusion lock that maintains ocular alignment. The results of Kertesz and Hampton show a way in which such an alignment may be accomplished by way of the motor and sensory components of fusional response.

CYCLOFUSIONAL RESPONSE

Definitions

The human cyclofusional response to orientation disparities (otherwise known as torsional disparities) shown in Figure 9.8 is composed of two components: (1) a motor response in the form of cyclovergent eye movements that are rotations in opposite directions about the lines of sight and (2) a sensory or nonmotor component limited to the extent of Panum's fusional areas.

If the initially horizontal stimulus lines are rotated in the direction shown in Figure 9.8, the resulting orientation disparity and the cyclofusional response are defined as positive. If the lines are rotated in the opposite direction the resulting disparity and response are negative. The cyclofusional amplitude corresponding to a particular stimulus configuration is determined by finding the largest orientation disparity in a given direction that can be presented to the subject without destroying the fused percept of the stimulus (a single, straight, horizontal line in the case of Figure 9.8).

Background

Nagel (1868) was first to suggest that torsionally disparate images of the type shown induce counterrotation of the eyes about the line of sight in the interest of binocular fusion. The response is referred to as a cyclofusional movement (Ogle and Ellerbrock, 1946; Ellerbrock, 1954) The initial assumption concerning the existence of these movements was based solely on subjective measurements. Brecher (1934) is sometimes mistakenly credited for the objective measurement of cyclofusional "movements." In fact, he only measured cyclorotations of the eyes in response to rotating discs and compared these results with cyclofusional responses obtained subjectively using a mirror haploscope. Hofmann and Bielschowsky (1900), Ames (1926), Verhoeff (1934), Ogle and Ellerbrock

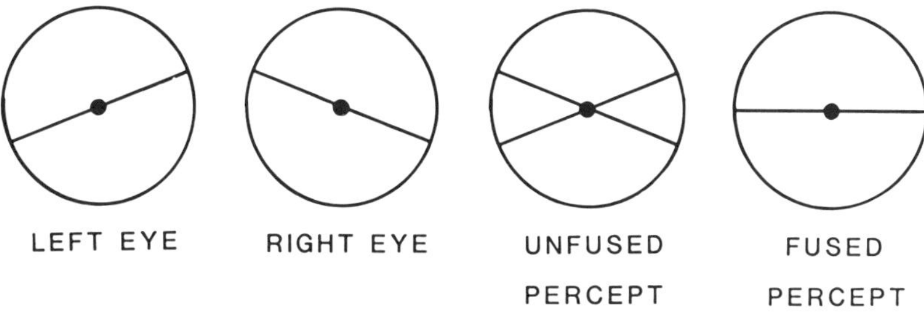

FIGURE 9.8. Presentation of a positive cyclofusional disparity.

(1946) and Ellerbrock (1954) have measured cyclofusional "movements" but in all cases subjectively. Ellerbrock reported the largest response of 23.7° in one direction and 10.2° in the opposite direction resulting in an overall range of 33.9°.

Kertesz and Jones (1970) were first to carry out objective measurements of cyclofusional response using stimuli subtending 10°. They found that subjects were able to fuse orientation disparities of several degrees without any apparent cyclofusional movements. These movements, if present, were indistinguishable from normal fixational movements and could not be correlated with introduction of disparity. The authors concluded that the responses were mediated by a sensory component rather than through actual movements of the eyes. These subjects who did not exhibit cyclofusional movements executed typical horizontal fusional movements and responded with cyclotorsional movements to nonfusional stimuli of rotating sectored discs.

Increasing stimulus complexity was found to result in a dramatic increase of cyclofusional amplitude, sometimes as much as fourfold, but this increase was realized solely by an increased sensory response (Kertesz, 1972). The greater cyclofusional amplitude resulting from increased stimulus complexity for the stimulus subtending 10° was realized by an increased sensory component, while compensatory eye movements, if they occurred, played a minor role. Kertesz (1972) therefore concluded that the extent of Panum's fusional areas should not be considered constant and their dependence on stimulus parameters should be recognized.

Wright and Kertesz (1974) investigated the way in which disparity information is detected or assessed within Panum's areas. In the case of torsionally disparate retinal images of the type shown in Figure 9.8, one could postulate two different neural mechanisms for assessing the disparity: a mechanism that is tuned to orientational disparities, or alternatively, one that is detecting positional disparities. The choice between the two mechanisms is dictated by what proves to be the effective stimulus parameter. Experiments show that in the case of torsionally disparate retinal images, it is not the orientational disparity between the two images of the stimulus but the positional disparity introduced by the stimulus at each pair of retinal points to which the fusional mechanism primarily responds. This conclusion is in agreement with the neurophysiological data of Nelson, Kato, and Bishop (1977).

Kertesz and Optican (1974) explored the nature of spatial interactions between adjacent retinal regions during cyclofusional response to stimuli subtending 10° of visual angle, which evoked a response consisting of the sensory component only. They investigated the effect of a disparity in one retinal region on the fusional range of adjacent regions. Their experiments revealed substantial interactions between adjacent regions. The ability of the sensory component to cope successfully with a disparity introduced in a given retinal region is a functon of the sign and magnitude of disparities present in adjacent regions. This bilateral interaction enhances the ability of the central neural mechanism to fuse disparities occurring in the same direction in neighboring retinal regions, and inhibits its ability to cope with disparities occurring in opposite directions. The results indicate that the extent of Panum's fusional areas is not only a function of stimulus size and complexity, but it is a function of the size and spatial distribution of disparities present in adjacent retinal regions as well.

In all the foregoing experiments, stimuli subtending 10° field of view were used. This should be emphasized at this point because it will soon become apparent how important stimulus size is in the characterization of cyclofusional response. These early objective measurements using stimuli subtending 10° field of view, did not document the existence of cyclofusional eye movements. These movements, if present, were indistinguishable from normal fixational movements and could not be correlated with the introduction of the torsional disparity.

It was only in 1975, a little over 100 years after Nagel postulated their existence, that cyclofusional eye movements were objectively recorded by Crone and Everhard-Halm (1975) in response to stimuli occupying a 25° field of view. They used a photographic technique to monitor initial and final eye positions and found cyclovergent movements of up to 5° in response to a 7° torsional disparity contained in the stimulus subtending 25°. All of Crone and Everhard-Halm's objective data were obtained during wide-angle (25° field of view) stimulation. They also proposed a subjective method for the measurement of cyclofusional eye movements, but it is difficult to see why their's would be more reliable than those proposed by others since it shares the principal shortcoming of all subjective methods, namely, inability to distinguish the effect of eye movements from sensory transformations brought about by the central neural mechanism involved in the sensory component of cyclofusional response.

Crone and Everhard-Halm's wide-angle data are extremely interesting, especially in the light of Kertesz's previously obtained narrow-angle (stimulus subtending 10°) results that were unable to elicit cyclofusional eye movements as part of the response. Clearly, it became necessary to assess the effect of stimulus size on the sensory and motor components of cyclofusional response.

Effect of Stimulus Size

Kertesz and Sullivan (1978) measured the effect of stimulus size on the sensory and motor components and examined for the first time the dynamic characteristics of cyclofusional eye movements. Eye positions were monitored continuously by an objective binocular technique that detected horizontal, vertical, and torsional components of movement of each eye with a resolution of 1 minute of arc. Each stimulus consisted of a circular region of 10°, 30°, or 50° diameter, filled with randomly segmented, initially horizontal lines (similar to that shown in Figure 9.7) surrounding a central fixation point (0.3° diameter) that served as a center of rotation of the stimulus. Equal and opposite rotations of the dichoptic stimuli presented a torsional (orientation) disparity between the two retinal images and evoked a cyclofusional response. The subject was instructed to fixate the center of the stimulus and use singleness, straightness, and horizontality of all stimulus lines as criteria for fusion.

Kertesz and Sullivan (1978) first determined the cyclofusional amplitudes that corresponded to stimuli of different sizes. A typical set of fusional amplitudes is shown in Table 9.1. Increasing the stimulus size from 10° to 50° resulted in a slight increase of fusional amplitude. The largest fusional amplitude for this subject corresponded to a negative

TABLE 9.1. Cyclofusional Amplitudes Measured with a Stimulus Consisting of Randomly Segmented Lines

Stimulus Size (°)	*Threshold* (°)
10	+5.1 ± 0.6[1]
	−10.3 ± 0.7
30	+6.7 ± 0.8
	−12.4 ± 0.7
50	+6.7 ± 0.7
	−12.4 ± 0.9

Each entry is an average of 10 observations.

[1] Standard deviation.

disparity contained in a stimulus subtending 50°. The data of Table 9.1 also show an asymmetry in fusional amplitudes. This particular subject had larger amplitudes to negative than to positive disparities for all three stimulus sizes. This asymmetry was observed for all subjects, but in different directions.

When Kertesz and Sullivan (1978) measured the motor response to these wide-angle (50° field of view) stimuli, they found that a −10° symmetric orientation disparity contained in the 50° stimulus evoked a 6.1° cyclovergent response shared more or less equally by the two eyes (the right eye contributed 3° and the left eye contributed 3.1° to the overall disjunctive component). The movements were slow both in response to the introduction of disparity as well as to its removal, requiring several seconds for completion. While the total motor compensation of 6.1° constituted a substantial portion of the response, it nevertheless fell short of compensating for the entire disparity by 3.9°, or 39%, thus allowing for a significant nonmotor or sensory component as well.

The effect of stimulus size on the composition of cyclofusional response as reported by Kertesz and Sullivan (1978) is summarized in Table 9.2. Samples of individual and averaged eye movement responses to introduction of a 5° torsional (orientation) stimulus disparity are shown in Figures 9.9 and 9.10. The data show that as the stimulus containing the fixed disparity was reduced in size from 50° to 10°, so was the magnitude of motor response. The total motor response to a −5° torsional disparity contained in a 50° stimulus was 3.5° (70% of total response, Figure 9.9), whereas the corresponding motor response to the same disparity contained in the 10° stimulus was only 1° (20% of total response, Figure 9.10).

TABLE 9.2. Average Cyclofusional Motor Responses to the Introduction of a Torsional Step Disparity

Stimulus Size (°)	*Disparity Magnitude* (°)	*Torsional Movement of Right Eye* (°)	*Torsional Movement of Left Eye* (°)	*Total Motor Response (R + L)* (°/%)
50	−5	−1.7	−1.8	−3.5/70[1]
30	−5	−1.7	−1.6	−3.3/66
10	−5	−0.3	−0.7	−1.0/20
50	+5	+1.2	+0.9	+2.1/42
30	+5	+0.8	+0.7	+1.6/32
10	+5	+0.9	+0.2	+1.1/22

Computed from five individual runs.

Positive sign denotes extorsional eye movements.

[1] Percentage of stimulus disparity compensated by the motor component.

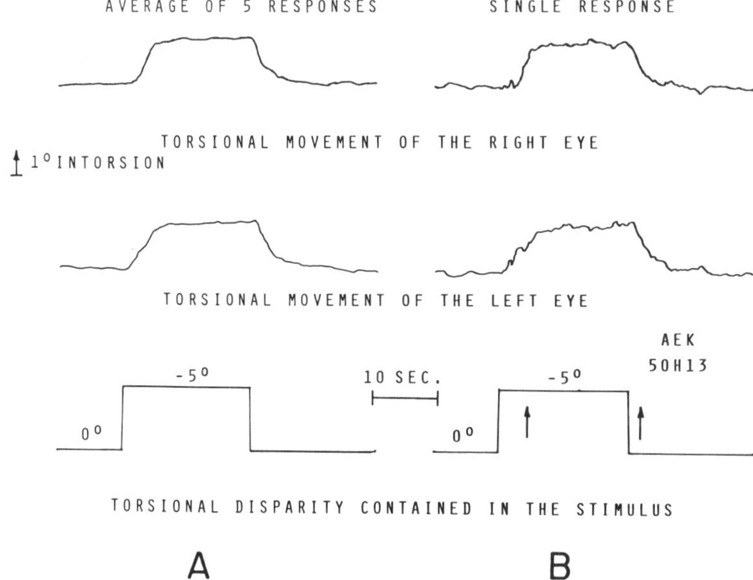

FIGURE 9.9. Torsional eye movements in response to introduction and removal of a −5° torsional step disparity contained in the 50° stimulus. The arrows at the bottom of B indicate the time at which the subject was able to fuse the stimulus subsequent to introduction or removal of the step disparity. Note that the magnitude of stimulus disparity as indicated in the figure was drawn to a different scale from that used for the eye-movement recordings. Reprinted with permission from Vision Research, 18, Kertesz AE, Sullivan MJ, Effect of stimulus size on human cyclofusional response, 1978, Pergamon Press, Ltd.

The sensory component continued to become more and more dominant at the expense of the motor component as stimulus size was reduced to less than 10°. The data thus show the importance of peripheral stimulation for evoking a significant motor component of cyclofusional response. These results are in agreement with the objective data of Crone and Everhard-Halm (1975) and of Hooten and associates (1979).

Sullivan and Kertesz (1979) commented on the different cyclofusional responses of the same subject to stimuli subtending 10°. As was discussed previously, Kertesz and Jones (1970) did not observe a cyclofusional motor response to 10°-diameter stimuli, whereas after many years of a null response, one of the subjects did exhibit a small motor response subsequent to wide-angle stimulation. Sullivan and Kertesz suggest a learning effect, that is, exposure to wide-angle cyclofusional stimuli that evoked a substantial motor response influenced response to narrow-angle stimulation. Experimental data were obtained suggesting that exposure to wide-angle stimulation aids in the development and maintenance of

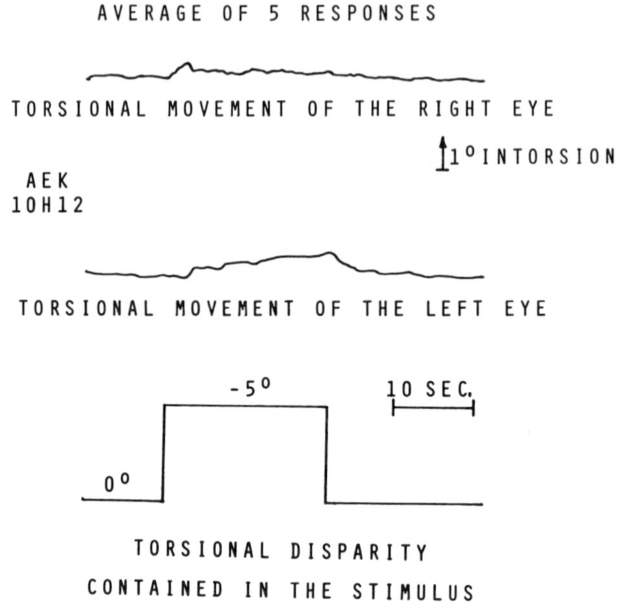

FIGURE 9.10. Torsional eye movements in response to the introduction and removal of a −5° torsional step disparity contained in the 10° stimulus. Note that the magnitude of stimulus disparity as indicated in the figure was drawn to a different scale from that used for the eye-movement recordings. Reprinted with permission from Vision Research, 18, Kertesz AE, Sullivan MJ, Effect of stimulus size on human cyclofusional response, 1978, Pergamon Press, Ltd.

the cyclofusional motor response. When wide-angle cyclofusional stimulation was deliberately not given to a subject for a month, his cyclofusional motor response to narrow-angle stimulation diminished with rest. After a few minutes of wide-angle stimulation, however, the motor response increased. This bit of evidence coupled with the subject's initial development of a motor response following wide-angle stimulation implies that the cyclofusional motor response is dependent on the history of exposure to wide-angle cyclofusional stimulation.

Symmetric Disparity Presentation

Sullivan and Kertesz (1978) studied the cyclofusional response to symmetric step disparity presentations (involving equal but opposite rotations of the dichoptic stimuli). All of the stimuli occupied a circular field subtending 50° and consisted of initially horizontal, randomly segmented lines surrounding a central fixation point.

Typical cyclofusional eye movements are shown in Figure 9.11. The averaged and single responses show that the settling time of intorsional response (left) to the 5.75° disparity is 10 to 12 seconds less than the settling time of the extorsional response (right). Intorsion proceeds smoothly, and unlike extorsional response, the eyes settle into a final position within 12 seconds after the introduction of torsional disparity. Intorsional movements of the right and left eyes show considerable similarity in amplitude and time course. Extorsional movements show differences: the left eye settled faster than the right eye and moved by a smaller amount. After torsional disparity was returned to zero, the return movements of both eyes were alike.

Table 9.3 summarizes the results of five different disparity presentations that indicate that torsional movements of the two eyes are similar

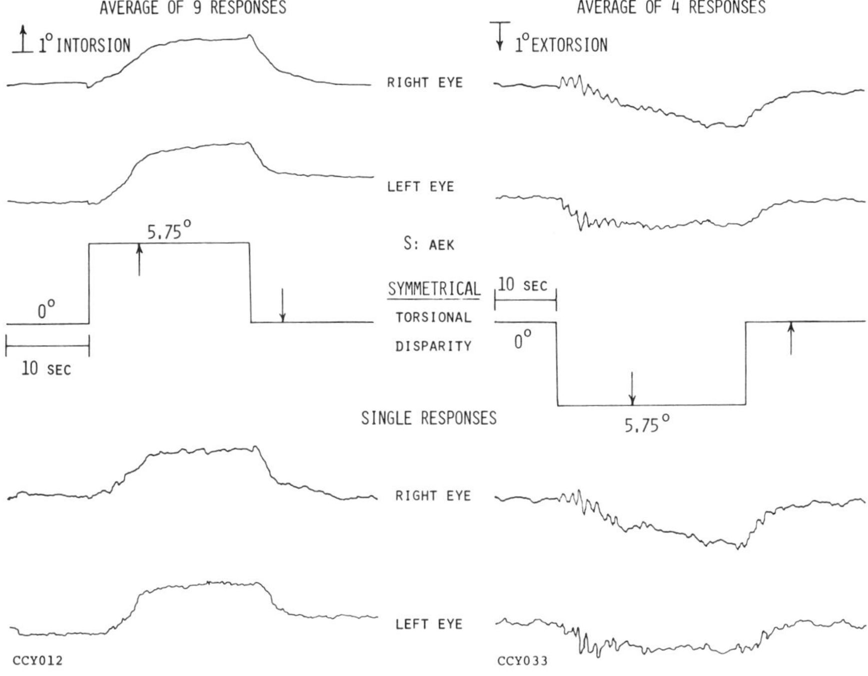

FIGURE 9.11. Intorsional eye movements (*left half*) and extorsional eye movements (*right half*) are shown in response to the presentation of 5.75° symmetric torsional step disparities. The stimulus plots located between the averaged and single response plots depict the time course of the torsional disparity contained in the stimulus. Small arrows are associated with the single responses and mark the time when the subject fused the stimuli after the disparity was changed to or from 0°. Reprinted with permission from Vision Research, 18, Sullivan MJ, Kertesz AE, Binocular coordination of torsional eye movements in cyclofusional response, 1978, Pergamon Press, Ltd.

TABLE 9.3. Summary of Averaged Responses to Symmetric Torsional Step Disparities

Disparity Size	$-2°$	$+2°$	$-5.75°$	$+5.75°$	$-10°$
Intorsion					
(R. eye/L. eye) deg	0.6/0.9		1.6/1.6		3.1/3.1
Extorsion					
(R. eye/L. eye) deg		0.6/0.6		1.6/1.2	
Initial velocity					
(R. eye/L. eye) deg/sec	0.28/0.28	0.12/0.06	0.14/0.19	0.15/0.11	0.62/0.62
Motor response					
(% total disparity)	75	60	56	48	62
Nonmotor response					
(% total disparity)	25	40	44	52	38

Positive sign signifies that the right stimulus was rotated clockwise and the left stimulus was rotated counterclockwise.

in magnitude and initial velocity. In general, excyclovergence was more slowly completed and less smoothly executed than incyclovergence. When the torsional disparities were returned to zero in a step, the return movement of the eyes was of approximately equal duration from a state of intorsion or extorsion. The results also show good concordance of cyclofusional movements with Hering's law of equal innervation. This judgment is based on the general features of the majority of response plots. Strong similarity of right and left eye movements in time course and amplitude is often apparent and this exemplifies the fundamental principles embodied in Hering's law.

The motor component compensated 48% to 75% of the stimulus disparity while the remaining 52% to 25% of the disparity was compensated by the sensory component. There has been some recent discussion concerning the existence and usefulness of a sensory component in cyclofusional response (Kaufman and Arditi, 1976; Kertesz and Sullivan, 1976). While these results do not shed new light on the usefulness of the sensory component they do offer additional evidence of its existence and of the substantial role it plays in fusional response. Bishop (1978, 1981) argues that orientation disparities are a common occurrence in everyday life. They assume a particular importance when we look downward during reading and walking, during which tasks the visual system is presented with a continuum of orientation disparities simultaneously. The simultaneous fusion of this wide range of orientation disparities can only be accomplished by the sensory component of cyclofusional response, since cyclovergent eye movements could not accomplish this.

Asymmetric Disparity Presentation

Sullivan and Kertesz (1978) also studied the cyclofusional response to asymmetric, 5.75° step disparity presentations resulting from the rotation of only the right or left eye's stimulus. The stimulus shown to the other eye was always a pattern of horizontally segmented lines. All of the stimuli occupied a circular field subtending 50° and consisted of initially horizontal, randomly segmented lines surrounding a central fixation point. All four possible stimulus configurations that result in a 5.75° asymmetric torsional disparity were tested. The percept that was reported when disparity had been fused was a single unified pattern of slightly inclined segmented lines. Fusion gave rise to the percept of a single pattern of segmented lines with an orientation that was spatially intermediate to the orientations of monocular stimuli.

Figure 9.12 shows cyclofusional motor responses to asymmetric 5.75° torsional disparities. Both eyes exhibit a motor response in each case. The response is cyclovergence with both eyes contributing substan-

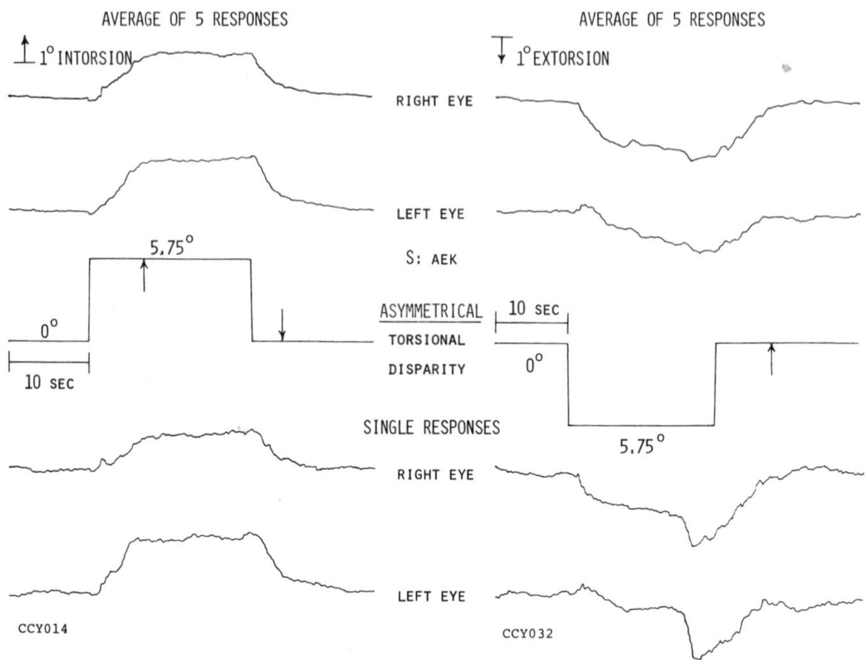

FIGURE 9.12. Intorsional eye movements (*left half*) are shown in response to the presentation of asymmetric torsional step disparities of 5.75° with clockwise rotation of the left stimulus only. Extorsional eye movements (*right half*) are shown in response to the presentation of asymmetric torsional step disparities of 5.75° with clockwise rotation of the right stimulus only. The stimulus plots that are located between the averaged and single response plots depict the time course of the torsional disparity contained in the stimulus. Small arrows are associated with the single responses and mark the time when the subject fused the stimuli after the disparity was changed to or from 0°. Reprinted with permission from Vision Research, 18, Sullivan MJ, Kertesz AE, Binocular coordination of torsional eye movements in cyclofusional response, 1978, Pergamon Press, Ltd.

tial torsional movements. The intorsional movement (left) is smoother and is completed more rapidly than the extorsional one (right). The extorsional responses do not show an equal amplitude in each eye but the time courses of the movements of the two eyes are similar. The subject required approximately seven seconds to fuse the disparate stimuli during intorsion but there was little or no diplopia experienced during the slower extorsional responses, and therefore no marker indicating a delay of fusion of the step disparity is present in the stimulus plot associated with extorsion. The single run in the lower half of Figure 9.12 was not typical in its time course because the movement seems to have two distinct phases during the presentation of the 5.75° disparity. This response is included because it shows how closely the two eyes often resemble one another's motor behavior during cyclofusion.

Table 9.4 presents the results based on averaged records from tests with all four of the asymmetric 5.75° disparities. Comparing right and left eyes, most averaged motor response amplitudes are equal or are almost equal. Once again, the results show concordance with Hering's law. The bilateral nature of the motor response during cyclofusion is supported by the results. The movements of the eyes were always such as to bring their images closer to corresponding retinal points. Accordingly, all of the asymmetric disparities induced a bilateral response that brought the two retinal images closer to correspondence even though the stimulus to only one eye was rotated. The subject always perceived a single fused image of intermediate orientation to the orientation of either component of the disparity, proving the binocular character of the cyclofusional response.

The range of the motor contribution was 49% to 70% of total disparity. This leaves a variable sensory component of fusional response, or equivalently, a broad range of values for the size of Panum's fusional areas.

Strictly Peripheral Stimulation

Sullivan and Kertesz (1979) investigated the effectiveness of macular versus peripheral stimulation during cyclofusional response. These experiments were motivated by the pronounced effect of wide-angle, full-field stim-

TABLE 9.4. Summary of Averaged Responses to 5.75° Asymmetric Torsional Step Disparities

Stimulus Rotation	CW Right Eye	CCW Right Eye	CW Left Eye	CCW Left Eye
Intorsion (R. eye/L. eye) deg		1.9/1.3	1.6/1.7	
Extorsion (R. eye/L. eye) deg	2.1/1.9			1.6/1.2
Initial velocity (R. eye/L. eye) deg/sec	0.13/0.16	0.26/0.11	0.21/0.18	0.15/0.11
Motor response (% total disparity)	70	56	57	49
Nonmotor response (% total disparity)	30	44	43	51

Stimulus: 50°-diameter randomly segmented lines.

The stimulus to only one eye was rotated by 5.75° in a clockwise or counterclockwise direction from the horizontal. The stimulus to the other eye remained horizontal.

ulation in eliciting a motor response during cyclofusion and were designed to determine whether stimulation with torsional disparities presented only in the peripheral visual field evoke torsional eye movements as does full-field stimulation that includes the central (macular) regions.

The stimuli consisted of either 50°-diameter circular discs or annuli of three different sizes (13° to 50°, 13° to 27°, or 30° to 50° diameters). The stimuli contained randomly segmented, initially horizontal lines with a fixation point at their center. The purpose of using annular stimuli was to confine the cyclofusional disparities to peripheral regions of the retina.

Table 9.5 presents the average torsional eye movements in response to the presentation of a −5.75° torsional step disparity. Substantial intorsional eye movements were obtained in response to disparities presented with each stimulus configuration. In particular, the annular patterns that stimulated only peripheral portions of the visual field elicited many of the largest movements. Over all stimuli tested, the subject compensated for 49% to 80% of the −5.75° disparity by the combined intorsional movements of the two eyes. This left the range of 51% to 20%, that was compensated by the sensory component. These results show that cyclofusional response may be elicited by torsional disparity confined to the peripheral visual field.

Kertesz and Sullivan (1979) also studied cyclofusional response when torsional disparities of opposite sign were presented in the central and peripheral retinal regions. An example of the stimuli used in this experiment is shown in Figure 9.13. The stimulus field of randomly segmented lines was divided into two regions: a center and a surround that were separated by a 3°-wide gap. Two cases were studied. In the first case, the center region was 27° in diameter, the surround was 30° to 50° in diameter; 4° torsional disparities of opposite sign were presented in each region or a 4° torsional disparity was presented in only one region while the other region contained zero torsional disparity. In a second case, torsional disparities were presented in the same combinations as above but the center region was reduced to 10° in diameter, the surround

TABLE 9.5. Intorsional Eye Movement Response to a −5.75° Torsional Step Disparity

	Average Intorsional Eye Movement	
Stimulus Diameter	*Left Eye (°)*	*Right Eye (°)*
50° disc	−1.5	−1.3
13°–50° annulus	−2.0	−1.5
13°–27° annulus	−2.1	−2.3
30°–50° annulus	−1.7	−1.9

Each entry represents an average of three to five responses.

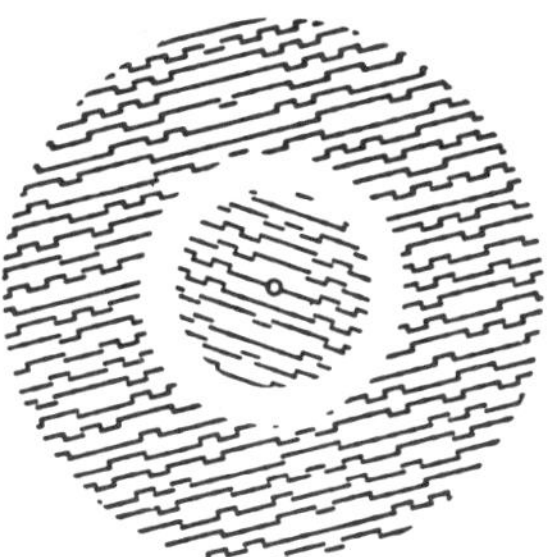

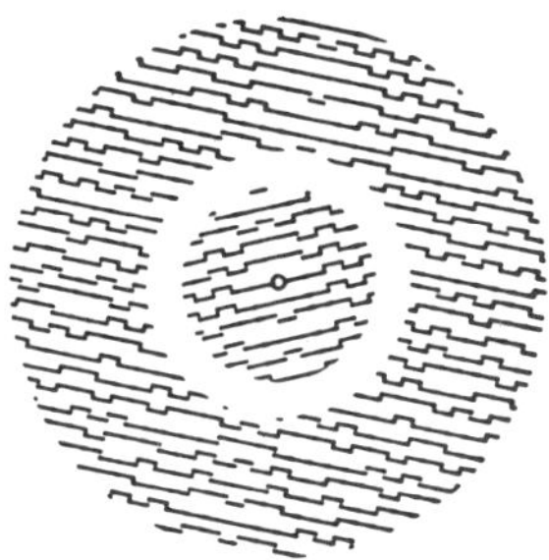

FIGURE 9.13. An example of randomly segmented line stimuli used for the study of regional interactions. The center and surround regions were not continuous but were separated by a gap of 3° width. Different torsional disparities were presented in each of the regions. Stimulus rotations in each region are exaggerated in the figure for the purpose of illustration. The different center-surround disparity combinations were those specified in Table 9.6. The fused percept of the disparate stimuli consisted of single, straight, horizontal segmented lines. (From Sullivan and Kertesz, 1979)

was changed to 13° to 50° in diameter, and the disparity size was fixed at 2°. The 4° and 2° sizes were chosen because they represented the largest disparities that the subject could fuse during the simultaneous presentation.

Table 9.6 contains the average amount and direction of torsional eye movement that resulted from each center-surround disparity combination. The data indicate opposite motor response trends associated with the large center (27°) stimulus and the smaller center (10°) stimulus. Motor response to the former was torsional eye movement that generally compensated for or reduced the torsional disparity in the center region while increasing the retinal image disparity in the surround. Torsional motor response of the eyes to the stimulus having the smaller center usually compensated for the disparity in the surround while increasing the retinal image disparity in the center.

These results provide clear objective evidence that the fusional mechanism can exhibit a motor response that reduces the disparity in the 13° to 50° region while increasing the retinal image disparity in the 10° central field. These compensatory eye movements were surprising and could not have been predicted. Their occurrence raises a number of questions concerning the relationship between the motor and sensory components of cyclofusional response. One would expect coordination between the two response components so that single vision would be facilitated primarily in the center of the visual field. There may, however, be instances of increased need for single vision in the visual periphery,

TABLE 9.6. Average Torsional Eye Movement Responses to Conflicting Torsional Disparities in Center and Surround Regions

	Torsional Disparity (°)		*Average Eye Torsion (°)*	
Stimulus	*Center*	*Surround*	*Left*	*Right*
	−4	+4	−0.6	−0.8
	+4	−4	+1.3	+1.1
Center: 27°	0	+4	0	+0.1
Surround: 30°-50°	0	−4	−0.1	−0.1
	−4	0	−0.7	−0.8
	+4	0	−1.2	+1.1
	−2	+2	+0.2	+0.3
	+2	−2	−0.4	−0.5
Center: 10°	0	+2	+0.6	+0.6
Surround: 13°-50°	0	−2	−0.4	−0.5
	−2	0	0	0
	+2	0	0	0

(+) Intorsion, (−) Extorsion. Each entry represents an average of three to five responses.

such as in cases of impaired central vision. The results imply that the relative contributions of motor and sensory components are not solely determined on the basis of minimizing torsional retinal image disparity uniformly across the visual field or in central retinal regions only, but that peripheral stimulation exercises a strong influence on both.

It should be noted that the sensory component plays a prominent role in this experiment. Since the disjunctive torsional eye movements partially compensated for only the torsional disparity presented in one of the regions, these same eye movements increased the retinal image disparity present in the other stimulus region. Nevertheless, the entire pattern was judged by the subjects to be fused. This plainly illustrates a complex operation of the sensory component of cyclofusional response that simultaneously provides opposite compensation in two regions of the visual field. When opposing stimulus disparties larger than those chosen for the experiment were used in center and surround, diplopia was experienced in one of the regions. This is consistent with Burian's (1939) finding that peripheral fusional stimuli could disrupt fusion near the center of the visual field.

Cyclofusional Stimulation that Contains Depth Cues

The interaction between the fusional and stereoptic mechanisms may be investigated by the use of cyclofusional stimuli that contain depth cues.

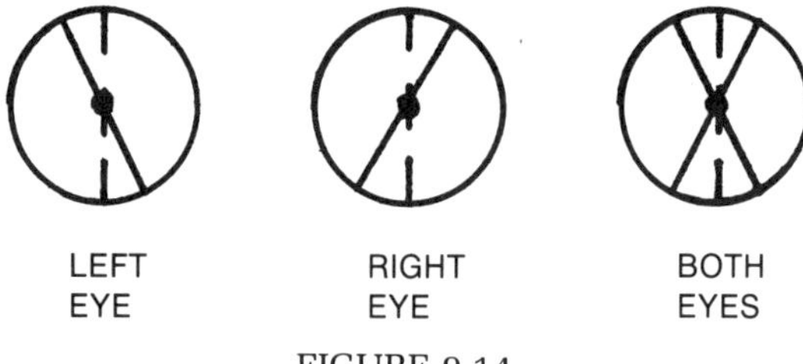

FIGURE 9.14

The visual system may interpret retinal image disparities as an indication of misalignment between the two monocular visual fields, requiring a fusional correction, or in the case of relative horizontal disparities, as a depth cue. The combined effect of these two strategies is to provide us with a single three-dimensional percept of the space around us.

Ogle and Ellerbrock (1946; Ellerbrock, 1954) conducted a series of experiments designed to measure the cyclofusional response by using stimuli that contained both cyclofusional and stereoptic cues. Subjects fixated the center of an initially vertical line that was subsequently rotated in opposite directions as seen by each eye (Figure 9.14). Ogle and Ellerbrock suggested that if the disparity introduced by the stimulus was not too large, the response could take one of three forms:

1. If the eyes undergo a cyclofusional movement equal to the magnitude of the orientation disparity, then a single vertical line is seen.
2. Without any cyclofusional eye movements, the continuum of crossed and uncrossed horizontal disparities contained in the stimulus will cause the line to appear tilted in space, with its top appearing farther away from the observer than its bottom.
3. If the cyclofusional eye movements are not large enough to eliminate the entire orientation disparity between the retinal images of the stimulus, but only succeed in bringing those images nearer to their corresponding meridians, then the remaining continuum of crossed and uncrossed horizontal disparities between the retinal images is used as a depth cue, and is translated into a fore-and-aft tilting of the stimulus line. The amount of tilt perceived with only partial cyclofusional motor compensation is smaller than the tilt perceived in case 2 with no cyclofusional compensation.

The implication in case 3 is that the cyclofusional response results in a reduction of the orientation disparity between the retinal images of the stimulus, and that only the relative horizontal disparities contained in this reduced orientation disparity serve as depth cues. Ogle and Ellerbrock found only partial cyclofusional compensation, but they did not measure cyclofusional eye movements and thus were unable to distinguish between the motor and sensory components of the response. Instead, the amplitude of the response was inferred from the difference between the physical disparity contained in the stimulus and the portion of the physical disparity that was used as a depth cue.

Hampton and Kertesz (1980) used an objective binocular technique to monitor eye positions during the response. They found that the response contained three components: (1) a cyclofusional motor component, (2) a nonmotor, sensory cyclofusional component, and (3) a stereoptic compensation in which the continuum of horizontal disparities contained within a portion of the orientation disparity was used as a depth cue. Therefore both the stereoptic and cyclofusional mechanisms contributed to the response. The cyclofusional response is composed of small compensatory eye movements as well as a substantial sensory contribution rather than consisting of torsional eye movements alone, as was suggested by Ogle and Ellerbrock (1946; Ellerbrock, 1954). The composition of the overall response is constant for changes in stimulus size, but is affected by changes in stimulus complexity. Increasing stimulus complexity brings about an increase of the magnitude of cyclofusional response and a corresponding decrease of the stereoptic contribution. Much of the increase in the cyclofusional amplitude is realized by a corresponding increase in torsional eye movements, while the magnitude of the sensory cyclofusional component remains relatively constant, compensating for approximately 50% of the stimulus disparity.

SUMMARY

The fusional response to retinal image disparity contains motor and nonmotor or sensory components. Substantial differences exist between the horizontal, vertical, and cyclofusional responses.

Horizontal fusional response is fastest. The response to a step change in disparity is completed within 1 second (Rashbass and Westheimer, 1961), whereas 8 to 10 seconds may be required for the completion of a vertical or cyclofusional step response (Perlmutter and Kertesz, 1979; Kertesz and Sullivan, 1978). The horizontal and cyclofusional responses exhibit a fairly good conformance to Hering's law of equal innervation during symmetric disparity presentations (Perlmutter and Kertesz, 1978; Sullivan and Kertesz, 1978), whereas the corresponding vertical fusional response exhibits clear violations of this law both in the time course and in the final monocular contributions to the overall motor response (Perlmutter and Kertesz, 1978). In fact, good concordance to Hering's law is observed for horizontal and cyclofusional responses even to asymmetric step disparity presentations.

Stimulus size, that is, the visual angle subtended by the stimulus, has a significant effect on the magnitude of both motor and sensory components of vertical and cyclofusional responses. For vertical fusional response, increasing stimulus size results in an increased fusional amplitude, that is realized by significant increases in both components (Kertesz, 1981). The results are even more interesting for the cyclofusional response, because its composition changes with increasing stimulus size. For stimuli subtending 10° or less the sensory component is the major factor and fusion occurs with relatively little eye rotation. For stimuli subtending greater than 10° there is a relative increase in the motor component, so that at 25° it becomes the major factor. Even torsional disparities that are confined to strictly peripheral retinal regions (annular stimuli of 30° to 50° in diameter) evoke a cyclofusional response with a substantial motor component.

REFERENCES

Ames A Jr. Cyclophoria. Am J Physiol Opt 1926;7:3–38.

Bishop PO. Orientation and position disparities in stereopsis. In: Cool SJ, Smith EL III, eds. Frontiers in visual science. New York: Springer-Verlag, 1978:336–50.

Bishop PO. Binocular vision. In: Moses RA, ed. Adler's physiology of the eye, clinical application. 7th ed. St. Louis: CV Mosby, 1981:575–649.

Brecher GA. Die Optokinetische Ausloesung von Augenrollung und Rotatorischem Nystagmus. Pflugers Arch Ges Physiol 1934;234:13–18.

Burian HM. Fusional movements: role of peripheral retinal stimuli. Arch Ophthalmol 1939;21:486–91.

Crone RA, Everhard-Halm Y. Optically induced eye torsion. I. Fusional cyclovergence. Albrecht Von Graefes Arch Klin Exp Ophthalmol 1975;195:231–39.

Ellerbrock VJ. Experimental investigation of vertical fusional movements. Am J Optom 1949;26:327–37; 388–99.

Ellerbrock VJ. The effect of aniseikonia on the amplitude of vertical divergence. Am J Optom 1952;29:403–15.

Ellerbrock VJ. Inducement of cyclofusional movements. Am J Optom 1954;31:553–56.

Fender DH, Julesz B. Extension of Panum's fusional area in binocularly stabilized vision. J Opt Soc Am 1967;57:819–30.

Hampton DR, Kertesz AE. Cyclofusional responses to stereoptic stimuli. J Opt Soc Am 1980;70:1634.

Hofmann FB, Bielschowsky A. Uber der Willkur entzogenen Fusions bewegungen der Augen. Pflugers Arch Ges Physiol 1900;80:1–40.

Hooten K, Myers E, Worrall R, Stark L. Cyclovergence: the motor response to cyclodisparity. Albrecht Von Graefes Arch Klin Exp Ophthalmol 1979; 210:65–68.

Houtman WA, Roze JH, Scheper W. Vertical motor fusion. Doc Ophthalmol 1977;44:179–85.

Kaufman L, Arditi A. The fusion illusion. Vision Res 1976;16:535–43.
Kertesz AE. The effect of stimulus complexity on human cyclofusional responses. Vision Res 1972;12:699–704.
Kertesz AE. Disparity detection within Panum's fusional areas. Vision Res 1973;13:1537–44.
Kertesz AE. The effect of stimulus size on fusion and vergence. J Opt Soc Am 1981;71:289–93.
Kertesz AE, Hampton DR. Motor response to peripheral fusional disparities. Invest Ophthalmol Visual Sci 1980;18(Suppl):79.
Kertesz AE, Jones RW. Human cyclofusional response. Vision Res 1970;10:891–96.
Kertesz AE, Optican LM. Interactions between neighboring retinal regions during fusional response. Vision Res 1974;14:339–43.
Kertesz AE, Sullivan MJ. Fusion prevails. Vision Res 1976;16:545–49.
Kertesz AE, Sullivan MJ. Effect of stimulus size on human cyclofusional response. Vision Res 1978;18:567–71.
Miller JM, Ono H, Steinbach MJ. Additivity of fusional vergence and pursuit movements. Vision Res 1980;20:43–47.
Nagel A. Uber das vorkommen von Wahren Rollungen des Auges um die Gesichtslinie. Albrecht Von Graefes Arch Klin Exp Ophthalmol 1868;188:231–88.
Nelson JI, Kato H, Bishop PO. Discrimination of orientation and position disparities by binocularly activated neurons in cat striate cortex. J Neurophysiol 1977;40:260–83.
Ogle KN. Binocular vision. New York: Hafner, 1964.
Ogle KN, Ellerbrock VJ. Cyclofusional movements. Arch Ophthalmol 1946;36:700–35.
Perlmutter AL, Kertesz AE. Measurement of human vertical fusional response. Vision Res 1978;18:219–23.
Perlmutter AL, Kertesz AE. Vertical fusional response to asymmetric disparity presentations. J Opt Soc Am 1979;69:1423.
Perlmutter AL, Kertesz AE. Vertical fusional response to stabilized disparity presentations. J Opt Soc Am 1980;70:1634.
Perlmutter AL, Kertesz AE. Vertical fusional response to open and closed loop disparity presentation. Proc Oculomotor System-81, Pasadena, Ca. In press.
Rashbass C, Westheimer G. Disjunctive eye movements. J Physiol 1961;159:339–60.
Sullivan MJ, Kertesz AE. Binocular coordination of torsional eye movements in cyclofusional response. Vision Res 1978;18:943–49.
Sullivan MJ, Kertesz AE. Peripheral stimulation and human cyclofusional response. Inves Ophthalmol Visual Sci 1979;18:1287–91.
Verhoeff F. Cycloduction. Tr Am Ophthalmol Soc 1934;32:208–28.
Winkelman JE. Peripheral fusion. Arch Ophthalmol 1951;45:425–30.
Wright JC, Kertesz AE. The role of positional and orientational disparity cues in human fusional response. Vision Res 1974;15:427–30.
Zuber BL, Stark L. Dynamical characteristics of the fusional vergence eye-movement system. IEEE Trans Systems Sci Cybernet 1968;SSC-4:72–79.

10

Model of the Disparity Vergence System

V. V. Krishnan
Lawrence Stark

The disparity vergence system has been studied by optometrists, physiologists, and more recently, by bioengineers and control engineers. The interests and approaches of these groups are quite different, as reflected by the nature of data obtained by them and by their subsequent analysis of these data. Optometrists have essentially been interested in formulating empirical relationships between the magnitudes of the input disparity and the magnitude of the resulting vergence eye movement, although they have been aware of latencies and dynamics of vergence eye movements. Physiologists are interested primarily in the nature and characteristics of the neuronal signals and the mechanisms by which they are generated. Control engineers view the system in yet another perspective and are interested in the dynamics of the system and its interactions with the other visual systems.

The control theory approach to biological systems is generally built up from an abstract point of view and usually indicates how a system could work. The mathematical model of a biological system as initially developed by the control engineer is generally a simple one based on the system's previously established characteristics. This model is then used to "predict" system behavior under various input conditions; it is constantly refined and possibly enlarged using information generated by the deviance, or agreement, between the predicted and the actual responses of the system to predetermined input. It is in this context that computer simulation of biological system models becomes an important and useful tool. Simulation is generally used for two purposes, synthesis and identification. In the case of synthesis, one simulates models with various topologies, all generally subject to a limited number of predetermined constraints, with a view of obtaining a desired response to a given input. Identification involves simulating systems models with different structures, again subject to constraints imposed by physical and physiological considerations, to obtain a model with a response that closely resembles the actual response of the given system to the given stimulus. This approach is particularly useful in developing and refining models of biological systems.

Modeling and identification of biological systems through simulation has been subject to some criticism as games played on computer without much resemblance to reality. This criticism is valid in the case of a few highly abstract and mathematical models, but can generally be avoided if the models are developed strictly to conform to known physiological and anatomic facts. It is important to note that a mathematical model is a simplification of the real system and is not, nor is it meant to be, a complete representation. With a model and its active simulation one can not only become familiar with the various behavioral aspects of the system, but can also suggest new physical experiments that can lead to a refined model that is both parsimonious and precise in its formulation (Stark, 1971).

There are two major components in dynamic human vergence eye movements that occur in normal binocular viewing: accommodative vergence and fusional or disparity vergence. Accommodative vergence movements are the result of strong coupling between the accommodation and vergence systems and are produced whenever there is a change in the level of accommodation. Disparity vergence movements, which will be our sole concern here, occur when there is retinal disparity between the images of the target in the two eyes (Westheimer and Mitchell, 1956; 1969; Stewart, 1961; Mitchell, 1970). These movements have conventionally been called fusional vergence movements because the objective of the disparity vergence system seems to be to obtain and maintain retinal correspondence so that the image of the target appears fused. Since the stimulus to these movements is probably the existence of retinal disparity rather than diplopia itself (Stark et al., 1980), we refer to the movements as disparity vergence movements and to the system as the disparity vergence system.

Descriptive Model of Disparity Vergence System

The system may be visualized in a descriptive block diagram form as shown in Figure 10.1. One of the three major components of the system

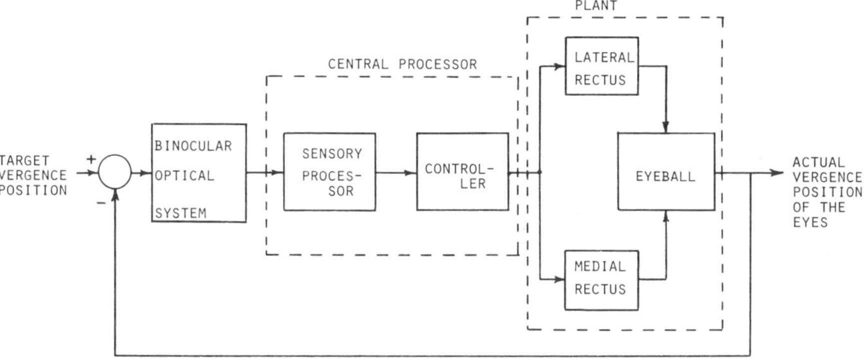

FIGURE 10.1. An elementary block diagram representation of the disparity vergence system. Reprinted by permission of the publisher, from Krishnan VV. A heuristic model for the human vergence eye movement system. Institute of Electrical and Electronics Engineers, Transactions in Biomedical Engineering, © 1977 IEEE.

is the binocular optical system, which compares the target position with the instantaneous vergence position of the eyeballs and produces the disparity signal from the retinal images in the two eyes. It should be clear that the binocular optical system may also include some neural processing to produce the disparity signal. The central processor includes both the sensory processing and the generation of the motor controller signal. In control system terminology, the binocular optical system is thought of as a comparator and the central processor as a controller. The neural signal generated by the controller rotates the eyeballs through the action of the associated musculature; in control terminology this portion of the system is called the plant or the process. The entire system operates as an automatic control system where response (actual vergence position of the eyes) is compared with reference input (appropriate vergence position as determined by the target location), and the plant is driven by the output of the controller, which in turn is processed from the error signal (retinal disparity).

Measurement of Disparity Vergence

To develop a mathematical model the first requirement is that data be available on the instantaneous values of both the target and the vergence positions. Two popular methods for measuring instantaneous angular positions are the photocell and electrooculography (EOG) techniques. Although each procedure has its own adherents, the photocell technique seems to be a little more accurate and reliable. It is simple, and takes advantage of the difference in reflectivity between the white scleral portion of the eye and the darker iris (Figure 10.2) Two infrared-sensitive photocells are mounted in front of the eye so that each of the viewing fields falls on the boundary between the iris and the sclera. An infrared light source is used and the amount of light received by each photocell is directly proportional to the amount of illuminated sclera in its field. The difference between the voltage output of the photocells is then a direct measure of angular rotation of the eye, but the apparatus has to be calibrated before each experimental run. This set-up and procedure have been widely reported in literature (Torok et al., 1951; Stark et al., 1962; Stark, 1968). There is some criticism of this method because it is sensitive to both rotational and translatory movements of the eyeball. It is important therefore to ensure that there is no translatory movement of the eyeball with respect to the photocells; this can be done by mounting the photocells on a spectacle frame worn by the subject, and by eliminating any head movement by having the subject bite into a bite-bar during the experiment. The actual translatory movement of the eyeball within its socket during vergence movements is quite small and negligible (Krishnan and Stark, 1977).

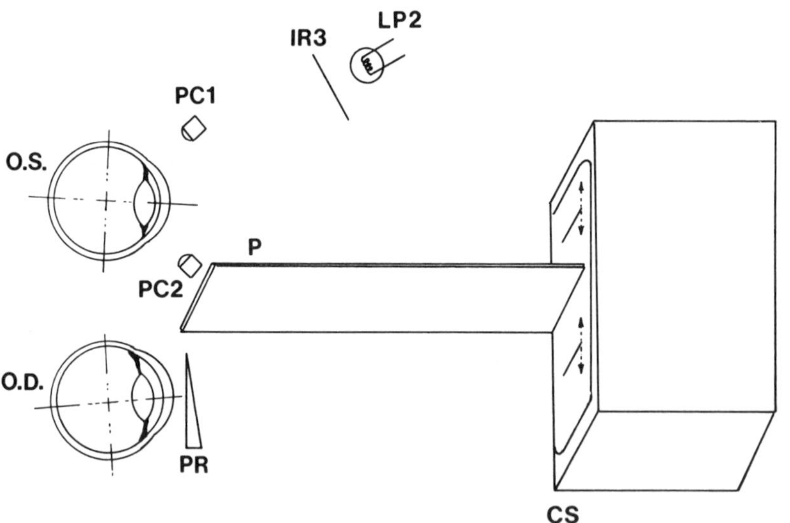

FIGURE 10.2. A schematic diagram of the experimental set-up for generating the disparity stimulus and measuring the fusional vergence response. CS = television screen on which the two vertical lines are generated; P = septum to ensure that the left eye sees only the left vertical line and the right eye the right line; PC_1, PC_2 = infrared-sensitive photocells; LP2 = a DC light source; IR3 = infrared filter; PR = base-out prism used with large-amplitude stimuli. Reprinted by permission of the publisher, from Krishnan VV. A heuristic model for the human vergence eye movement system. Institute of Electrical and Electronics Engineers, Transactions in Biomedical Engineering, © 1977 IEEE.

Input to the disparity vergence system has to be generated with some care so as not to contaminate the system response with either saccadic or versional components, or more important, with an accommodative vergence component. The stimulus generally consists of two identical images, each presented to one eye, so that each eye views a separate but identical target at the same time. The horizontal separation between the targets is varied with respect to time so that external input to the system can be made to follow any desired time-dependent function. The most common and simple method is to use two coupled cathode ray oscilloscopes to generate the targets viewed by the two eyes. Studies on the characteristics of stimuli that elicit a vergence response (Westheimer and Mitchell, 1969; Mitchell, 1970) show that there is a substantial latitude in the shape, size, and luminance characteristics of acceptable targets. Contamination by versional eye movements can be avoided by ensuring that the two targets are always symmetric with respect to the midline or the "cyclopian axis." Contamination by accommodative vergence is more difficult to avoid; the common methods are to use small target excursions so that the accommodation induced is within the accommodation dead-band, or to use a target with poorly defined edges so that the large resulting target-blur acts as a very poor accommodation stimulus. The ideal solution is to use a pin-hole pupil but this generally poses mechanical problems. It would be very valuable from the point of view of modeling to measure intermediate signals as well. It is, of course, not possible at present to monitor neural signals in the visual cortex but even electromyographic studies of ocular muscles during vergence movements have not so far yielded reliable and quantifiable data.

Modeling Approaches

There are two approaches to developing a model for the disparity vergence system. The first is to rely solely on measured input-output data and develop a mathematical model that approximates the input-output relationship by a mathematical equation—generally a differential equation in the case of dynamic systems. This "black-box" approach is quite useful and popular where the primary goal of the model is to mimic the response of the system to a given input. However, it is generally not of much use if the goal is to help understand the underlying mechanisms or, as in the case of the disparity vergence system, to study and understand the nature of its interaction with other systems.

The other approach assumes that individual elements of the system and their interconnections are known to a sufficient degree of accuracy, and that using certain basic rules of systems theory, a mathematical relationship can be obtained between input and response. This method is particularly useful when the objective is to predict the system's response to some given input or to determine the effect of changing the properties of some element of the system on its overall response. In the case of the disparity vergence system one has to follow an intermediate approach, since the musculature involved in eye movement can be currently modeled at a detailed elemental level, whereas so little is known about the central processor or controller that it has to be treated essentially as a black box.

PLANT MODEL

We start by examining available models for the ocular muscles involved in vergence movements and developing a detailed model of the plant. It is well known that horizontal rotational movement of the eye is carried out by the lateral rectus and the medial rectus, which are reciprocally innervated. It is believed that this reciprocal innervation is also characteristic of the horizontal vergence movements (Alpern, 1969). Although the versional and the vergence systems operate through the same pair of muscles, they have different response characteristics. The versional movements are generally very fast whereas the vergence movements are almost an order of magnitude slower. It has been suggested that there could be two distinct sets of fibers in the rectus muscles that could be respectively responsible for the two types of movements (Alpern and Wolter, 1956; Jampel, 1967). That there exist at least two physiologically classifiable fibers in the extraocular mammalian muscles has been shown by others as well (Bach-y-Rita, 1971; Hess and Pilar, 1963) but it has not been conclusively established that "slow" fibers are exclusively responsible for slow movements and "twitch" fibers for fast movements. Studies of firing patterns of neurons that innervate the lateral and medial rectus do not seem to support the theory that different fiber types serve different movements (Fuchs and Luschei, 1970; Robinson, 1970). In fact, studies suggest that the firing rates of neurons appear to be proportional only to the position and velocity of the movement (Keller and Robinson, 1972). It would seem that the same mathematical model can be used to model the plant for both vergence and versional systems.

There have been two important models to describe the extraocular muscular system associated with horizontal eye movements, although both were developed in connection with versional system. In the simpler, earlier model of Robinson (1964) the active elements of the two rectus muscles are represented by a single force-generator element in parallel with a viscous damping element and in series with an elastic element. A schematic mechanical network representation of this model is shown in Figure 10.3. The passive elements of the two muscles are together

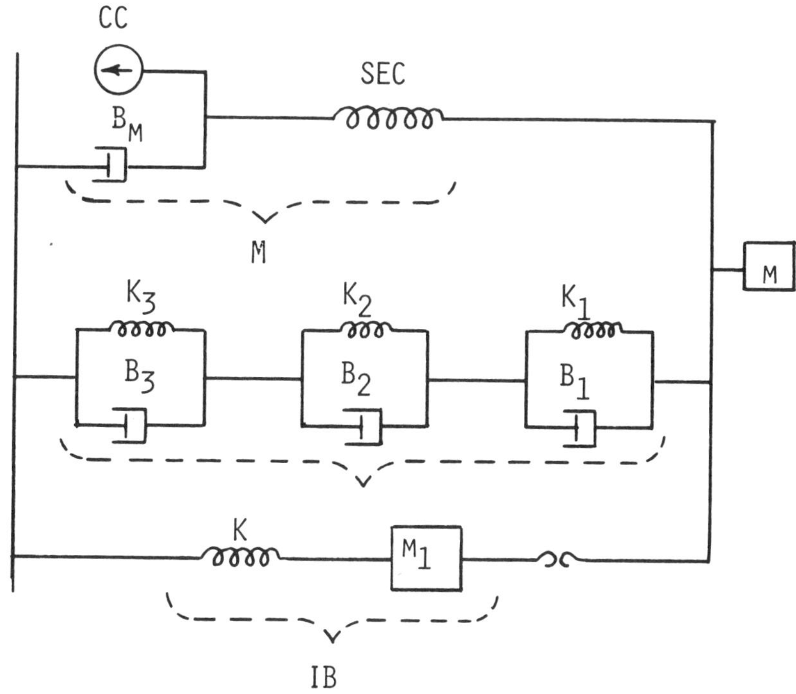

FIGURE 10.3. Robinson's model for the horizontal eye movement plant. The active portion of the muscles (M) is divided into a contractile component (CC) and a series elastic element (SEC). The passive elements of the muscle and the orbit are grouped into three viscoelastic components with short, intermediate, and long time constants. The isometric beam (IB) is included for the simulation of isometric tension experiments performed by Robinson.

represented by a set of three viscoelastic or first-order elements in series. This is essentially a black-box model of the plant since there is no means of distinguishing the action of the lateral rectus from that of the medial rectus; it also does not take into account reciprocal innervation to the muscles. The validity of this model has never been established using vergence data, possibly because of the slow nature of vergence movements (Robinson, 1966).

A later model incorporating the idea of reciprocal innervation and explicitly identifying elements of the muscles and the eyeball was developed by Cook and Stark (1967, 1968). The mechanical network representation of this model is shown in Figure 10.4. Its validity has been established by a number of studies involving the analysis of the versional saccadic and smooth pursuit systems (Clark and Stark, 1974; Bahill et al., 1975). In addition, sensitivity analysis has been carried out on this model to study the effect of its different elements on its overall behavior (Hsu

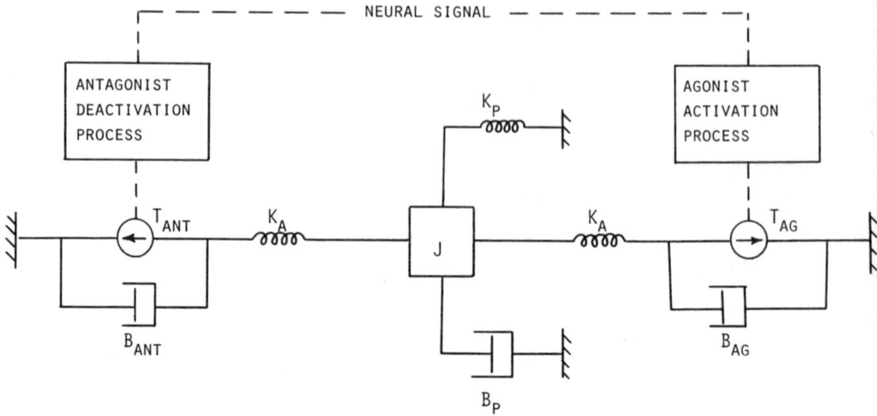

FIGURE 10.4. Cook-Stark model for the horizontal eye-movement plant. J = moment of inertia of the eyeball; the actual value of J is small and has negligible effect on the plant dynamics; K_P = passive elastic elements of the rectus muscles and the orbital tissues; B_P = damping between eyeball and socket; K_A = series elastic element of the rectus muscles; B_{AG} = parallel viscous damping of the agonist muscle; B_{ANT} = parallel viscous damping of the antagonist muscle; T_{AG}, T_{ANT} = forces developed by the agonist and the antagonist muscles respectively.

et al., 1976). These studies show that the effect of the moment of inertia of the eyeball is insignificant and that this parameter may be conveniently ignored. If F_e and F_k are the respective forces produced by the viscous and elastic elements in a direction opposing any change in their position, and x_B and x_k are their respective relative displacements, then their governing mathematical relationships are

$$F_B = B\frac{dx_B}{dt} \tag{a}$$

and

$$F_k = Kx_k \tag{b}$$

where B = damping coefficient of the viscous element;
and K = spring constant of the elastic element.

Combining these relationships with the mechanical equilibrium equations leads to a systems model of the plant as shown in Figure 10.5. There are two inputs to this plant model because of the dual reciprocal innervation to the lateral and the medial rectus. Since they act as an agonist-anatagonist pair, when one of them is activated the other is simultaneously deactivated. The time constants associated with activation and deactivation are different and are respectively indicated by T_a and T_d in Figure 10.5. This difference between them is much too small compared to the overall speed of response of the vergence system so that it can, in general, be ignored while modeling the disparity vergence system; however, this difference is crucial when modeling the very fast saccadic eye movements.

If the forces generated by the contractile elements in the agonist and antagonist muscles are respectively labeled T_{ag} and T_{an}, then elementary rules of block-diagram reduction (Beachley and Harrison, 1978) can be used to obtain the vergence position of the eye, θ, as

$$\theta(s) = \frac{\left(\frac{K_a}{B_{ag}S + K_a}\right) T_{ag}(s) - \left(\frac{K_a}{B_{an}S + K_a}\right) T_{an}(s)}{(B_pS + K_p) + S\left(\frac{B_{ag}K_a}{B_{ag}S + K_a} - \frac{B_{an}K_a}{B_{an}S + K_a}\right)}.$$

The numerical values of the different parameters are indicated in Figure 10.5. To obtain the time course of the vergence eye position, $\theta(t)$, given T_{ag} and T_{an}, one can find the inverse Laplace transform of the above expression. It is much easier, however, to find $\theta(t)$ by numerical com-

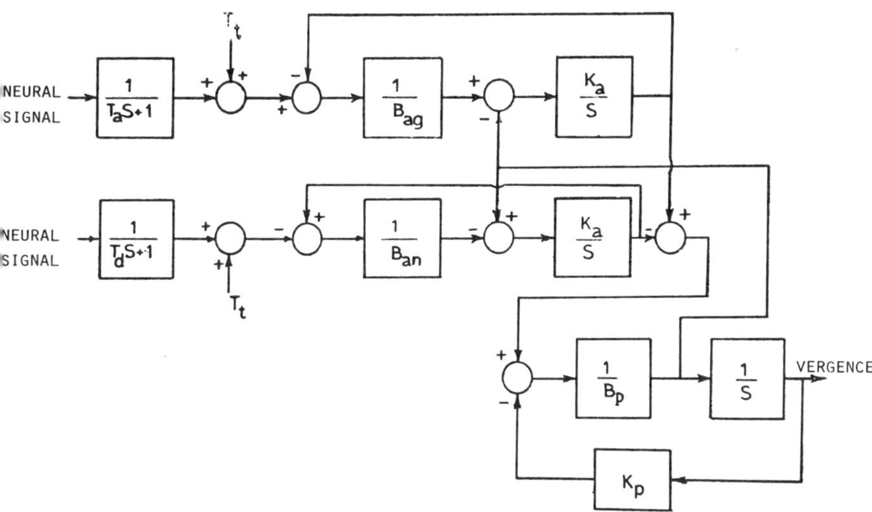

FIGURE 10.5. Systems representation of the modified Cook-Stark plant model used in simulations. K_a = 1.8 g/o; K_p = 1.5 g/o; B_p = 0.018 g = sec/o; T_a = 0.004 sec; T_d = 0.008 sec; $B_{ag} = \frac{1.25T_{ag}}{(900 + \phi)}$ $B_{an} = \frac{3T_{ant}}{900}$; T_t = tonic tension level of 37.5 g; T_{ag} = force generated by the agonist; T_{ant} = force generated by the antagonist; ϕ = vergence movement in degrees. Reprinted by permission of the publisher, from Krishnan VV. A heuristic model for the human vergence eye movement system. Institute of Electrical and Electronics Engineers, Transactions in Biomedical Engineering, © 1977 IEEE.

putation rather than by analytic methods. Numerical simulation of the plant model shows that the vergence plant can be modeled approximately by a single first-order element with a time constant of about 40 to 50 msec. A note of caution should be made here concerning the numerical simulation of the Cook-Stark plant model. Because of the nonlinear viscous damping coefficient of the agonist, B_{ag}, and because of the small time constants involved, the stability of the numerical computation technique is very sensitive to step increments of time, Δt, used in the computation; to ensure stability and avoid erroneous results, it is necessary to maintain Δt less than 0.1 millisecond during simulation. If the central purpose of the modeling process is simply to generate the appropriate vergence response and the appropriate controller output to a given input, without any consideration toward accurately modeling the plant, it is much more efficient computationally to replace the entire plant model by a simple first-order transfer function of the form $\frac{1}{\tau S + 1}$ where τ = 40 to 50 msec.

MODEL OF DISPARITY VERGENCE CONTROLLER

Modeling the controller block of the disparity vergence system has to be approached from a black-box point of view at present since no quantitative data are available on the individual elements that together comprise the controller. In fact, the neuroanatomic pathway of the system is known only in vague descriptive terms; the specific neuronal elements and their relative locations and functions have not yet been identified with certainty. The development of the controller model has therefore to be based on data collected on the input-response characteristics of the whole system. We begin with a simple linear model of the system and gradually refine it by incorporating into it experimentally determined characteristics.

The first modeling decision that needs to be made is whether the controller operates in a continuous mode or in a sampled-data mode. It is well established that the saccadic system, which uses the same plant, operates in a sampled-data mode (Stark et al., 1962; Young and Stark, 1963; Stark, 1968); it is not unreasonable to suspect that vergence eye movement may do so as well. This assumption is tested by observing the response of the disparity vergence system to short pulse inputs to the system. The duration of the input pulses typically ranges from 50 msec to about 500 msec, although experimental results (Zuber and Stark, 1968) show that the system consistently responds to pulses of duration as short as 20 msec. This implies that the system operates in a continuous mode, that is, the controller monitors the sensory input continuously, unlike in the case of the saccadic controller that samples the input approximately at 200-msec intervals. The disparity vergence system may therefore be modeled as a continuous control system.

It has long been known through static clinical studies that the system has a negligible steady-state error, that is, the final vergence position of the eyes is almost equal to that demanded by the target position. The steady-state error is less than a few minutes of arc for both convergence and divergence (Riggs and Niehl, 1960; Ogle, 1964). In linear system theory it is well known that a type 1 system, i.e., a system with a pure integrator element in its forward path, leads to a zero steady-state error for step inputs. On the other hand, type 0 systems that do not have pure integrator elements can also lead to very small steady-state errors if the gain of the controller is very large. Rashbass and Westheimer (1961) postulated the existence of an integrator element in the system based on the open-loop step response of the vergence system, which is obtained by canceling out the effect of the inherent physiological negative feedback by means of parallel, positive electronic feedback; this results in clamping of the disparity input at a fixed value. Experimental results show that the vergence position of the eyes show a ramp-type response to a fixed disparity stimulus. This result has been confirmed by later investigators (Zuber and Stark, 1968). Experimental investigation of the open-loop response to sinusoidal inputs also tends to support this idea (Rashbass and Westheimer, 1961; Zuber and Stark, 1968).

Based on their open-loop investigations, Rashbass and Westheimer (1961) suggested a system model described by the equation

$$\frac{dV_r}{dt} = KV_t \text{ or } V_r(s) = \frac{K}{s} V_t(s) \qquad \text{(d)}$$

where V_r = vergence response;
V_t = vergence stimulus;
and K = controller gain.

The other well-known characteristic of the disparity vergence system is its latency. Studies have shown that this varies from about 130 to 250 msec for different subjects when using unpredictable inputs such as random step stimuli. When simple periodic inputs such as sinusoids are used the latency drops down to very small values, possibly because of some higher-level prediction operator (Krishnan et al., 1973).

The first feedback model for the disparity vergence system was proposed by Toates (1969). It incorporated both the integrator and the latency, but modeled the plant by means of a simple first-order system. Toates did not simulate the model numerically since it was proposed as a part of a more complex model of the near response triad. A slightly modified version is shown in Figure 10.6(A). Figure 10.6(B) shows the closed-loop step

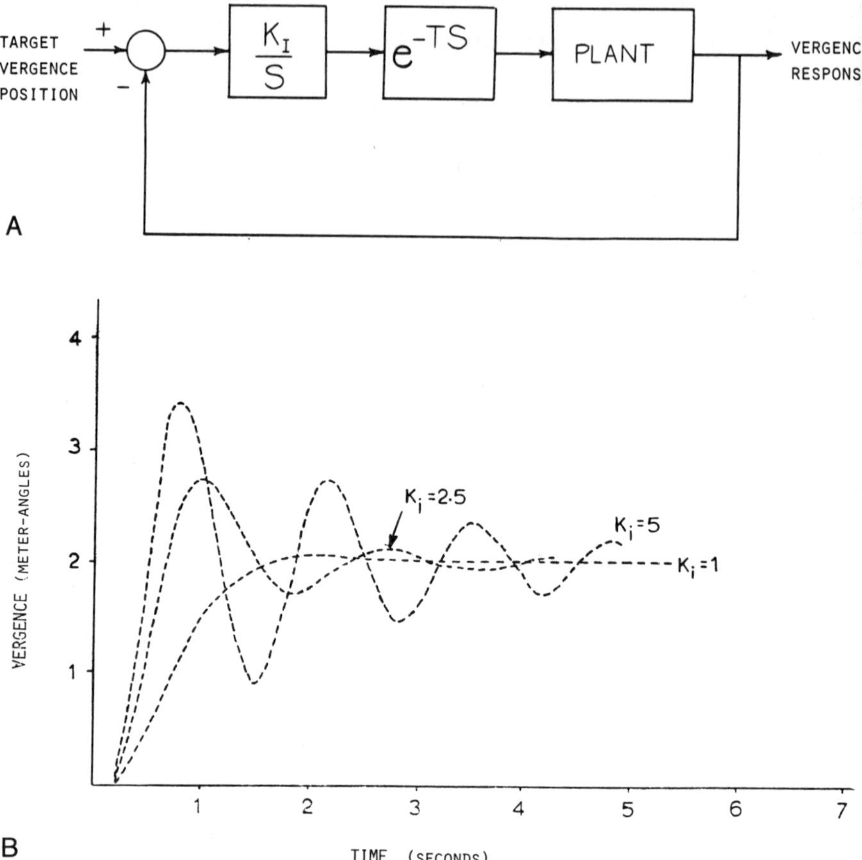

FIGURE 10.6. A Simple integral controller model. The value of time-delay T was 160 msec. B Responses of the integral controller model for different values of integrator gain, K_I. Figure 6B reprinted by permission of the publisher, from Krishnan VV. A heuristic model for the human vergence eye movement system. Institute of Electrical and Electronics Engineers, Transactions in Biomedical Engineering, © 1977 IEEE.

response of this model to a step of two meter-angles for various values of the controller gain, K_i. The value of the latency used is 160 msec for all three simulations.

The step response of the model shows oscillatory behavior for large values of K_i. Experimentally observed step responses of the disparity vergence system do not exhibit any oscillatory behavior, although convergence responses show a small amount of overshoot. When $K_i = 1$ or less the model response is very stable but much slower than experimentally observed step responses. The model response reaches its peak at approximately 1.9 seconds and does not settle down to its final steady-state value until almost 3 seconds. In contrast, the experimental step response to a convergence input of 2 meter angles reaches its peak at about 0.7 seconds and settles down to its steady-state value at about 1.4 seconds.

Comparison between the model response and the step response shows that the output of a simple integral controller is much too slow, but that its steady-state value is appropriate; this suggests the presence of a parallel controller element that would contribute only to the fast initial response but would have no steady-state contribution. A possible controller configuration that satisfies the above requirement is the proportional integral controller (PI control) where the controller output is the sum of the outputs of a proportional and an integral element. Such a controller can be described by the equation

$$m(t) = K_p e(t) + K_i \int_o^t e(t)dt \qquad (e)$$

or

$$m(s) = K_p e(s) + \frac{K_i}{s} e(s) \qquad (f)$$

where $m(t)$ is the output of the controller element and $e(t)$ is the value of the disparity at time t (see Appendix).

Computer simulation of the disparity vergence system model with PI control shows that this model suffers from the same problem as the pure integral controller model. Although the speed of initial response of the system is slightly improved, the oscillatory behavior and the long setting time still persist. It is clear that the parallel control element should not only provide a large initial response to a step change in the disparity level, but that this component of response should decay very rapidly with time.

A derivative element is the obvious choice to fulfill the above requirements. However, since pure differentiation is unlikely to occur in a real physiological system, a pseudoderivative element may be assumed. The new configuration of the controller is called ID control and is described by the relationship

$$m(s) = K_d \cdot \frac{s}{s + a} e(s) + \frac{K_i}{s} \cdot e(s). \qquad (g)$$

The model of the disparity vergence system with this controller is shown in Figure 10.7. It adequately simulates both the step response and the frequency response of the vergence system. Numerical sensitivity analysis shows that the most crucial parameters in the model are the time delay

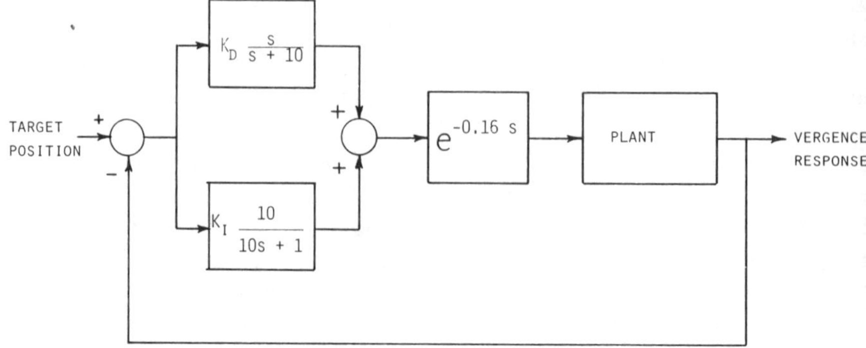

FIGURE 10.7. A parallel integral-derivative controller model for the human disparity vergence system.

or latency, T_d, and the gain of the integrator element K_i (Krishnan, 1972). The response is most sensitive to changes in the value of the latency. Although the model performs adequately in the commonly encountered latency values of 160 to 250 msec, its response becomes oscillatory for larger latencies and is much too slow for latencies under 100 msec. This is a particularly important and thorny problem since latencies as low as 10 msec are frequently observed when the subject is presented with a predictable input such as a pulse train at a frequency of around 1.5 Hz (Krishnan et al., 1973). Simulations have shown that the experimentally observed responses under predictable input conditions can be matched by the model responses, but only if the gains K_i and K_d are altered drastically from their normal values. It is possible that under predictable input conditions some higher-level controller comes into play and alters the value of the parameters in the system but there are no studies available that address this question.

The model's sensitivity to variations in latency remains one of its shortcomings. Very low values of K_i lead to a slow step response while very large values of K_i lead to an oscillatory behavior. Both very low and very high values of the derivative gain, K_d, lead to oscillatory behavior. These results are in keeping with those obtained through control theory analysis.

The integrator element in the controller can be modified further to account for the experimentally observed no-target response, where the target is suddenly switched off after the disparity vergence system has reached a steady-state level. Under this condition the controller does not receive any disparity input; since the target is removed completely, there is no reference level for the sensory processor to compute a disparity signal. The disparity vergence system responds by slowly drifting back to the resting position of the eyes. The dynamics of this no-target response is very much slower than the dynamics of a typical step response (Figure 10.8). If the controller is assumed to be a pure integrator as proposed earlier, one should expect that the eye position would not show any drift. The slow dynamics of the drift indicates that the controller element can be better modeled by a pseudointegrator element of the form $\frac{T}{Ts + 1}$, T being greater than 1. Such an element would also show a dynamic behavior that is very close to the open-loop behavior observed by Rashbass and Westheimer (1961) and Zuber and Stark (1968), in addition to accounting for the no-target response of the system. The value of the parameter T can be estimated from the no-target response of Figure 10.8 and is approximately 10 seconds.

The final model of the vergence system obtained using the above approach is shown in Figure 10.9. The step response of this model is compared with the experimentally observed step responses for convergence and divergence in Figure 10.10. Comparison of the frequency characteristics of the model and experimental responses are shown in Figure 10.11. The fits between the model responses and the experimental responses appear acceptable in both cases.

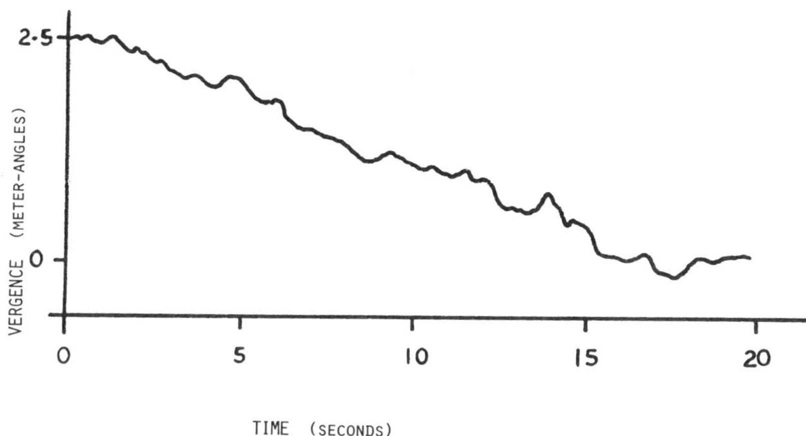

FIGURE 10.8. The no target experimental response of the disparity vergence system. Note that the system takes almost 16 seconds to reach 0 meter angles under no target conditions, compared to the 2 seconds settling time for the normal closed-loop divergence response shown in Figure 9.10. Reprinted by permission of the publisher, from Krishnan VV. A heuristic model for the human vergence eye movement system. Institute of Electrical and Electronics Engineers, Transactions in Biomedical Engineering, © 1977 IEEE.

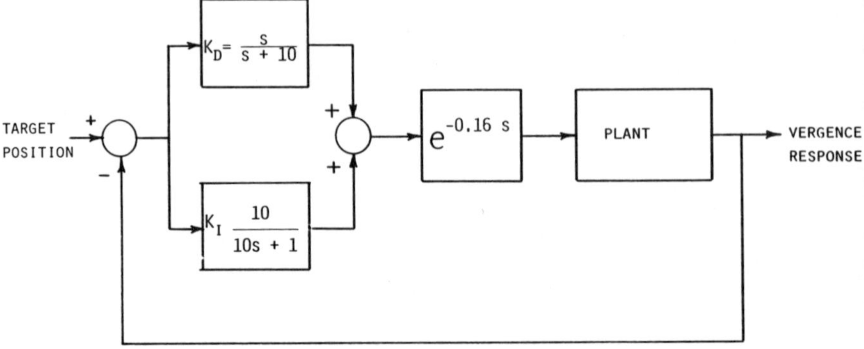

FIGURE 10.9. A pseudointegral-derivative controller model for the disparity vergence system. $K_I = 2.5$, $K_D = 0.4$ for convergence response and $K_I = 1.25$, $K_D = 0.2$ for divergence response. Reprinted by permission of the publisher, from Krishnan VV. A heuristic model for the human vergence eye movement system. Institute of Electrical and Electronics Engineers, Transactions in Biomedical Engineering, © 1977 IEEE.

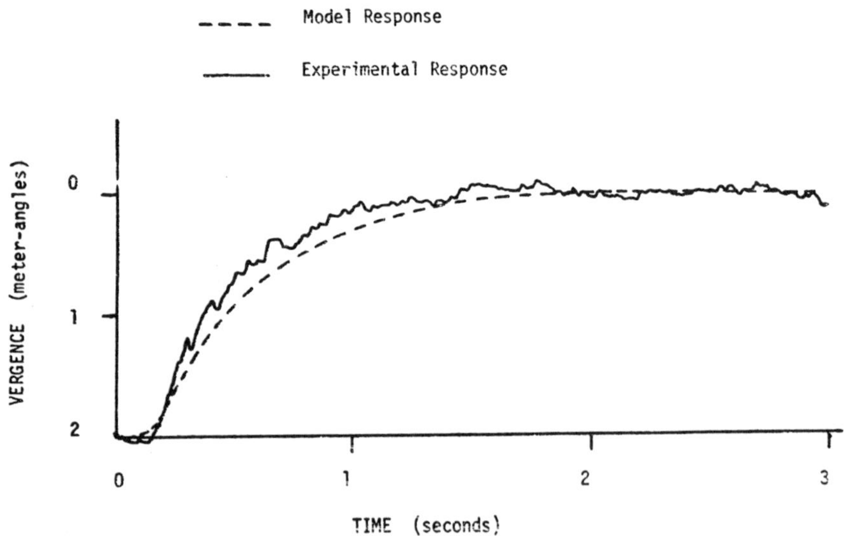

FIGURE 10.10. A Convergence step response. The continuous line indicates the actual convergence response of a 29-year-old subject to a 2-meter-angle step stimulus. The broken line indicates the response of the model shown in Figure 9.9 for a similar stimulus. B Divergence step response. The continuous line indicates the actual response of a subject to a divergence step of 2 meter angles. The broken line shows the response of the model of Figure 9.9 to a similar stimulus. Reprinted by permission of the publisher, from Krishnan VV. A heuristic model for the human vergence eye movement system. Institute of Electrical and Electronics Engineers, Transactions in Biomedical Engineering, © 1977 IEEE.

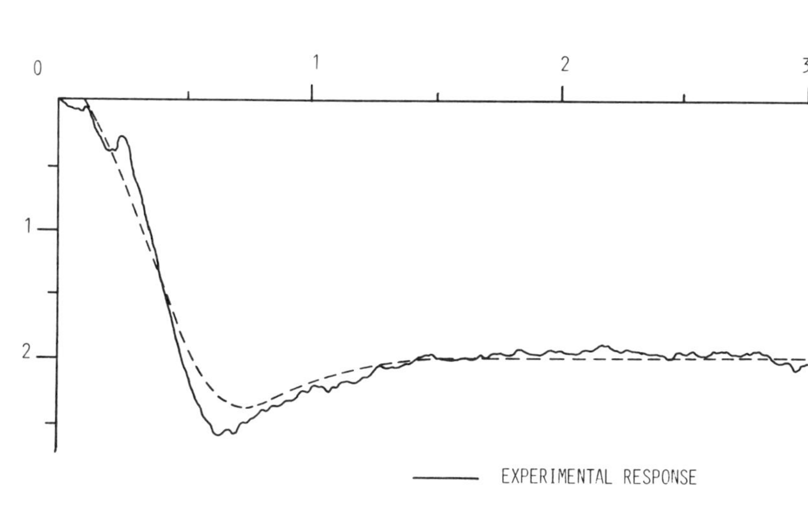

FIGURE 10.10. (*Continued*)

Nonlinearities in Disparity Vergence System

The most important nonlinearity in the disparity vergence system is asymmetry between the convergent and divergent step responses. The former are generally faster than the latter. The model incorporates this feature by altering the controller gains for convergent and divergent disparity inputs; in this sense, this model is nonlinear. There is yet another nonlinearity in the system that has not been incorporated into this model. The maximum velocity attained during disparity vergence movements reaches a saturation level, but since there is no agreement on the value of this maximum velocity it is not possible to include it in the present model.

Directions for Future Modeling

The model developed above adequately represents the system in its response to unpredictable inputs. When the inputs are predictable and periodic, latency drops to very low values and the model dynamics no longer match the actual dynamics of the system. The nature of the higher-level prediction operator involved in the control of the system under predictable input conditions is at present not clearly understood. One possible future direction in disparity vergence modeling is to incorporate

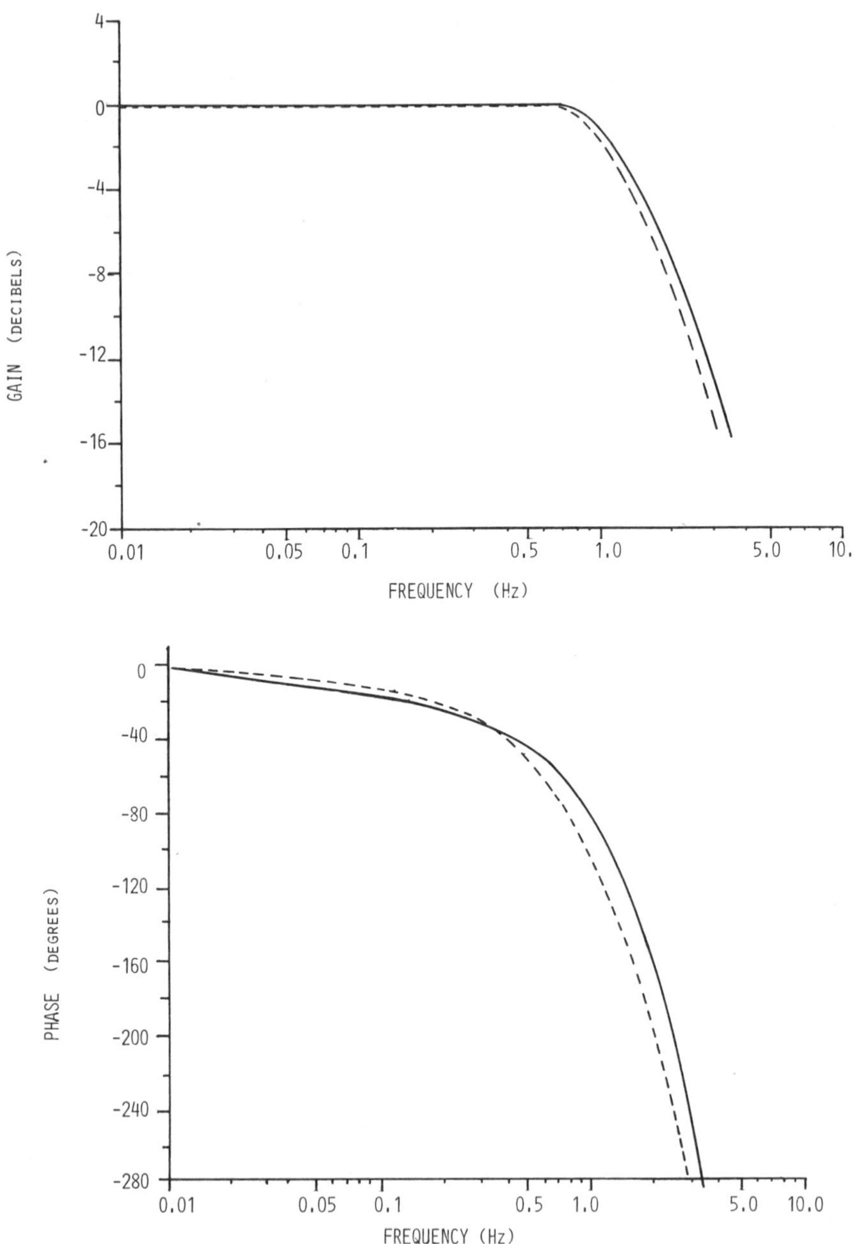

FIGURE 10.11. Comparison of the closed-loop frequency characteristics of the actual disparity vergence system and the model of Figure 9.10. The continuous lines indicate the closed-loop frequency response to the actual system and the broken lines show the model closed-loop frequency plots. Reprinted by permission of the publisher, from Krishnan VV. A heuristic model for the human vergence eye movement system. Institute of Electrical and Electronics Engineers, Transactions in Biomedical Engineering, © 1977 IEEE.

the prediction operator into the model. Since the prediction operator appears to be stochastic, incorporating it would alter our model from a deterministic to a stochastic model.

Another possible direction for future modeling is to consider alternate controller structures. The derivative controller used in the present model assumes that there is a neural network that is sensitive to the rate of change of disparity rather than to the actual magnitude of the disparity. While it is possible to construct simple neural models that can accomplish this, there is no direct physiological evidence yet to indicate that such a network actually exists. The closest physiological evidence points to a neuron that is sensitive simply to directional changes in disparity (Pettigrew, 1973) rather than to the actual rate of change. An alternate model structure can be developed that does not use the pseudoderivative controller element; it would use the output of the direction-sensitive element to reset the integral controller gain, K_i. Initial simulations have shown promising transient response results, but the model response appears to be overly sensitive to the value of K_i.

A third, far more interesting direction for future modeling is to study triadic interactions. The disparity vergence system is an important component of the near-response triad; in fact, Fincham (1951) believed that vergence stimulus is actually the primary stimulus to accommodation under binocular viewing conditions. Since the disparity vergence system has a latency of only 130 to 250 msec compared to the accommodation latency of 300 to 400 msec, this theory seems quite plausible. Coupling the models of these two systems through accommodative vergence and vergence accommodation raises several interesting questions and may lead to a better understanding of the triadic near response. Semmlow and Hung report some new developments in triadic modeling in Chapter 6.

REFERENCES

Alpern M, Wolter JR. The relation of horizontal saccadic and vergence movements. Arch Ophthalmol 1956;56:685–90.

Alpern M. The anatomy of eye movements. in: Dawson, H, ed. The eye. Vol. 3. New York: Academic Press, 1969.

Bach-y-Rita P. Neurophysiology of eye movements. In: Bach-y-Rita P, Collins CC, Hyde JC, eds. The control of eye movements. New York: Academic Press, 1971.

Bahill AT, Clark MR, Stark L. Glissades—eye movements generated by mismatched components of the saccadic motoneural control signal. Math Biosci 1975;26:303–18.

Beachley NH, Harrison HL. Introduction to dynamic system analysis. New York: Harper & Row, 1978.

Clark, MR, and Stark L. Control of human eye movements. Math Biosci 1974;20:191–265.

Cook G, Stark L. Derivation of a model for the human eye-positioning mechanism. Bull Math Biophys 1967;29:153–75.

Cook G, Stark L. Dynamic behavior of human eye-positioning mechanism. Comm Behav Biol 1968;1:197–204.

Fincham EF. Accommodation reflex and its stimulus. Br J Ophthalmol 1951;35:381–93.

Fuchs AF, Luschei ES. Firing patterns of abducens neurons of alert monkeys in relationship to horizontal eye movements. J Neurophysiol 1970;33:383–92.

Hess A, Pilar G. Slow fibers in the extraocular muscles of the cat. J Physiol 1963;169:780–98.

Hsu FK, Bahill AT, Stark L. Parametric sensitivity of a homeomorphic model for saccadic and vergence eye movements. Comp Prog Biomed 1976;6:108–16.

Jampel R. Multiple motor systems in the extraocular muscles of man. Invest Ophthalmol 1967;6:288–93.

Keller EL, Robinson DA. Abducens unit behavior in the monkey during vergence movements. Vision Res 1972;12(3):369–82.

Krishnan VV. Control mechanisms for distance vision in man. Ph.D thesis, University of California, Berkeley, 1972.

Krishnan VV, Farazian F, Stark L. An analysis of latencies and prediction in the fusional vergence system. Am J Optom Arch Am Acad Optom 1973;12:933–39.

Krishnan VV, Stark L. A heuristic model for human vergence eye movement system. IEEE Trans Biomed Eng 1977;BME-24,1:44–49.

Mitchell DE. Properties of stimuli eliciting vergence eye movements and steriopsis. Vision Res 1970;10:145–62.

Ogle KN. Researches in binocular vision. New York: Hafner, 1964.

Pettigrew JD. Binocular neurons which signal change of disparity in area 18 of cat visual cortex. Nature New Biol 1973;241:123–24.

Rashbass C, Westheimer G. Disjunctive eye movements. J Physiol 1961;159:339–60.

Riggs L, Niehl EW. Eye movements recorded during convergence and divergence. J Opt Soc Am 1960;50:913–20.

Robinson DA. The mechanics of saccadic eye movements. J Physiol 1964;174:245–64.

Robinson DA. The mechanics of human vergence movement. J Pediatr Ophthalmol 1966;34:31–37.

Robinson DA. Oculomotor unit behavior in the monkey. J Neurophysiol 1970;393–404.

Stark L. Neurological control systems. New York: Plenum Press, 1968.

Stark L. The control system for versional eye movements. In: Bach-y-Rita P, Collins CC, Hyde JC, eds. The control of eye movements. New York: Academic Press, 1971.

Stark L, Voissius G, Young LR. Predictive control of eye tracking movements. IRE Trans 1962;HFE-3:52–57.

Stark L, Kenyon RV, Krishnan VV, Ciuffreda K. Disparity vergence: a proposed name for a dominant component of binocular vergence eye movements. Am J Optom Phys Optom 1980;57:606–9.

Stewart CR. Jump vergence response. Am J Optom 1961;38:57–86.

Toates FM. Accommodation and convergence in the human eye. Measurement & control 1969; 3:29–33.

Torok N, Guillemin V, Barnothy JM. Photoelectric nystagmography. Ann Otol Rhinol Laryngol 1951;60:917–27.

Westheimer G, Mitchell AM. Eye movement responses to convergence stimuli. Arch Ophthalmol 1956; 55:848–56.

Westheimer G, Mitchell DE. The sensory stimulus for disjunctive eye movements. Vision Res 1969; 9:749–55.

Young LR, Stark L. Variable feedback experiments testing a sampled-data model for eye tracking movements. IEEE Trans Hum Factors Electron 1963;HFE-4:38–51.

Zuber BL, Stark L. Dynamical characteristics of the fusional vergence system. IEEE Trans Systems Sci Cybernet 1968;SSC-4:72–79.

APPENDIX

An automatic control system may be thought of as a feedback control system that is driven by the error between the desired response and the actual response of the system. As we have seen, the disparity vergence system fits this definition, with the binocular disparity being the error between the "desired" vergence as required by the target position and the actual vergence position of the eyes at any given instant. A crucial element of the automatic control system is the controller, which uses the error signal as its input and generates the actuating signal, which in turn becomes the input to the plant or the process. For the horizontal fusional vergence system, the error signal is the retinal disparity, the central processor (Figure 10.1) is the controller, and the eyeball and the lateral and medial recti form the plant. The actuating signal would then be the neural input to the agonist-antagonist action of the lateral and medial rectus muscles.

The complete control action of the central processor is quite complex and is probably arranged as a hierarchical sequence of control actions. At the lowest level of this hierarchy, one expects that the controller performs relatively simple processing of the disparity signal. At this level, the control action can be described as proportional, integral, derivative, proportional-integral, proportional-derivative, or integral-derivative, depending on the control action postulated in the model.

If $e(t)$ and $m(t)$ are the instantaneous values of the disparity signal and the neural signal to the rectus muscles respectively at time t, then we have:

a proportional controller (P-control) if

$$m(t) = K_p e(t) \qquad (a)$$

where K_p = constant; an integral controller (I-control) if

$$m(t) = K_i \int_o^t e(t)dt + m(o) \tag{b}$$

where K_i is a constant and $m(o)$ is the actuating signal at time $t = 0$; a derivative controller (D-control) if

$$m(t) = K_d \frac{d}{dt} e(t) \tag{c}$$

where K_d is a constant; a proportional-integral controller (PI-control) if

$$m(t) = K_p e(t) + K_i \int_o^t e(t)dt + m(o); \tag{d}$$

a proportional-derivative controller (PD-control) if

$$m(t) = K_p e(t) + K_d \frac{d}{dt} e(t); \tag{e}$$

and an integral-derivative controller (ID-control) if

$$m(t) = K_d \frac{d}{dt} e(t) + K_i \int_o^t e(t)dt + m(o). \tag{f}$$

In nonmathematical terms, the output of a P-controller at any instant of time depends solely on the value of the error signal at that instant, that is, the neural signal to the musculature at any given instant is dependent only on the disparity at that instant, and not on previous disparities. This type of controller is unlikely to exist in the binocular vergence system for two reasons: (1) given the model of the musculature and eyeball, this type of controller will lead to a significant steady-state error in the vergence position of the eyes and we know from experimental observations that the steady-state error in the fusional vergence position is negligible. Also, (2) because of the delay associated with the system, a proportional controller with a value K_p greater than 1 will lead to a sustained oscillatory vergence response, which again, is not substantiated by experimental observations.

The output of the I-controller depends not only on the current value of the disparity but on its past values as well. In other words, the current instantaneous output of the I-controller depends on the sum (integral) of the disparity up to the present, rather than on the current disparity alone. An I-controller will yield a zero steady-state error for the fusional vergence system and is therefore feasible. Its major drawback is that it leads to a slower and more oscillatory response than is observed experimentally.

The output of a D-controller is not related to the value of the disparity signal itself but is dependent solely on the rate of change of the disparity signal at the particular instant. Because of the rules of causality, it is unlikely that such a controller exists in this exact form in neural systems. It is possible, however, to envision neural circuits that could provide an approximate version of such a controller. A D-controller by itself will not provide the zero steady-state error, but can speed up the response and reduce the oscillatory behavior when used in parallel with a proportional or integral controller.

The PI, PD, ID controllers provide outputs that are equal to the sum of the outputs of the component controllers. For instance, the output of an ID-controller in our system would depend both on the integral of the disparity signal up to the current time and on the rate of change of the disparity signal at the current time. Such a controller can provide both the zero steady-state error and the nonoscillatory behavior of the fusional vergence response that is observed experimentally.

A pseudointegral controller behaves very much like an I-controller, but unlike an I-controller, its output gradually decays to zero when the error signal is maintained at a zero value over a long period of time. A pure I-controller will indefinitely maintain the same output level as existed when the error signal was set to zero. In theory, the pseudointegrator will always have a non-zero steady-state error, but this error would be exceedingly small. Similarly, a pseudoderivative controller behaves almost like a D-controller, except that its output changes more gradually with time as compared to a pure D-controller. Both the pseudointegrator and pseudoderivative controllers also have the added advantage that they are physically feasible control elements in neural control systems.

11
The Combination of Version and Vergence

Hiroshi Ono

It is said that Hering's many insights are neither appreciated nor recognized, but his contributions to the theory of eye movement are exceptions (Hurvich, 1969). His theory of binocular eye movement deals with the combination of version and vergence, and is well known as the law of equal innervation. A perusal of the literature, however, indicates that his theory is often misunderstood even by some of the most respected investigators of eye movements. Thus, the first part of this chapter is devoted to a restatement of Hering's theory. What follows is a discussion of its testability, and a comparison of some experimental results with predictions from the theory.

HERING'S THEORY OF BINOCULAR EYE MOVEMENT

A Restatement of Hering's Hypothesis

Hering's general idea was that the two eyes see and move together as if they were one; his theory of binocular vision postulates that although we have two eyes, we see as though we have one cyclopean eye. Similarly, his theory of binocular eye movement, often called the law of equal innervation, postulates that the two eyes move as though there was only one. Hering's hypothesis of equal innervation describes the processes causing these movements. The two quotations that follow give the flavor of Hering's writings. They also show how he emphasized the unity of the two eyes and how he related the concept of the cyclopean eye to binocular eye movements.

> By this theory therefore, the eyes are treated . . . as a single organ. To the motivating will however, it is a matter of indifference, that this organ in reality consists of two separate members, since it is not necessary to guide and move each of these parts by itself. Rather does one and the same impulse of the will control both eyes, as a team of horses is guided by a single pair of reins. (1879, p. 153)

> . . . we can think of both eyes as a single imaginary eye which lies midway between the two real eyes. If such an eye had to be innervated to turn to the left, right, above or below, the two real eyes would always be equally innervated, and if such an eye had to be innervated to accommodate for greater nearness or distance, both eyes would be innervated not only for an internal accommodation but also for an external bifixation of both lines of sight for nearness or distance. (1868, p. 19)

Notice that two kinds of innervation are postulated: one for conjunctive movement and another for disjunctive movement and accommodation. The first causes eye muscles to pull the two eyes equally to the right, to the left, upward, or downward. The second causes eye muscles to pull the two eyes equally inward or outward. For either type of movement, the amount of innervation to the two eyes is equal; thus the term equal innervation. A change in the point of fixation can be the outcome of either type of innervation or it can be the outcome of both. When the fixation point is changed to a target in a different direction but at the same distance, version innervation is involved and the two eyes will move through equal angular extents and with equal velocities in the same direction. When fixation is changed to a target at a different distance but in the same direction, vergence innervation is involved and the two eyes move through equal extents in opposite directions. When fixation is changed to a target in a different direction and at a different distance, both types of innervation are involved, and the two eyes will move through unequal extents and with unequal velocities.

(Throughout this chapter, version and vergence refer to the hypothesized underlying process, and conjunctive and disjunctive movements refer to actual eye movements.)

Hering thought that the combination of version and vergence innervation was additive and he used this idea to explain unequal lateral movements of the two eyes. For example, consider a version innervation to the eyes to move rightward and an equal amount of vergence innervation to move inward. If both innervations occur simultaneously, the left eye will move rightward because the innervation to move inward and the innervation to move rightward are congruous. The extent of the movement should be twice that from the innervation for version alone or for vergence alone. The right eye should remain fixed because the innervation to move rightward and the innervation to move inward cancel each other. Hering sometimes observed a "quiver" of the right eye in this situation but he explained it by the competing innervations "which do not necessarily desist at the same time" (1879).

To support his hypothesis, Hering cited cases that were best explained by the presence of two kinds of innervation equal for the two eyes. For instance, version innervation was illustrated in the case of monocular blindness or when one eye was closed, because the eyes continued to move together despite the lack of vision in one. Hering argued that if the eyes were independently innervated, one would not expect coordinated movement in the unseeing eye. He also demonstrated that the distant field of vision was wider than the near field, and he argued that this phenomenon was due to the two kinds of innervation. His method was this: he established a strong, centered afterimage of a vertical line. Holding his head in a fixed position, he looked through a clear window to the distance and as far to the left as he could. He noted the distant object to which he could align the afterimage and marked on the glass the line of sight to that object. He then focused on the window glass and again looked as far to the left as he could. He was unable to move the afterimage as far to the left as the mark on the glass. Hering argued that for the near fixation distance, vergence innervation to move the eyes inward should be greater. Therefore the left eye should be receiving greater vergence innervation competing against its version innervation to move leftward, and so it should not be able to rotate as far to the left.

Misinterpretations of Hering's Hypothesis

Hering's hypothesis as stated here is simple, and one may wonder why it has been misinterpreted. One reason may be Hering's writing style, which in contrast to Helmholtz's, was neither clear nor direct. (See Bridgeman's Translator's Note in Hering, 1868).

It is claimed and often implied that Hering's hypothesis was meant to be invoked for version but not for vergence. Westheimer (1976; 1981) made this interpretation because Hering's statement that "a team of horses being guided by a single pair of reins" makes it "difficult to visualize a pair of horses in a convergence situation" (Westheimer, personal communication). Another factor contributing to this misinterpretation may be that most of the evidence cited by Hering to support the idea that the two eyes work together is related to version. Perhaps because of this interpretation it has also been written that when one eye remains fixed while the other eye moves, or when the two eyes move by different amounts, Hering's hypothesis is "violated." Alpern and Ellen (1956) implied that accommodative vergence movement violates Hering's hypothesis. In their experimental situation, measurements showed that one eye remained fixed during such movements. Howard and Templeton (1966) stated that the hypothesis does not apply to slow pursuit eye movements because the two eyes moved different amounts when the target movement required it. Clark and Crane (1978) and Steinman and Collewijn (1980) said that it does not apply to saccades when the two eyes move different amounts. It has been suggested (Howard, 1982) that these misinterpretations probably stem from Hering's statement that "the two eyes are so related to one another that one cannot be moved independently of the other; rather, the musculature of both eyes reacts simultaneously to one and the same impulse of will" (1868).

The point emphasized here is that Hering did not consider unequal movement of the two eyes to be inconsistent with his hypothesis; observations of unequal movements are not sufficient to refute it. Movements such as accommodative vergence or unequal abrupt movements can be considered violations only if one makes some additional assumptions. To discuss what constitutes a violation we need to examine the formal structure of the hypothesis.

Analysis of Hering's Hypothesis

Despite its usual label as a law, Hering's hypothesis is not a law in the sense that there is ample evidence supporting it. In fact, what does constitute support or falsification is not entirely clear. Thus we examine the formal aspects of his hypothesis to make explicit its testable deductions. The concepts of version and vergence are defined, and then the hypothesis that specifies how the two combine are stated. This discussion is restricted to lateral eye movements because the combination of version and vergence applies only to such movements.

Formal Statement of the Hypothesis

Let Θ represent the angular magnitude of the conjunctive movement "intended" by a given version innervation. Positive version by itself would move the eyes clockwise as viewed from above, and negative version would move them counterclockwise. When only version is involved in an eye movement, the value of Θ corresponds to the extent of the angular rotation of each eye. Let μ represent the angular magnitude of the disjunctive movement "intended" by a given vergence innervation. Positive vergence is convergence and negative vergence is divergence. The extent of a disjunctive movement produced by a given μ is equal to the change in the angle subtended by the two visual axes. When only vergence is involved in an eye movement, the value $\mu/2$ corresponds to the extent of rotation of each eye.

According to Hering, binocular eye movement consists of these two components and they are hypothesized to be additive. Thus the relationship between them and the actual movement of each eye can be expressed by equations (*a*) and (*b*):

$$\Theta + \mu/2 = M_L \quad (a)$$

$$\Theta - \mu/2 = M_R \quad (b)$$

where M_R represents the angular rotation of the right eye, and M_L the rotation of the left eye. Hering himself used equations very similar to these to explain unequal eye movements (see Hering, 1868, pp. 17 and 21; 1879, pp. 153 and 155). Since equations (*a*) and (*b*) are linear and contain both variables, *any* binocular eye movement (or any stimulus movement) can be described in terms of Θ and μ. Thus instead of describing the magnitude and direction of each eye separately, one can always use Θ and μ to describe a binocular eye movement whether Hering's hypothesis is valid or not.[1] This point is important for examining the testability of the hypothesis, and will be elaborated shortly.

Regardless of the validity of Hering's hypothesis, Θ and μ can describe any eye movement and any stimulus movement. Thus the formal structure of the hypothesis can be used to check agreement between stimulus movement and binocular eye movement or simply to describe either movement. That is, if a target moves from one point to another point, this movement and the corresponding eye movement can be described in terms of Θ and μ. For an example of such use, see Rashbass and Westheimer (1961).

Geometric Correlates of Θ *and* μ

Specification of the points in space using this formal structure has been called the "oculomotor map" of visual space by Carpenter (1977), and it

[1] Rashbass and Westheimer (1961) used another description of binocular eye movement, which appears different from equations (*a*) and (*b*) but is, in fact, similar (Ono, 1980; Nakamizo and Ono, 1978). They defined the conjunctive eye position, ϕ, as $\frac{1}{2}(\alpha_R + \alpha_L)$, and the disjunctive eye position, γ, as $\alpha_L - \alpha_R$, where α_R and α_L represent the right and left eye positions, respectively. Any eye movement can be described as changes in ϕ and γ. Because the two descriptions are equivalent, obviously Rashbass and Westheimer have defined the two types of eye movement in the same way as did Hering, and their idea is a restatement of Hering's hypothesis. Furthermore, although Hering is not mentioned in their article, their conclusion that the two types of eye movements are independent is in agreement with Hering's hypothesis.

is the same geometry of binocular vision used to discuss the loci in space that stimulate corresponding points on the two retinas. The same geometry also applies to the description of a binocular eye movement and its stimulus. For any purely conjunctive movement all the points of intersection of the two visual axes will fall on a circle called the Vieth-Müller circle. The circle passes through the centers of rotation of the two eyes and the points of intersection. In other words, when the point of intersection of the two visual axes remains on a given Vieth-Müller circle, a change from one point on the circle to another corresponds to angular rotations of the eyes that are equal in direction and magnitude. For any purely disjunctive movement, however, the points of intersection form one hyperbola from the family of Hillebrand hyperbolas. In this case, when the intersection of the visual axes remains on a given hyperbola, a change from one point on the hyperbola to another corresponds to angular rotations of the two eyes that are equal in magnitude but opposite in direction. Both types of loci appear in Figure 11.1. A movement of the intersection of the two visual axes from the top left corner of any enclosed region to the bottom right corner corresponds to an eye movement in which $\Theta = 10°$ and $\mu = 10°$.

It might be helpful here to give concrete examples of the linear shifts in the point of fixation that would result from these angular values of Θ

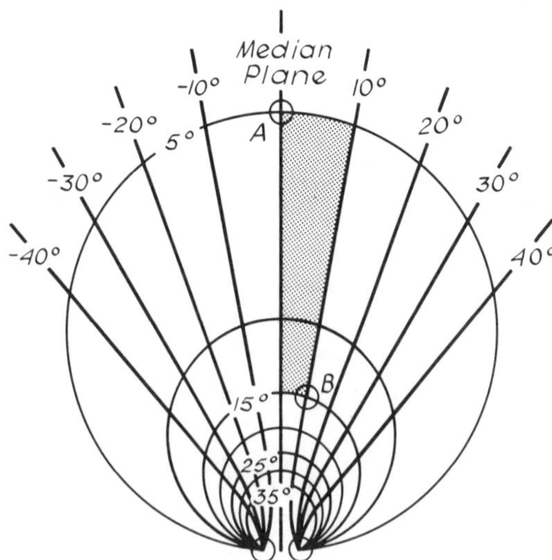

FIGURE 11.1. Geometric representation of the two components of eye movements by locations of the intersections of the two visual axes. The value in degrees marked on each circle denotes the convergence angle and the value in degrees marked on the hyperbola denotes the visual direction when a line is not very close to the eyes.

and μ. Conjunctive movement of 10° corresponds to a 10-cm change in the direction of gaze at a viewing distance of 57 cm, and to a 20-cm change in the direction of gaze of 114 cm. The extent of a disjunctive movement is measured by the change in the angle subtended by the two visual axes. For a subject with an interocular distance of 6 cm, 10° of disjunctive movement corresponds to a change in fixation distance from 11 cm to 17 cm, from 17 cm to 34 cm, or from 34 cm to optical infinity.

Figure 11.2 represents the positions of the two eyes in a Cartesian coordinate system. Because binocular eye movements will be mapped onto such coordinates in the next section, the relationships between the points of fixation shown in Figure 11.1 and the positions of the eyes shown in Figure 11.2 are discussed briefly here. In Figure 11.2, the angular position of the right eye is represented on the abscissa and the angular position of the left eye is represented on the ordinate. In this figure, straight lines with a slope of +1 indicate conjunctive movement without vergence and correspond to the Vieth-Müller circles in Figure 11.1. Straight lines with a slope of −1 indicate disjunctive movement without version and correspond to the Hillebrand hyperbolas in Figure 11.1. Thus an eye movement in which $\Theta = 10°$ and $\mu = 10°$ could be the movement from A to B in Figure 11.2. This eye position shift compares with the fixation shift from A to B in Figure 11.1. The different shaded areas in

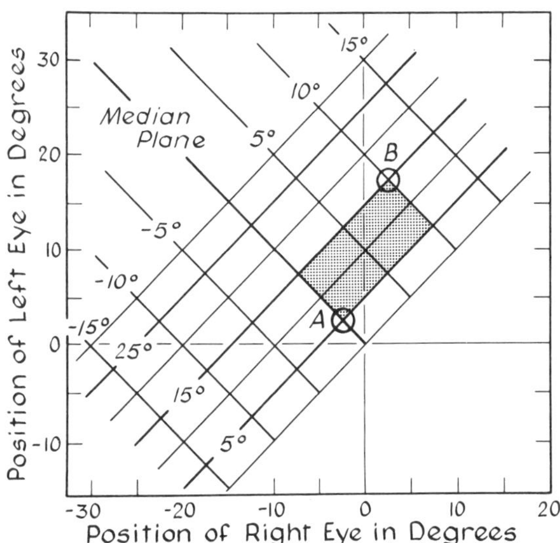

FIGURE 11.2. Representation on Cartesian coordinates of the two components of eye movement. (There is an error on the version scale of the similar figure presented in Ono, 1980, which was brought to my attention by E. Peli.)

each figure indicate corresponding regions in the two figures. Note that all the curved lines in Figure 11.1 correspond to straight lines in Figure 11.2. Mapping of a binocular eye movement on Cartesian coordinates (also called a Lissajous figure) can be useful in separating or identifying the two mathematical components. For an example, see Rogers, Steinbach, and Ono (1974) and Ono and Steinbach (1982).

Testability of the Hypothesis

As mentioned before, any binocular eye movement can be described in terms of Θ and μ. This mathematical description of Hering's hypothesis cannot be falsified, and in fact, Θ and μ may not correspond to any underlying processes. That an eye movement may be described as the sum of two mathematical components does not necessarily mean that there are two actual additive components that control eye movements. By analogy, one can separate mathematically the northern and eastern components of a northeast wind, but from the results of such an analysis one does not conclude that there are two origins for the wind.

It is not clear whether or not Hering was aware of the non-falsifiability of his mathematical equation, but obviously he wanted to say more than simply that all binocular eye movements can be described as the sum of two additive components. The word innervation in the hypothesis suggests that he was concerned with the underlying physiological processes, even though he was unable to observe them directly. To repeat what has been mentioned previously, his hypothesis states that the innervation to move both eyes together to the right or left is equal for each eye and that the innervation to rotate the eyes inward or outward is also equal for each eye. Furthermore, it states that the two kinds of innervation are additive.

As the foregoing discussion implies, the validity of this hypothesis may depend ultimately on neurophysiological data. (For a discussion of the relationship between neurophysiology and Hering's hypothesis, see Howard, 1982). An argument can be made that Hering himself used a "systems approach," and that direct observation of eye movements can provide greater insight than neurophysiological data (see Stark's commentary on Part 1 in Hering, 1868). Regardless of whether the neurophysiological or the systems approach is more appropriate, only behavioral studies of eye movements are considered in the next section, because most of the studies that address Hering's hypothesis are not neurophysiological but behavioral. While examining the results of these studies, we will treat the hypothesis as dealing with constructs or intervening variables, namely Θ and μ of equations (*a*) and (*b*), and not with actual physiological innervation.

When we deal with behavioral data, another issue must be considered. There can be other processes between the level of the hypothesized process and actual eye movement. Consequently, even if the hypothesis is correct at one level, the prediction may fail at the behavioral level. For example, Kenyon, Ciuffreda, and Stark (1980) and Ono and Saida (1981) obtained results apparently incompatible with Hering's hypothesis, but noted that the incompatibility might be due to an additional process at the biomechanical level rather than at the innervation level. No doubt the future theory that explains the combination of version and vergence will detail the different levels. Speculations on this matter will not be made in this chapter because they do not serve to summarize existing data. It is hoped, however, that the data summarized will aid in such speculation and lead to further experimental work.

Hering's hypothesis, considered at only one level, may be separated into three propositions (Ono, 1980): (1) there are two actual (rather than mathematical) innervation components which produce eye movements—version and vergence; (2) the magnitude of the version component is equal for each eye and the magnitude of the vergence component is equal for each eye; and (3) the signed components of version and vergence are additive for each eye. In the rest of this chapter (1) will be referred to as the two-components proposition, (2) as the equal-components proposition, and (3) as the additivity proposition.

EXPERIMENTAL RESULTS

Two points will be noted before dealing with the experimental data. The first concerns the kind of stimulus used to study eye movements and the second concerns a problem associated with their measurement.

In many of the studies reported here, stimulus movement is simulated with a stereoscope. Figure 11.3 illustrates a typical stereoscope setup. Stereoscopic stimuli can be arranged so that they are equivalent to real stimuli with regard to retinal disparity, but when a distance shift is simulated, there is not the accompanying required change in accommodation or in retinal image size that would occur with a real stimulus. Since accommodation and image size are known to affect eye movements (for a summary, see Toates, 1974), there must be some difference between the movements to real and stereoscopic stimulus presentations. These differences are not the main focus of the following discussion, but the reader should be aware that there may be limitations on the extent to which we can generalize from one presentation method to the other.

In the measurement of eye movements one must assume that a subject correctly fixates on a calibration stimulus. In binocular studies the experimenter usually asks a subject to fixate on each of several points in a frontoparallel plane and adjusts the readings of an eye movement mon-

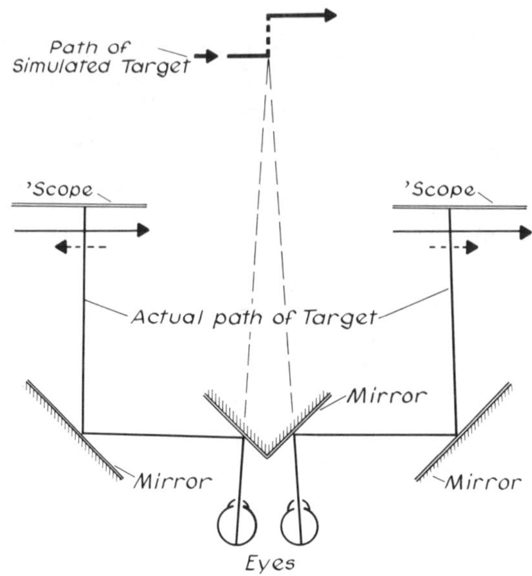

FIGURE 11.3. Mirror stereoscope through which stimuli are viewed. Stimuli moving at the same velocity but in different directions on the scopes (*dotted arrows*) appear as a single stimulus moving toward or away from the viewer. Stimuli moving at the same velocity in the same direction (*solid arrows*) appear as a single stimulus moving to the left or right in front of the viewer.

itor so that the outputs from the two eyes for each fixation point are equal. In using this procedure, the experimenter implicitly assumes that Hering's hypothesis about equal innervation for version is valid. Strictly speaking, when a statement concerning equality or inequality is made, what is referred to is the difference between the eye movements to a stimulus shift in a different direction and the eye movements to a shift to a different distance and/or a different direction.

Results Related to the Two-Components Proposition

It is generally accepted that the distinction between version and vergence is viable when there are changes in fixation among discrete stimuli. A clear distinction can be based on the differences in the time courses of the two kinds of movement. For example, when a subject changes fixation from one stationary target to another that is 3° away, or changes fixation to a target that steps (jumps) 3° to the left or to the right, each eye moves with a latency of about 200 milliseconds, a peak velocity of about 150° per second, and a duration of about 30 milliseconds (Fuchs, 1971). Saccades of the two eyes are closely synchronized (for a recent study see Williams and Fender, 1977), and profiles are similar (for the slight difference see Bahill et al., 1976). In contrast, if a stimulus is stepped in the median plane toward or away from the subject so that the movement required of each eye is also 3°, the eyes move with a latency of about 175 milliseconds, a peak velocity of only 10° per second, and a duration of about 2 seconds (Robinson, 1966). Under these two conditions, the profiles of the two movements are obviously different. Furthermore, if a subject changes fixation to a target that is in a different direction and also at a different distance, the two movements can still be identified (Alpern and Ellen, 1956; Riggs and Niehl, 1960; Westheimer and Mitchell, 1956; Yarbus, 1965–67). A sample eye movement record for this latter stimulus situation is shown in Figure 11.4. On the left, time is represented on the abscissa and eye position on the ordinate. A conjunctive movement appears as the abrupt saccade and a disjunctive movement appears as the gradual change. On the right, right eye position is represented on the abscissa and left eye position is represented on the ordinate. Eye movement begins at the right and moves to the left of the graph. If we had used an example of divergent eye movement, the trace would move from left to right. Here, the saccade produces a trace with a slope of approximately +1, and the disjunctive movement produces a trace with a slope of about −1. Because of these differences the existence of the two components seems indisputable.

When the terms version and vergence are applied to eye movements that pursue a continuously moving target, the question of the validity of the two-components proposition is complicated. A target that moves

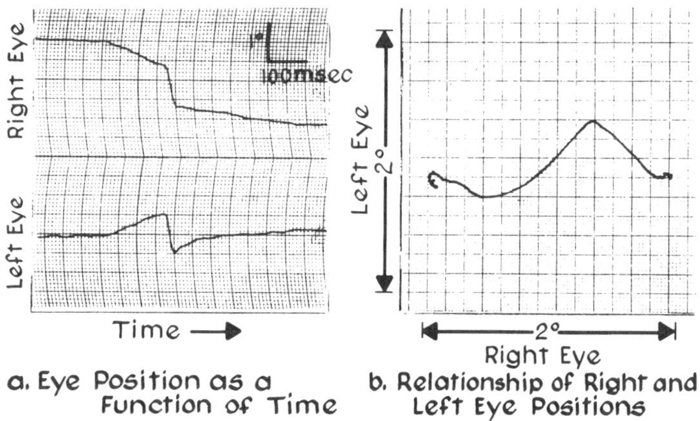

FIGURE 11.4. a) Sample record of eye movement when the target is abruptly moved to a different distance and different direction. b) Representation of the same eye movement on Cartesian coordinates.

smoothly along a Vieth-Müller circle, along a Hillebrand hyperbola, or on any other path, can within certain limits be accurately tracked. Unlike eye movements for a stepped stimulus, pursuit movements match the stimulus movement and the two components of eye movement cannot be distinguished.

There is one experiment directly relevant to the two-components proposition for pursuit movements. Using a stereoscope, Rashbass and Westheimer (1961) presented a smoothly moving target for which version and vergence components had been mathematically described. They found cases in which eye movement followed the version component of the stimulus movement but not the vergence component, and they concluded that the two systems were dissociated.

These findings are held to confirm the two-components proposition for pursuit movement, but the authors made an assumption that can be questioned. They assumed that stimuli for the two hypothesized movement systems were such that both systems could have operated during the "dissociation." In their stimulus arrangement, however, it is very likely that their subject could not maintain binocular fusion of the stimuli. The subject would thus perceive two separate targets moving laterally, and the stimulus for vergence movement would be inadequate. We have often obtained a similar sort of eye movement in stimulus situations in which there is only mathematically defined vergence but not version. When oscillating movement in the median plane is simulated in a stereoscope, the eye movements consist initially of disjunctive movements but later only of pure conjunctive movements. This pattern occurs despite the absence of a formal stimulus for version. An alternative and parsimonious interpretation for our results, or those of Rashbass and Westheimer, is that the subject was tracking the apparent movement of one of the diplopic images.

Given this alternative interpretation, the two-components proposition as it applies to pursuit movements remains unsubstantiated, and some questions remain unanswered. Does the common mechanism for lateral pursuit eye movement and for slow control suggested by Robinson (1975), Murphy, Kowler, and Steinman (1975), and Kowler and Steinman (1979) also control disjunctive pursuit movement? Does this control mechanism also control the disjunctive movement to a stimulus in depth? The most basic question: how should one test the two-components proposition for smooth eye movements?

The foregoing discussion implies that the two-components proposition is a good working hypothesis, but it may be too simple. Additional considerations also indicate that it needs to be further developed. For instance, the results of the well-known experiments of Rashbass (1961), which suggest that the pursuit and saccadic systems are independent (cf. Jurgens and Becker, 1975), dictate that two types of version be considered:

saccadic and pursuit. If we incorporate this notion into Hering's hypothesis we must consider at least three components rather than two. Moreover, the titles of many of the chapters in this book also suggest that there are different types of vergence, hence eventually we may be considering more than four.

Results Related to the Equal-Components and Additivity Propositions

The equal-components and additivity propositions are discussed together because in the experiments to be cited they are studied together. Usually, one of them is being assumed while the other is being examined. We discuss the propositions under the four different stimulus conditions that result from the combination of two *rates* of stimulus movement: smooth or stepped movement, and two *paths* of stimulus movement: along a Vieth-Müller circle or along a Hillebrand hyperbola. Movement along a Vieth-Müller circle is referred to as a shift in direction, while movement along a Hillebrand hyperbola is referred to as a shift in distance. One of the four situations has generated more studies than the other three; that situation is discussed last.

Target Moves Smoothly to a Different Direction and a Different Distance

The validity of the first proposition has already been questioned for this stimulus situation in which a target moves smoothly to both a different direction and a different distance. Because the validity of the second and third propositions depends on that of the first, evaluation is difficult until the uncertainty is removed. Apparently, it is also difficult to test any of the propositions in terms of physiological hypotheses. Tamler, Jampolsky, and Marg (1958) found electromyographical evidence that supports additivity of the two components at the muscle level, but Breinin (1955) and Blodi and Van Allen (1957) did not. The status of the two propositions for this stimulus situation remains uncertain.

Target Steps to a Different Direction but Moves Smoothly to a Different Distance

When a target steps to a different direction but moves smoothly to a different distance, the stimulus condition is similar to that used to study the superimposition of saccadic and conjunctive pursuit movements (Jurgens and Becker, 1975; Rashbass, 1961). The step and smooth movements of the target may be accompanied by corresponding abrupt and smooth eye movements. If the subject is tracking the stimulus, the smooth eye movement should be disjunctive with equal velocities for the two eyes.

The abrupt portion of the record is of interest because it can be examined to make inferences about the additivity proposition, if we make certain assumptions. For example, if this abrupt movement is equal in magnitude and velocity for the two eyes, we must conclude that the saccadic system has shut off the disjunctive pursuit movement and that the two components are not additive. This inference would be like that of Jurgens and Becker, who maintained that saccadic movement shuts off conjunctive pursuit. If there are two additive components for the two eyes, then the abrupt movements should differ by a predictable amount. There is no published study dealing with this stimulus arrangement that tests for additivity, but Saida and Ono are now working on it.

Saida and Ono are simulating in a stereoscope a moving target that changes distance smoothly and direction abruptly. A sample record is shown in Figure 11.5. Notice that during the abrupt change, an eye movement that is in the same direction as the pursuit movement is larger than an eye movement in the opposite direction. This difference has been found in almost all the abrupt portions of the record, which indicates that the saccadic system has not shut off the on-going disjunctive pursuit movement. Although the direction of the difference between the eye movements in Figure 11.5 is consistent with the additivity proposition, the extent of the difference is larger than that predicted by it. For example, when the target stepped 3° to the side while it approached or receded at the rate of 1.6° per second, the mean duration of the abrupt movements

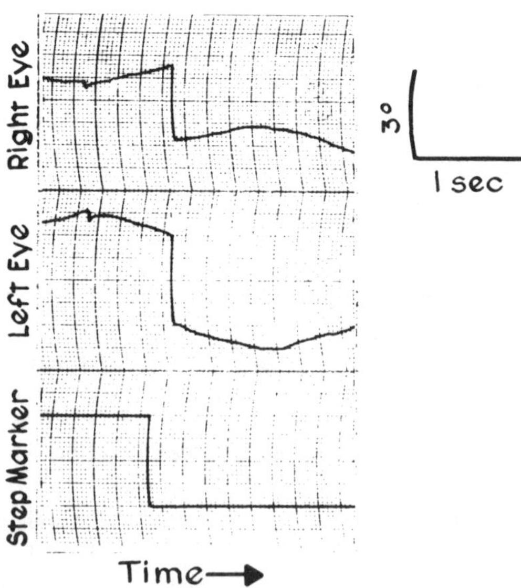

FIGURE 11.5. Sample record of eye movement when the target moves smoothly to a new distance but changes direction abruptly.

was 35.9 milliseconds. For this time interval the additivity proposition predicts a difference in rotation of 0.11° for the two eyes, but the obtained mean difference was 0.27°. We have tentatively concluded that the difference between the combined movements of the two eyes is too large to be explained by the additivity proposition.

Target Moves Smoothly to a Different Direction but Steps to a Different Distance

When the target moves smoothly to a new direction and steps to a new distance, the dimensions in which the target steps and moves are reversed from the condition discussed in the previous section. The expected eye movement is unlike the previous one because the step should evoke a slow, smooth disjunctive movement. As in the first situation, the two components (if they exist) cannot be easily distinguished from each other in the eye movement record alone. Thus in the following study the additivity proposition is tested with the assumptions that the two components exist and that they are equal for the two eyes. One can test the additivity proposition here but not in the first situation because a combined eye movement, if one occurred, would appear after the step is introduced.

Miller, Ono, and Steinbach (1980) simulated a stimulus moving smoothly in a given direction but stepped in distance. In this study, the onset and the end point of the combined eye movement are not easily identified so it is difficult to make a statement concerning the magnitude of the movement. We can, however, examine velocity. A sample record from the study (Figure 11.6) shows the eyes converging during pursuit movement to the right. For the left eye, disjunctive movement is in the same direction as conjunctive pursuit, and the velocity of the combined eye movement is faster than the velocity of the pursuit movement alone (broken line). For the right eye, disjunctive movement is in a direction opposite to conjunctive pursuit and the combined movement is slower. This pattern was found in all of the records we analyzed and suggests additivity. The analysis indicated that in general, additivity holds for the eye for which pursuit and disjunctive movements are in opposite directions, but not for the eye for which the movements are in the same direction. When they are in the same direction, the maximum speed of the combined eye movements is on average 11% less than the sum of the separate version and vergence components.

Target Steps to a Different Direction and to a Different Distance

Eye movements in which the target steps to both a different direction and a different distance are the types discussed most frequently in the literature. For this condition, it is often claimed that both the equal-compo-

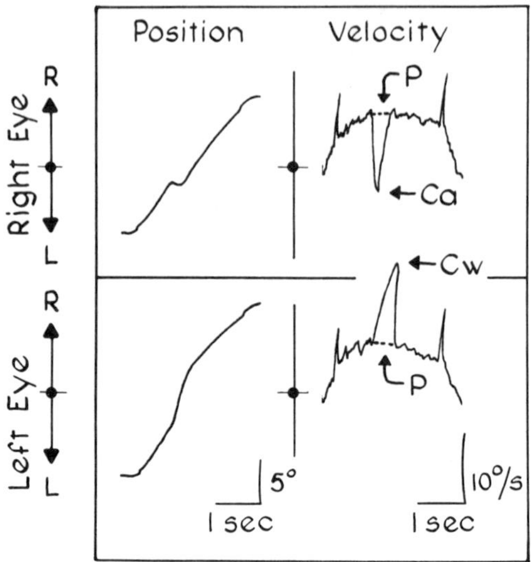

FIGURE 11.6. Sample record showing position and velocity of eye movemen when the target moves smoothly to a new direction but changes distance abruptly Reprinted by permission of the publisher, from Miller JM, Ono H, Steinbach MJ Additivity of fusional vergence and pursuit eye movements. Vision Research 1980.

nents and the additivity propositions are valid (Alpern, 1969; Yarbus 1965–67; Zuber, 1971). If we make certain assumptions we can examine the equal-components and additivity propositions separately, thus the two are discussed in two different subsections. As mentioned in the discussion of the two-components proposition, the eye movement that occurs for this stimulus situation has three parts: (1) an initial slow disjunctive movement, (2) a saccade (on which conjunctive movement is presumed to be superimposed), and (3) a final stage of slow disjunctive movement (see Figure 11.4). Because saccadic latency is longer and its duration shorter than that of disjunctive movement, the saccade occurs during the disjunctive movement. The disjunctive portion is examined with respect to the equal-components proposition and the abrupt portion with respect to the additivity proposition.

The equal-components proposition. Eye movements that approximate the movements predicted by the equal-components proposition are obtained with several different kinds of target presentation: with real targets located in two different positions (Ono and Nakamizo, 1977; Riggs and Niehl, 1960; Yarbus, 1965–67), with stereoscopic targets (Ono, Nakamizo, and Steinbach, 1978; Westheimer and Mitchell, 1956), and with real targets that shift their apparent position when a prism is placed in front of one eye (Alpern, 1957). The saccades of the two eyes are said to be directed toward the visual direction of the destination target (Yarbus, 1965–67) or toward the bisector of the angle of convergence at the destination target (Westheimer and Mitchell, 1956). Both descriptions are consistent with predictions derived from the equal-components proposition for version as well as for vergence, because the disjunctive portions for the two eyes will be approximately equal if the combined movements are also approximately equal. (The reason for the qualification "approximately" is that the combined portion is not expected to be equal according to the additivity proposition.)

This description is given in many secondary texts as a typical eye movement for the stimulus situation (Alpern, 1971; Carpenter, 1977; Howard and Templeton, 1966; Richards, 1975). The portrayal is a nice one, because it seems to be a case in which modern technology for measuring eye movements confirms a century-old prediction. Unfortunately, results in our laboratory indicate that it does not always apply. Ono and Nakamizo (1978) recorded eye movements in which two stimuli were aligned to one eye. There were four conditions that differed according to possible reliance on accommodation:

1. Constant accommodation, in which the accommodation requirement was the same for the two stimuli. This condition was conceptually equivalent to the conditions of Alpern (1957) and Westheimer and Mitchell. In our study the method of stimulus presentation was closer to that of Westheimer and Mitchell since a Polaroid filter was used instead of a prism. Westheimer and Mitchell call this condition the Panum-Wheatstone-limiting case.

2. Peripheral accommodation, in which the far target was occluded by the near target for one eye and provided accommodation cues peripherally to only one eye. This condition is often called the Panum-limiting case.

3. Disparity accommodation, in which concordance existed between the accommodation required and the convergence required for each stimulus. This condition is conceptually equivalent to that of Riggs and Niehl (1960) and to one of the stimulus situations of Alpern and Ellen (1956). The far target was placed slightly above the near one so that the two targets could be seen.

4. Accommodation, which is the traditional accommodative vergence situation. This condition consisted of one eye being occluded, and is sometimes referred to as the Johannes Müller experimental situation. The four conditions are illustrated in Figure 11.7.

Most of the eye movements in the first two conditions fit the textbook portrayal well and were very much like those shown in Figure 11.4. That

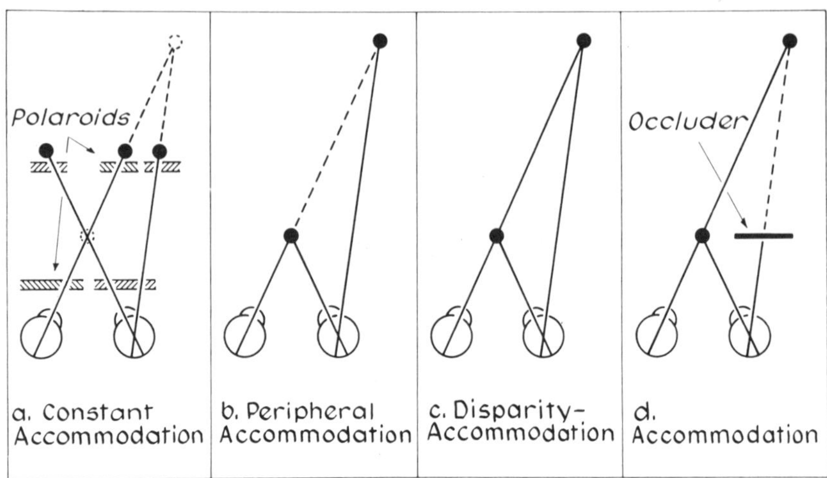

FIGURE 11.7. Illustrations of four stimulus conditions in which two stimuli are aligned with one eye. Reprinted by permission of the publisher, from Ono H, Nakamizo S. Changing fixation in the tranverse plane at eye level and Hering's law of equal innervation. Vision Research, 1978.

these eye movements conformed is not surprising. Our results are consistent with those of other studies that have used similar experimental conditions. They cannot, however, be generalized completely to eye movements in a more normal situation such as the disparity accommodation condition, in which there were noticeable individual differences in eye movements. For some subjects, eye movements sometimes conformed closely to the portrayal, but at other times appeared to be accommodative vergence (Figure 11.8). Note that half of the eye movement in Figure 11.8 looks very similar to that in Figure 11.9, which shows accommodative vergence obtained from the accommodation condition. The other subjects produced almost no movements that conformed to the portrayal. Their saccades were generally too small, and many of the movements were like those of accommodative vergence.[2]

Eye movements said to conform to the predictions of the equal-components proposition are most likely to occur when (1) the accommodation required for the two stimuli is held constant or (2) the accommodation stimulus is not on the fovea. When the accommodation and convergence

[2] During accommodative vergence, the eye with which the two stimuli are aligned was thought to remain fixed (Alpern, 1969; Alpern and Ellen, 1956), but we have classified as accommodative vergence many eye movements that show the aligned eye has moved slightly. We did this because we noticed that there were movements of the aligned eye during almost all trials in the accommodation condition. Also see Kenyon, Ciuffreda, and Stark (1978).

required are in concordance, however, some eye movements conform to the portrayal and others resemble accommodative vergence. Whether accommodative vergence or slow asymmetric disjunctive movements contradict the equal components proposition is discussed shortly, but these movements are not the ones that are usually ascribed to Hering's hypothesis. Nevertheless, one might expect that these stimulus conditions would produce movements that conform to Hering's hypothesis. Knowing Hering's idea was that one kind of innervation is for vergence (which he called "internal accommodation"), one would think that a retinal disparity or an unfocused image would produce the same response. In fact, the eye movement commonly ascribed to Hering's hypothesis occurs infrequently when the two kinds of distance information are available and not at all when only the accommodation cues are available.

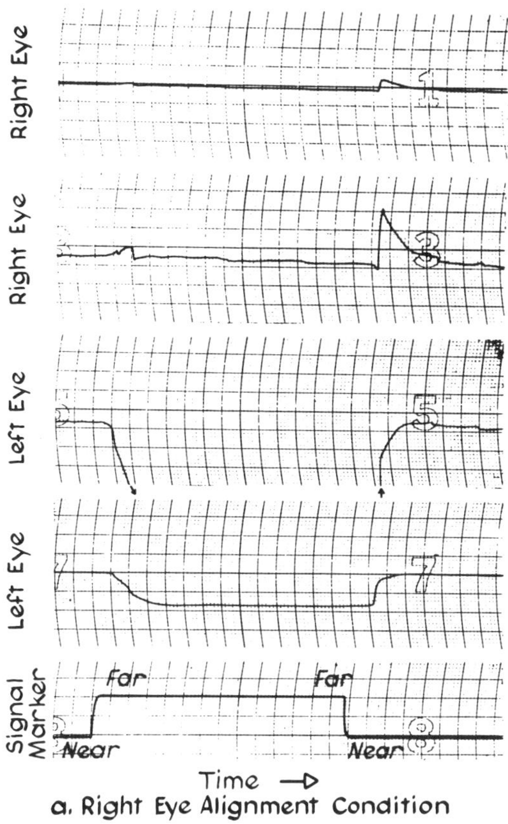

FIGURE 11.8. Sample record of eye movement from one subject obtained in the disparity accommodation condition. Reprinted by permission of the publisher, from Ono H, Nakamizo S. Changing fixation in the tranverse plane at eye level and Hering's law of equal innervation. Vision Research, 1978.

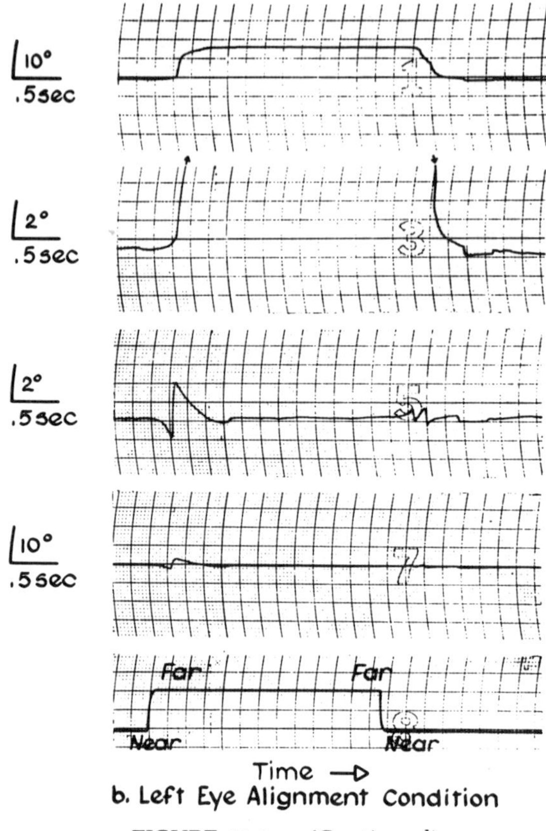

FIGURE 11.8. *(Continued)*

These results suggest that in a situation where both target points are not on the visual axis, eye movements will not fit the usual portrayal because both disparity and accommodation information are available. Ono and Tam (1981) therefore compared eye movements that occur when both targets are not on the axis with the movements that occur when the targets are on the axis. For this analysis we counted the frequencies of four different kinds of eye movements that occurred during the target position shift: (1) no saccade (disjunctive movement only), (2) single saccade (the textbook portrayal), (3) unidirectional multiple saccades (several in the same direction during a single target position shift), and (4) bidirectional multiple saccades (in different directions during a single target position shift). Because we were concerned with the overall pattern of eye movement, we ignored the very small so-called corrective saccades that sometimes occur. Based on Yarbus's description, saccades less than 0.75° were not counted.

Figure 11.10 shows the relative frequencies of these four types of

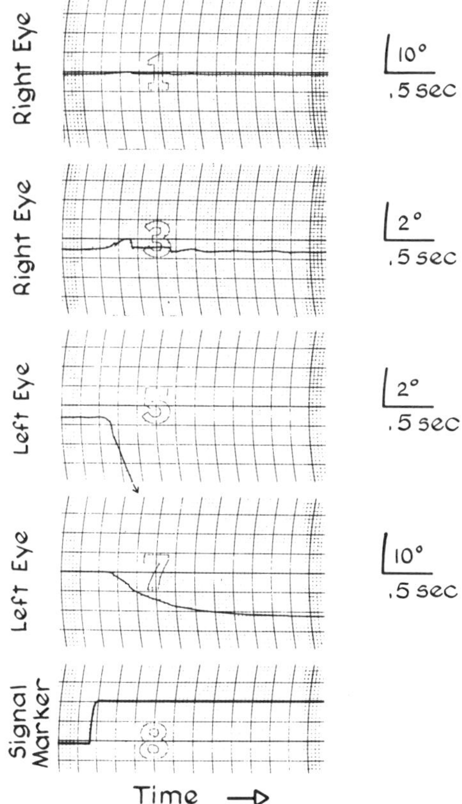

FIGURE 11.9. Sample record of eye movement obtained for one subject in the accommodation condition. Reprinted by permission of the publisher, from Ono H, Nakamizo S. Changing fixation in the tranverse plane at eye level and Hering's law of equal innervation. Vision Research, 1978.

eye movements as a function of the extent of shift in target direction. The results for convergence and divergence conditions are presented separately because there were striking differences between the two. The figure shows that the eye movement consisting of a single saccade superimposed on a disjunctive movement occurred reliably only in the Panum-limiting case (or when the required version is about 6°). In other stimulus arrangements there occurred asymmetric disjunctive movements and bidirectional saccades when the required version was small, and multiple saccades when the required version was larger. Because the relevance of the two kinds of multiple saccades or the convergence-divergence difference to Hering's hypothesis is not clear, it is not discussed further. The points to be emphasized here are the poor fit of the usual textbook portrayal for

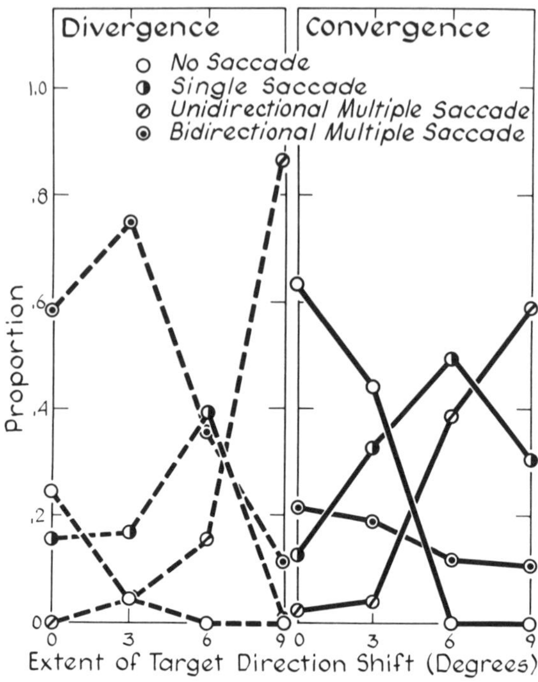

FIGURE 11.10. Mean proportion of the four types of eye movements as a function of target direction shift. Reprinted by permission of the publisher, from Ono H, Tam WJ. Asymmetrical vergence and multiple saccades. Vision Research, 1981.

eye movement to a target not in the Panum-limiting case, and the asymmetry of the disjunctive movement.

Figure 11.10 shows that some eye movements under the convergence condition when the target was displaced 3° occurred without saccades. This means that subjects can rotate their eyes smoothly in opposite directions even when the difference in extent of rotation is as much as 6°. A further experiment in the same study showed that the extent can be as large as 8° (Figure 11.11). Whether to consider these unequal and disjunctive smooth eye movements an outcome of vergence is a matter of definition. There is no logical need to assume that vergence leads to movements equal in magnitude and opposite in direction, but in the context of Hering's hypothesis, it is postulated to do just this. Therefore the existence of disjunctive movements of different magnitudes and the accommodative vergence noted before poses a theoretical problem.

Whether this movement violates or conforms to the equal-components proposition depends on certain assumptions. Asymmetrically smooth disjunctive movement is a violation of Hering's hypothesis if one considers only saccades to be appropriate for version in our stimulus

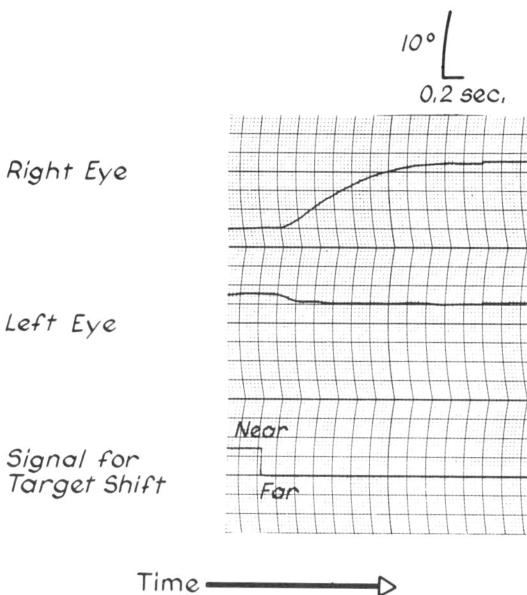

FIGURE 11.11. Sample eye movement record from the 4° shift condition showing symmetric disjunctive movement. The difference in the magnitudes of the smooth movement between the eyes is 8°. Reprinted by permission of the publisher, from Ono H, Tam WJ. Asymmetrical vergence and multiple saccades. Vision Research, 1981.

situation. As noted earlier, when the hypothesis was first proposed by Hering the distinction between saccadic and pursuit eye movements had not been made, and he thought that unequal movements were consistent with his hypothesis. He assumed that they were the outcome of the addition of version and vergence. Accordingly, if one argues that a slow version component is somehow adding to the vergence component, the asymmetric smooth movement of the two eyes does not violate Hering's hypothesis. (For such an argument see Peli and Comerford, 1982). Another possible argument is that smooth asymmetric disjunctive movements are the result of the imprecision of the vergence system. It is not obvious to us what kind of experimental results would support either argument.

Every time the saccades are not directed to the visual direction of the target as specified from the cyclopean eye, the smooth portions of the movement will be unequal for the two eyes and the movement will deviate from the portrayal ascribed to Hering's hypothesis. Pickwell (1972) hypothesized the deviation exists because the cyclopean eye is not located midway between the eyes. This idea is attractive because it appears to explain eye movements that seem to violate the equal-components proposition within Hering's theoretical framework. Pickwell equated the location of the cyclopean eye to the location of the dominant eye and predicted that the magnitude of the saccade would be larger when two stimuli are aligned to the nondominant eye than when aligned to the dominant eye. (If they were aligned to the dominant eye there should be no saccade.) Our data (Ono and Nakamizo, 1978) do not support this. The prediction should hold whether fixation is changed from near to far or from far to near, and our data suggested that the occurrence of larger saccades depends on whether eye movement is toward the right or toward the left and not on which eye is dominant.

An example of the larger magnitude of the rightward saccades can be seen in Figure 11.8. When both targets are aligned to the right eye and the subject changes fixation from the near to the far left stimulus, eye movements similar to accommodative vergence occur, but when fixation shifts from the distant to the near stimulus a large saccade occurs. In contrast, when both targets are aligned with the left eye and fixation shifts from the near to the far target, there is a large saccade, and when fixation shifts back to the near target the eye movement is similar to accommodative vergence movement. For these eye movements to be consistent with Pickwell's hypothesis, we must assume that the eye that is dominant is a function of whether the change in fixation is from near to far or from far to near. It is more parsimonious to say that the oculomotor system of a given subject has a preference for making saccades in one direction.

The additivity proposition. In the traces we have shown, the portion of the eye movement that consists of a saccade combined with a smooth slow movement is easy to identify. As before, we can examine this combined portion for the validity of the additivity proposition if we assume that the equal-components proposition holds for this stimulus situation. Three studies are addressed to the additivity proposition for this stimulus situation.

Using a stereoscope, Ono and Nakamizo (1978) and Ono, Nakamizo, and Steinbach (1978) studied the combination of saccade and disparity-produced disjunctive movement with accommodation held constant. The magnitudes and velocities of the combined eye movements for which saccades and disjunctive movements were in the same direction were larger than those of the combined movements in which they were in opposite directions. The larger movements were 1.8 times larger than the smaller movements and 1.9 times faster. The direction of this difference is consistent with the additivity proposition, but the magnitudes of the differences are too large. We arrived at this conclusion by several different analyses, of which two are reported here. First, we considered the velocity of the disjunctive movement before the onset of combined eye movements, as well as the duration of the combined movement, and computed the difference in magnitude for the two eyes. The obtained difference was 1.9

times larger than predicted. Second, we computed the predicted difference in the peak velocities of the combined movements for the two eyes. The obtained difference was 5 times larger than predicted.

Kenyon, Ciuffreda, and Stark (1980) also examined this inequality in a different stimulus situation. Their targets were placed in the median plane and they examined what we have called bidirectional saccades, the frequency of which is shown in Figure 11.10. Near the onset of disjunctive movement, the combined eye movements in which saccades and disjunctive movements were in the same direction were over three times larger than movements in which the components were in the opposite direction. This difference diminished near the end of the disjunctive movement. These authors also reported that combined movements of saccades and accommodative vergence followed the same function; the inequality was again largest near the onset of the accommodative vergence.

SUMMARY

Hering's hypothesis concerning lateral eye movement is the only one that deals directly with the combination of version and vergence. It states that each eye moves as the result of the sum of two types of eye movement. In a purely formal way, the hypothesis can describe any binocular eye movement. Thus a mathematical separation of the version and vergence components says nothing about the validity of Hering's hypothesis in its empirical form, and one must make explicit the possible empirical propositions.

Consequently, three propositions were derived from the hypothesis: (1) there exist two components, (2) both the version component and the vergence component are equal for both eyes, and (3) the signed components are additive. These components can be examined for the eye movements to a target changing location abruptly. In accordance with the two-components proposition, both saccades and disjunctive movements occur, but the velocities and magnitudes of the latter are not always equal for the two eyes. Whether this inequality contradicts the equal-components proposition depends on the assumption that a slow version component is not involved. When the disjunctive movement combines with slow conjunctive movement, the difference in velocities for the two eyes is slightly less than that predicted from the additivity proposition. When the disjunctive movement combines with saccadic movement, the differences in magnitude and velocity are larger than those predicted. The validity of all three propositions is yet to be substantiated or falsified for eye movements to a smoothly moving target.

REFERENCES

Alpern M. The position of the eyes during prism vergence. Arch Ophthalmol 1957;57:345–53.

Alpern M. Types of movement. In: Davson H, ed. The eye. 2nd ed. New York: Academic Press, 1969:65–174.

Alpern M. Effector mechanisms in vision. In: Kling JW, Riggs LA, eds. Woodworth and Schlosberg's experimental psychology. 3rd ed. New York: Holt, Rinehart & Winston, 1971:369–94.

Alpern M, Ellen P. A quantitative analysis of the horizontal movements of the eyes in the experiment of Johannes Müller. I. Method and results. Am J Ophthalmol 1956;42:289–303.

Bahill AT, Ciuffreda KJ, Kenyon RV, Stark L. Dynamic and static violations of Hering's law of equal innervation. Am J Optom Physiol Opt 1967;53:786–96.

Blodi FC, Van Allen MW. Electromyography of extraocular muscles in fusional movement. I. Electric phenomena at the breakpoint of fusion. Am J Ophthalmol 1957;44:136–44.

Breinin GM. The nature of vergence revealed by electromyography. Arch Ophthalmol 1955;54:407–409.

Carpenter RHS. Movements of the eyes. London: Pion, 1977.

Clark MR, Crane HD. Dynamic interactions in binocular vision. In: Senders JW, Fisher DF, Monty RA, eds. Eye movements and the higher psychological functions. Hillsdale, N.J.: Erlbaum, 1978:77–88.

Fuchs AF. The saccadic system. In: Bach-y-Rita P, Collins CC, eds. The control of eye movements. New York: Academic Press, 1971:343–62.

Hering E. Spatial sense and movements of the eye (1879). Radde CA, trans. Baltimore: American Academy of Optometry, 1942.

Hering E. The theory of binocular vision (1868). Bridgeman B, Stark L, eds, trans. New York: Plenum Press, 1977.

Howard IP. Human visual orientation. Chichester: Wiley, 1982.

Howard IP, Templeton WB. Human spatial orientation. New York: Wiley, 1966.

Hurvich LM. Hering and the scientific establishment. Am Physiol 1969;24:497–514.

Jurgens R, Becker W. Is there a linear addition of saccades and pursuit movements? In: Lennerstrand G, Bach-y-Rita P, eds. Basic mechanisms of ocular motility. Oxford: Pergamon Press, 1975:525–29.

Kenyon RV, Ciuffreda KJ, Stark L. Binocular eye movements during accommodative vergence. Vision Res 1978;18:545–55.

Kenyon RV, Ciuffreda KJ, Stark L. Unequal saccades during vergence. Am J Optom Physiol Opt 1978;57:586–94.

Kowler E, Steinman RM. The effect of expectations on slow oculomotor control. II. Single target displacements. Vision Res 1979;19:633–46.

Miller JM, Ono H, Steinbach MJ. Additivity of fusional vergence and pursuit eye movements. Vision Res 1980;20:43–47.

Murphy BJ, Kowler E, Steinman RM. Slow oculomotor control in the presence of moving backgrounds. Vision Res 1975;15:1263–68.

Nakamizo S, Ono H. Changing fixation and Hering's law. Shinrigaku Hyoron (Jpn Psychol Rev) 1978;21:166–90.

Ono H. Hering's law of equal innervation and vergence eye movement. Am J. Optom Physiol Opt 1980;57:578–85.

Ono H, Nakamizo S. Saccadic eye movements during changes in fixation to stimuli at different distances. Vision Res 1977;17:233–38.

Ono H, Nakamizo S. Changing fixation in the transverse plane at eye level and Hering's law of equal innervation. Vision Res 1978;18:511–19.

Ono H, Saida S. Accommodative-vergence and Hering's law of equal innervation. Paper read at the Annual Meeting of the Association for Research in Vision and Ophthalmology, Inc., 26 April-1 May 1981, Sarasota, Fla. Abstract in Suppl Invest Ophthalmol Visual Sci. 1981;20:191.

Ono H, Steinbach MJ. Eye movements during the Pulfrich phenomenon. Paper read at the Annual Meeting of the Association for Research in Vision and Ophthalmology, Inc., 2-7 May 1982, Sarasota, Fla. Abstract in Suppl. Invest Ophthalmol Visual Sci. 1982;22:84.

Ono H, Tam WJ. Asymmetrical vergence and multiple saccades. Vision Res 1981;21:739–43.

Ono H, Nakamizo S, Steinbach MJ. Nonadditivity of vergence and saccadic eye movement. Vision Res 1978;18:735–39.

Peli E, Comerford JP. Dynamics of eye movements in unilateral cover test. Paper read at the Annual Meeting of the Association for Research in Vision and Ophthalmology, Inc., 2-7 May 1982, Sarasota, Fla. Abstract in Suppl. Invest Ophthalmol Visual Sci. 1982;22:266.

Pickwell LD. Hering's law of equal innervation and the position of the binoculus. Vision Res 1972;12:1499–1507.

Rashbass C. The relationship between saccadic and smooth tracking eye movements. J Physiol 1961;159:326–38.

Rashbass C, Westheimer G. Independence of conjugate and disjunctive eye movements. J Physiol 1961;159:361–64.

Richards W. Visual space perception. In: Carterette EC, Friedman MP, eds. Handbook of perception. Vol. 5. New York: Academic Press, 1975:351–86.

Riggs LA, Niehl EW. Eye movements recorded during convergence and divergence. J Opt Soc Am 1960;50:913–20.

Robinson DA. The mechanics of human vergence eye movement. J Pediatr Ophthalmol 1966;3:31–37.

Robinson DA. Oculomotor control signals. In: Bach-y-Rita P, Lennerstrand G. Basic mechanisms of ocular motility. Oxford: Pergamon Press, 1975:337–78.

Rogers BJ, Steinbach MJ, Ono H. Eye movements and the Pulfrich phenomenon. Vision Res 1974;14:181–85.

Steinman RM, Collewijn H. Binocular retinal image motion during active head rotation. Vision Res 1980;20:415–29.

Tamler E, Jampolsky A, Marg E. An electromyographic study of asymmetric convergence. Am J Ophthalmol 1958;46:174–82.

Toates FM. Vergence eye movements. Doc Ophthalmol 1974;37:153–214.

Westheimer G. Donders', Listing's and Hering's laws and their implications. In: Zuber BL, ed. Models of oculomotor behavior and control. Boca Raton, Fla.: CRC Press, Inc., 1981:149–59.

Westheimer G. Oculomotor control: the vergence system. In: Monty RA, Senders

JW, eds. Eye movements and psychological processes. Hillsdale, N.J.: Erlbaum, 1976; pp. 55–70.

Westheimer G, Mitchell AM. Eye movement responses to convergence stimuli. Arch Ophthalmol 1956;55:848–56.

Williams RA, Fender DH. The synchrony of binocular saccadic eye movements. Vision Res 1977;17:303–306.

Yarbus AL. Eye movements and vision. Riggs LA, Haigh B, eds, trans. New York: Plenum Press, 1965–67.

Zuber BL. Control of vergence eye movements. In: Bach-y-Rita P, Collins CC, eds. The control of eye movements. New York: Academic Press, 1971:447–71.

V

CASE ANALYSIS OF BINOCULAR DISORDERS, EXCLUDING STRABISMUS AND CENTRAL NERVOUS SYSTEM DISORDERS

12

Basic Concepts Underlying Graphical Analysis

Glenn A. Fry

Graphical analysis as described by Hofstetter in Chapter 13 has its roots in the assumptions made about the relation between accommodation and convergence. As Hofstetter points out, the relation involves five variables:

1. Distance phoria.
2. AC/A ratio.
3. Positive fusional convergence.
4. Negative fusional convergence.
5. Amplitude of accommodation.

The distance phoria is well understood and is assumed to be the position of the eyes when the two eyes are dissociated and accommodation is maintained at its maximum relaxation. It is necessary to consider the reflex nature of positive and negative fusional convergence and the relation between accommodation and the convergence and pupil constriction associated with it. This is known as the triad response. It is important to know the significance of the blur break-range in normal subjects and to know how voluntary use of the triad response can supplement reflex fusional movements in maintaining single vision. Finally, it is necessary to understand the relation between accommodation and convergence at the upper limit of accommodation, and in particular why the amplitude and the AC/A ratio change with age.

HERING'S LAWS OF EQUAL INNERVATION

At the outset, let us affirm Hering's laws of equal innervation (1868). In a normal observer the pupil responses and accommodative responses of the two eyes are always nearly equal even though the stimuli may be confined to one eye or may be unequal for the two eyes.[1]

Furthermore, conjugate movements of fixation of the two eyes are nearly equal and disjunctive movements like convergence also involve equal innervation to the muscles of the two eyes. I will not attempt to prove the validity of these laws or recite the evidence that may be offered in support of them.

RELATION BETWEEN ACCOMMODATION AND CONVERGENCE

Various investigators have made assumptions about the relation between accommodation and convergence. Sheard (1917) like Maddox (1893) proposed that there is only one kind of accommodation and several kinds of convergence including tonic convergence. Accommodation and accommodative convergence are tied together so that whenever one accommodates, this brings along with it a certain amount of accommodative convergence. The graph in Figure 12.1 illustrates the relation between accommodation and the different types of convergence as conceived by Sheard (1930). The amount of convergence (A) in play at the zero level of accommodation when the eyes are dissociated represents the tonic convergence. The phorias at the different levels of accommodation create the phoria line (AB). This shows the relation between accommodation and the associated accommodative convergence. In 1938 I called the reciprocal of the slope of the phoria line the AC/A ratio. The base-in and base-out to blur points fall on lines EF and CD, which are parallel to the phoria line and which represent the limits of positive and negative fusional convergence. These two forms of reflex convergence provide the zone of play or independence between accommodation and convergence.

When I began my investigations of the relation between accommodation and convergence in 1935, I had to choose between the analysis given by Sheard and that given by Cross (1911). Cross proposed that there is one kind of convergence and that there are two kinds of accommodation, convergent and supplementary. The relation proposed by Cross is shown in Figure 12.2. Supplementary accommodation provides the independence between accommodation and convergence. Convergence always brings with it convergent accommodation.

[1] Strictly speaking, Hering's laws apply only to disjunctive and conjugate eye movements, but may be extended to include accommodation and pupil constriction.

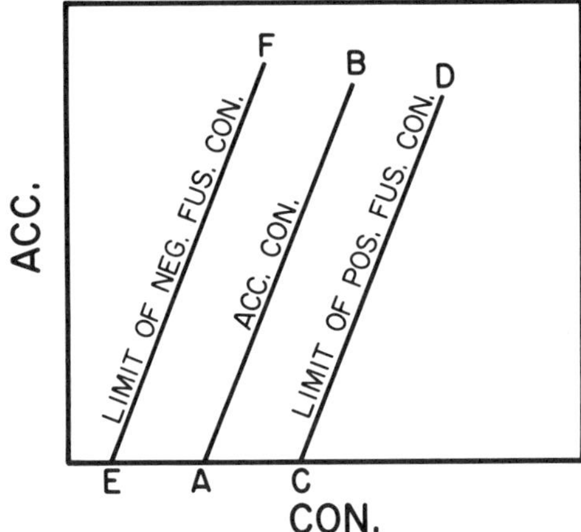

FIGURE 12.1. Sheard's analysis of the accommodation convergence relation. Reprinted by permission of the publisher, from Fry GA. Further experiments on the accommodation convergence relationship. American Journal of Optometry, © (1939), American Academy of Optometry per The Williams & Wilkins Company (agent).

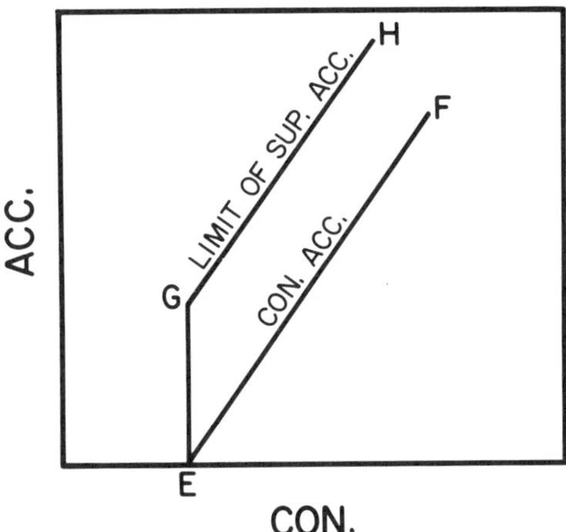

FIGURE 12.2. Cross' analysis of the accommodation convergence relation. Reprinted by permission of the publisher, from Fry GA. Further experiments on the accommodation convergence relationship. American Journal of Optometry, © (1939), American Academy of Optometry per The Williams & Wilkins Company (agent).

If the Cross analysis were correct, one would expect a finite range of relative accommodation at the far point of convergence. In 1937 I demonstrated that the range at this level of convergence is zero and this is what is predicted by Sheard's theory (see Figure 12.1).

In the case of prism base-in and base-out to blur tests, the eyes will compensate the prism by reflex fusional convergence or divergence that responds to disparity. Between the blur points and the break points the eyes have to throw themselves out of focus to maintain fusion. This means that accommodative convergence is being substituted for fusional convergence.

In the case of relative accommodation, convergence is kept fixed and plus and minus lenses are added to determine how much the accommodation can be increased or decreased with a fixed amount of convergence. Many investigators, even prior to Sheard and Maddox, had studied relative accommodation and convergence. Hofstetter (1945) has presented a review of these studies.

This was the state of the art when I began my investigations of the relation between accommodation and convergence around 1935. My first study (1937, 1939) of the relation was designed to demonstrate what happens between the blur points and the break points in the base-in and base-out tests. To carry out this study, I built a device that would measure precisely the amount of accommodation when the stimulus to accommodation was kept constant and the stimulus to converge was set at various levels. It was also noted at what level of convergence the targets would blur and at what level they would break apart. Various lenses were placed before the two eyes to vary the stimulus to accommodation. For each combination of stimuli to accommodation and convergence, the amount of accommodation in play in the right eye was measured with an optometer that uses the Scheiner principle. This was done without affecting the stimulus to accommodation.

The graph in Figure 12.3 shows the data for one subject. The curved lines represent the amounts of accommodation in play for different amounts of convergence for fixed levels of stimulus to accommodation. Between the blur points and the break points, the curves acquired a slope parallel to the phoria line, which indicates that beyond the blur point the fusional convergence is replaced by accommodative convergence. The dashed lines tangent to the solid lines represent the limits of positive and negative fusional convergence.

Base-In and Base-Out Blur-Break Ranges

The real problem about the blur-break range is how a person makes the transition at the blur point from fusional to accommodative convergence. The transition occurs without the person's being aware of the switch.

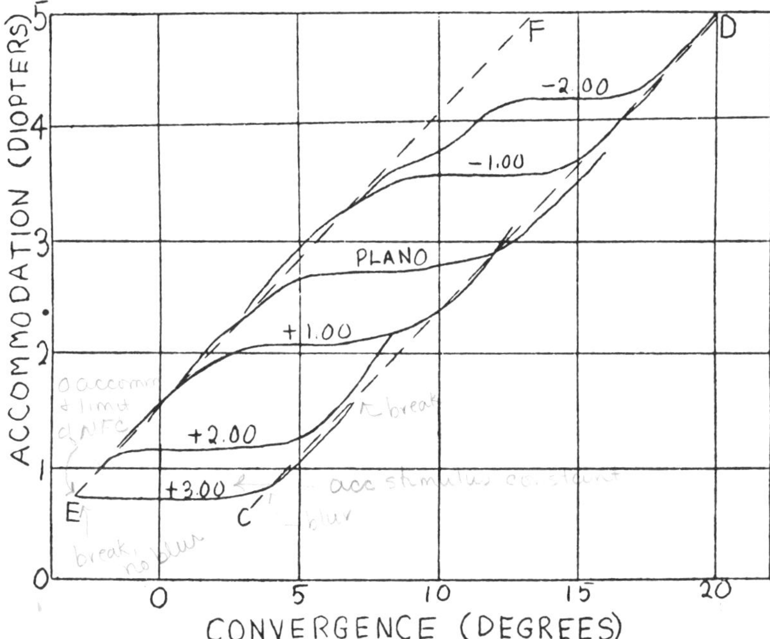

FIGURE 12.3. Relative convergence curves at different levels of stimulus to accommodation. The stimulus to accommodation is varied by viewing targets at 40 cm through various plus and minus lenses. Reprinted by permission of the publisher, from Fry GA. Further experiments on the accommodation convergence relationship. American Journal of Optometry, © (1939), American Academy of Optometry per The Williams & Wilkins Company (agent).

Let us assume in a base-in or base-out to blur test that the prisms are gradually changed in power and in equal amounts for the two eyes. My first guess about the mechanism controlling fusion was that the eyes did not respond to the prisms until the retinal disparity exceeded a certain amount and then made a fusional response to restore fusion. It was supposed that after the first fusional movement the eyes had to wait until again the retinal disparity exceeded the critical amount, and so on. This appears not to be the case.

Rashbass and Westheimer (1961) used a method of recording eye rotations that made it possible for them to demonstrate responses to jump fusional stimuli as low as 15 minutes of arc, and they believed that there was no level of disparity below which the eyes would not respond. They also found a latent period of about 160 msec in the case of jump stimuli. The speed of the movement slows down as fusion becomes restored. At each moment the speed of the movement is proportional to the amount of disparity 160 msec before.

They were able to immobilize the disparate stimuli presented to the two eyes and showed that with a constant amount of disparity, the fusional response has a constant speed that depends on that amount (Figure 12.4). They did not determine the upper limit of disparity beyond which the reflex movement would not occur, nor did they examine what happens at the base-in and base-out blur points.

During the first part of a base-in or base-out to blur test we may suppose that the eyes lag behind the prisms just enough to generate a fusional movement that tends to compensate the change in prism power. When a balance can no longer be maintained, the amount of disparity increases and produces the stereo effect of an object moving forward or backward. The eyes can respond to this perceived change in distance by changing accommodation and the associated accommodative convergence. The break occurs when at some point the disparity exceeds a certain amount or when the absolute limit of convergence or divergence is reached. Once fusion is broken, the eyes drift toward the phoria position.

It may be noted in Figure 12.3 that each of the solid lines at the midlevels of accommodation shows a slight slope between base-in to blur

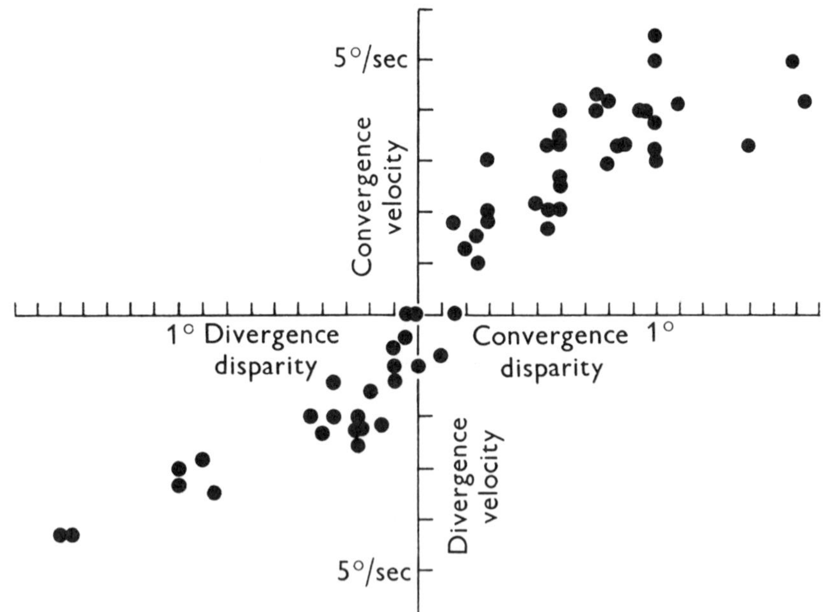

FIGURE 12.4. Relation between the magnitude of constantly maintained disparity and velocity of eye vergence induced by it. Reprinted by permission of the publisher, from Rashbass C, Westheimer G. Disjunctive eye movements. Journal of Physiology, 1961.

and base-out to blur. This slope indicates a gradual drift toward a higher or lower level of accommodation that does not exceed the depth of focus of the eyes. This means that a balance is being struck between the use of accommodation and accommodative convergence, on the one hand, and fusional convergence, on the other, to maintain single vision. An effort is being made to keep the eyes as sharply focused as possible and this depresses the amount of possible change in accommodation and accommodative convergence.

At the zero stimulus to accommodation, the solid curve in Figure 12.3 terminates at the limit for negative fusional convergence, indicating that there can be no further relaxation of accommodation and accommodative convergence and no further activation of negative fusional convergence. A break point occurs instead of a blur point. This terminal point represents the absolute limit of divergence. This limit is not imposed by check ligaments because both eyes can still move to the right or left.

The fact that the lines representing the zero level of accommodation and the limit of negative fusional convergence cross at a sharp point constitutes proof that accommodation, accommodative convergence, and positive and negative fusional convergence are sufficient to explain the flexible relation between accommodation and convergence. It demonstrates the falseness of the notion that there are two kinds of accommodation as proposed by Cross, because if there were a form not associated with convergence, the zone of single clear binocular vision would be bounded by a vertical line on its left side.

Relative Accommodation

It must be assumed that any accommodative response must be associated with accommodative convergence. It is therefore necessary to explain relative accommodation as an indirect involvement of changes in fusional convergence. When the stimulus to convergence is kept constant, adding plus or minus lenses changes the amount of accommodation and the associated accommodative convergence in play, but the change in accommodative convergence is neutralized by a change in fusional convergence. Since the subject is unaware of any diplopia during the entire process, it has to be assumed that fusional convergence can be a reflex response to a small amount of disparity that falls within Panum's limit for single vision. At the limit of relative accommodation, the use of the large amount of fusional convergence inhibits further changes in accommodation and the target is seen as blurred rather than doubled. Sometimes it is actually seen as double.

It may be argued that if the experience of stereopsis can be generated by a difference in disparities produced by two objects without any awareness of diplopia, the disparity can also initiate a fusional movement without awareness of diplopia.

Negative Fusional Convergence

There was some controversy as to whether there were two kinds of fusional movements in the lateral direction, namely, convergence and divergence. The alternative was to regard divergence, or negative convergence, as a kind of inhibition or relaxation of positive convergence. The argument against a single kind of lateral vergence was based on the comparison with vertical divergence where there was no basis for calling right and left supravergence positive and negative or vice versa.

Mechanisms Underlying Fusional Movements

Although convergence and divergence and right and left supravergence can all arise from disparate images from the two retinas arriving at the same part of the cortex, it is still not clear how the motor impulses are generated and distributed to the extraocular muscles.

Nature of the Tie-up between Accommodation and Accommodative Convergence

There has been a lot of controversy about the nature of the tie-up between accommodation and accommodative convergence. One notion is that of a chain reflex in which accommodation is the primary response. It generates a sensory feedback that initiates accommodative convergence. This seemed inappropriate from the outset because of the timing of the two responses but the relative timing was not precisely assessed until sometime later. (See the section Timing of the Accommodation and Accommodative Convergence Responses.)

Most of the people who talked about accommodative convergence being a reflex did not think in terms of a chain reflex but merely of a relation in which accommodation and accommodation convergence are tied together in such a way that both respond when accommodation is stimulated. We need, however, to be more specific.

Helmholtz (1925) proposed that the tie-up is a learned response similar to the relation between raising the hand and opening the mouth in eating. The independence between the functions is derived from the ability to suppress one response while activating the other. According to this concept, we could have accommodative convergence, convergent accommodation and relative accommodation, and relative convergence. The difficulty with this proposal is that it does not recognize the reflex nature of positive and negative fusional convergence.

A third kind of assumption is that there is a single brain center (triad center), which when activated will produce simultaneously accommodation and convergence (Figure 12.5). The combination may be called accommodation and accommodative convergence if the center is activated by the desire to see clearly or the effort to focus attention at some far or near point. It is always a voluntary response. The combination may be called convergence and convergent accommodation if it involves a voluntary effort to converge a given amount and if the capability of responding to changes in blur is eliminated.

This is the assumption advocated by the writer and, in addition, it is proposed that positive and negative fusional convergence are separate reflex forms of vergence responding to retinal disparity. In addition to fusional movements in the horizontal direction, it is necessary to recognize positive and negative vertical divergence as forms of fusional movements. Furthermore, we must recognize cyclofusional movements.

The Jampel Center

Although the need for a brain center mediating accommodation and convergence simultaneously appeared to be needed, it took time for such a

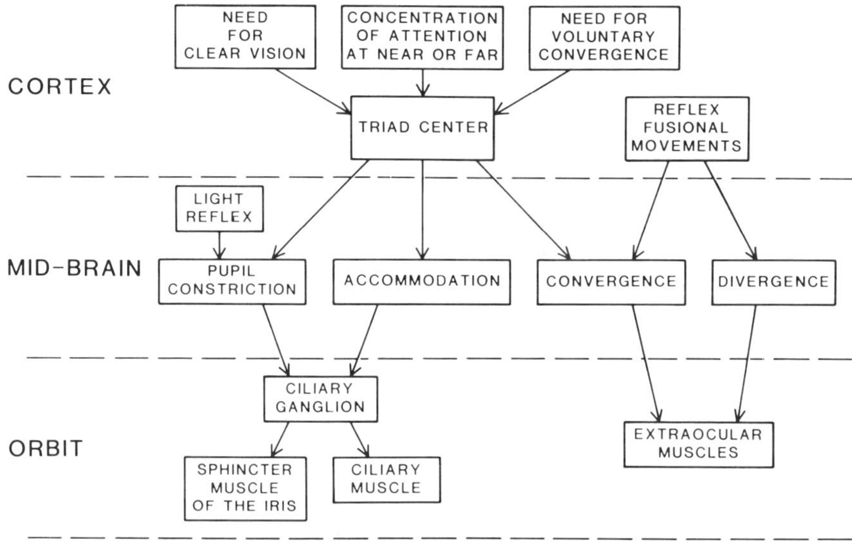

FIGURE 12.5. Neural mechanisms involved in accommodation, convergence, and pupil constriction.

center to be discovered. In the early days of my career, anatomists and physiologists had not located it. Weaver (1937) claimed that accommodation was a reflex mediated by a center in the midbrain similar to that for the light reflex. I argued that the response to blur was too complicated to be mediated by a center in the midbrain and that awareness of nearness also required complicated mechanisms at the cortical level. For example, stereopsis, which requires pathways from the two eyes to be channeled through the cortex to generate information about relative distances can be used to guide accommodation in focusing on a specific target.

Most of the responses produced by stimulating the cortex electrically, like movements of the limbs, can be easily detected but one would not expect a change in the refractive state to show up unless the experimenter were uniquely prepared to detect such changes. Alpern and Hendley, around 1949, used a retinoscope to look for such responses to stimulation of a cat's cortex but found none. Alpern later suggested that Jampel should look for such a response produced by stimulation of a macaque's cortex, and a center now known as the Jampel center was found (Jampel, 1960), which when stimulated produced accommodation, convergence, and pupil contraction (Figure 12.6).

The next question to be concerned about is how impulses from the Jampel center are distributed to the centers in the brain stem that control

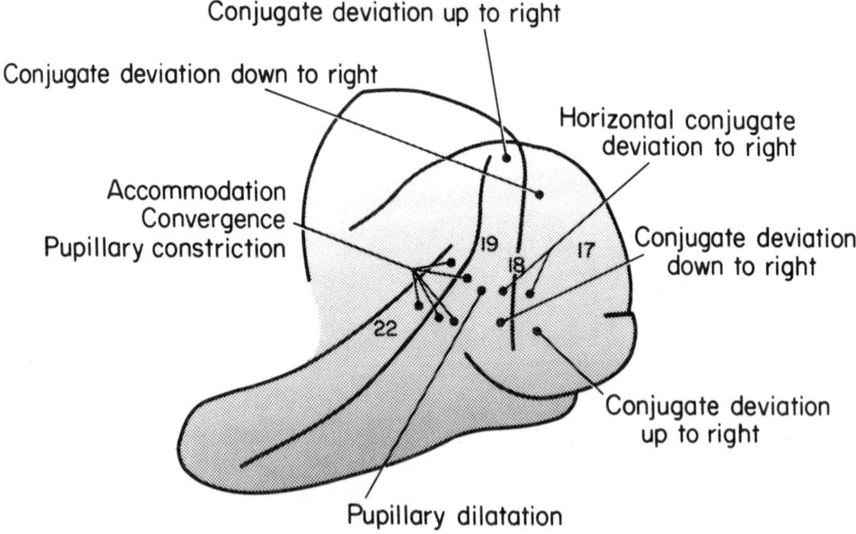

FIGURE 12.6. Left posterior hemisphere. A drawing of the left occipital eye field of *Macaca mulatta*. Reprinted by permission of the publisher, from Jampel RS. Convergence, divergence, pupillary reactions and accommodation of the eyes from farradic stimulation of the macaque brain. Journal of Comparative Neurology, 1960.

accommodation, convergence, and pupil size. Are they distributed directly to the separate centers or are they directed to one of the centers and relayed to the other two? Since there are two kinds of pupil contraction (accommodation and light responses) and at least two kinds of convergence responses (fusional and accommodative), it is more than likely that if a redistribution is carried out in the midbrain it is done at the center for accommodation. This is also unlikely because separate centers for accommodation and convergence are needed to explain the spike phenomenon (this will be taken up later in the chapter).

Although we do not recognize two kinds of accommodation, we can recognize two kinds of input to the Jampel center that are involved in focusing the eyes. One is awareness of nearness and the other is the desire to clear up blur. See Figure 12.5.

Fusional Convergence vs Triad Convergence

We ought to call the convergence produced by voluntary activation of the Jampel (or triad) center by the name *triad convergence*. This can be clearly differentiated from fusional vergence, which is reflex and produced by an entirely different mechanism. If we want to discover the characteristics of fusional vergence, it is better to study these movements in a vertical direction where the situation is not complicated by the triad response. If the two eyes are converging and accommodating on a 2° disk and all of a sudden a base-up prism is placed over one eye, the eyes will respond with a vertical fusional movement to overcome the diplopia.

On the other hand if base-out prisms of equal power are placed in front of the two eyes, there are two ways the eyes can overcome the diplopia. One way is to let the two eyes make the necessary lateral fusional movements and this is likely to happen, if the prisms are weak. If the prisms are strong, the triad mechanism can become involved. The prisms not only produce a momentary diplopia but also, through stereopsis, they cause the disk to move toward the observer. The subject shifts his attention to the new position of the disk and this evokes a triad response which temporarily throws the eyes out-of-focus and also makes the eyes converge. If needed, fusional convergence completes the job. And then as the accommodation relaxes to get the image clear again, the triad convergence, which also relaxes, is replaced by fusional convergence.

When the stereogram in Figure 12.7 is viewed in a stereoscope, the eyes can voluntarily switch convergence from the disk to the star and vice versa. Stereopsis provides awareness of a difference in distance so that the observer can switch concentration of attention from far to near or vice versa. At each switch there is a change in triad convergence and accommodation but if time is allowed between switches to clear up the

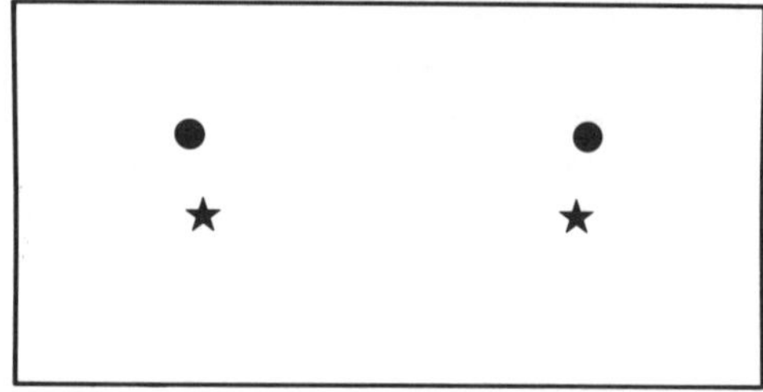

FIGURE 12.7. Stereogram for demonstrating the use of voluntary convergence to switch convergence from far to near or vice versa.

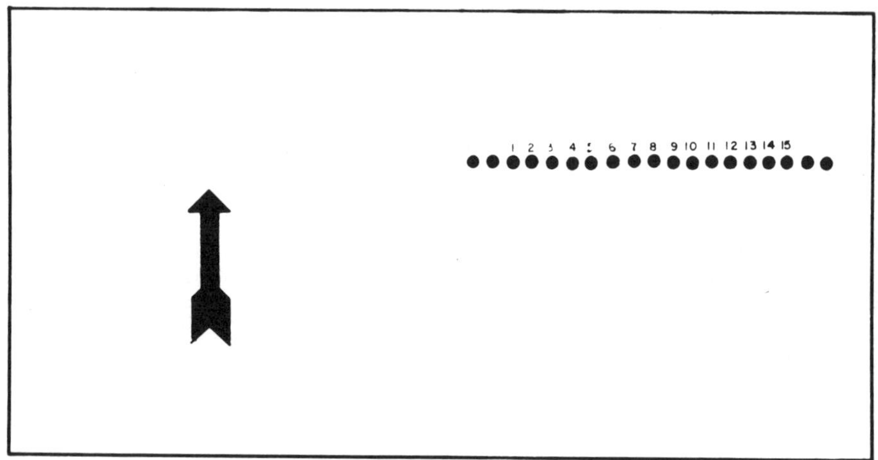

FIGURE 12.8. Stereogram for demonstrating the voluntary control of convergence. Reprinted from *Master Orthorater and Modified Orthorater Instructions*, 3rd. ed. New York: Bausch and Lomb, Inc.

blur, the accommodative convergence is gradually replaced by fusional convergence.

There is also the possibility that the observer can fixate the center of one of the stars or the center of one of the disks and then the placement of a given pair of images in the foveas will result in a reflex fusional movement and a fusion of that pair of images. The fusion reflex is stronger for foveal stimuli than for peripheral stimuli. Since the targets all lie in the same plane, no changes in accommodation are required and none are made.

When the stereogram in Figure 12.8 is viewed in a stereoscope, a person who has been trained to converge the eyes voluntarily can do so to line up the arrow with any of the dots. Fusional convergence is out completely. It is a matter of what strategy can be used to activate the triad response. The subject can voluntarily switch concentration of attention from far to near and vice versa and he will find that the arrow will move to the right or left, and then use this kind of maneuver and its feedback to bring the arrow to rest under a given dot. This activation of the triad center brings about not only changes in convergence but also changes in accommodation and pupil constriction.

Convergent Accommodation vs Accommodative Convergence

Discovery of the Jampel center for the triad response provided an answer to the controversy about accommodative convergence and convergent accommodation. Those who had emphasized the role of convergent accommodation regarded convergence as the primary response and convergent accommodation as a secondary response that follows as a reflex from the first. Those who had emphasized accommodative convergence regarded accommodation as the primary response and accommodative convergence as secondary.

If we accept the concept of a single center like the Jampel center that simultaneously evokes changes in accommodation, in convergence, and in pupil size, there is no need for regarding any of these responses as primary. All we have to do is to say that the Jampel center can be activated in different ways. Accommodation becomes primary only when a change in accommodation or maintaining it at a given level is the primary objective of the voluntary effort that activates the triad mechanism. Convergence becomes primary only when a change in convergence or maintaining it at a given level is the primary objective of the voluntary effort that activates the triad mechanism.

To illustrate accommodative convergence, we place before one eye a group of small Snellen letters and ask the subject to bring them into focus. This is done by activating the Jampel center and this brings along with it constriction of the pupil and the so-called accommodative convergence, which is pure triad convergence.

To illustrate convergent accommodation, we place a number of dots before one eye and an arrow before the other (see Figure 12.8). We must also place a small artificial pupil in front of each eye so that neither can accommodate on the target. We then ask the subject to converge both eyes so that the arrow falls under, let us say, dot number 9. This voluntarily activates the Jampel center to produce pure triad convergence and brings along with it convergent accommodation and also a change in pupil size.

To illustrate the use of the Jampel center to produce a change in pupil size, one can cover one eye and concentrate attention on an imaginary near point. The pupil shrinks, distant targets go out of focus, and the eye under cover turns in. Using a Broca Pupillometer, a subject can

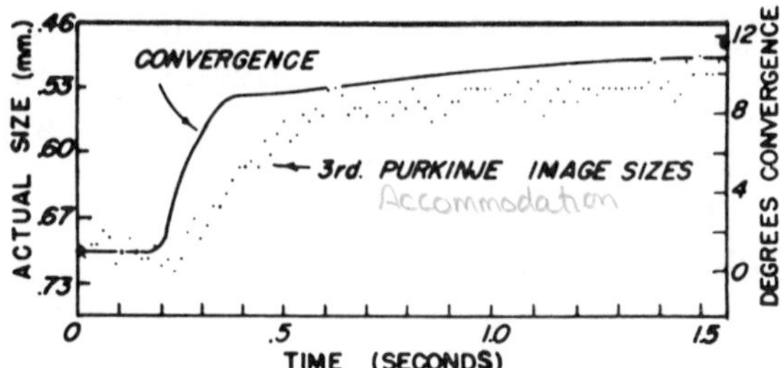

FIGURE 12.9. Simultaneous recording of changes in accommodation and accommodative convergence. Reprinted by permission of the publisher, from Allen MJ. An objective high speed photographic technique for stimultaneously recording changes in accommodation and convergence. American Journal of Optometry and Archives of American Academy of Optometry, © (1949), American Academy of Optometry per The Williams & Wilkins Company (agent).

see a pair of shadows of the pupil of one of the eyes formed on the retina of that eye and can manipulate the triad mechanism to produce a pupil of any given size.

Timing of Accommodation and Accommodative Convergence Responses

Allen (1949) studied the time relations between the accommodative response and the accommodative convergence response. He measured changes in accommodation by means of the third Purkinje image and convergence movements by means of the first Purkinje images in the two eyes. Figure 12.9 shows the changes in each mechanism as a function of time. Convergence appears to be a little faster and this may be attributed to the lag of the lens behind the contraction of the ciliary muscle. The two responses cannot involve a chain reflex.

PROXIMAL CONVERGENCE

Hofstetter (1942) differentiated between proximal convergence and the other forms of convergence and reviewed the history of this topic. Clinically, it was encountered in two ways. If the distance phoria finding was taken with +2.50 lenses and a near (16-in) target, it was found to yield a higher level of convergence than could be found with the distance correction and a 20-foot target. If an attempt was made to measure the distance lateral phoria with an ordinary stereoscope, the phoria found involved a higher level of convergence than that found when the phoria was measured with a target at 20 feet.

An effort was made to relate this phenomenon to instrument myopia in which a person with one eye looking into an instrument such as a microscope would exert accommodation that had to be neutralized by adjusting the eyepiece. The effect appeared to depend on the objects being perceived as closer to the eye than the optical image, and the optical image had to be adjusted to bring it into focus.

It must be recognized that there are two kinds of stimuli to accommodation: (1) awareness of nearness and (2) blur. The accommodative response in both cases can be associated with accommodative convergence, however, and we can hang on to the idea that there is only one motor center through which all accommodative responses must be channeled. If proximal convergence is induced by the effect of awareness of nearness on accommodation and the associated accommodative convergence, one would expect to find the eyes overaccommodated during phoria measurement, but not enough to produce a noticeable blur.

Hofstetter (1951) found the base-in and base-out blur points as well as the phoria to be shifted on the accommodation convergence graph and concluded that there is in fact a form of convergence that is not accommodative convergence. This has never created a problem clinically because target distances have been selected that avoid the problem. In connection with stereoscopes the problem can be solved by using bright points and lines in a dark field.

THE SPIKE

The original haploscope was limited because it could not deal with high levels of accommodation and convergence. The typical young subject can converge between 50° and 60° and accommodate more than 10 diopters. With a new haploscope it was possible to produce stimuli to accommodation and convergence that would exceed these maximal responses.

The set of relative convergence curves for a typical subject is shown in Figure 12.10. At the maximum level of accommodation, the tolerance for base-out prism exceeds the limit of positive fusional convergence found at lower levels of accommodation. This phenomenon has come to be known as the spike. The problem of the spike was pointed out by Hofstetter (1945).

In Figure 12.11 the line RS represents the maximum level of accommodation as determined by the measurement of the amplitude of accommodation. The point P represents the limit of positive fusional convergence at 2.50 diopters of accommodation. The line through P parallel to the phoria line represents the limit of positive fusional convergence. In attempting to do the base-out to blur at the maximum level of accommodation, the target does not blur at point R but remains

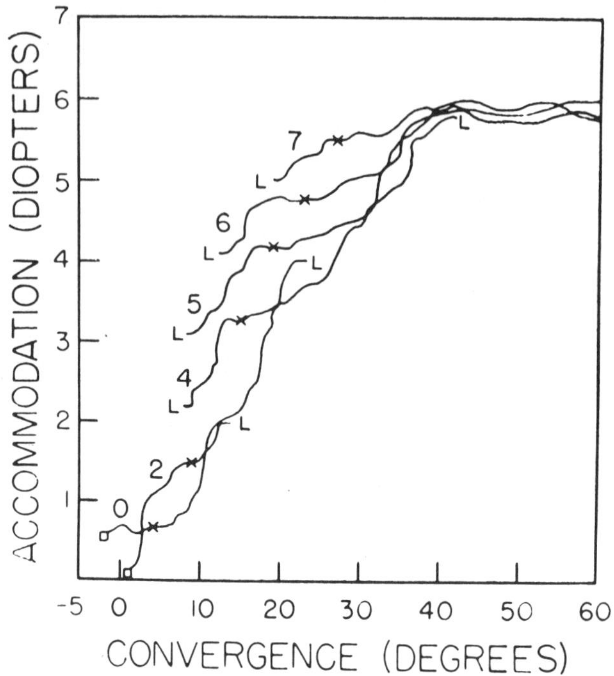

FIGURE 12.10. A set of relative convergence curves similar to that in Figure 11.3 except that this set includes curves at the upper levels of accommodation. Reprinted by permission of the publisher, from Van Hoven RC. Partial cyclopegia and the accommodation-convergence relationship. American Journal of Optometry and Archives of American Academy of Optometry, © (1959), American Academy of Optometry per The Williams & Wilkins Company (agent).

clear and single until it breaks at the point S, which represents the near point of convergence.

Alpern (1950) used a device called a proximometer to study the characteristics of the spike.

My first interpretation of this phenomenon was that the spike indicated latent fusional convergence that could not be expressed until the maximum accommodation had been reached and it was no longer possible to substitute accommodative convergence for positive fusional convergence.

An alternative explanation may be based on the concept of latent accommodation offered by Flieringa and van der Hoeve (1924). They claimed that the upper level of accommodation as measured by clinical tests did not represent the maximum level of contraction of the ciliary muscle, but the level at which the lens stopped responding to reduction of tension in the zonule. The spike therefore must indicate the extent to

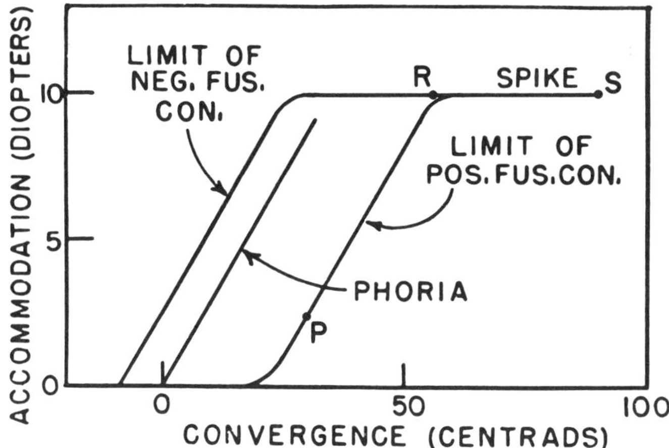

FIGURE 12.11. The spike phenomenon. Reprinted by permission of the publisher, from Fry GA. The image-forming mechanism of the eye. In: J. Field, ed. Handbook of Physiology, Neurophysiology I. American Physiological Society, 1959.

which the ciliary muscle and the associated accommodative convergence keep increasing after the lens has lost its capability of responding to the decreased tension in the zonule. By extending the line representing the limit of positive fusional convergence to the point at which it crosses the vertical line through the near point of convergence, one can locate the level the accommodation would have reached if the lens could have responded to the reduced tension in the zonule (Figure 12.12).

There are two facts that do not gibe with this theory. First, by using eserine it is possible to raise the level of accommodation above that produced in the normal eye by exerting the effort to accommodate to its limit. This was shown by Fincham (1955). Second, the persons who participate in this kind of experiment are very much aware that a great deal of voluntary effort is being expended. The amount of convergence at the near point oscillates and produces what is known as end-point nystagmus. It is difficult to identify any of this activity as related to reflex fusional convergence.

Van Hoven (1959) has made an exhaustive study of this phenomenon. He paralyzed the accommodation of one eye and at various times during recovery measured the AC/A ratio and the amplitude of accommodation for each eye. He showed that during recovery from atropine, the AC/A gradually decreased as the amplitude of accommodation increased, and reached its minimum at the same time that accommodation reached its maximum level. The limit of convergence remained unaf-

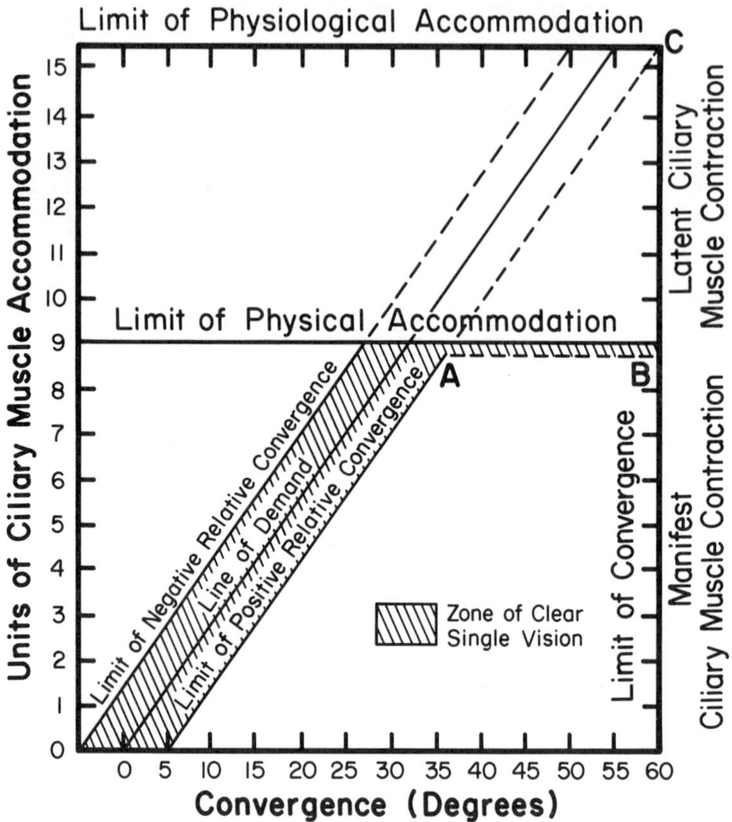

FIGURE 12.12. The concept of latent accommodation. Reprinted by permission of the publisher, from Van Hoven RC. Partial cyclopegia and the accommodation-convergence relationship. American Journal of Optometry and Archives of American Academy of Optometry, © (1959), American Academy of Optometry per The Williams & Wilkins Company (agent).

fected. It may be deduced from this that at a certain level of excitation of the Jampel center, the midbrain center for accommodation saturates and no further ciliary response is possible, although output from the convergence center in the midbrain continues to increase. This gives good reason for concluding that the output from the Jampel center to the convergence center in the midbrain is not relayed through the center for accommodation.

Fry (1959a) made a study of the role played by voluntary effort. He presented the large disc in Figure 12.13 to the right eye and the small disks to the left eye. The arms of the haploscope were set so that various amounts of convergence were required to bring the targets into alignment and then the targets were moved in a fore-and-aft direction to determine

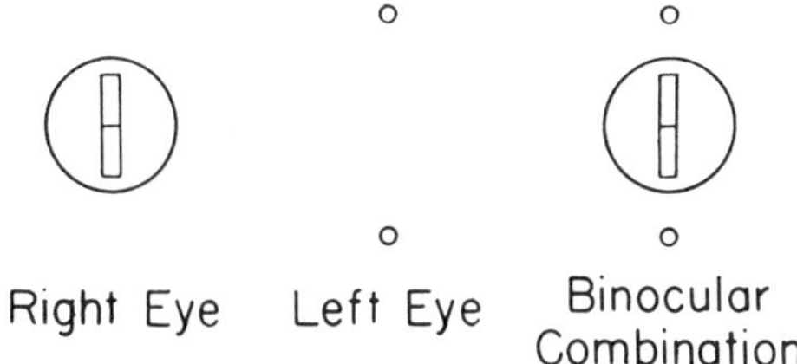

FIGURE 12.13. Targets for measuring the convergent accommodation associated with pure voluntary triad convergence. Reprinted by permission of the publisher, from Fry GA. The effect of homatropine on accommodation-convergence relations. American Journal of Optometry and Archives of American Academy of Optometry, © (1959), American Academy of Optometry per The Williams & Wilkins Company (agent).

the amount of accommodation. The two rectangles were used to assess when the eyes were in or out of focus. The curve representing the accommodation at different levels of convergence follows the phoria line at low levels of convergence, but at the maximum level of accommodation the curve levels off and extends along the spike all the way to the near point of convergence. In this case, the convergence represents accommodative vergence produced by voluntary alignment of the targets, and fusional convergence is not involved in bringing convergence to its maximum level. In the usual procedure for studying the spike, the two eyes are allowed to converge on a target and hence either fusional convergence or accommodative convergence could be involved, but near the end of the spike the fusional convergence is making little or no contribution.

BASE-IN AND BASE-OUT BLUR-BREAK RANGES IN DIFFERENT PERSONS

With the revised haploscope it is possible to vary the stimulus to convergence all the way from the far limit to the near limit of convergence. With this equipment it is possible to find patients with relative convergence curves such as are shown in Figures 12.3 and 12.10 that extend all the way on the base-out side to the near limit of convergence and on the base-in side all the way to the far limit of divergence (Figures 12.14, 12.15, and 12.16).

There are a few people who cannot throw accommodation out of focus to supplement fusional convergence and hence the blur-break range is zero. This is likely to occur in cases of very small AC/A ratios. The phenomenon can occur on either the base-in (Figure 12.17) or the base-out side or both (Figure 12.18).

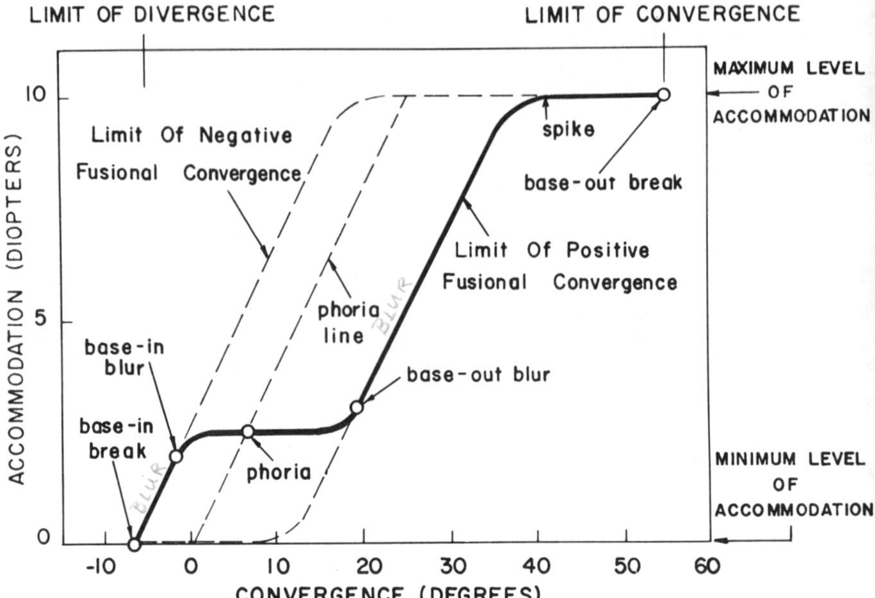

FIGURE 12.14. Relative convergence curve for a 2.50-D stimulus to accommodation. The target is seen as blurred when the amount of accommodation exceeds or falls short of the stimulus by about 0.5 D. A skilled observer can maintain fusion all the way from the absolute limit of divergence to the absolute limit of convergence.

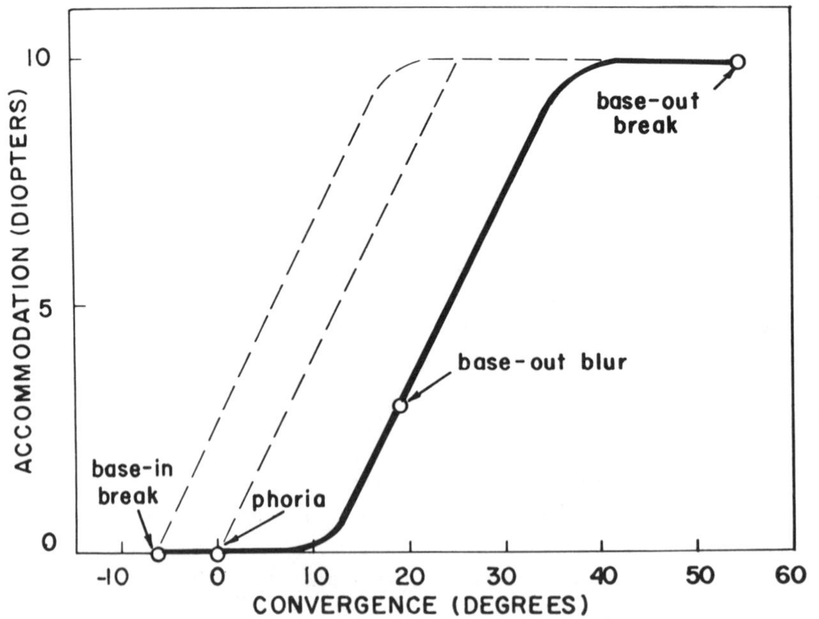

FIGURE 12.15. Relative convergence curve for a zero stimulus to accommodation.

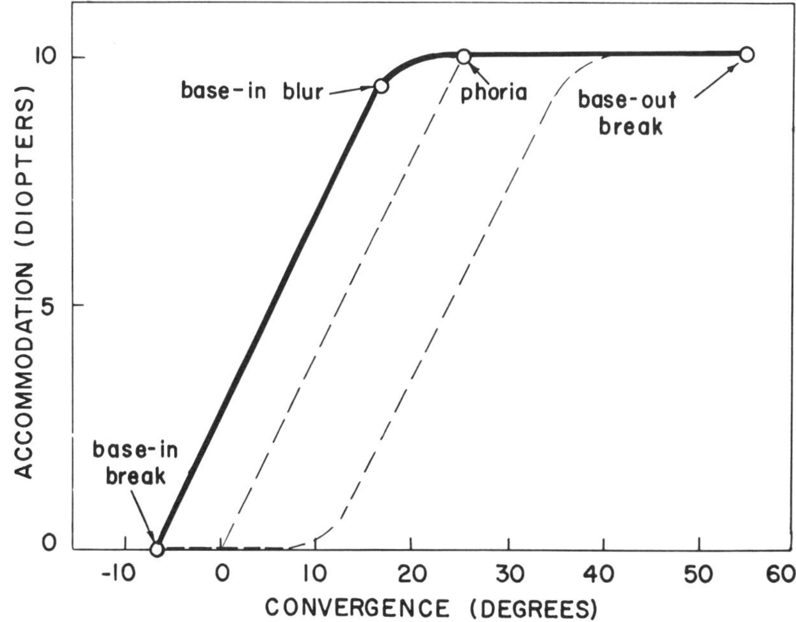

FIGURE 12.16. Relative convergence curve for a stimulus that evokes the maximum level of accommodation.

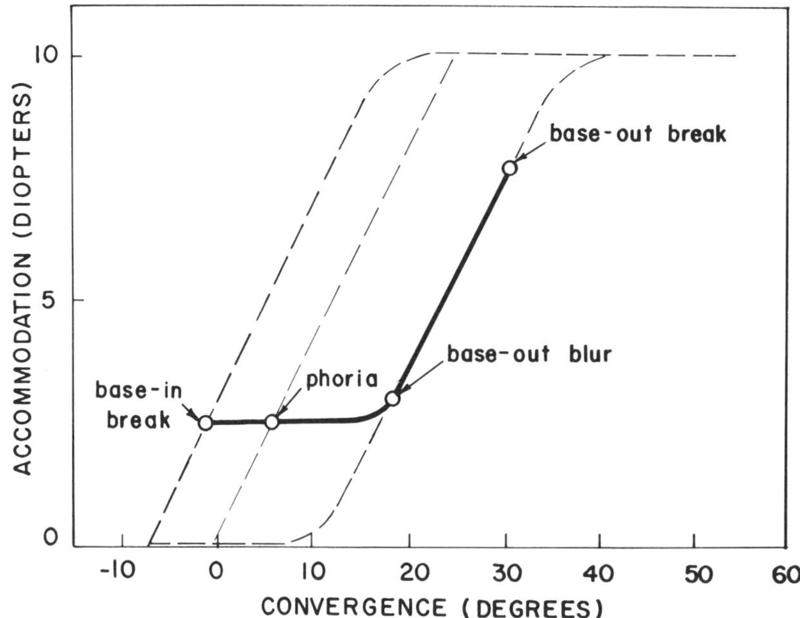

FIGURE 12.17. Relative convergence curve for a 2.50-D stimulus to accommodation for a person who cannot relax accommodation to extend relative convergence in the base-in direction. Also in the base-out direction, the relative convergence does not extend to the absolute limit of convergence.

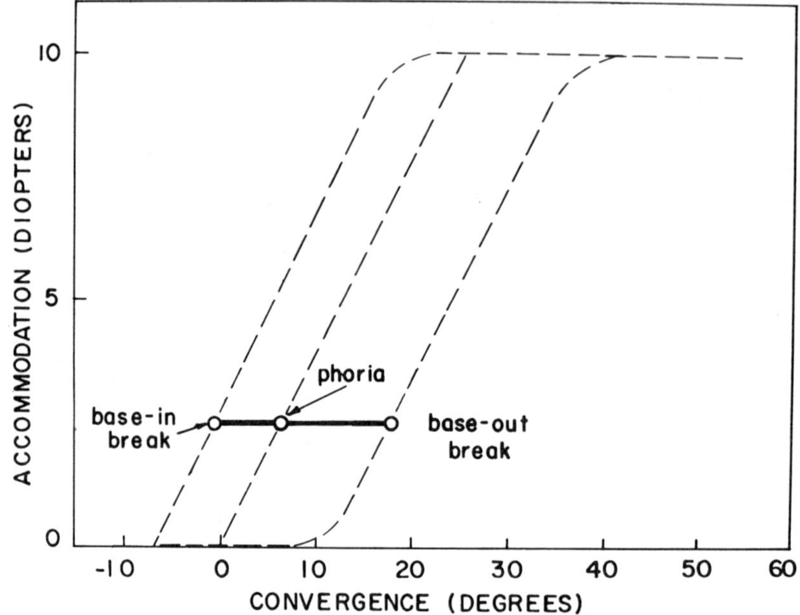

FIGURE 12.18. Relative convergence curve for a 2.50-D stimulus to accommodation for a person who cannot throw his eyes out of focus in either direction to extend relative convergence.

FUSION REFLEX

The recovery findings for base-up and base-down as well as base-in and base-out provide us with information about the fusion reflex. If the recovery finding is made immediately following the break, we have to assume that the eyes drift back to the phoria position. In many cases sufficient time is not allowed for this to happen. To interpret the finding it is also necessary to know whether the subject is fixating the image seen with the left eye or the one seen with the right.

If the test is made properly it indicates how far the image of the target can be displaced in an up, down, right, or left direction from the fovea on the nonfixing eye and still evoke a movement that will make it fuse with the image seen by the fovea of the fixing eye.

It is easier to understand these findings when they are made with a campimeter. The two halves of the campimeter chart are shown in Figure 12.19. A small disk that serves as the fixation point for the right eye is set at the straight ahead position. It is called the stationary target. Let us assume that target for the left eye is brought in from the periphery from different directions to determine the points at which fusional movements are evoked. The line connecting these points is the boundary of the fusion field for the left eye. The phoria point for the left eye can also be located, which indicates the position of the fovea of the left eye at the beginning of the fusional movements.

The fusion field is elliptical and the major axis should correspond to the plane of the horizontal recti of the nonfixing eye. The fusion field for the right eye can be mapped out in a similar way by keeping the stationary target at the straight ahead position for the left eye.

The fusion fields described above are the foveal fusion fields. Peripheral fusion fields can be studied in a similar way by keeping the fixation target at the straight ahead position for the fixing eye and placing the stationary fusion target at some point in the periphery. The fusion reflex is stronger at the fovea than in the periphery.

The recovery test is similar to a jump test in which a person recovers fusion after a prism has been placed before one eye. When the two eyes are suddenly confronted with a sizable disparity they will respond with a fusional movement. Stewart (1961) studied this problem using an ophthalmograph. His data are shown in Figure 12.20. At the outset, the two eyes were converging on a target at three meters when suddenly the eyes were confronted with a pair of targets that required a decrease or increase in convergence.

The ophthalmograph does not properly record the eye movements because it does not eliminate displacements of the eyes with respect to the head. These movements are not differentiated from eye rotations. A part of the noise in the records was introduced in processing the data. Because of this contamination it was not possible for Stewart to detect responses to small changes in the stimulus to convergence. When the change is large enough to produce an identifiable response, it shows that the response has a latent period of about 160 msec and is very rapid at first but slows down when a new stable position is found. This fits in with the principle laid down by Rashbass and Westheimer (1961) that as the eyes approach fusion, the disparity shrinks and the speed of movement

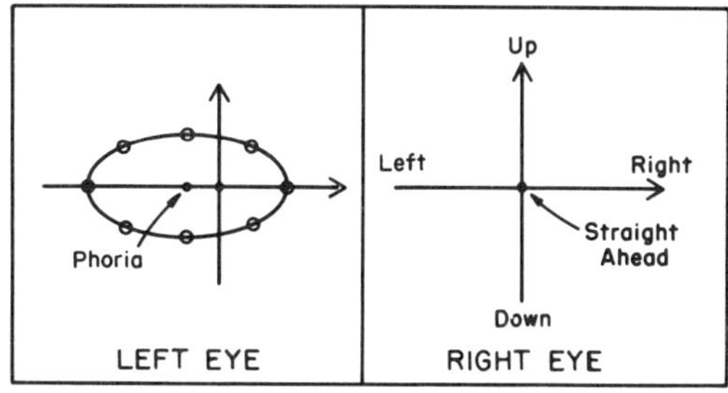

FIGURE 12.19. A plot of the phoria and the limits of the foveal fusion field for the left eye as mapped out with a campimeter.

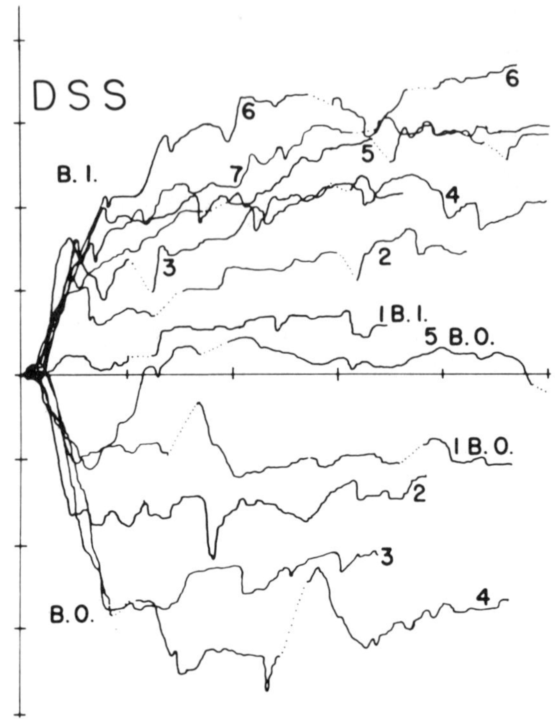

FIGURE 12.20. Change in convergence in recovering fusion after a sudden change in the stimulus to convergence. Each division of the vertical scale represents one prism diopter and each division of the horizontal scale represents one second. The number for each curve represents the change in the stimulus to convergence (prism diopters). Reprinted by permission of the publisher, from Stewart CR. Jump vergence responses. American Journal of Optometry and Archives of American Academy of Optometry, © (1961), American Academy of Optometry per The Williams & Wilkins Company (agent).

slows down. As long as the subject is passive, the response is a recording of the fusion reflex, but if the subject tries to recover fusion voluntarily, this introduces accommodative convergence that gradually gives way to fusional convergence.

Stewart also recorded the changes in convergence that occurred when the stimulus to convergence was suddenly removed after the eyes had been made to converge or diverge from the phoria position for a period of time. During this time the eyes compromised on the mixture of fusional convergence and triad convergence required for single vision with as little sacrifice of clear vision as possible. It took about two seconds for the eyes to return to the phoria position. In this kind of situation Semmlow and Hung (1980) and Semmlow and Heerema (1979) have tried to isolate the roles played by the mechanisms responsible for clear vision and those responsible for single vision.

THE TRIAD PUPIL RESPONSE

Since the triad response involves only accommodative convergence and not fusional convergence, it should be possible to demonstrate that the pupil response associated with convergence is associated with accommodative but not fusional convergence.

Fry (1945), Marg and Morgan (1949, 1950), and Knoll (1949) have investigated this problem. Accommodation and associated accommodative convergence produce a sizable pupil response. Fusional convergence produces a small response in some people but in others no effect on the pupil is found. Further study of this relation is needed.

In the case of a presbyopic person blind in one eye, it is possible to monitor the use of the triad response by measuring the phoria position of the blind eye or by measuring pupil size. Even when one eye is enucleated, one can still use pupil size to monitor use of the triad response.

AGE AND THE AC/A RATIO

Age has two effects on the relation between accommodation and convergence. It lowers the maximum level of accommodation and increases the AC/A ratio. According to Hamasaki, Ong, and Marg (1956) the amplitude drops to zero at about age 54. The increase in the AC/A comes about because the ratio of innervation to accommodation and that to convergence remains constant with age, but the ability of the lens to respond to tension of the zonule decreases. This is difficult to demonstrate by the usual clinical measurements because the depth of focus becomes relatively large with respect to the total range of accommodation in older subjects. It is necessary to carry out the measurements with equipment with which precise measurements of accommodation can be made.

I had occasion to measure the amplitude of my accommodation and to make an assessment of my AC/A ratio at various ages; the data are plotted in Figure 12.21. The curve is based partly on two assumptions: (1) that the amplitude drops to zero at the age of 54 in accordance with the findings of Hamasaki, Ong, and Marg (1956) and (2) that the ratio is inversely proportional to amplitude.

There is, of course, the long-standing controversy as to whether a presbyope requires more ciliary effort to produce one diopter of accommodation than a younger person. Those who claim he does not also have to claim that at the maximal level of accommodation the lens stops re-

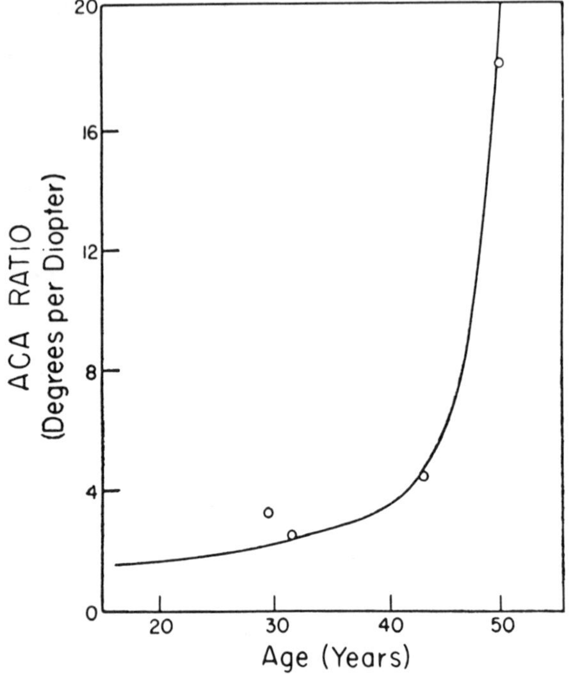

FIGURE 12.21. The relation between the AC/A ratio and age. Reprinted by permission of the publisher, from Fry GA. The effect of age on the AC/A ratio. American Journal of Optometry and Archives of American Academy of Optometry, © (1959), American Academy of Optometry per The Williams & Wilkins Company.

sponding to changes in the ciliary muscle and that there exists a considerable amount of contraction of the muscle that has no effect on the lens. Van Hoven's (1959) study described above indicates that the range of the latent ciliary muscle contraction does not exist and that more effort is required for older people to accommodate.

Hofstetter (1945) pointed out that if a presbyope requires no more effort for one diopter of accommodation than a younger person, there is no reason why one-half of a presbyope's accommodation should be held in reserve while doing near work. This is known as Donder's rule. If no effort is involved, from where does the discomfort come?

MEASUREMENT OF CONVERGENT ACCOMMODATION

Convergence accommodation represents the accommodation associated with a given amount of convergence when there is no stimulus to accommodation. It has always appealed to refractionists that at the near point (16 in) the amount of convergent accommodation that is found in play should be allowed to remain in play for performing tasks at that distance. The usual procedure is to create a stimulus to convergence at 16 inches and measure the accommodation without stimulating it.

One procedure is to place a skiascope and a course target in a plane 16 inches in front of the spectacle plane and find a combination of lenses placed in front of the eyes that will neutralize the reflex. This does not achieve the result desired because the stimulus to accommodation is not completely eliminated and the refractive state changes as the lenses are changed (Fry, 1950).

Another approach is the binocular cross-cylinder test in which the eyes look at the target through crossed cylinders and cannot see the horizontal and vertical lines clearly at the same time. Generally, the accommodation comes to rest at a point in between and hence neither eye is focused on either set of lines. It is assumed erroneously that the stimulus to accommodation is eliminated. A combination of lenses for each eye is found that will make the vertical and horizontal lines equally clear. Here again the refractive state of the eye is not constant during the test and it is difficult to evaluate the final equilibrium that is achieved (Fry, 1940).

The technique devised by Luckiesh and Guth (1949) called sensitometric refraction illustrates a more appropriate procedure for measuring convergent accommodation. A target such as that shown in Figure 12.22 is placed at 16 inches. The vertical line is so blurred that it cannot serve as a stimulus to accommodation but is used as a stimulus for convergence. A gradient neutral filter is placed before each eye and also a plus cylinder with the axis horizontal. These render the biconcave bar invisible for each eye and hence the bar cannot constitute a stimulus to accommodation. The lens in front of one eye is very strong and the biconcave bar is never seen by that eye. The lenses before the other eye, which is being tested, are much weaker and that eye can see the bar when the density of gradient filters is reduced. The filters are rotated until the black bar is visible. As soon as it becomes visible, the test is over and hence the black bar cannot stimulate accommodation. This is repeated for various lenses, and the lens that yields the lowest threshold indicates the amount of accommodation in play.

RELATION OF ACCOMMODATIVE CONVERGENCE TO CONVERGENT ACCOMMODATION

What is the relation of convergent accommodation to accommodative convergence? Theoretically, these two responses are interrelated because

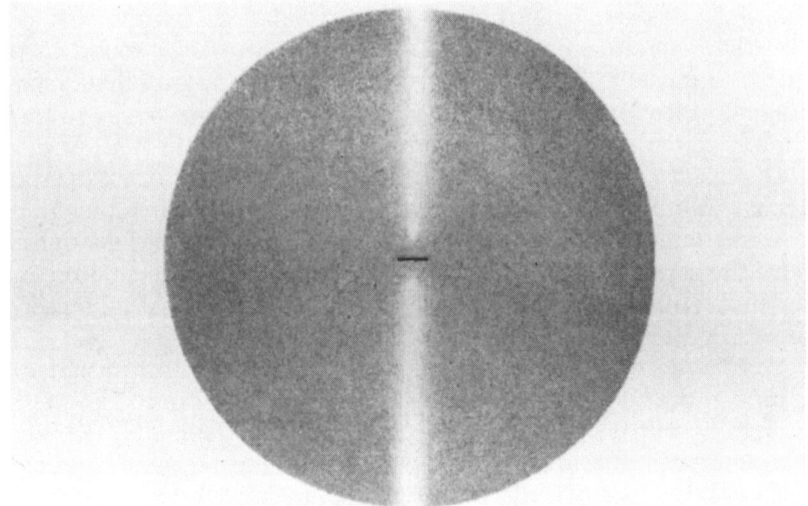

FIGURE 12.22. The target used by Luckiesh and Guth for measuring convergent accommodation. The bright vertical bar is the stimulus for convergence. The black biconcave bar at the center is used for measuring the amount of accommodation in play. Reprinted by permission of the publisher, from Luckiesh M, Buth SK. A sensitometric method of refraction—theory and practice. American Journal of Optometry and Archives of American Academy of Optometry, © (1949), American Academy of Optometry per The Williams & Wilkins Company (agent).

both involve the triad response, and the phoria line representing accommodative convergence on an accommodation convergence graph should conform to the convergent accommodation line when convergent accommodation is produced by pure voluntary triad convergence.

Balsam and Fry (1949) devised a haploscope arrangement that measures both the phoria and convergent accommodation produced by a fusion stimulus. For measuring phoria, the targets shown in Figure 12.23 were used. The Snellen chart was seen by the left eye and the two small disks by the right eye. Two bright vertical lines (not shown in Figure 12.23), which were seen by the left eye to be superimposed on the Snellen target, were used to measure the amount of accommodation. When the Snellen chart is made to fall between the two small disks by moving the arms of the haploscope, the amount of convergence corresponds to the lateral phoria.

The targets for measuring convergent accommodation are shown in Figure 12.24. The large disk is seen by both eyes with a fixed amount of convergence. The large disk and the two small disks are seen through very small artificial pupils to prevent the disk from stimulating accommodation. Two vertical lines (not shown in Figure 12.4) were seen by the

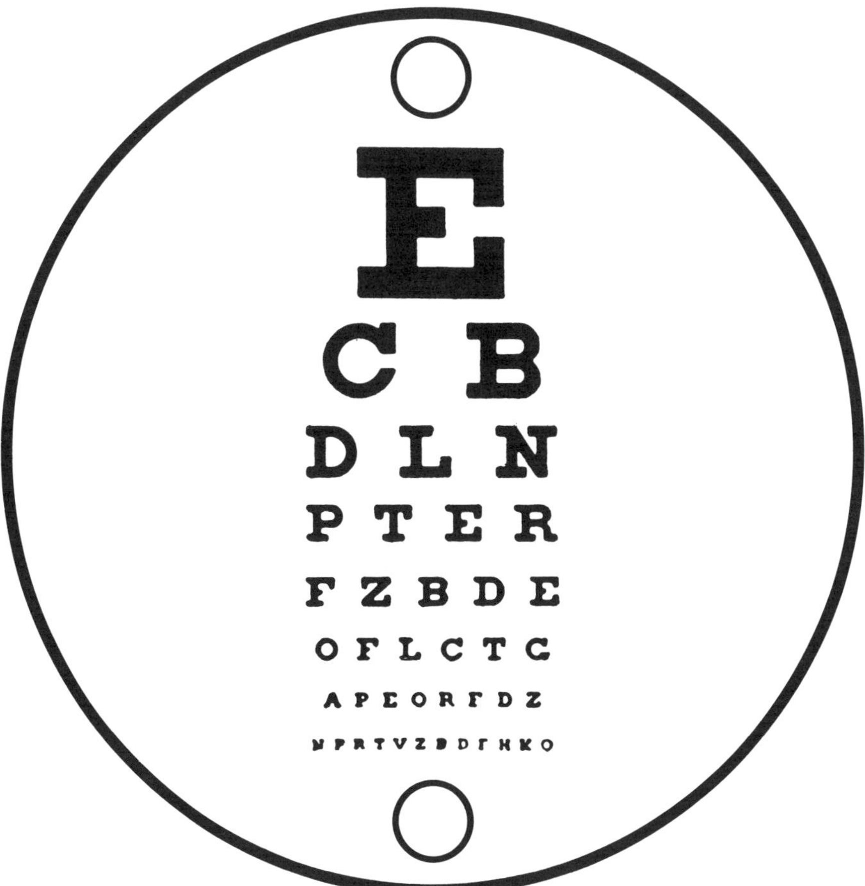

FIGURE 12.23. Targets for measuring accommodative convergence. Reprinted by permission of the publisher, from Balsam MH, Fry GA. Convergence accommodation. American Journal of Optometry and Archives of American Academy of Optometry, © (1959), American Academy of Optometry per The Williams & Wilkins Company (agent).

left eye superimposed on the disk and were used to measure the amount of accommodation in the left eye. The alignment between these vertical lines and the small disks permits a check on the amount of convergence.

Figure 12.25 shows a plot of the findings for one subject. The phoria line is straight and the convergence accommodation line is sigmoid. The lower end of the convergent accommodation line should fall at the limit of divergence at the zero level of accommodation.

Because of the increased depth of focus there is no blur to stimulate

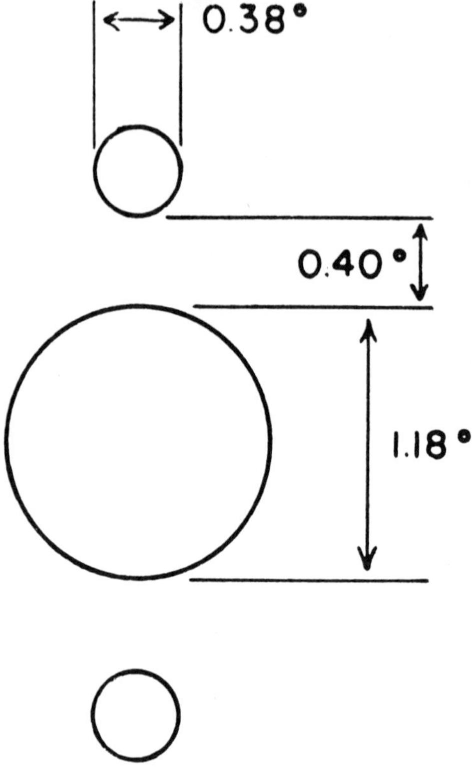

FIGURE 12.24. Targets for measuring convergent accommodation. Reprinted by permission of the publisher, from Balsam MH, Fry GA. Convergence accommodation. American Journal of Optometry and Archives of American Academy of Optometry, © (1959), American Academy of Optometry per The Williams & Wilkins Company (agent).

the eyes to relax accommodation to the usual zero level. At the point of maximum divergence, however, the maximum relaxation of accommodative convergence is required and accommodation should also drop to zero. At the upper level of accommodation, the convergent accommodation curve becomes continuous with the spike.

Failure of the convergent accommodation curve to coincide with the phoria line at intermediate levels of accommodation is probably due to the fact that the curve involves more than pure triad convergence; it includes also some fusional convergence. If the targets in Figure 12.13 had been used that require pure triad convergence for alignment, the two curves should have coincided at the intermediate levels of accommodation.

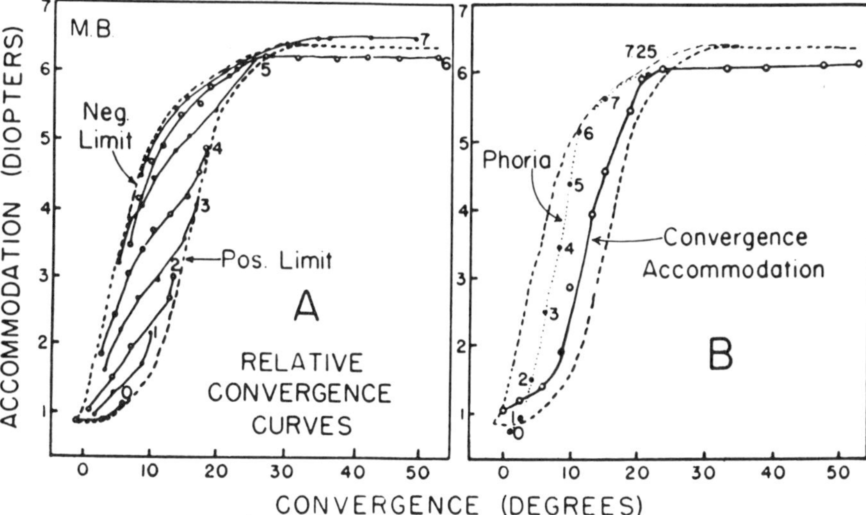

FIGURE 12.25. The relation between accommodative convergence (phoria line) and convergent accommodation. The relative convergence curves in the left graph were used to establish the limits of positive and negative fusional convergence. Reprinted by permission of the publisher, from Balsam MH, Fry GA. Convergence accommodation. American Journal of Optometry and Archives of American Academy of Optometry, © (1959), American Academy of Optometry per The Williams & Wilkins Company (agent).

PATIENT-TO-PATIENT VARIATIONS IN THE AC/A RATIO

The AC/A ratio varies widely from patient to patient. The distribution has been investigated by Fry and Haines (1940); the data are shown in Figure 12.26. Each of the 100 subjects had an amplitude of accommodation in excess of five diopters.

This wide variation is often used as an argument that the AC/A ratio cannot involve an anatomic center such as the Jampel center, but must involve a learned relation such as that suggested by Helmholtz.

Efforts at changing the ratio by training have not been demonstrated to be effective when the results are measured with equipment that provides precise measures of accommodation and convergence. This suggests that the relation is determined by the distribution of elements in the Jampel center and is fixed for a given individual except for changes that occur with age and drugs, which produce their effects at lower levels in the visual system.

Hofstetter (1946) compared the distribution of AC/A ratios in a group of squinters with that for a group of persons with binocular vision and

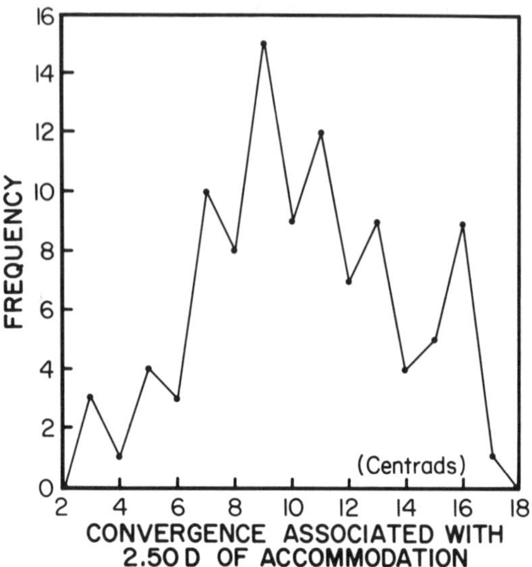

FIGURE 12.26. Distribution of AC/A ratios for 100 subjects. Each subject had an amplitude of accommodation in excess of 5 D.

found the two distributions to be very similar. Hofstetter (1948) also found that the ratios of identical twins are more nearly alike than those of pairs of persons chosen at random, even though the variation from one pair of twins to another is similar to that for unrelated groups of subjects.

CYCLOROTATION ASSOCIATED WITH CONVERGENCE

It has been found that convergence is associated with excyclorotation of the eyes and this occurs with both accommodative and fusional convergence (Allen, 1954). This would imply that a single center in the midbrain subserves both kinds of convergence.

RECIPROCAL INNERVATION AND COMFORT

Reciprocal innervation is found to occur in the case of conjugate movements of fixation. Muscles with actions that oppose each other contract and relax reciprocally. Co-contraction of opposing muscles might lead to increased tension and pain or discomfort. Fixating with one eye while the other is covered is relatively free from discomfort and this is explained by reciprocal innervation.

The fusional innervation involved in compensating vertical phoria does lead to discomfort and the question may be raised whether this kind of innervation leads to co-contraction. The movement involved in overcoming the phoria is small in comparison to the 45° or more that the eyes can turn up or down in conjugate movements of fixation. The same problem occurs with horizontal fusional movements, but here the problem is complicated by the simultaneous occurrence of triad convergence. The triad convergence is disjunctive in the same sense as fusional convergence and divergence, but at low levels of convergence it produces no discomfort.

People blind in one eye converge whenever they accommodate, but are notably free from discomfort. We must therefore suppose that discomfort found in using both eyes must be derived from the fusional convergence or divergence superimposed on the triad convergence. A person with esophoria at distance must use pure fusional divergence to overcome the esophoria, but this is the only instance in which fusional vergence in a horizontal direction occurs without a concurrent involvement of triad convergence.

In the special case of the near point of convergence that involves pure triad convergence, the convergence does produce discomfort, and it must be supposed that at this maximum level of triad convergence a certain amount of co-contraction does exist. This occurs in spite of the fact that at lower levels discomfort is not encountered.

It should be noted that when both eyes turn in at the same time, the total amount that each eye can turn in is about 30° even though each eye can turn in as much as 60° when the opposite eye turns out. This limiting value for convergence cannot therefore depend on check ligaments or on limits of contraction or relaxation of the muscles.

REFERENCES

Allen MJ. An objective high speed photographic technique for simultaneously recording changes in accommodation and convergence. Am J Optom Arch Am Acad Optom 1949;26:279–89.

Allen MJ. The dependence of cyclophoria on convergence, elevation and the system of axes. Am J Optom Arch Am Acad Optom 1954;31:297–301.

Alpern M. Zone of clear single vision at the upper limits of accommodation and convergence. Am J Optom Arch Am Acad Optom 1950;27:491–513.

Balsam MH, Fry GA. Convergence accommodation. Am J Optom Arch Am Acad Optom 1959;36:567–75.

Cross AJ. Dynamic skiametry in theory and practice. (pp 80–3) New York: AJ Cross Optical Co., 1911.

Fincham EF. The proportion of ciliary muscular force required for accommodation. J Physiol 1955;128:99–112.

Flieringa HJ, van der Hoeve J. Accommodation. Br J Ophthalmol 1924;8:97–106.
Fry GA. An experimental analysis of the accommodation-convergence relation. Am J Optom 1937;14:402–14.
Fry GA. Further experiments on the accommodation convergence relationship. Am J Optom 1939;16:325–34.
Fry GA. Significance of the fused cross cylinder test. Optom Weekly 1940;31:16–19.
Fry GA. The relation of pupil size to accommodation and convergence. Am J Optom Arch Am Acad Optom 1945;22:451–65.
Fry GA. Skiametric determination of the near point correction. Optom Weekly 1950;41:1469–72.
Fry GA. The effect of homatropine on accommodation-convergence relations. Am J Optom Arch Am Acad Optom 1959a;36:525–31.
Fry GA. The image-forming mechanism of the eye. In: Field J, ed. Handbook of physiology. Neurophysiology I. Washington: American Physiological Society, 1959b:647–70.
Fry GA. The effect of age on the AC/A ratio. Am J Optom Arch Am Acad Optom 1959c;36:299–303.
Fry GA, Haines HF. Tait's analysis of the accommodative-convergence relationship. Am J Optom 1940;17:393–401.
Hamasaki D, Ong J, Marg E. The amplitude of accommodation in presbyopia. Am J Optom Arch Am Acad Optom 1956;33:3–14.
Helmholtz H. Treatise on physiological optics. (Vol. III, pp 54–8) Southall JPC, ed. Optical Society of America, 1925.
Hering E. Die lehre vom binocularen sehen. (pp 2–14) Leipzig: Engleman, 1868.
Hofstetter HW. The proximal factor in accommodation and convergence. Am J Optom Arch Am Acad Optom 1942;19:67–76.
Hofstetter HW. The zone of clear single binocular vision. Am J Optom Arch Am Acad Optom 1945;22:301–33; 361–84.
Hofstetter HW. Accommodative convergence in squinters. Am J Optom Arch Am Acad Optom 1946;23:417–37.
Hofstetter HW. Accommodative convergence in identical twins. Am J Optom Arch Am Acad Optom 1948;25:480–91.
Hofstetter HW. The relationship of proximal convergence to fusional and accommodative convergence. Am J Optom Arch Am Acad Optom 1951;28:300–308.
Jampel RS. Convergence, divergence, pupillary reactions and accommodation of the eyes from farradic stimulation of the macaque brain. J Comp Neurol 1960;115:371–99.
Knoll HA. Pupillary changes associated with accommodation and convergence. Am J Optom Arch Am Acad Optom 1949;26:346–57.
Luckiesh M, Guth SK. A sensitometric method of refraction—theory and practice. Am J Optom Arch Am Acad Optom 1949;26:367–78.
Maddox EE. The clinical use of prisms. 2nd ed. (pp 83–106) Bristol, England: John Wright & Sons, 1893.
Marg EP, Morgan MW Jr. The pupillary near reflex. Am J Optom Arch Am Acad Optom 1949;26:183–98.
Marg EP, Morgan MW Jr. Further investigation of the pupillary near reflex. Am J Optom Arch Am Acad Optom 1950;27:217–25.
Rashbass C, Westheimer G. Disjunctive eye movements. J Physiol 1961;159:339–60.

Semmlow JL and Heerema D. The synkinetic interaction of convergence accommodation and accommodative convergence. Vision Res 1979;19:1237–42.

Semmlow JL, Hung GK. Binocular interactions of vergence components. Am J Optom Physiol Opt 1980;57:559–65.

Sheard C. Dynamic ocular tests. (pp 58–85) Columbus: Lawrence Press, 1917.

Sheard C. Zones of ocular comfort. Am J Optom 1930;7:9–25.

Stewart CR. Jump vergence responses. Am J Optom Arch Am Acad Optom 1961;38:57–86.

Van Hoven RC. Partial cycloplegia and the accommodation-convergence relationship. Am J Optom Arch Am Acad Optom 1959;36:21–39.

Weaver AM. Optometrical anatomy. (pp 68, 69) Columbus: HL Hedrick, 1937.

13

Graphical Analysis

H. W Hofstetter

HISTORY

The Coordinates

Use of the Cartesian coordinate system to illustrate relationships between accommodation and convergence of the eyes appears to have been initiated by Donders's doctoral student MacGillavry (1858). Later his graphs were published in Donders's book (1864). Convergence was represented on the abscissa scale in degrees and minutes, and accommodation on the ordinate in Parisian inches[1] on a scale of equal reciprocal intervals.

The choice of the abscissa for convergence and of the ordinate for accommodation seems logically to have been due to the aim of MacGillavry's research, namely, to determine the effect of convergence on the amplitude of accommodation, rather than to any consideration of whether it is convergence or accommodation that serves the primary functional role in the interrelationship. Except in one instance (Hofstetter, 1967, 1968), all subsequent users of the Cartesian coordinates for evaluation of the interrelationship have followed the MacGillavry-Donders precedent of representing convergence and accommodation on the abscissa and ordinate, respectively (Nagel, 1880; Landolt, 1886; Pereles, 1889; Schmiedt,

[1] One Parisian inch = 27.07 mm.

1893; Howe, 1900, 1907, 1908; Hess, 1901, 1903; Roelofs, 1913; Flieringa and van der Hoeve, 1924; Weymouth et al., 1925; Sheard, 1930; Lesser, 1933; Fry, 1937; Haines, 1938; Hofstetter, 1945; Westheimer, 1955; Flom, 1960).

Accommodation and Convergence Units

Introduction of the diopter by Monoyer in 1872 (Duke-Elder and Abrams, 1970) quickly added to the ease of specification of accommodation, but there were inconsistencies in the choice of the ocular reference point, with varying preferences for the anterior nodal point, anterior principal point, entrance pupil, and the spectacle plane. The last of these, if only by default, is now by far the overwhelming choice inasmuch as optometric test lenses are routinely placed in, or effectively calculated for, the spectacle plane. Similarly, the specification of convergence underwent several changes, none of which is unanimously favored today. In 1880 Nagel proposed the meter angle, a unit that resembles the diopter in that the number of meter angles of convergence is equal to the reciprocal of the distance in meters between a binocularly fixated object in the median plane and the center of rotation of each eye. The actual angle is of course not the same for different interpupillary distances, nor do the obtained values precisely equal the diopter values, which are not measured from the center of rotation. Also, meter angles are not linearly additive or easily transformed into optical prism scale units.

A few years later two new angular units were introduced almost simultaneously: the prism diopter by Prentice in 1890 (Prentice, 1907), and the centrad by Dennett in 1891 (Emsley and Swaine, 1951). The prism diopter, or prism dioptry as Prentice preferred to call it, is conventionally symbolized by the Greek letter delta, Δ, and is mathematically equal to 100 times the tangent of the angle. Because measurements of prism deviations, phorias, and vergences are typically made on a tangential scale they may be made directly in prism diopters, although they are not linearly additive for large angles.

The centrad, also called arc centune, is conventionally symbolized by the inverted delta, ∇, and is equal to one one-hundredth of a radian, or 0.573°. It has all of the favorable and unfavorable attributes of a degree scale except that the number of centrads of deviation produced by an ordinary ophthalmic glass prism closely approximates the refracting angle of the prism in degrees, that is, a 1° glass prism produces approximately 1^{∇} of light deviation. For small angles the centrads and prism diopters are practically equal.

Uses of the Graph

For about 80 years the Cartesian coordinate system was used in this connection to illustrate only statistical and research data involving accommodation and convergence, as in published research reports and textbooks. The measurement criterion for convergence was the presence or absence of diplopia, and that for accommodation was the presence or absence of blurredness. In each case the responses were presumed to be respectively equal to the stimulus to convergence and to the stimulus to accommodation whenever the binocularly fixated object was seen singly and clearly.

A suggestion that the graph be used by refractionists as a routine clinical aid appears to have been made initially by Lesser in 1933. He included a somewhat unique design in his textbook for practitioners, calling it a "neurological chart," but it suffered from inadequate explanation. In about 1938 the basic graphical form was adapted by Fry for use in optometry classrooms and clinics at the Ohio State University to analyze the accommodation/convergence findings of individual patients. The adaptation consisted of (1) labeling and numbering the ordinate scale at the left to represent the stimulus to accommodation, (2) a supplementary ordinate scale at the right to represent lens additions to the distance correction for testing at 40 cm, (3) labeling and numbering the abscissa scale at the bottom to represent convergence of the lines of sight from parallelism in terms of measurement on an ophthalmic prism scale at 6 m or infinity, and (4) a supplementary abscissa scale at the top to represent prism scale readings when testing at 40 cm. This graph is illustrated in Figure 13.1.

During the next decade the same graphical form with various minor adaptations came into wide use as a clinical tool and classroom aid in optometry schools in the United States and Canada and subsequently in a number of other countries.

CONSTRUCTION AND DESIGN

Assumptions and Approximations

In the design of the graphical form in Figure 13.1 a number of assumptions and approximations were made to be convenient for clinical measurements at the test distances of 6 m and 40 cm. The conventional optometric testing distance at or about six meters was considered reasonably equivalent to infinity. A fixed allowance of 15^{Δ} was made for the required convergence at the distance of 40 cm regardless of the patient's inter-

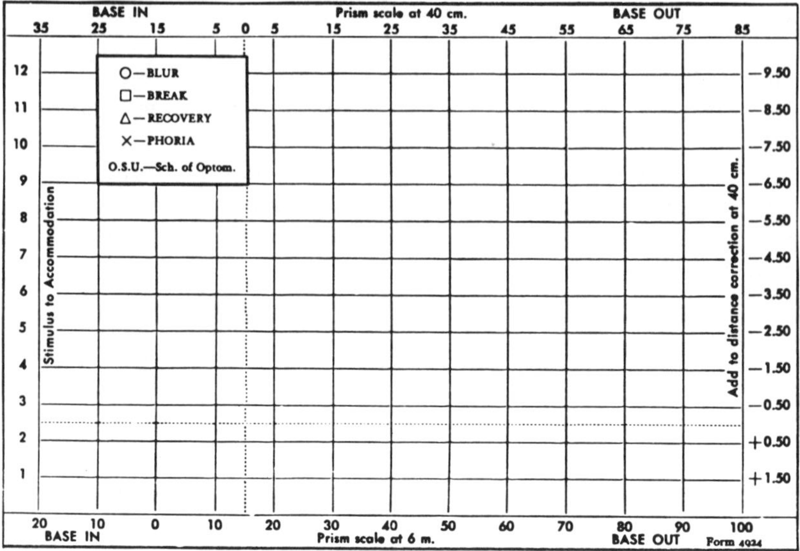

FIGURE 13.1. Graph form introduced by Fry at the Ohio State University in 1938.

pupillary distance, as shown by the 15^{Δ} displacement of the upper scale with respect to the lower scale. For purposes of reckoning accommodation and convergence stimulus values, the test object distance for each was assumed to be from the same ocular plane of reference, that is, that the ocular center of rotation and the spectacle plane were approximately coincident. In addition, representation of convergence in terms of the "prism scale at 6 m" made no allowance for the effectivity of the measuring prism in terms of the center of rotation of the eye.

These errors, however, are rarely of serious magnitude in terms of the purposes and interpretations of routine optometric findings on individual patients, especially if the examiner is aware of their nature and mode of occurrence. Familiar with the influence of such errors on the measurements, the examiner can still judge both the validity and reliability of individually plotted data points from knowledge of certain firmly established interrelationships in much the same way that one can ascertain all cardinal directions on the horizon if at least one is known.

The "Demand" Line

A secondary construction feature often included in the design of the graph is the "demand," "orthophoria," or "Donders" line, an oblique line or curve extending from the zero-zero coordinate point through about the 2.50 D&15^{Δ} coordinate point and beyond. This is the locus of points representing accommodation and convergence stimulus values of a fixation object at various distances along the observer's midline. Originally it was used by MacGillavry and Donders to illustrate the mechanically ideal relationship between accommodation and convergence. It has been adapted in recent years to compensate for variations of interpupillary distances, shown as families of curves in Figures 13.2 and 13.3. To compute these curves the reference plane for convergence was assumed to lie 2.7 cm posterior to the spectacle plane, the reference plane for accommodation.

The demand lines or curves serve as well to facilitate easy plotting of clinically obtained optometric data (Pitts and Hofstetter, 1959). To do so for each clinical datum it is first necessary to locate the point that represents the testing distance on the demand curve for the appropriate interpupillary distance. This point is at the intersection of the accommodative stimulus dioptric equivalent of the test target distance and the demand curve. From this point, in Figure 13.2 the datum is plotted up (for minus lenses) or down (for plus lenses) according to the number of

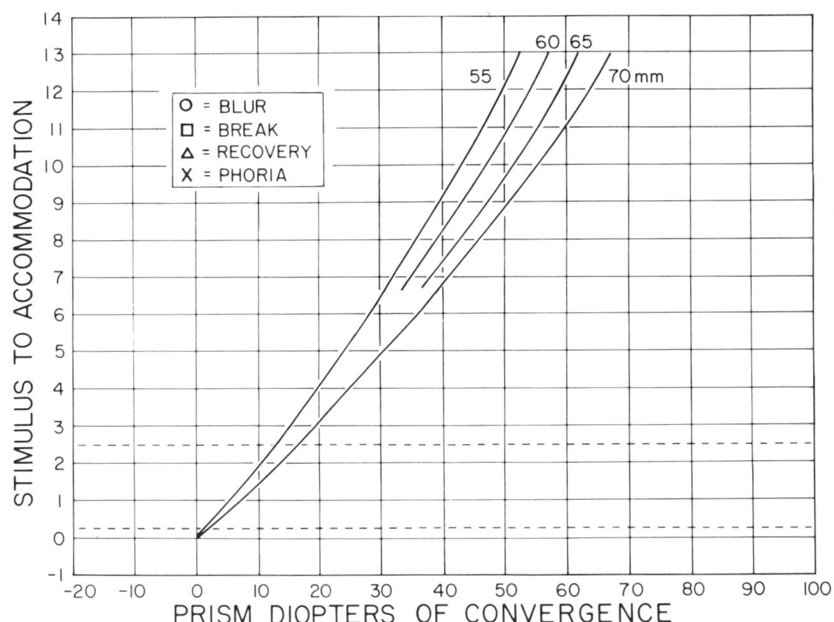

FIGURE 13.2. Conventional graphical analysis form. The dotted horizontal lines represent the accommodative stimulus values of test targets at 4 m and 40 cm. The numbers adjacent to the demand curves are interpupillary distance values. The ordinate values are with reference to the spectacle plane, and the abscissa with reference to the ocular centers of rotation. The spectacle plane is assumed to be 52 mm anterior to the plane of the centers of rotation.

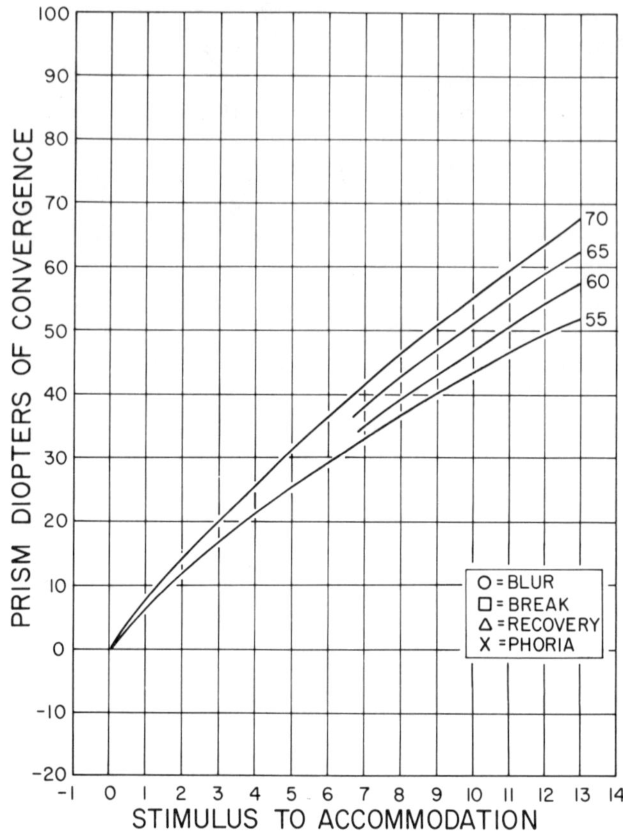

FIGURE 13.3. The inverse of Figure 13.2, i.e., with accommodation on the abscissa and convergence on the ordinate.

diopters of auxiliary lenses in place, and to the right (for base-out) or left (for base-in) according to the number of prism diopters of lenses in place. In Figure 13.3 the minus and plus lens additions would be plotted to the right and left, and the base-out and base-in upward and downward, respectively.

The actual stimulus values, including effects of both target distance and auxiliary lenses, are coordinate values on the abscissa and ordinate scales of the graph itself in either Figure 13.2 or 13.3.

Correction of Convergence Measurement Errors

When, as in many clinical settings, virtually all optometric testing is done at 4 m (Hofstetter, 1973) and 40 cm, and an average interpupillary distance of about 63 or 64 mm (Hofstetter, 1972) is assumed for each patient, the two reference demand points may be considered to be at 1.5^{Δ}, 0.25 D for

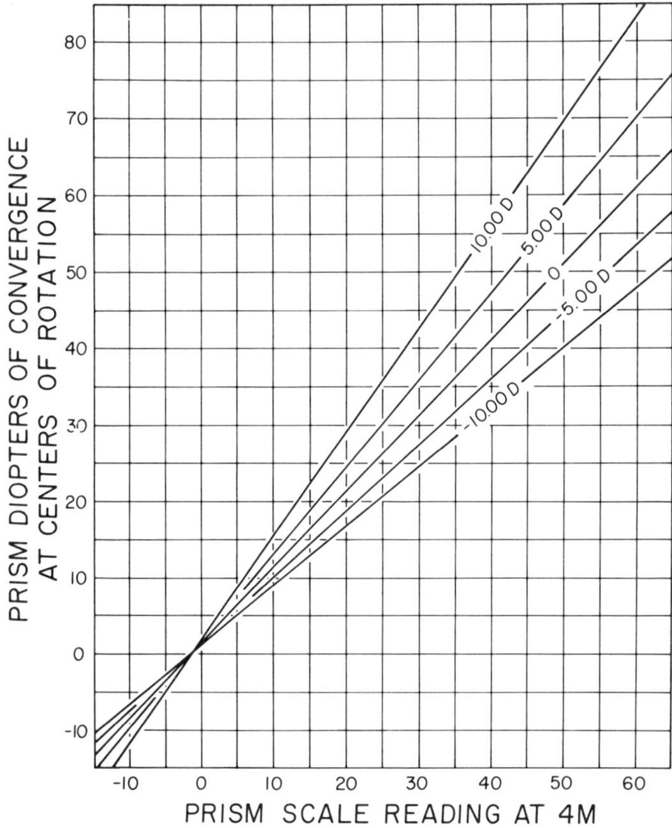

FIGURE 13.4. The effective convergence at the centers of rotation represented by prism scale readings obtained through various powers of lenses when the test target is 4 m anterior, the measuring prisms 25 mm anterior, and the center of rotation 27 mm posterior, to the spectacle plane. The oblique lines correspond to their indicated lens powers in the horizontal meridian. (See page 446 for textual explanation.)

the 4-m distance and 15^{Δ}, 2.5 D for the 40-cm distance, with reasonably small and infrequent error. When, however, the interpupillary distance is quite extreme, or the lens correction for the refractive error is quite large, or the prism scale reading is unusually high, such simplified approximations can result in significant error even for individual case analysis. For statistical purposes a resultant error of lesser magnitude may take on significance.

These sources of error may be almost completely eliminated by use of the following formula:

$$A = \frac{d\Delta - S\Delta + 100p}{C + d - CDd} \qquad (a)$$

where: A = angle of convergence in prism diopters;
d = distance from spectacle plane to target in meters;
Δ = prism scale reading in prism diopters (base-in negative);
S = separation of spectacle and prism planes in meters;
p = the interpupillary distance in meters;
C = distance from plane of the centers of rotation to the spectacle plane in meters;
D = power of lenses in the spectacle plane in diopters.

Graphical representations of this formula are shown in Figures 13.4 and 13.5 for the respective test distances of 4 m and 40 cm, for which C and S are assumed to be 27 and 25 mm, respectively. The test distances

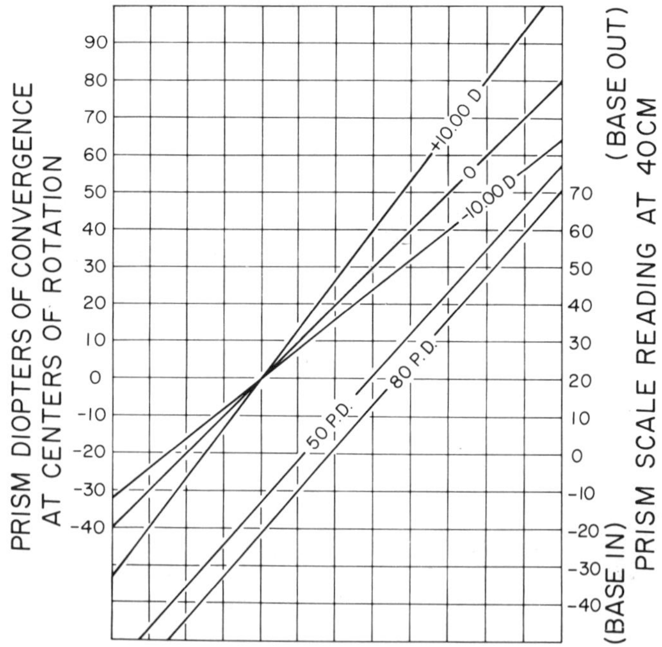

FIGURE 13.5. Nomograph showing the effective convergence at the centers of rotation (scale at left) represented by prism scale readings (scale at right) obtained through various powers of lenses and for different interpupillary distances when the test target is 40 cm anterior, the measuring prisms 25 mm anterior, and the centers of rotation 27 mm posterior, to the spectacle plane. The two parallel oblique lines correspond to the extreme interpupillary distances (*PD*) of 50 and 80 mm. The three oblique lines intersecting at zero convergence correspond to their indicated lens powers in the horizontal meridians. Effective convergence is obtained by moving leftward from the given prism scale reading to the appropriate interpupillary distance (*PD*) value, then upward to the appropriate lens value, and finally leftward again to the effective convergence scale value.

comply with recent recommendations of the National Academy of Sciences—National Research Council (Working Group 39, 1980).

In Figure 13.4 the interpupillary distance is ignored because the errors attributable to its normal variations are negligible at the testing distance of 4 m. The lens power in the spectacle plane, however, as represented in the family of oblique lines, can introduce substantial prismatic effect. The graph shows, for example, that a prism scale reading of $+20^{\Delta}$ (base-out) can represent 19^{Δ} of convergence when measured through -5.00-D lenses, or 24.5^{Δ} through $+5.00$-D lenses.

Figure 13.5 is a nomograph designed to include corrective allowance for differences of interpupillary distance, which take on significance at the 40-cm test distance, and with increasing magnitude at shorter distances as is apparent in formula (*a*). The nomograph shows, for example, that for the very extreme interpupillary distances of 50 and 80 mm a $+20^{\Delta}$ prism scale reading through plano lenses would represent 29^{Δ} and 36^{Δ} of convergence from parallelism, respectively. For this test distance each interpupillary distance difference of 4 mm produces an effective convergence difference of approximately 1^{Δ}.

DATA TO BE PLOTTED

In terms of conventional clinical tests and measurements the data indicative of relationships between accommodation and convergence are of four types based on four different psychophysical criteria: blurs, breaks, recoveries, and phorias, represented graphically by the symbols ○, □, △, and X, respectively, as shown in Figures 13.2 and 13.3.

Blurs, Breaks, and Recoveries

A blur may be induced by the binocular addition of plus or minus spherical lenses, or of base-in or base-out prism in or near the spectacle plane while the subject is fixating an otherwise clearly seen object at some empirically determined distance in the midsagittal plane. If a blur is not induced when the lenses or prisms are added, a break or doubling of the fixated object can be expected to occur in its stead. Either the blur or the break-without-a-preceding-blur may be regarded quite equivalently as a limit of clear single binocular vision, often abbreviated CSBV.

A break or diplopia may be induced by the binocular addition of base-in or base-out prism whether or not it is preceded by a blur. A break may also be induced by the binocular addition of plus or minus lenses in certain circumstances when the decreased or increased accommodative response invokes too little or too much accommodative convergence, respectively. A break that is preceded by a blur is an indication of the limit of single (but not clear) binocular vision and can be plotted on the graph in terms of its accommodation and convergence stimulus values, but its position on the accommodation scale (the ordinate in Figure 13.2) is quite meaningless as a measure of accommodative response.

A recovery is obtained by reduction of the binocular addition of prisms or lenses that previously induced a break until the diplopia images are again fused into one. If the subject accommodates during the test so as to keep the diplopic images clear, and therefore also the resultant fused image clear, and if he can invoke his full fusional response during the diplopia, the recovery finding is also a kind of measure of the limit of clear single binocular vision. Without meeting these conditions, however, the recovery finding is quite meaningless as a direct measure of either the accommodative or convergence function. Nevertheless, this finding, like the break-preceded-by-a-blur, may be plotted in terms of its coordinate stimulus values as a kind of statistical reinforcement of the reliability and validity of the companion blur and break-without-a-preceding-blur.

Phorias and Other Tests

A (lateral) phoria measurement is obtained by any of numerous techniques in which the binocular fusion stimulus is absent or rendered inadequate, and the convergence or divergence component of the measuring stimulus is varied by means of prisms or mirrors until both retinal images fall on their respective foveas or in apparent vertical alignment with each other. Probably most common in optometric practice is the dissociation by means of base-up or base-down prism in front of one eye and the vertical alignment of the resultant two perceived images of a test object by varying the amount of base-in or base-out prism in front of the other eye. If the subject maintains clarity of the test target, that is, of one of the diplopic images, and if his/her retinal correspondence is normal, the phoria indicates the convergence of the lines of sight associated with accommodation in play in the absence of any stimulus to fusion.

A fifth kind of test indicative of the functional relationship between accommodation and convergence is the measurement of accommodation while the convergence stimulus is in effect but the accommodative stimulus is absent. Insofar as a visible convergence stimulus cannot be presumed to be without some accommodative stimulus value, this test is not totally feasible. Certain ordinary clinical procedures, such as the crossed cylinder and bichrome tests (Cline, Hofstetter, and Griffin, 1980), are sometimes presumed to approach the desired conditions, but such data have not been used for routine clinical analysis of accommodation-convergence relationships.

Computation of Stimulus Values

For each of these tests and measurements ordinate and abscissa values in Figures 13.2 and 13.3 can be derived from the distance of the real test object and the dioptric and prism power of the lenses in front of the eyes. In conventional graphing the dioptric lens values affecting the stimulus to accommodation are the lens values supplementary to those that correct the subject's ametropia. For example, a 2-diopter myope looking at a test object at 40 cm through a pair of −3.00 diopter spherical lenses is considered to have a stimulus to accommodation of 3.5 diopters. This is according to the formula

$$S = \frac{1}{d} - D + R \qquad (b)$$

in which S = stimulus to accommodation;
d = distance from spectacle plane to test object in meters;
D = total power of the lenses in front of the eye (in the spectacle plane);
R = power of lenses that correct the ametropia.

The amplitude of accommodation can be reckoned from the same formula. When it is measured monocularly by a push-up technique the accompanying convergence is not known, in which case the finding may be plotted simply as a straight line perpendicularly intersecting the accommodation scale at the amplitude value.

Plotting of convergence values is usually approximated by merely adding $1\frac{1}{2}^{\Delta}$ to the lateral prism scale readings at 4 m, or 15^{Δ} at 40-cm testing. The more precise techniques are described in the preceding section on construction and design.

The near point of convergence obtained by a direct push-up technique with no prisms or lenses in place may be converted to prism diopters by the formula

$$A = \frac{100p}{C + d} \qquad (c)$$

derived directly from formula (a). Because the accompanying accommodation is not known this finding should be plotted as a straight line perpendicularly intersecting the convergence scale at the prism dioptric value of A.

CLINICAL INTERPRETATION

Purposes

The basic values of graphing accommodation versus convergence findings are those of graphing any quantitatively expressible data, namely, the enhanced visibility of trends and interrelationships; the ease of quantification, interpolation, and extrapolation of such trends and relationships by direct inspection; and the improved identifiability of spurious findings in terms of both reliability and validity.

Apparently because the technique of graphical analysis of clinical data is routinely taught to optometry students in association with diagnostic and prescribing methods, there occurs frequently the misconception that graphical analysis is per se a doctrinal concept to be accepted or rejected on the basis of philosophical criteria. It needs therefore to be emphasized that graphical analysis as applied to optometric data is simply analogous to graphic techniques used in every other field in which quantifiable data are viewed. It is a mode of data handling, not a theoretical approach based on one or another eclectic concept.

Errors to Consider

Interpretation of plotted clinical findings is of course dependent in large part on an awareness of certain fundamental relationships that are more perfectly demonstrable only under rigorous experimental controls. Such influences as changes of the perceived distance of the test object, variation of pupil size or of angular subtense of the test object, and of inadequate elimination of fusion stimuli, are all sources of error for which allowances must be made for best interpretation.

Changes of the perceived distance of the test object are quite normally associated with routine clinical testing at near and distance. On the other hand the changes are relatively negligible with increases and decreases of dioptric lens powers. Perceived distance changes have been found to result in average (and widely variant) positive displacements of 1.5^{Δ}, 7.6^{Δ}, and 2.6^{Δ} of the base-in and base-out limits of clear single binocular vision and of the phorias, respectively, for identical levels of the accommodation stimulus at 6 m and 33 cm testing distances (Hofstetter, 1951). This phenomenon is variously called proximal, psychic, or directional convergence.

Pupil size itself is covariant with accommodation and may also be altered by differences in test target luminance. The angular subtense of the test object, unless specifically compensated for by systematic changes of test object size, will vary with test distance and the power and placement of the test lenses. Each of these factors will vary the magnitude of the depth of focus, the subject's ability to detect out-of-focus blurredness, and therefore the accommodative accuracy of any given data point.

Inadequate elimination of fusion stimuli may derive, for example, from the vertically oriented borders of a test target enclosure or frame that may be too long to be completely separated vertically by a nominal amount of dissociating prism. This can provide an unintended lateral fusion stimulus during phoria measurement.

The Double Parallelogram Model

When these various sources of measurement error are eliminated or minimized, the relationships between accommodation and convergence can be represented by a double parallelogram, the zone of clear single binocular vision (Hofstetter, 1945) illustrated schematically in Figure 13.6. These relationships may then be quantitatively specified in terms of five fundamental variables (Fry, 1943) as follows:

1. The distance phoria (or tropia), which serves as a point of reference to identify the position of the graph on the convergence scale. It is located at zero on the accommodation scale when the distance of the test is infinite and the subject is corrected for ametropia.
2. Amplitude of accommodation, the height of the parallelogram.
3. The accommodative convergence to accommodation (AC/A) ratio, corresponding to the inclination of the parallelogram. In Figure 13.6 the ratio is $4^{\Delta}/1$ D, approximately a population average.
4. Positive fusional convergence (PFC), the lateral distance from the phoria line (median oblique line) to the base-out limit (righthand border).

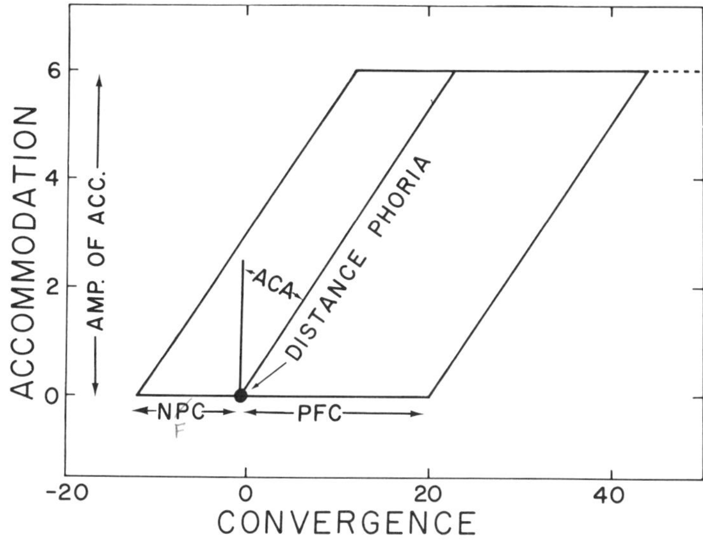

FIGURE 13.6. Schematic representation of the zone of clear single binocular vision in terms of Fry's (1943) five fundamental variables.

5. Negative fusional convergence (NFC), the lateral distance from the phoria line to the base-in limit (lefthand border).

The dotted line at the upper right corner of the parallelogram merely calls attention to the fact that there is conflicting evidence as to whether or not the maximum attainable convergence in some subjects extends beyond the limit of the upper right corner of the parallelogram (Hofstetter, 1945; and Alpern, 1950). In terms of graphical analysis of clinical findings, however, this involves only the interpretation of the near point of convergence.

It is the above set of relationships that an examiner attempts to deduce from clinically determined findings for a given subject. Knowing that the magnitude of each of the five fundamental variables is not derivable from knowledge of the magnitudes of the other four, but that they must form a double parallelogram, one can pursue graphical analysis quite methodically, much as one might solve a puzzle of a structural nature for which only the sought-after shape is known.

Depth of Focus Effects

The effect of a given depth of focus on this kind of analysis is illustrated schematically in Figure 13.7 in which a depth of focus of a full diopter is represented by a series of arrows. In terms of pure detectability of blurredness, one diopter is certainly an excessive assumption, but it may not be so in test procedures requiring that the subject report blurredness only when he or she is certain of its occurrence. No allowance is made for variation of depth of focus at different levels of accommodation.

It can be seen in Figure 13.7 that the depth of focus does not affect the lateral position of the absolute convergence and divergence limits, but that it does affect the intermediate convergence and divergence limits of clear single binocular vision as lateral vectors of the vertical expansions of the zone. The fundamental parallelogram is the interior zone, delineated by subtraction of depth-of-focus values, the arrows, from the clinically measured outer limits. Exceptions are the lower right and upper left corners, shown as dashed lines, where subjects characteristically show inability, respectively, to relax or exert accommodation fully. These suggest that near the limits of positive and negative fusional convergence there are induced tendencies to invoke accommodation as if to anticipate the need for accommodative convergence or divergence.

Blur and Break Interrelationships

This suggestion is supported by the solid sigmoid curves in Figure 13.8. These curves are schematic representations of haploscopic tracings of the

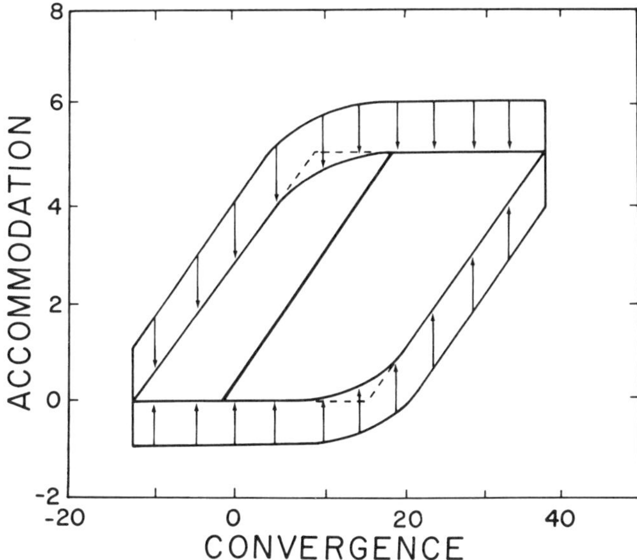

FIGURE 13.7. Schematic representation of the relationship of the fundamental (inner) and clinically measured (outer) limits of the zone of clear single binocular vision in which the depth of focus is arbitrarily assumed to be one diopter.

accommodative response to different levels of accommodative stimulus while the fusional convergence stimulus is continuously varied from one extreme to the other (Fry, 1937, 1938; Hofstetter, 1945). In the neighborhood of the phoria each curve is quite horizontal, showing no change of accommodation with change of convergence. As the limit of positive fusional convergence is approached, however, accommodation increases, and may continue to do so until its amplitude is reached, and a blur is reported when the accommodation and its stimulus are a diopter apart (depth of focus). If accommodation continues to increase into greater and greater blurredness the absolute maximum of convergence, represented by the squares, may be reached at every accommodative stimulus level.

Similarly, but inversely as the limit of negative fusional convergence is approached, accommodation may reduce until it reaches zero, and a blur is reported when the depth of focus is exceeded. If relaxation of accommodation continues to the zero level, the blurredness increases further and the absolute maximum of divergence may be attained at every accommodative stimulus level.

The absolute maximum of convergence, or divergence, may not be attained, however, if after a blur is reported the subject chooses not to accept an increasingly greater blur or attempts to recover the clarity of the test object, whereupon the accommodative convergence, or divergence, ceases and diplopia occurs.

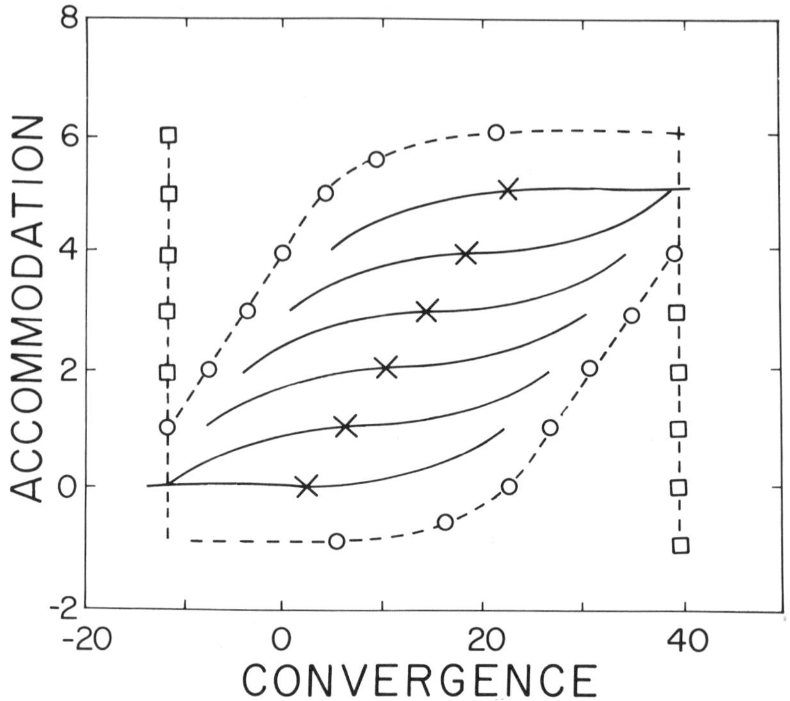

FIGURE 13.8. Schematic representation of the relationship of blurs (○), breaks (□ and +), phorias (*X*), and accommodative responses (*sigmoid curves*) to each of several accommodative stimulus levels as the fusional convergence stimulus is varied.

If the subject chooses not to accommodate, or not to relax accommodation, in order to prevent a break, the break then occurs as soon as the limit of fusional convergence, or divergence, is reached, and no blur is reported. In most such cases, i.e., where no blurs, only breaks, are obtained, the accommodative response tracings are more typically straight horizontal lines rather than sigmoid curves. Such subjects can be taught to increase or decrease their accommodation to prevent diplopia as the fusional limit is reached, in which instances the accommodation response tracings then take on the sigmoid curvature of those in Figure 13.8.

A SAMPLE PLOTTING

Figures 13.9 and 13.10 are plots of 10 reasonably typical clinical findings on an emmetrope with an interpupillary distance of 63 mm, identified

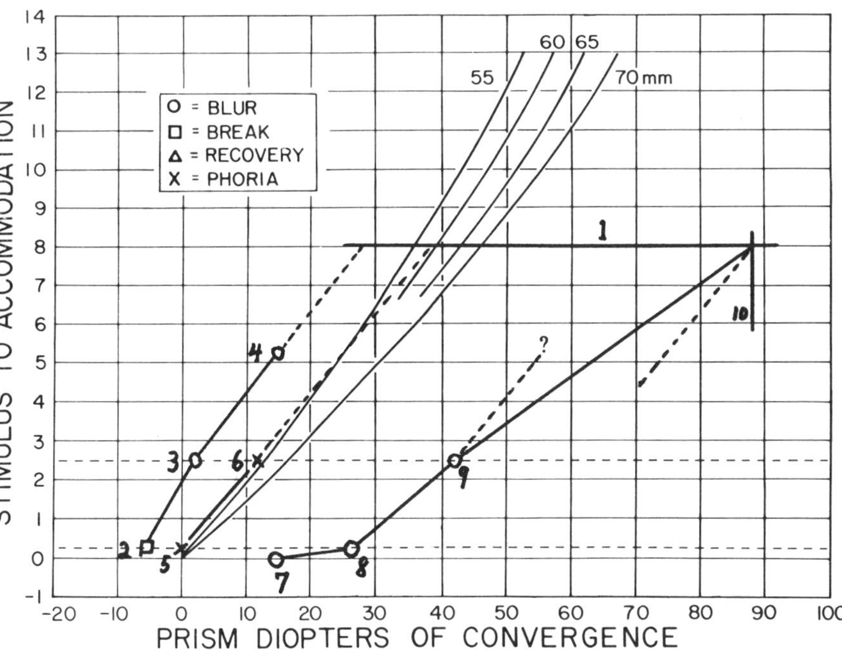

FIGURE 13.9. A sample set of 10 conventional clinical optometric data plotted to illustrate their roles in determining the zone of clear single binocular vision. See text for comments on each of the findings.

in the graphs as follows:

1. Amplitude of accommodation—8D
2. Base-in prism limit (break) at 4 m—-8^{Δ}
3. Base-in prism limit (blur) at 40 cm—-13^{Δ}
4. Binocular minus lens limit (blur) at 40 cm—-2.75 D
5. Phoria at 4 m—-1.5^{Δ} (exo)
6. Phoria at 40 cm—-3^{Δ} (exo)
7. Binocular plus lens limit (blur) at 40 cm—2.50 D
8. Base-out prism limit (blur) at 4 m—25^{Δ}
9. Base-out prism limit (blur) at 40 cm—27^{Δ}
10. Near point of convergence from spectacle plane—45 cm (87.5^{Δ})

The amplitude of accommodation, measured as a near point of accommodation at 12.5 cm from the spectacle plane, is represented in Figure 13.9 by a heavy horizontal line labeled 1, long enough to serve as the total upper border or limit of the zone of clear single binocular vision.

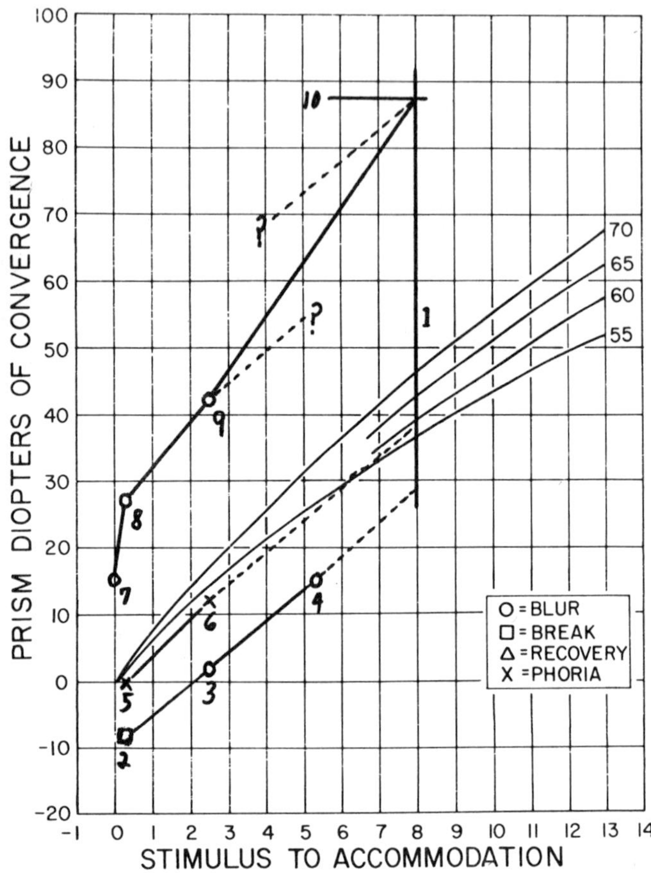

FIGURE 13.10. The same data as in Figure 13.9, with ordinates reversed to reflect accommodation instead of convergence as the primary variable.

Negative Fusional Convergence Limits

The base-in limit at 4 m is identified as #2 and plotted as a square because it is a break rather than a blur. A prior blur would not be expected here because there is only one-quarter diopter or less of accommodation available to be relaxed, not enough to place the test target detectably out of focus. This also means that there can be no further reduction of accommodative convergence to enable the eyes to diverge more. It is therefore the absolute limit of divergence, corresponding to a point on the vertical line segment at the lower left of the diagram in Figure 13.7, or a + symbol at the lower left in Figure 13.8.

The base-in limit at 40 cm, #3, is a blur, indicating that accommodation was relaxed to an out-of-focus level as negative fusional convergence was depleted. This then corresponds to a point at the 2.5-diopter level on the outer left border of the diagram in Figure 13.7, or to a circle (O) symbol at the sloping left border in Figure 13.8. This may explain in part why the line segment that connects findings #2 and #3 does not lean as much as the line segment between #3 and #4. That the difference of their slopes is as small as it is, however, may in part be attributable to the subject's awareness that the test object for #3 was closer than that for #2, that is, that greater proximal convergence occurred for #3 than for #2. For these two reasons, the depth-of-focus and proximal effects, the slope of the 2-3 line segment may not be a very valid measure of the accommodative convergence to accommodation (AC/A) ratio, although each of the findings #2 and #3 shows high statistical reliability.

The next finding, #4, is a blur, the most typical end response to increasing additions of minus lenses, representing simple cessation of an increase of accommodation after the limit of clear single binocular vision is reached. Had the subject closed one eye, had the vision in one eye been blocked inadvertently, or had the vision of one eye been suppressed as in strabismus, the blur might not have been reported until the full 8 diopters of accommodative amplitude were depleted, thus to show a −5.50-D lens addition. An alternative response could have been simply that of letting the test target double, an uncrossed diplopia produced by the accommodative convergence accompanying the increased accommodation. For the purposes of graphical analysis, the so-reported "break" or "double" would have the same quantitative significance as a reported blur.

Since the physical target distances in #3 and #4 are the same, 40 cm, and the effect of 2.75 additional diopters of accommodation on pupil size is small, the differential proximal convergence and depth-of-focus effects on these two findings may be presumed to be small, if not negligible. Accordingly, the slope of the line segment connecting #3 and #4 should be the most valid single measure of the AC/A ratio. On this basis, and because the slope is reasonably approximated by that of the 2-3 line segment, the 3-4 line segment may quite reliably be extrapolated upward, shown by a dashed line, to meet the upper limit of the zone at 8 D. The slope of the 3-4 line in this instance is that of an accommodative convergence to accommodation (AC/A) ratio of $5^{\Delta}/1$ D.

Phorias

The 1.5^{Δ} exophoria at 4 m, plotted point #5, turns out in this instance to be parallelism of the lines of sight. It may be extrapolated that at true infinity the dissociated divergence of the lines of sight would be 5 ×

0.25, or 1.25$^{\Delta}$ exophoria. As pointed out previously, this datum may be regarded as the fundamental variable or point of reference that specifies the position of the double parallelogram on the abscissa scale, thereby identifying this subject as an exophore. This is analogous to specifying the position of a race horse by the location of its nose, or the starting position of a foot-race contestant by the placement of his or her more forward toe. The subject is therefore regarded as an exophore irrespective of the magnitudes or locations of the other nine findings.

The phoria at 40 cm, plotted as item #6, suggests an AC/A ratio slightly greater than 5/1 inasmuch as the deviation of line segment 5-6 from the vertical may be slightly greater than that of line segment 3-4. It is reasonable to suspect, however, that the phoria at 40 cm was influenced a bit more by the awareness of nearness than was the 4-m phoria. Differences of pupil size on the other hand would have negligible effect.

A not infrequent measurement-invalidating effect is that of the subject's failure to keep the test target in sharp focus at the moment that alignment of the dissociated target images is reported. This usually transient failure is typically manifested as underaccommodation for the dioptric stimulus with concomitant reduction of accommodative convergence, and therefore a spurious reading of more exophoria or less esophoria. When it occurs this measurement error tends to be quite large, in unusual instances resulting in an almost vertical 5-6 line segment. Control for this type of error is the insistence or procedural requirement that the subject keep the fixated target image in sharp focus during the moment of making his or her judgment of alignment of the diplopic images.

Positive Fusional Convergence Limits

Plotted point # 7, when measured from either of the conventional near test distances of 33 or 40 cm, rarely meets the convergence border of the zone of clear single binocular vision, meeting instead the horizontal base of the zone, the zero level of accommodation. For the same reason it is extremely rare that a break instead of a blur would occur, although theoretically possible for a subject with a combination of substantial exophoria, low positive fusional convergence, and an average or high AC/A ratio. The line segment 7-8 therefore has no diagnostic significance beyond the fact that it connects two neighboring limit values in the convergent area of the zone, that is, that positive fusional convergence is being used, in part or in full, in both test responses. The slope of this segment can only be thought of as an artifact resulting from lack of precise information as to where the oblique righthand border of the zone of clear single binocular vision intersects the horizontal or zero base line.

Number 8, in contrast, is quite invariably a direct determination of the range of positive fusional convergence near the zero level of accommodation. However, especially when it manifests itself as a blur, it is a finding that will usually demonstrate considerable increase of magnitude upon repetitive testing until a plateau is reached, suggesting that the manifestation of blur in a single trial or two is a "premature" accommodative response in that it occurs before the limit of positive fusional convergence is reached. This induced tendency, referred to earlier in the section on clinical interpretation, corresponds to the curved border in the lower right corner of Figure 13.7. The clinical examiner therefore must repeat the base-out-to-blur test at distance several times, reducing the base-out prism each time from the consecutively increased prism-to-blur level to an again clear image until no further increase is manifested, in order to consider the finding a valid measure of the maximum available positive fusional convergence.

Because accommodation tends to be so readily induced at or near the zero level of accommodation and in apparent response to the depletion of positive fusional convergence, the expectation of a break instead of a blur would be small in a base-out-prism limit test at four or more meters. In fact it occurs almost exclusively among only the very few subjects who never learned the "trick" of invoking a change of accommodation, and therefore of accommodative convergence, to supplement fusional convergence.

Plotted point #9, a base-out prism limit at 40 cm, has all of the psychophysical attributes of #8, but with a lesser tendency for accommodation to be invoked before positive fusional convergence is exhausted. It manifests itself as a break with greater frequency than does the base-out-prism limit at four meters. It shows less increase of magnitude with repetitive trials than does the distance test. Therefore the connecting line segment 8-9 will show a greater tilt than that of the subject's true AC/A line, extended upward from point #9 in Figure 13.9 by the dashed line ending at a question mark. Nevertheless, it is this prism finding that may be the best single clinical measure of the available positive fusional convergence, that is, its distance from plotted point #6. Incidentally, there are good psychophysical arguments for making this clinical determination at a test distance nearer than 40 cm, but the optical and mechanical disadvantages of shorter testing distances with conventionally available clinical testing equipment probably outweigh such arguments.

The Near Point of Convergence

The near point of convergence is represented by #10 in Figure 13.9 as a short vertical line segment which, if extended downward, would intersect the abscissa at 87.5^{Δ}. Its intersection of the 8-D amplitude of accommodation line, #1, is of course the upper right limit of the zone of clear single binocular vision and for that reason may properly be connected by a line segment with point #9 to complete the enclosure of the zone as measured.

As pointed out in the section on clinical interpretation, there is conflicting evidence as to whether the upper right area of the zone of clear single binocular vision terminates in the shape of an acute corner of a parallelogram or extends as a horizontal line or "tail" in manifestation of additional convergence, presumably "myodioptric" accommodative convergence (van der Hoeve and Flieringa, 1924). If the former is true it would be reasonable to extend the oblique dashed line downward from point #10 in Figure 13.9 to represent the true AC/A slope and the absolute limit of positive fusional convergence at all levels. If the latter is true, the limit of positive fusional convergence would be represented more correctly by the oblique dashed line extended upward from point #9 in Figure 13.9. Its intersection with line #1 would then demarcate the upper right corner, and the continuation of line #1 to the right would constitute the "tail."

Linearity Considerations and Diagnosis

The above representations of the true AC/A ratio by straight lines rather than by nonlinear curves obviously ignore the fact that instances of significant nonlinearity have been reported (Hofstetter, 1945; Westheimer, 1955; Flom, 1960) and that linearity depends as well on the choice of convergence units, whether degrees, prism diopters, meter angles, or centrads. There appears, however, to be no single type of curve more generally compatible with data of the population at large than the straight line. Flom (1960) concluded, " . . . observed nonlinearities are not of practical significance and the assumption of linearity is good and valid."

The clinical diagnostic decision in this instance depends on whether or not there is ample positive fusional convergence to meet the functional and comfort needs of the subject for the distance at which clear single binocular vision must be sustained. This patient happens to meet these needs adequately by the criteria of Sheard, Percival, and others (Abel and Hofstetter, 1952) whether the limit of fusional convergence is presumed to be indicated by finding #9 or #10. If this were not the case the prescribing optometrist then might consider the use of compensating base-in prism in the spectacle correction or the possibility of extending the base-out limits, namely #8 and #9, by exercises.

All of the discussion relative to the points plotted in Figure 13.9 applies simultaneously to identical data in Figure 13.10 with allowance for the fact that the ordinate and abscissa are reversed.

CLINICAL CRITERIA OF ADEQUACY

Reference was made in the preceding section to certain commonly used clinical diagnostic criteria, the best known two of which are identified especially with Sheard (1917, 1928, 1930) and Percival (1892, 1928). These and similar criteria have been in use for many decades as rules of thumb to guide the prescribing optometrist in recommending prism, spherical power, exercises, monocular occlusion, change of work habits, or even surgery.

Such rules of thumb lend themselves conveniently to graphical analysis since they use the relationship of the limits of the patient's zone of clear single binocular vision to the sustained working demand on accommodation and fusional convergence. The essence of Percival's rule is that, for sustained comfort, the point of demand—the intersection of the demand line with the accommodative stimulus level—should be in the middle one-third of the combined range of positive and negative fusional convergence. This rule is sometimes called the "middle third" criterion. Sheard's rule on the other hand includes consideration of the phoria, the magnitude of which is called the "demand." The range of opposing fusional convergence measured from the demand line to the limit of clear single binocular vision at the same accommodative stimulus level is called the "reserve." Sheard said that for sustained comfort the reserve should be equal to at least twice the demand. Stated in clinical testing terms, the base-out prism limit should be at least twice the exophoria, or the base-in prism limit should be at least twice the esophoria.

Other empirical clinical rules of thumb employ degrees of balance between binocular plus-lens and minus-lens limits, or ratios between various combinations of dimensions of the zone, including the phoria. This means therefore that each such rule can be represented geometrically or algebraically in terms of Fry's five fundamental variables.

On a statistical basis the various criteria seem to effect similar diagnostic conclusions, that is, most patients who meet or fail to meet one criterion respectively meet or fail to meet the other criteria. This has made it difficult to evaluate the relative merits of the several criteria, suggesting that each may merely identify persons whose findings deviate greatly from population means.

GRAPHICAL ANALYSIS IN STRABISMUS

Except that fusional convergence is absent in most cases of concomitant strabismus, the graphical representation is the same as for a subject with normal binocular vision (Hofstetter, 1946, 1947; Alpern and Hofstetter, 1948; Heath and Hofstetter, 1952). The same holds true for a subject with one blind eye (Hofstetter, 1946). In either case, that of the blind eye or that of the squinting eye, the nonseeing eye will manifest measurable accommodative convergence in its directional relationship to the fixating eye. When fusional convergence is absent the relationship between accommodation and convergence will be represented by a single line rather than by a parallelogram. This then would more properly be called the tropia line instead of a phoria line.

ORTHOPTICS SPECIFICATION

The graphical technique has useful application in the specification of the area of the zone of binocular vision in which orthoptic training is given (Hofstetter, 1949). Training can be indicated by means of an arrow or some comparable directional symbol on the graph itself. The location of the tip of the arrow would show the region of the zone to be exercised; the direction of the arrow would identify the kind of exercising stimulus, that is, whether base-in or base-out prism, plus or minus lenses, or binocular push-up or recession training; and the length of the arrow could arbitrarily represent quantitative values to be attained.

REFERENCES

Abel A, Hofstetter HW. The graphical analysis of clinical optometric findings. Los Angeles: Los Angeles College of Optometry, 1952.

Alpern M, Hofstetter HW. The effect of prism on esotropia. A case report. Am J Optom Arch Am Acad Optom 1948;25:80–91.

Alpern M. The zone of clear single binocular vision at the upper limits of accommodation and convergence. Am J Optom Arch Am Acad Optom 1950;27:491–513.

Cline D, Hofstetter HW, Griffin J. Dictionary of visual science. 3rd ed. Radnor, Pa.: Chilton Book Co., 1980.

Donders FC. On the anomalies of accommodation and refraction of the eye. London: New Sydenham Society, 1864.

Duke-Elder, S, Abrams, D. System of ophthalmology. Vol. 5. St. Louis: CV Mosby, 1970.

Emsley HH, Swaine W. Ophthalmic lenses. London: Hatton Press, 1951.

Flieringa HJ, van der Hoeve, J. Arbeiten aus den Gebiete der Akkommodation. Albrecht Von Graefes Arch Ophthalmol 1924;114:1–46.

Flom C. On the relationship between accommodation and accommodative convergence. I. Linearity. Am J Optom Arch Am Acad Optom 1960;37:474–82.

Fry GA. An experimental analysis of the accommodation-convergence relation. Am J Optom 1937;14:402–14.

Fry GA. Further experiments on the accommodation-convergence relationship. Trans Am Acad Optom 1938;12:65–74.

Fry GA. Fundamental variables in the relationship between accommodation and convergence. Optom Weekly 1943;34:153–55; 183–85.
Haines HF. An experimental analysis of the factors affecting the relationship between accommodation and convergence. MS thesis, Columbus, Ohio: The Ohio State University, 1938.
Heath G, Hofstetter HW. The effect of orthoptics on the zone of binocular vision in intermittent exotropia. A case report. Am J Optom Arch Am Acad Optom 1952;29:12–31.
Hess C. Die relative Akkommodation. Albrecht Von Graefes Arch Ophthalmol 1901;52:143–74.
Hess C. Die Anomalien der Refraction und Akkommodation des Auges mit einleitender Darstellung der Dioptrik des Auges. Graefe-Saemisch Handbuch der Gesamten Augenheilkunde. 1903;8:458–518.
Hofstetter HW. Zone of clear single binocular vision. Am J Optom Arch Am Acad Optom 1945;22:301–33; 361–84.
Hofstetter HW. Accommodative convergence in squinters. Am J Optom Arch Am Acad Optom 1946;23:417–37.
Hofstetter HW. Certain variations in the angle of deviation in concomitant squint. Am J Optom Arch Am Acad Optom 1947;24:463–71.
Hofstetter HW. Orthoptics specification by a graphical method. Am J Optom Arch Am Acad Optom 1949;26:439–44.
Hofstetter HW. The relationship of proximal convergence to fusional and accommodative convergence. Am J Optom Arch Am Acad Optom 1951;28:300–308.
Hofstetter HW. Verbessertes Schema für die grafische Analyse des Akkommodations-Konvergenz-Verhältnisses. Augenoptik 1967;84:103–105.
Hofstetter HW. A revised schematic for the graphic analysis of the accommodation-convergence relationship. Can J Optom 1968;30:49–52.
Hofstetter HW. Interpupillary distances in adult populations. J Am Optom Assoc 1972;43:1151–55.
Hofstetter HW. From 20/20 to 6/6 or 4/4? Am J Optom Arch Am Acad Optom 1973;50:212–21.
Howe L. Concerning relative accommodation and convergence, with description of an instrument for their measurement. Trans Am Ophthalmol Soc 1900;36th annual meeting. p 92.
Howe, L. The muscles of the eye. Vol. 1, Vol. 2. New York: GP Putman's Sons, 1907, 1908;309–47; 22–58.
Landolt, E. The refraction and accommodation of the eye. Edinburgh: YJ Pentland, 1886.
Lesser SK. Fundamentals of procedure and analysis in optometric examination. Fort Worth, Tex.: published by author, 1933.
MacGillavry TH. Onderzoekingen over de Hoegrootheid der Accommodate. PhD thesis, Utrechtsche Hoogeschool, Utrecht, 1858.
Nagel A. Die Anomalien der Refraktion und Akkommodation. Graefe-Saemisch Handbuch der Gesamten Augenheikunde 1880;6:257–503.
Percival A. The relation of convergence to accommodation and its practical bearing. Ophthal Rev 1892;11:313–28.
Percival A. The prescribing of spectacles. 3rd ed. Bristol, England: John Wright & Sons, 1928.

Pereles H. Ueber die relative Accommodationsbreite. Albrecht Von Graefes Arch Ophthalmol 1889;35:84–115.

Pitts DG, Hofstetter HW. Demand line graphing of the zone of clear single binocular vision. J Am Optom Assoc 1959;31:51–55.

Prentice CF. Ophthalmic lenses. Philadelphia: Keystone, 1907.

Roelofs CO. Der Zusammenhang zwishen Akkommodation und Konvergenz. Albrecht Von Graefes Arch Ophthalmol 1913;85:66–136.

Schmiedt W. Über die relative Fusionsbreite bei Hebung und Senkung der Blickebene. Albrecht Von Graefes Arch Ophthalmol 1893;39:233–56.

Sheard C. Dynamic ocular tests. Columbus, Ohio: Lawrence Press, 1917.

Sheard C. Zones of ocular comfort. Trans Am Acad Optom 1928;3:113–29.

Sheard C. Zones of ocular comfort. Am J Optom 1930;7:9–25.

van der Hoeve J, Flieringa HJ. Accommodation. Br J Ophthalmol 1924;8:97–106.

Westheimer G. The relationship between accommodation and accommodative convergence. Am J Optom Arch Am Acad Optom 1955;32:206–12.

Weymouth FW, Brust PR, Gobar, FH. Ocular muscle balance at the reading distance and certain related factors. Am J Physiol Optics 1925;6:184–205.

Working Group 39, National Academy of Science—National Research Council Committee on Vision. Recommended standard procedures for the clinical measurement and specification of visual acuity. Adv Ophthalmol 1980;41:1–45.

14

Fixation Disparity and Vergence Adaptation

Clifton M. Schor

HISTORY

During binocular fixation small vergence errors can occur without causing diplopia as long as they do not exceed Panum's fusional limit (1858). Vergence errors have been referred to by a variety of terms. The errors were first observed by Hoffmann and Bielschowsky (1900) who reported that previously aligned fiducial marks became misaligned during forced convergence stimulated with a haploscope. They referred to the discrepancy between single vision and the error in convergence as residual disparity. Judd (1907) observed "residual vergence errors" objectively by photographing the right eye's position during monocular and binocular fixation. Lau (1921) observed vergence errors with subjective measurements taken during studies of the horopter. He determined that nonius lines were physically misaligned while they were perceived one above the other and that the misalignment increased with forced convergence. He concluded that this discrepancy resulted from inexact bifoveal fixation. Lewin and Sakuma (1924) using the haploscope with card targets (4 and 5 of diamonds), found that although the corner diamonds were fused, the center diamond changed its position with convergence demand. Ames and Glidden (1928) made an extensive study of vergence errors, which they called

Preparation of this chapter was supported by NEI grant EY-02573.

retinal slip. They found the magnitude of slip varied with heterophoria, convergence, divergence, cyclovergence, accommodative convergence, and the proximity of binocular fusion stimuli to the fovea. Ogle, Mussey, and Prangen (1949) referred to the inexactness of binocular fixation as fixation disparity. Since that time other concepts and terms have been suggested such as "an intermediate step between normal binocular vision and strabismus or microstrabismus" (Jampolsky, Flom, and Fried, 1957) and vergence discrepancy (Hebbard, 1960); however, the term fixation disparity continues to be used to describe the inexactness of binocular fixation.

SUBJECTIVE AND OBJECTIVE MEASUREMENT

Typically, fixation disparity is measured subjectively by an observer who aligns two vertical nonius lines, one above the other, while fusing binocular targets that surround the central lines (Figure 14.1). The amount of lateral displacement needed to obtain perceived alignment of the nonius targets is believed to measure the horizontal vergence error or horizontal fixation disparity. This assumption relies on an invariance of binocular corresponding retinal points. Several investigators have compared subjective and objective measures of fixation disparity. Hebbard (1962) used a contact lens mirror stalk to measure eye movements and observed

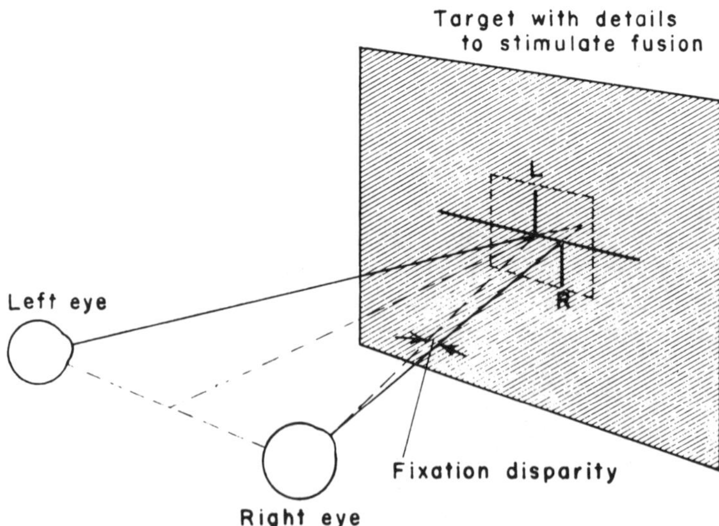

FIGURE 14.1. Nonius lines within the central square are adjusted by the subject to appear in vertical alignment. Peripheral pattern stimulates binocular fusion. Reprinted by permission of the publisher, from Martens TG, Ogle KN. Observations on accommodative convergence. American Journal of Ophthalmology, 1959.

close agreement (within experimental error) between subjective and objective measurements. In contrast, Clark (1936) and Stewart (1951) obtained objective measures of fixation disparity at the fovea that were an order of magnitude greater (2° to 4°) than values obtained with subjective techniques. This apparent discrepancy raises a question concerning the stability of normal binocular retinal correspondence. Perhaps it varies in a way similar to that reported with strabismus (Hallden, 1952; Alpern and Hofstetter, 1948) in which single binocular vision occurs in spite of large vergence errors that exceed Panum's area. Indeed, Diner (1978) has observed changes in binocular correspondence as evidenced by changes in the location of a Panum's area that corresponded to a fixed point in the contralateral eye. If correspondence varies in a way to minimize diplopia, the usual subjective measures of fixation disparity would underestimate actual vergence errors.

FUNCTIONAL SIGNIFICANCE OF FIXATION DISPARITY

There are two basic interpretations of fixation disparity: one is that it is a symptom of stress on the disparity vergence system and the other is that it is a purposeful error that provides a stimulus to the vergence system. Both of these interpretations may be correct under specific circumstances. The first concept was proposed by Ogle and Prangen (1953) and Mallett (1974), and may be interpreted from Jampolsky (1956). The vergence response is believed to lag behind the stimulus in proportion to stimulus load. This load or stress is the product of the amplitude of vergence stimulus and the quality or strength of fusional vergence response. The maximum slip that can occur with stress is limited in normal binocular vision by the threshold disparity for perception of diplopia (Panum's area) at the retinal site receiving the image of the fixation target. Hebbard (1960), and more recently, Woo (1974), Fender and Julesz (1967), and Schor and Tyler (1981) have shown that the amplitude of Panum's area can vary with the spatial and temporal characteristics of the stimulus. Panum's area is much larger when measured with slowly moving coarse detail than with abrupt changes in depth of fine detail. The maximum amplitude of fixation disparity will depend on the size, spatial frequency content, and motion of the target under fixation. In abnormal binocular vision central suppression and/or anomalous binocular correspondence will extend the singleness range (Jampolsky, 1956) so that unusually large vergence errors can occur without causing diplopia. These errors are detectable in a clinical examination with the unilateral cover test and are referred to as monofixation syndrome (Parks, 1971), microstrabismus (Jampolsky, 1956), and flick (Flom, 1958). They are characterized by an ocular deviation that is larger when measured by the alternate than by the unilateral cover test. It is believed that the large deviation found by the alternate cover test is the source of stress manifested as macrofixation disparity shown by the unilateral cover test in monofixation syndrome.

Fixation disparity has also been considered as a stimulus to the fusional vergence system. Ogle and colleagues (1951) and later Crone (1973) proposed that to maintain a given angle of convergence the vergence system required a constant driving force or torque that was stimulated by fixation disparity. The torque stimulated was proportional to the vergence error or fixation disparity. This stimulus-response characteristic is classified in systems analysis as a proportional controller (Toates, 1975; Crone and Hardjowijoto, 1979). As will be shown, however, the vergence system is operated by a leaky integrator rather than proportional controller (Schor, 1979b, 1980a). That is, the innervation required to maintain a given amplitude of convergence is stored in a manner similar to the storage of voltage across a capacitor. It has been shown that the convergence response decays (Ludvigh et al., 1964), presumably as a result of leakage of the stored innervation. Fixation disparity provides a stimulus (steady-state error) to replenish the decaying source of innervation (Schor, 1979b, 1980a). The steady-state error is proportional to the amplitude of the fusional vergence response (Schor, 1979b). Both the stress and stimulus hypotheses predict that the maximum fixation disparity that can provide a stimulus to maintain a vergence response is limited by sensory factors including the amplitude of Panum's area and suppression and variations in retinal correspondence. Other parameters that determine the amplitude of the steady-state error are considered in a later section of this chapter.

HETEROPHORIA

Heterophoria constitutes a vergence error that is corrected by fusional vergence. The functions of fixation disparity described in the preceding section predict that the direction and magnitude of fixation disparity should be related to the direction and magnitude of heterophoria. Ames and Glidden (1928) reported that a correlation existed between the direction of fixation disparity and the direction of heterophoria. Ogle (1954) confirmed this, but found that the magnitude of fixation disparity could not be predicted by the magnitude of heterophoria. Jamplosky, Flom, and Fried (1957) and Ogle (1954) both observed that when tested at remote viewing distances esofixation disparity increased at a rate of approximately 1-minute arc per prism diopter of esophoria but that fixation disparity remained nearly zero for most amplitudes of exophoria (Figure 14.2). Interestingly, at near test distances both studies reported that fixation disparity increased with both esophoria and exophoria (Figure 14.3). These results have been confirmed by McCullough (1978), but rejected by Palmer and von Noorden (1978) who state that the direction and mag-

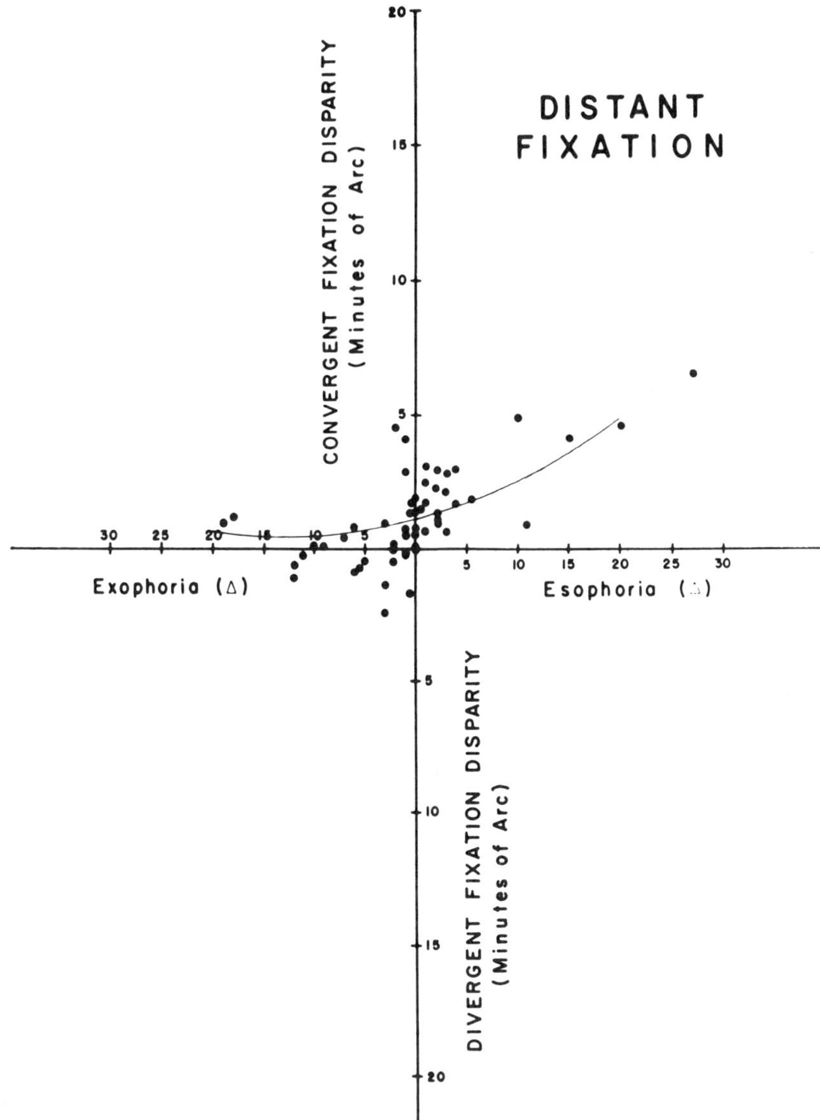

FIGURES 14.2 and 14.3. Scatter plots of fixation disparity as a function of heterophoria measured at 40-cm and 6-m viewing distances. Reprinted by permission of the publisher, from Jampolsky A, Flom B, Freid A. Fixation disparity in relation to heterophoria. American Journal of Ophthalmology, 1957.

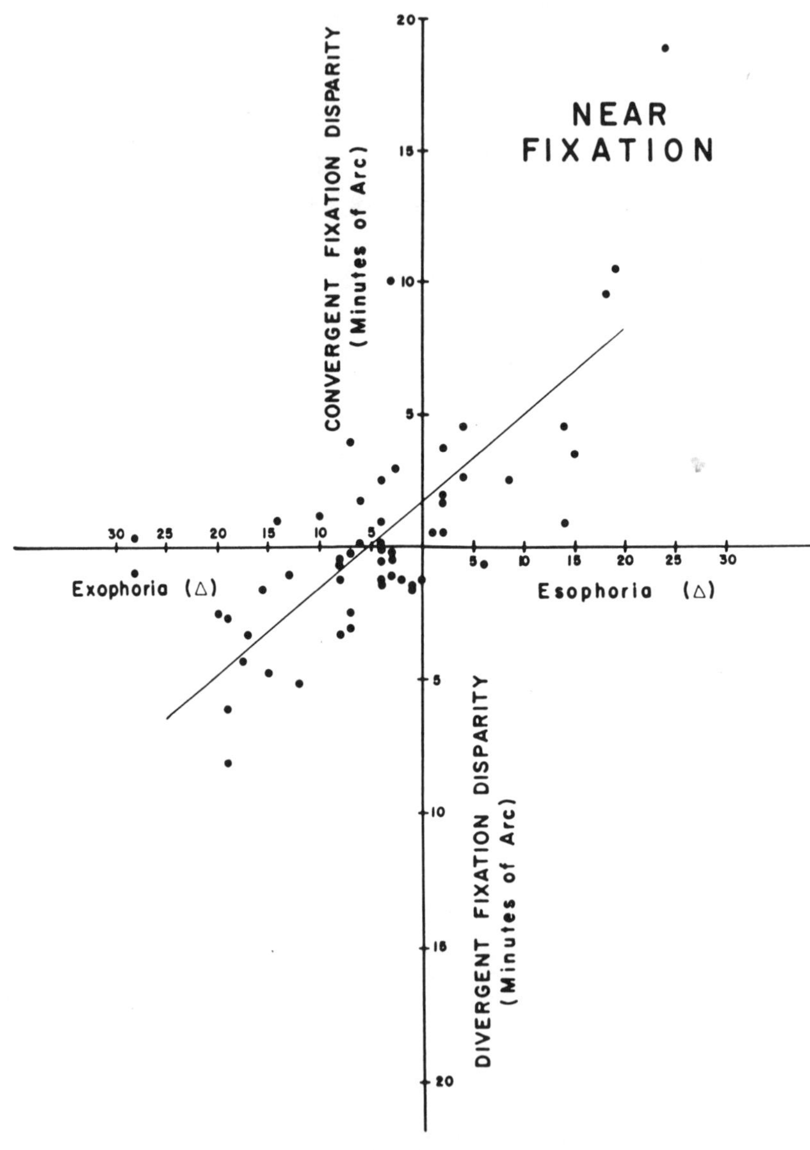
NEAR
FIXATION
CONVERGENT FIXATION DISPARITY
(Minutes of Arc)
DIVERGENT FIXATION DISPARITY
(Minutes of Arc)
Exophoria (Δ)
Esophoria (Δ)
20
15
10
5
30
25
20
15
10
5
5
10
15
20
25
30
5
10
15
20

FIGURE 14.3.

nitude of fixation disparity are uncorrelated with the direction and magnitude of heterophoria. Also in contradiction are three studies that report cases of paradoxical fixation disparity in which retinal slip and heterophoria are in opposite directions (Ogle, 1954; Jampolsky et al., 1957; Palmer and von Noorden, 1978).

Dissociated and Associated Heterophoria

Comparisons have also been made between the typical dissociated phoria and the prism amplitude that reduces fixation disparity to zero (associated phoria). Ames and Glidden (1928) and Ogle, Martens, and Dyer (1967) observed that the associated and dissociated phorias were usually of the same direction and similar magnitude. That magnitude of the former is usually less than that of the latter by a factor of 20% to 25% (Tubis, 1954). Differences between the amplitudes of the two phorias appear to result from prism adaptation, which is only active during binocular (associated) viewing conditions (Schor, 1980a). Lack of control of prism adaptation may also account for these reports of reduced correlation between amplitudes of fixation disparity and heterophoria. Variations in prism adaptation can be minimized by rigorous control of accommodative stimulus and response (Semmlow and Hung, 1979; Schor, 1980b), exposure duration to binocular stimuli prior to measurement of fixation (Schor, 1979a), and consistent preadaptation to zero prism to eliminate aftereffects of adaptation to previous prism stimuli or other test distances than the one currently being tested (Schor, 1980b).

Previous studies of heterophoria and fixation disparity were of asymptomatic normal subjects with either orthophoria or heterophoria. Prism adaptation appears to reduce the stress or load placed on the vergence system by the heterophoria under binocular viewing conditions. This adaptation is believed to be a characteristic of normal binocular vision (Ogle and Prangen, 1953; Carter, 1965). Carter has suggested that symptomatic persons with heterophoria may have deficient prism adaptation. In these abnormal cases a high correlation between fixation disparity and heterophoria would be expected. Orthoptics or visual rehabilitation increases prism adaptation in persons with occasional strabismus (Schor, 1979a). In some cases this learned ability to adapt to prism leads to a paradoxical relationship between direction of fixation disparity and heterophoria. After orthoptics therapy 28% to 38% of exophores show esofixation disparity (Vaegan, 1979). Excessive adaptation appears to overcompensate for heterophoria and place an inverse load or stress of opposite sign to the dissociated phoria during binocular fusion. The following section describes several factors that determine the amplitude of the fusional vergence response and its associated fixation disparity.

DISPARITY VERGENCE AND FIXATION DISPARITY

Horizontal Fixation Disparity

Ever since the discovery of fixation disparity it has been known that its amplitude varies with the magnitude of the stimulus disparity to fusional vergence. Ogle and co-workers (1967) have quantified various relationships between fixation disparity and the amplitude of the stimulus to convergent and divergent disparity vergence (Figure 14.4). They observed that the response of vergence to prism was slightly less than stimulus

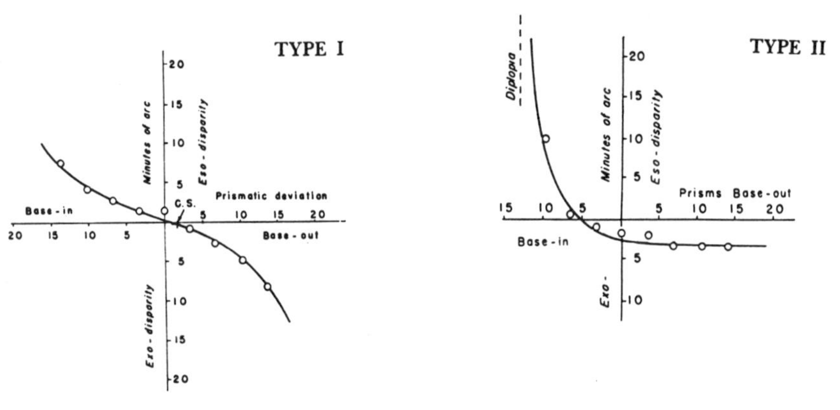

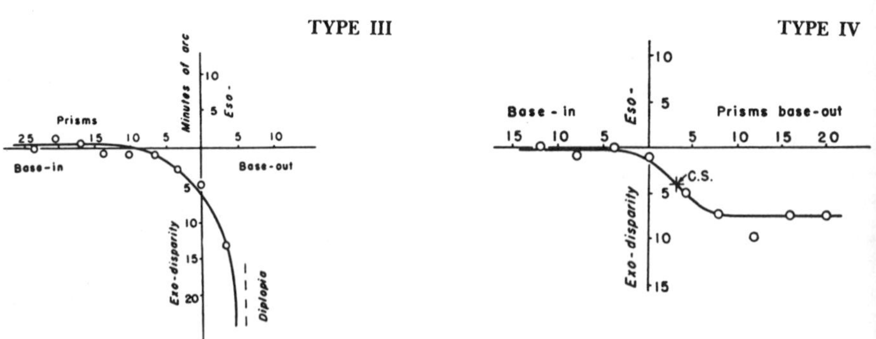

FIGURE 14.4. Fixation disparity stimulated by prism vergence has been classified by Ogle into four types of curves. Reprinted by permission of the publisher, from Carter DB. Parameters of fixation disparity. American Journal of Optometry and Physiological Optics, © (1980), American Academy of Optometry per The Williams & Wilkins Company (agent).

amplitude and that this lag increased with amplitude of stimulus. The lag of convergence and divergence responses are termed exofixation and esofixation disparity, respectively.

Curve Types

Ogle has classified horizontal fixation disparity plotted as a function of lateral prism vergence stimulus (Figure 14.4) as type I when the amplitude of fixation disparity increases in response to both divergent and convergent stimuli about equally. Thus as prism power is increased and the limiting amplitude of vergence response is approached, fixation disparity becomes large and is followed by the sudden appearance of diplopia. Prism-induced fixation disparity curves are classified as type II when errors of convergence are smaller than errors of divergence. Type III describes fixation disparity that is greater with convergent than with divergent stimuli. Type IV, which is found in some persons with abnormal binocular vision, is characterized by nearly a constant fixation disparity and an abnormally small amplitude of vergence responses to prism.

Vertical Fixation Disparity

Fixation disparity also occurs vertically in response to prisms placed base-up or base-down before one eye (Ogle and Prangen, 1953). Vertical forced duction fixation disparity curves take the form of a single straight line (Figure 14.5), demonstrating a linear relationship between vertical fixation disparity and vertical vergence stimuli. Hyperductions result in hypofixation disparity and hypoductions result in hyperfixation disparity. The vertical fixation disparity curves are remarkably similar among subjects, the slopes of fixation disparity curves derived for different subjects are more similar in response to vertical than to horizontal vergence stimuli (Ogle and Prangen, 1953). The maximum vertical fixation disparity induced with prism is 5 to 6 minutes of arc in comparison to 20 minutes of arc in the horizontal meridian (Ogle and Prangen, 1953). These differences in vertical and horizontal fixation disparity correspond to the vertical-horizontal anisotropy of Panum's area (Schor and Tyler, 1981).

PANUM'S FUSIONAL LIMIT

It has been stated repeatedly that the upper limit for fixation disparity equals Panum's area. Two studies provide evidence to support this statement. Charnwood (1951) observed that when vergence eye movements

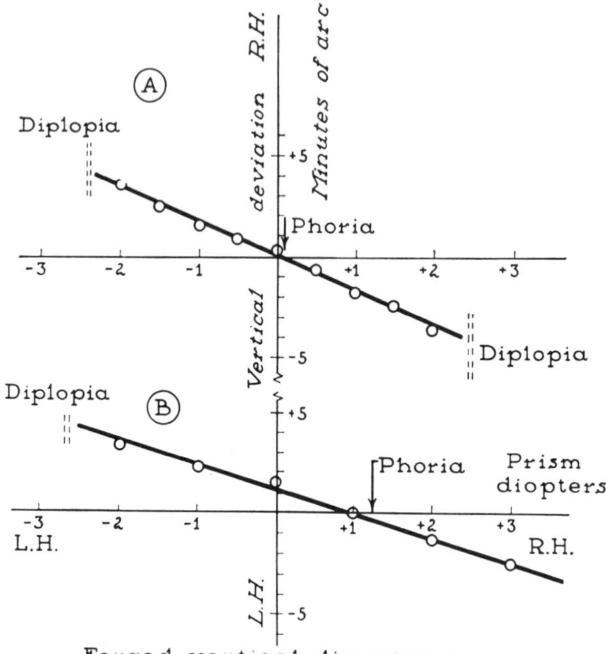

FIGURE 14.5. Fixation disparity in the vertical meridian when vertical divergences are enforced by prisms. Reprinted by permission of the publisher, from Ogle KN, Prangen A. Observations of vertical divergence and hyperphorias. Archives of Ophthalmology, 49:313–34. Copyright 1953, American Medical Association.

were stimulated with prism, the maximum fixation disparity achieved equaled Panum's area. Larger disparities resulted in diplopia. Hebbard (1964) found that blurring vergence stimuli resulted in increased fixation disparity, and Schor and Tyler (1981) provided evidence that blur could increase the size of Panum's area. Other factors than blur also increase the area and accordingly will increase the maximum limit of fixation disparity.

Retinal Eccentricity

Panum's area increases with retinal eccentricity (Ogle, 1964) and as a result, the maximum limit to fixation disparity increases as binocular fusion stimuli are moved away from the fovea. Ogle, Martens, and Dyer (1967) varied the central blanked-out area that contains the nonius lines for measuring fixation disparity from 0.5° to 6° (Figure 14.6). By doing so they increased the predominance of peripheral over central fusion cues.

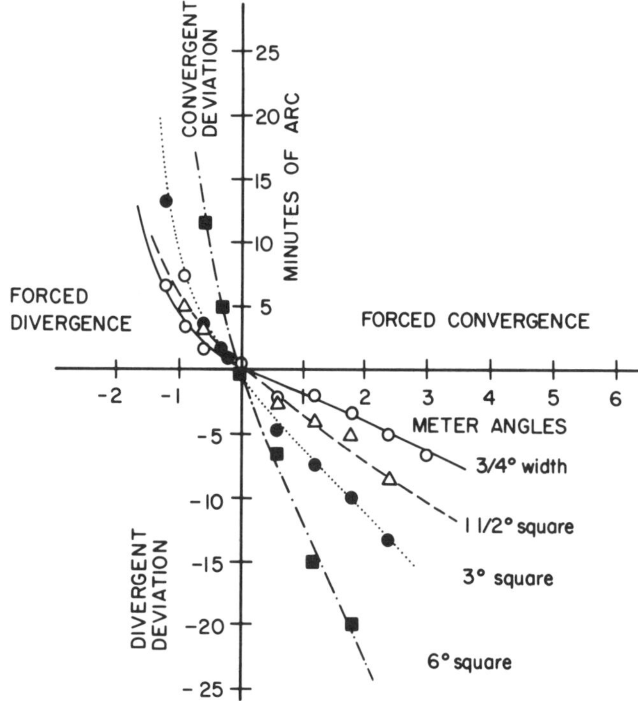

FIGURE 14.6. Ogle, Mussey, and Prangen (1949) show the progressive increase in slope of the fixation disparity curves as the size of the central blanked-out area is increased. Reprinted by permission of the publisher, from Ogle KN, Mussey F, Prangen A. Fixation disparity and the fusional processes in binocular single vision. American Journal of Ophthalmology, 1949.

With a 6° blanked-out region they found that fixation disparity increased markedly with increasing prism vergence stimuli, whereas with a small blanked-out region fixation disparity remained small over a broad range of prism vergence stimuli. As the blanked-out region decreased, the curve changed from a steep type I to a type II having a constant flat portion in the center of the curve. Thus changes of fixation disparity resulting from forced vergence were reduced by placing binocular fusion contours near the fovea.

Carter (1964) examined fixation disparity in the presence of central fusion (foveal) contours. He observed that with foveal fusion, fixation disparity rarely exceeded 6 minutes of arc with forced vergence in comparison to 20 minutes of arc with peripheral fusion contours. Fixation disparity curves resulting from forced ductions with foveal fusion contours were similar in shape but smaller in amplitude to groups I, II, and III found by Ogle and associates (1967) with peripheral fusion stimuli.

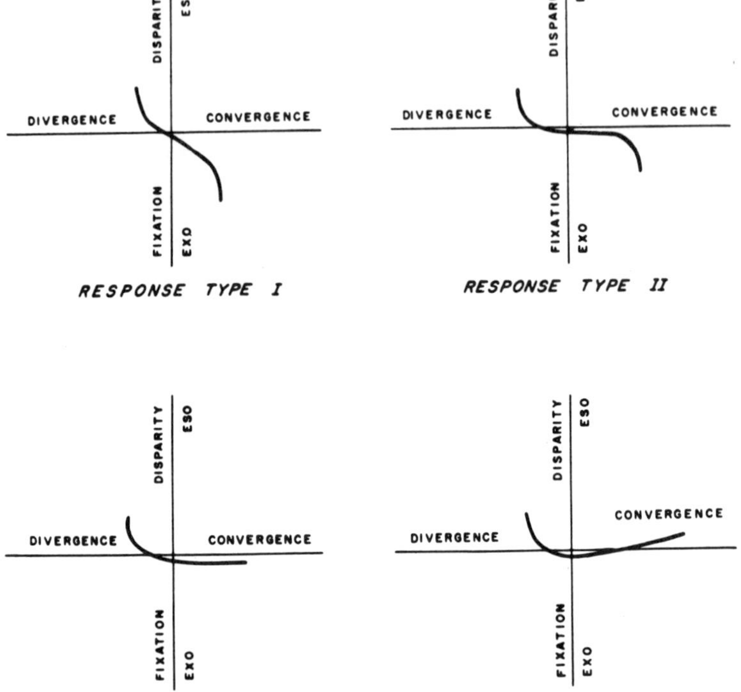

FIGURE 14.7. Four curve types of forced duction fixation disparity measured by Carter (1964) with foveal fusion contours. Reprinted by permission of the publisher, from Carter DB. Fixation disparity with and without foveal contours. American Journal of Optometry, 1964.

Carter found a new fourth curve in which both convergent and divergent vergence stimuli resulted in esofixation disparity at the limits of motor fusion but exofixation disparity with small vergence stimuli (Figure 14.7). The esofixation disparity noted with large convergence stimuli is similar to the paradoxical esofixation disparity found in some persons with exophoria. Both paradoxical responses appear to result from the same factors discussed earlier, that is, overconvergence in response to a high convergence demand. The source of this response is believed to originate from excessive adaptation of the vergence system to prism (Schor, 1980a).

ADAPTATION PHENOMENON

Changes in the vertical and horizontal phoria can result from wearing vertical or horizontal prism, respectively (Schubert, 1943). Similarly forced duction (vergence amplitude) tests have been shown to cause residual tonicity that alters the horizontal (Morgan, 1947) and vertical (Ellerbrock, 1950) fusion-free positions of the eyes (phorias). These changes in phoria can persist as long as 30 minutes after removal of vertical prism worn for several hours (Ellerbrock, 1950). This unrelaxed portion of the fusional vergence response is identified as prism adaptation or slow fusional vergence (Schor, 1979a). The amplitude of prism adaptation depends on how long the prism is worn. If prior to occlusion of one eye horizontal prism is worn for short duration (5 seconds), the horizontal fusional vergence response will completely relax in 15 seconds (Ludvigh et al., 1964). The temporal course of relaxation has been described as a decaying exponential with a time constant of 10 seconds (Krishnan and Stark, 1977). If horizontal fusional vergence is stimulated for longer durations (15 minutes), relaxation of fusional vergence on occlusion of one eye is incomplete for several hours or until binocular fixation is reinstated (Carter, 1965; Schor, 1979a). The temporal decay function of vertical vergence stimulated for several hours has two components: rapid decay, which is interrupted after 10 minutes by a slower decay function with a time constant of several hours (Ellerbrock, 1950). These examples of incomplete relaxation of fusional vergence have been interpreted by Ogle and Prangen (1953) as modifications of tonic convergence (Maddox, 1893).

The amount of adaptation that results from horizontal prism can be asymmetric for convergent and divergent stimuli. Figure 14.8 illustrates

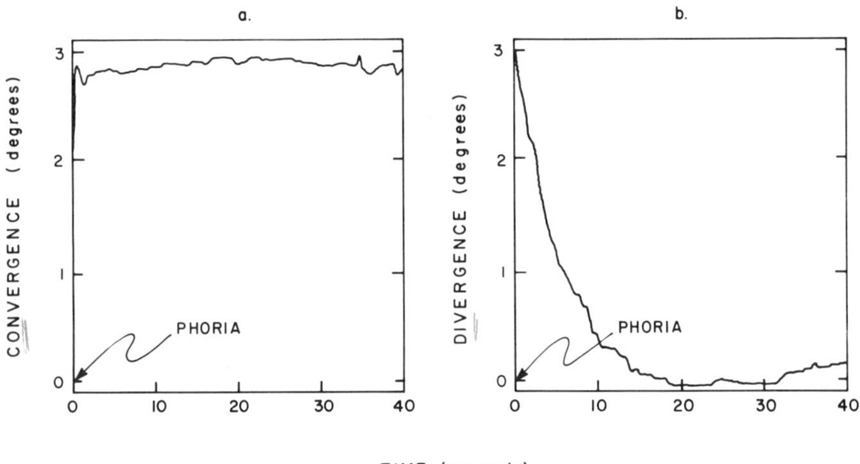

FIGURE 14.8. Averaged records of relaxation of fusional vergence following occlusion of one eye. a Total adaptation to a convergence stimulus persists 40 seconds after disrupting binocular fixation. b Total relaxation of the fusional vergence response. The decay is exponential and has a time constant of 10 seconds. Reprinted by permission of the publisher, from Schor CM. The influence of rapid prism adaptation upon fixation disparity. Vision Research, 1979.

unequal adaptation to base-in and base-out prism for a given individual. Marked prism adaptation to 3° convergent stimulus disparity is shown in Figure 14.8. No change occurs in vergence posture after one eye has been occluded for 40 seconds. There is an exponential decay of the fusional divergence response to a base-in prism for the same person. The curve has a time constant of 10 seconds and becomes asymptotic at 15 seconds to a vergence angle equal to this person's heterophoria. In a study of 14 normal subjects prism adaptation was quantified from recordings such as those shown in Figure 14.8 as the difference between prism amplitude stimulating fusional vergence for 30 seconds and the reduction or amount of decay of vergence response after 40 seconds of monocular occlusion.

The amplitude of this rapid (30-second) prism adaptation (Henson and North, 1980) for individual subjects is plotted in Figures 14.9 and 14.10 as a function of the amplitude of fusional vergence stimulus. The diagonal line in each graph represents total adaptation or no relaxation of fusional vergence, and points falling along the X axis represent an absence of prism adaptation or complete relaxation of fusional vergence. Every subject demonstrated unequal adaptation to base-in and base-out prism and was classified according to the direction of maximum prism adaptation as type B (Figure 14.9) or type C (Figure 14.10). Eight subjects showed marked adaptation to base-out prism and the remaining six had marked adaptation to base-in prism. In cases of partial adaptation, amplitude of adaptation after 40 seconds of monocular occlusion increased in proportion to the vergence stimulus amplitude. This suggests that the rate of prism adaptation is related to the amplitude of fusional vergence stimulus.

Influence of Prism Adaptation on Curve Type

The phenomenon of rapid prism adaptation appears to determine the shape or curve type of the forced duction fixation disparity curves described earlier. There is high negative correlation between the amplitude of fixation disparity and prism adaptation (Schor, 1979b). Fixation disparity forced duction curves were obtained from the same 14 subjects described above. Figures 14.11, 14.12, and 14.13 show type I, II, and III curves. Type II was the most prevalent response, followed by type III and type I. The relative incidence of these curve types varies with the size of the central blanked-out area (1.5° in this study) (Ogle et al., 1967). Large blanked-out areas yield a high incidence of type I curves, and foveal fusion contours reduce fixation disparity to nearly zero in response to all stimuli (Carter, 1964). A blanked-out area of 1.5° is ideal because it makes it possible to observe the marked asymmetries in fixation disparity re-

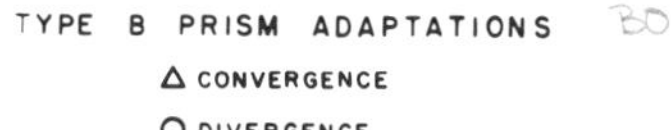

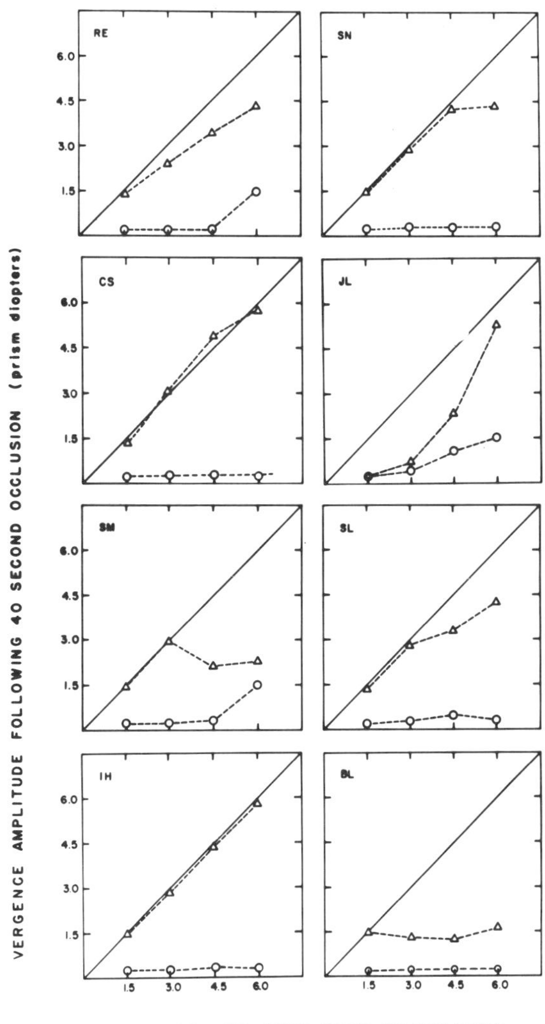

FIGURES 14.9 and 14.10. Amplitude of prism adaptation plotted as a function of the stimulus to convergence (△) and divergence (○). Data points along the diagonal line indicate total adaptation. Points along the X axis indicate an absence of adaptation, or total relaxation of fusional vergence. Points between these extremes indicate partial prism adaptation. Subjects showing marked adaptation to base-out prism or base-in prism are grouped in Figures 14.9 and 14.10, respectively. Reprinted by permission of the publisher, from Schor CM. The influence of rapid prism adaptation upon fixation disparity. Vision Research, 1979.

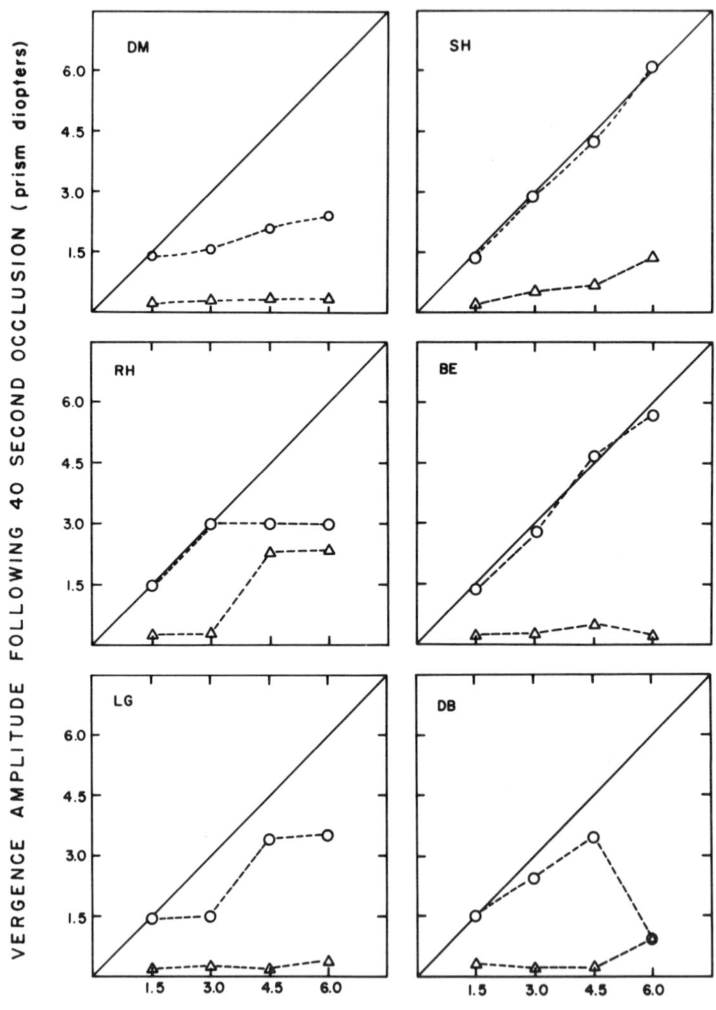

FIGURE 14.10.

sulting from convergent and divergent stimuli. Comparison of these prism-induced curves with prism adaptation reveals that low values of fixation disparity in one direction are associated with high prism adaptation in the same direction. Occasionally, equally low values of fixation disparity occur for both base-in and base-out prisms, even though the associated prism adaptation is unequal. Thus it is not always possible to predict the shape of the prism-induced curves by observing prism adaptation. Other factors must also influence the amplitude of fixation disparity resulting from forced vergence. It is tempting to relate reports by Richards (1975) of stereoblindness for either crossed or uncrossed disparity with the motor vergence asymmetries reported here. Richards observed that uncrossed-disparity and crossed-disparity stereoblind subjects had type II and type III fixation disparity curves, respectively. Examination of stereopsis in the 14 subjects described above with 80-msec pulsed disparities revealed normal stereopsis for both crossed and uncrossed disparities in spite of their marked difference of fixation disparity and adaptation.

Prism Adaptation and Exposure Duration

Other evidence of the influence of prism adaptation comes from comparisons of fixation disparity following short-term and long-term wearing of prism. Mitchell and Ellerbrock (1955) observed that the shape of the forced duction fixation disparity curve changed depending on how long

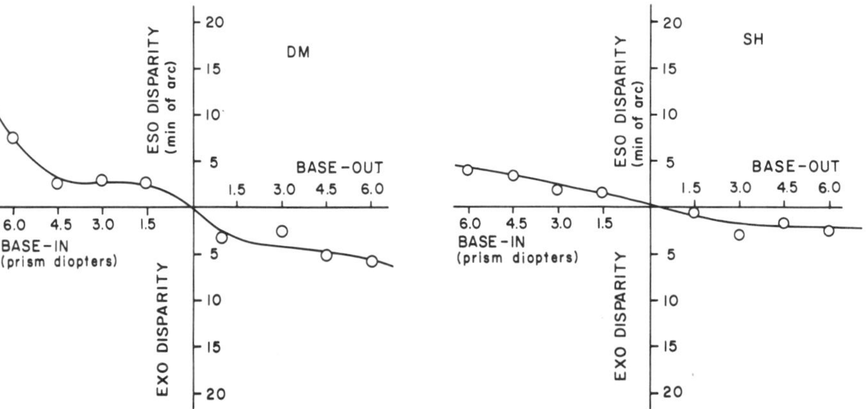

FIGURES 14.11, 14.12, and 14.13. Fixation disparity in minute of arc plotted for individual subjects as a function of amplitude of the stimulus to fusional vergence in prism diopters. Convergent stimuli (base-out prism) and divergent stimuli (base-in prism) are represented respectively to the right and left of the Y axis on each graph. Convergent (eso)fixation disparity and divergent (exo)fixation disparity are plotted respectively above and below the X axis. Reprinted by permission of the publisher, from Schor CM. The influence of rapid prism adaptation upon fixation disparity. Vision Research, 1979.

TYPE II FIXATION DISPARITY

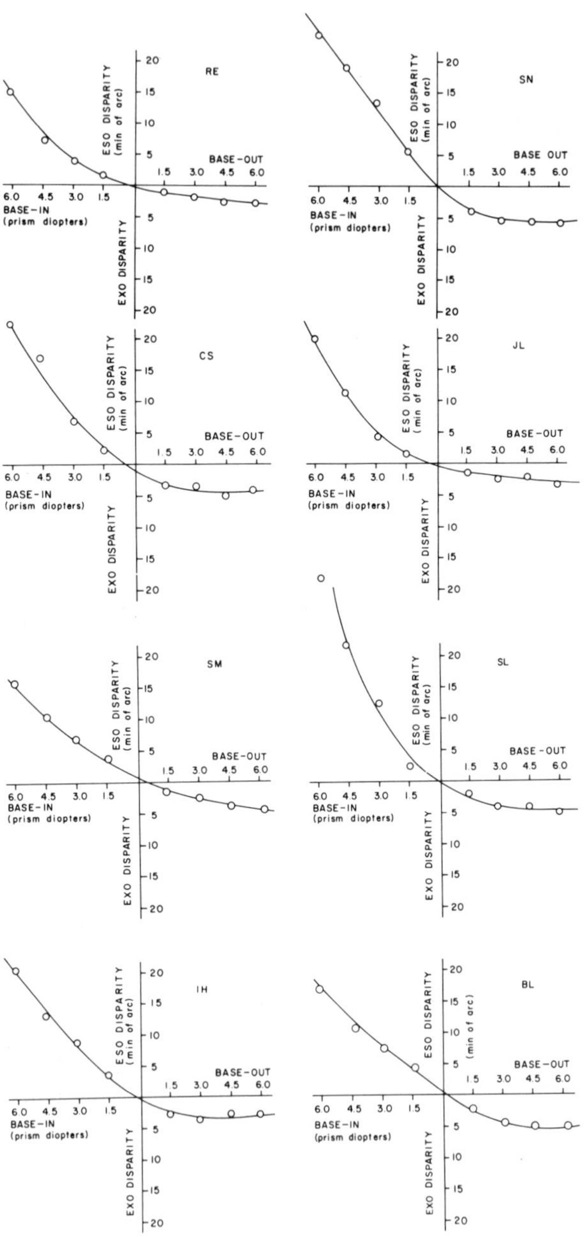

FIGURE 14.12.

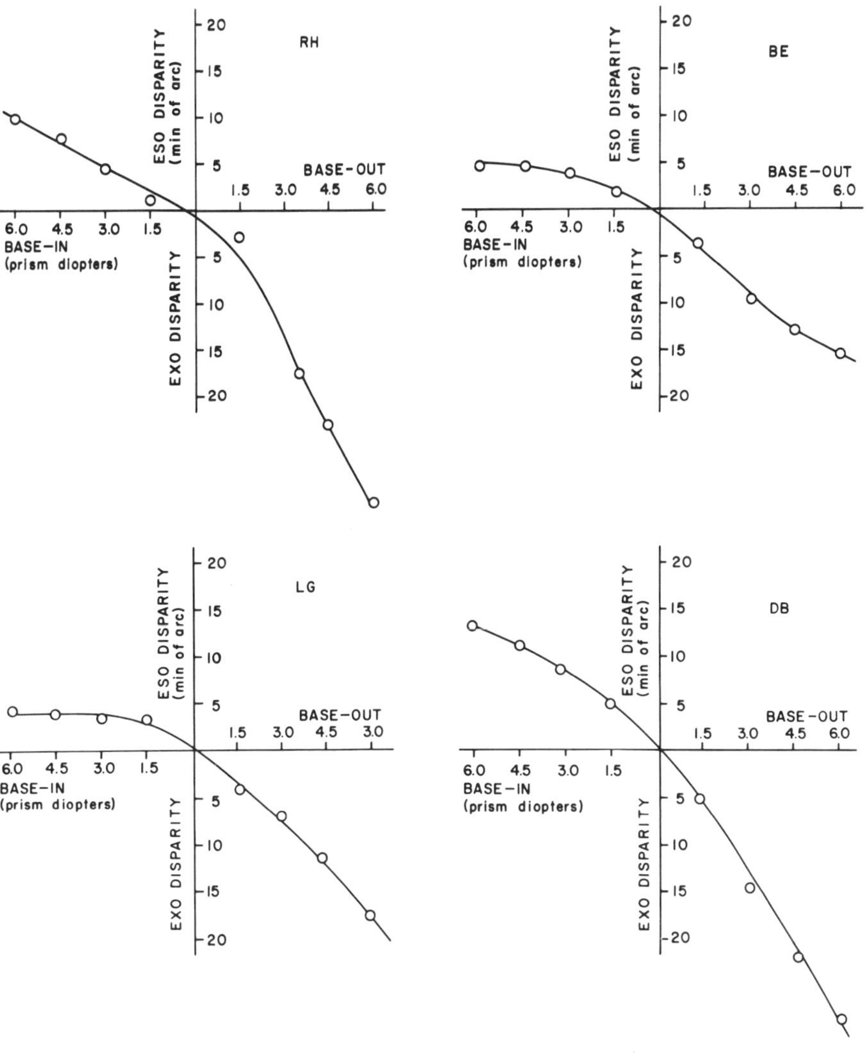

FIGURE 14.13.

prism vergence was stimulated. They found marked reductions in esofixation disparity that occurred after prolonged wearing of base-in prism; however, no changes were found for exofixation disparity after prolonged wearing of base-out prism. The different effects of stimulus duration on esofixation and exofixation are interpreted as unequal rates of prism adaptation. Their subject showed rapid prism adaptation to base-out prism that could not be detected by their experimental paradigm, and much slower adaptation to base-in prism. Subsequently, Carter (1965) and Ogle, Martens, and Dyer (1967) have reported that both esofixation and exofixation disparity can be reduced with long-term wearing of prism. Ogle and Prangen (1953) observed a reduction in vertical fixation disparity after subjects wore a vertical prism for two hours. After adapting to the prism, vertical fixation disparity had the same amplitude that was measured before the prism was worn. The time course for the reduction of vertical fixation disparity is approximately 15 minutes for a 2^{Δ} vertical prism (Ogle and Prangen, 1953) and 15 minutes for 32^{Δ} horizontal prism or any horizontal prism amplitude within the range of horizontal fusional vergence (Ogle et al., 1967; Carter, 1965).

Fast and Slow Fusional Vergence

Ogle and Prangen (1953) suggested that the reduction of fixation disparity with prolonged binocular fixation was due to a slow fusional process. They proposed that slow fusional vergence responded to stress on a faster form of fusional vergence. The sum of the fast and slow mechanisms equaled the total disparity-induced vergence response such that when slow fusional vergence increased there was an equal reduction of fast fusional vergence. This reduction would occur as a result of the negative feedback loop of the fusional vergence system. Thus output of the slow fusional mechanism relieves stress on the fast fusional mechanism, making it possible for fast fusional vergence to respond to subsequent stimulus disparities. Assuming that fixation disparity results from stress on fast fusional vergence, slow fusional vergence could account for the reduction of horizontal fixation disparity following prolonged wearing of a lateral prism.

The fast and slow vergence mechanisms appear to be responses to different stimuli or inputs. The stimulus for fast fusional vergence is retinal image disparity, which is derived from the error (difference) between the angle subtended at the entrance pupils by the fixation target and the angle of convergence of the eyes. Slow fusional vergence appears to be stimulated by the output, or effort, of the fast fusional vergence control mechanism. This arrangement is suggested by two observations. First, it is clear that the stimulus to slow fusional vergence is not retinal image disparity. Fast fusional vergence is capable of reducing retinal image disparity within one second (Rashbass and Westheimer, 1961) to less than 28 seconds of arc (Riggs and Niehl, 1960; Hebbard, 1962). The shortest reported duration of disparity-induced vergence that has resulted in prolonged changes in the phoria is 30 seconds (Schor, 1979a; Henson and North, 1980). Thus slow fusional vergence occurs well after retinal image disparity has been nulled by fast fusional vergence. Second, Carter

(1965) has observed a lack of prism aftereffect on the phoria in response to diplopia stimulated with a large prism. This provides further support for the hypothesis that the stimulus to vergence adaptation is the effort, or output, of the fast fusional vergence controller.

A MODEL OF PRISM ADAPTATION AND FIXATION DISPARITY

Evidence has been presented that supports the existence of two separate control mechanisms for fusional or disparity vergence. The first mechanism, fast fusional vergence, has been modeled as a leaky neural integrator. The leakage term describes the 10- to 15-second rapid decay of convergence following monocular occlusion (Ludvigh et al., 1964; Krishnan and Stark, 1977). The integrator term describes observations by Rashbass and Westheimer (1961) of large-amplitude vergence responses to small disparities presented under stabilized retinal image (open-loop) viewing conditions. The second mechanism, slow fusional vergence, has been modeled by Schor (1979b, 1980a) as a neural integrator with a very long-decay time constant (greater than 30 seconds). Figure 14.14 diagrams the inputs to fast and slow fusional vergence and the interaction between their controllers. The input to the system is target distance in meter angles, and the output is convergence in meter angles. The difference between these constitutes the error signal, retinal image disparity. This error must exceed a threshold of less than 28 seconds of arc (Riggs

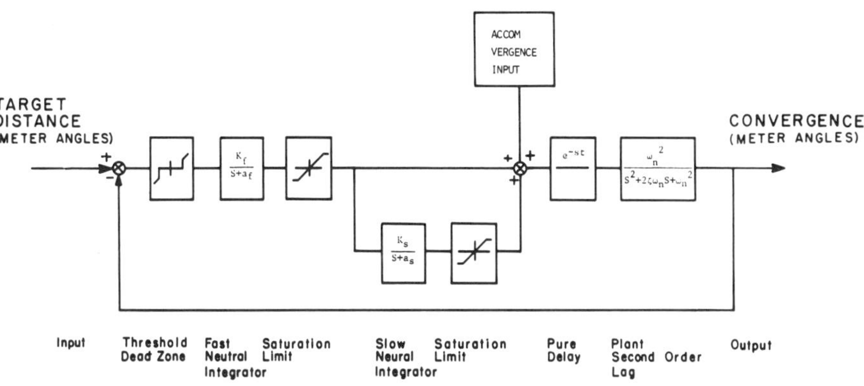

BLOCK DIAGRAM OF THE FUSIONAL VERGENCE SYSTEM

FIGURE 14.14. System model representation of the dual control mechanism of the fusional vergence motor system. Reprinted by permission of the publisher, from Schor CM. The relationship between fusional vergence and fixation disparity. Vision Research, 1979.

and Niehl, 1960) before activating convergence. This threshold is far less than Panum's fusional area at the fovea, which is reported to be 10 minutes of arc (Ogle, 1964). The error signal drives the fast neural integrator, which has a gain (k_f) of 2.5 and a time constant (l/a) of 10 seconds (Krishnan and Stark, 1977). The gain is defined as the initial velocity of the vergence response to a one-degree step change in disparity (Rashbass and Westheimer, 1961). The slow fusional vergence controller is in parallel with the output of the fast vergence controller, and the outputs of both controllers are summated in the forward path of the loop. Each controller is followed by a saturation limit, which indicates the peak amplitude of the controller's operating range. The two blocks that remain describe the latency of convergence and the dynamic properties of the extraocular muscles. The unique feature of this model is the arrangement of the fast and slow neural integrators controlling fusional vergence.

Computer Simulations

Dynamic interactions between the fast and slow vergence controllers were examined with an analogue circuit of the model in Figure 14.14. The gain of the fast neural integrator (k_f) and the reciprocal of its decay time constant (a_f) were set at empirical values of 2.5 and 0.1, respectively, derived by Ludvigh and colleagues (1964) and Krishnan and Stark (1977). The gain of the slow neural integrator (k_s) was set at 3 and its reciprocal time constant (a_s) at 0.03 on the basis of empirical values derived by Schor (1979a). Figure 14.15 illustrates the closed-loop simulated response of the two integral controllers and of the output of the whole system. The step response of the total system was completed in one second and then remained at a constant amplitude. The total response was made up of the sum of the two integral controllers. The fast integral controller carried out the initial step response. Gradually the slow integral controller took over the response and relieved the fast integrator, making it available for a rapid response to subsequent stimuli.

The static (steady-state) amplitude of the slow fusional vergence response need not equal total response, as it does in Figure 14.15. The relative amplitudes of the slow and fast neural integrator outputs depend solely on the gain (k) and time constant (T) of the slow neural integrator where $T = l/a$. The output of the slow neural integrator drives down the output of the fast neural integrator via the negative feedback loop of the vergence servo. Under closed-loop conditions steady-state equilibrium is reached between these two integrators when the ratio of outputs of the slow and fast neural integrators equals the absolute gain of the slow neural integrator (k_sT_S) (equation [a]). Total prism adaptation was simulated by setting the gain of the slow integrator (k_sT_S) at a high value. For example, in Figure 14.15 the absolute gain of the slow integrator was set at 100, so

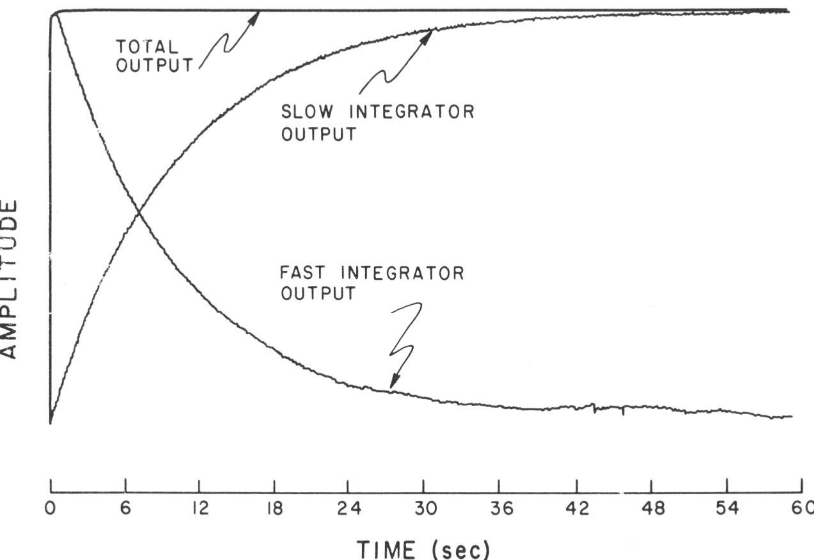

FIGURE 14.15. Total prism adaptation illustrated by an analogue computer simulation of the closed-loop response of the two neural integral controllers of fusional vergence and the output of the total vergence system. $K_f = 2.5$; $T_f = 10$; $K_s = 3$; $T_s = 33$; $K_sT_s = 100$. Reprinted by permission of the publisher, from Schor CM. The relationship between fusional vergence and fixation disparity. Vision Research, 1979.

that the ratio of the outputs for the slow and fast integrators was 100:1. Partial or incomplete prism adaptation was simulated by setting the gain of the slow integrator (k_sT_s) to a low value. In Figure 14.16 it was set at a value of one. As a result, the steady-state outputs of the slow and fast integrators were equal.

Equations describing the amplitudes of fast and slow integrator outputs are given. The total system output, which equals the sum of the outputs from the two integral controllers, has been designated as a value of one in equation (*b*). Outputs of the slow and fast neural integrators are indicated by *S* and *F* respectively. Given

$$S/F = k_sT_s \quad (a)$$

and

$$S + F = 1, \quad (b)$$

then

$$F = \frac{1}{1 + k_sT_s} \quad (c)$$

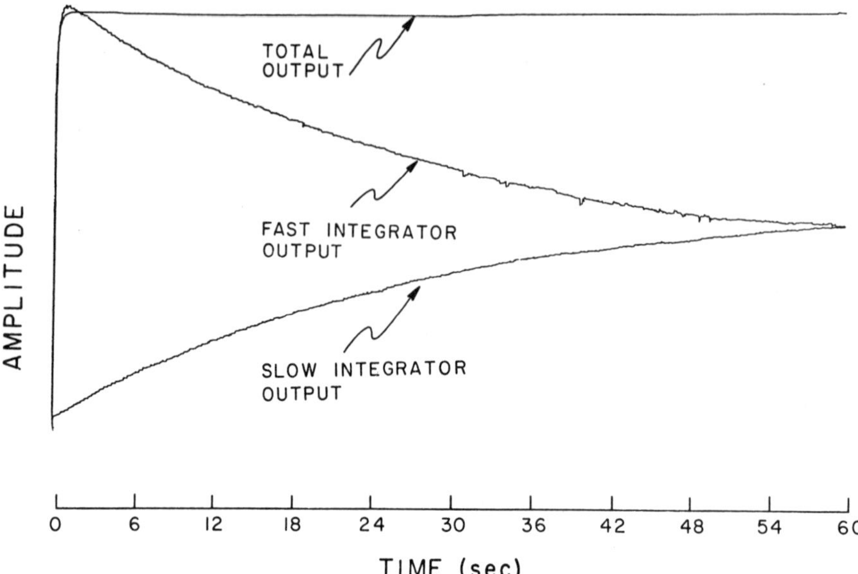

FIGURE 14.16. Partial prism adaptation illustrated by an analogue computer simulation of the closed-loop response of the two neural integral controllers of fusional vergence and the output of the total vergence system. $K_f = 2.5$; $T_f = 10$; $K_s = .03$; $T_s = 33$; $K_s T_s = 1.0$. Reprinted by permission of the publisher, from Schor CM. The relationship between fusional vergence and fixation disparity. Vision Research, 1979.

is the amplitude of the fast neural integrator and

$$S = \frac{1}{1 + k_s T_s} \tag{d}$$

is the amplitude of the slow neural integrator. The temporal course of the simulated interaction is consistent with prior reports of the temporal course and magnitude of changes in phoria resulting from disparity-induced vergence eye movements (Ogle and Prangen, 1953; Ellerbrock, 1950; Carter, 1965; Schor, 1979a; Alpern, 1969; Morgan, 1947).

Predictions of Fixation Disparity from Modeling

The mathematical model that describes integral controllers of the fusional vergence system is a valuable tool for illustrating the source of small errors of the vergence system referred to as fixation disparity. The model predicts that fixation disparity will be limited by either the threshold for fusional vergence or the steady-state error of the integral controllers, whichever of the two is larger. The threshold sets a lower limit for the error signal, or disparity, to which fast fusional vergence can respond. Error signals that are below threshold are effectively zero. A steady-state error is a small error of convergence that acts as a stimulus to maintain convergence under binocular viewing conditions. The small error drives the fast leaky integral controller to compensate for the leakage, or decay of convergence, that becomes manifest when one eye is occluded. The amplitude of the steady-state error depends on the gain and decay time constants of the two neural integrators. If fusional vergence were controlled exclusively by the fast neural integrator, the steady-state error would be expressed by the equation

$$fd = \frac{x}{kT + 1} \qquad (e)$$

where fd = fixation disparity;
x = disparate stimulus for vergence;
k = gain of integral controller;
T = open-loop decay time constant.

Equation (e) predicts a linear relaxation between the stimulus amplitude of disparity-induced vergence (x) and fixation disparity. Such a relation is illustrated by the straight lines in Figure 14.17 for convergent and divergent disparities. The plot was derived from empirical values of 2.5 for the gain of convergence, 1.25 for the gain of divergence, and 10.0 seconds for T (Krishnan and Stark, 1977). The computed linear relation for a single integral controller predicts much greater values for horizontal fixation disparity than are typically found (Ogle et al., 1967) with empirical measures of fixation disparity (open circles in Figure 14.17). Empirical values of fixation disparity normally increase at a low rate with low-amplitude vergence stimuli and more rapidly as the limits of convergence or divergence are approached (Ogle et al., 1967). The slopes of the extreme portions of the forced duction fixation disparity curve are similar to the slopes predicted by equation (e), suggesting that steady-state errors near the limits of the fusional vergence system are determined by characteristics of the fast neural integrator. The flat portion in the center of the forced duction fixation disparity curve appears to be a characteristic of the slow neural integrator that effectively reduces the stimulus to fast fusional vergence. The width of the central flat region of the curve in Figure 14.17 indicates the operating range and saturation limits or peak amplitudes of the slow neural integrator. The empirically derived forced duction fixation disparity curve can be approximated by reducing the stimulus amplitude (x) in equation (e) by the amount of prism adaptation (PA) caused by the slow neural integrator. This equation is based on a Maddox-like assumption that the total vergence response equals the sum

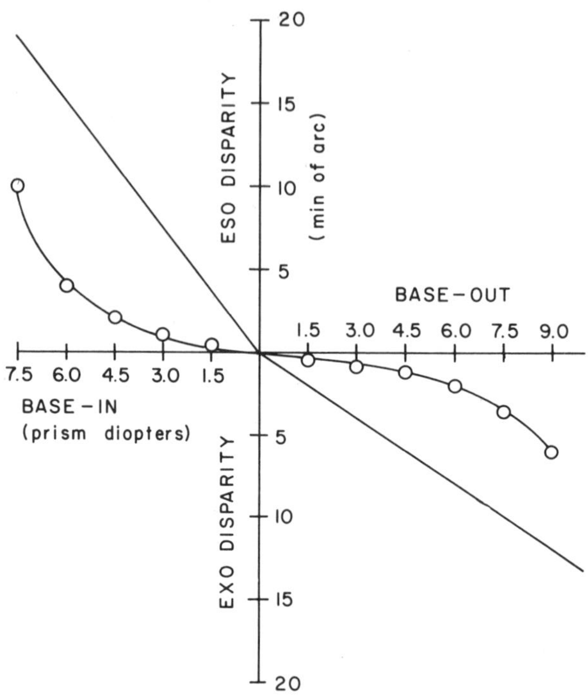

FIGURE 14.17. Straight lines illustrate fixation disparity predicted for various stimulus disparity amplitudes by equation (e), and empirical values of fixation disparity (*open circles*) are plotted as a function of stimulus disparity amplitude.

of disparity vergence and prism adaptation:

$$fd = \frac{x - (PA)}{kT + 1}. \tag{f}$$

A more precise equation based on the interaction described in Figure 14.4 is developed from the polynomial transfer function (equation [g]) describing the closed-loop output of the sum of the fast and slow neural integrators.

$$H(s) = \frac{K_f(S + [a_s + K_s])}{(S + a_f)(S + a_s) + K_f(S + [a_s + K_s])} \tag{g}$$

where a equals the reciprocal of the leakage time constants of the slow (s) and fast (f) neural integrators. Steady-state equations are derived by solving the transfer function for $S = O$.

$$H(O) = \frac{K_f a_s + K_f K_s}{a_f a_s + K_f a_s + K_f K_s}. \tag{h}$$

The steady-state unit step error equals $1 - H(O)$ where

$$1 - H(O) = \frac{1}{1 + k_f/a_f(1 + k_s/a_s)}. \qquad (i)$$

Let $T = l/a$. Then

$$1 - H(O) = \frac{1}{1 + K_f T_f(1 + k_s T_s)}, \qquad (j)$$

steady-state error of the fusional vergence system.

Applications to Horizontal and Vertical Fixation Disparity

The relationship between fixation disparity and prism adaptation described by equations (*f*) and (*j*) provides a tool for examining slow and fast fusional vergence using measures of forced duction fixation disparity curves. The equations illustrate quantitatively how the shapes of the forced duction fixation disparity curves described by Ogle are influenced by a variety of factors including prism adaptation, which flattens the curves or minimizes fixation disparity.

The same tools make it possible to examine slow and fast fusional vergence in the vertical meridian. As described earlier, fixation disparity resulting from vertical prism increases linearly and over a much smaller range than the nonlinear response to horizontal prism. The flat regions of the horizontal fixation disparity curves were shown to result from rapid prism adaptation to a small range of vergence stimuli. The absence of this flat range from the center of the vertical curves (Figure 14.5) indicates that there is no rapid adaptation to vertical prism, and assuming the model proposed in Figure 14.14, the slope of the curve is determined primarily by the gain and open-loop decay time constant of fast fusional vergence. An alternative explanation for the straight curve is that there is rapid prism adaptation that occurs over a range of prism equal to or greater than the operating range of fast vertical fusional vergence. A slow adaptation to vertical prism has been demonstrated, however, by reduction of vertical fixation disparity after vertical prism had been worn for several hours (Ogle and Prangen, 1953). Additional evidence comes from comparisons of the associated and dissociated phorias. The associated horizontal phoria is usually 25% smaller than the dissociated horizontal phoria due to the reduction of stress on fast fusional vergence by rapid prism adaptation. Ogle and Prangen (1953) observed that the vertical associated and dissociated phorias were identical, which suggests an absence of rapid adaptation to vertical prism.

FUNCTIONAL SIGNIFICANCE OF PRISM ADAPTATION

Orthophorization

Given the enormous number of mechanical, neural, and sensory variables that determine the position of the eyes, it is remarkable that the fusion-free vergence posture (phoria) is nearly zero in most normal persons (Hirsch et al., 1948). This high incidence of orthophoria has been compared to the high incidence of emmetropic refractive states (Crone and Hardjowijoto, 1979). Like the emmetropization process that coordinates the optical components that determine refractive state of the eye, it has been suggested that a similar process of orthophorization might coordinate the neuromuscular mechanisms that control binocular alignment (Crone and Hardjowijoto, 1979). A mechanism that could underlie orthophorization is prism adaptation (Ogle and Prangen, 1953; Carter, 1965). A disturbance of this mechanism could result in large heterophorias and possibly strabismus (Ogle and Prangen, 1953; Carter, 1965). Persons lacking the mechanism could benefit from prescription of prisms to adjust the directions of the lines of sight to a single object of regard. The benefits of prism would be longlasting, since recipients lack the adaptive mechanism that could reduce the effectiveness of prism therapy (Carter, 1965). There are, however, some persons with abnormal vertical or horizontal phorias who do adapt to prism so that their associated and dissociated phorias and fixation disparity are unchanged by the addition of prism. A classical example of adaptation returning the phoria to its original abnormal value is provided by Ogle and Prangen (1953). Their patient had 1.75 prism diopters of hyperphoria before and after compensation to 2 diopters and then 4 diopters of vertical prism. The patient's associated phoria and forced duction vertical fixation disparity curve remained the same before and after wearing vertical prism (Figure 14.18). Similar adaptation of vertical and horizontal heterophorias to prism was found by Schubert (1943). These observations suggest that prism adaptation may not serve the process of orthophorization in these examples, but rather the maintenance of some preestablished heterophoria (Carter, 1965; Crone and Hardjowijoto, 1979). This process is referred to as phorization.

Stability of Binocular Correspondence

It is assumed, but has not been demonstrated objectively, that prism adaptation returns the fusion-free vergence angle to the original phoria. The magnitude of phoria during and after adaptation is not measured objectively by cover test but is inferred from subjective measures using, for example, the Maddox-rod prism neutralization (Ogle and Prangen, 1953).

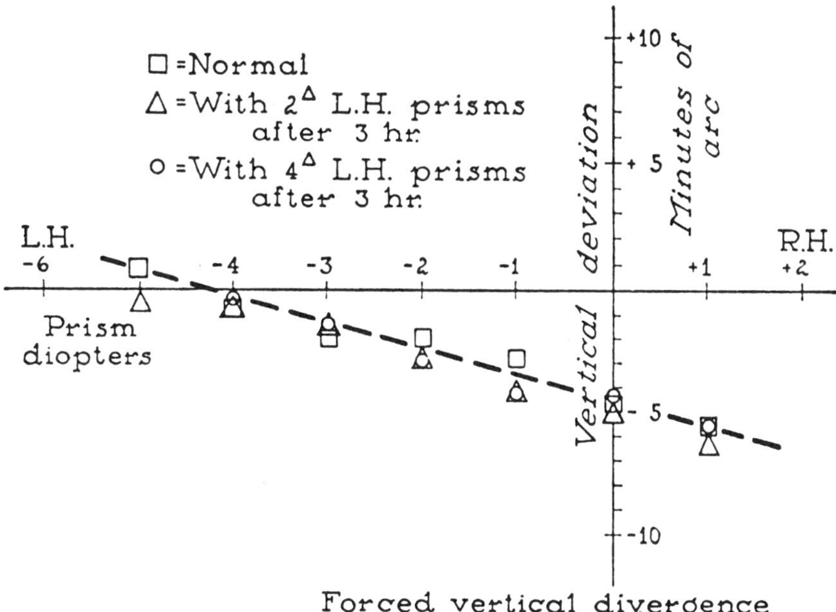

FIGURE 14.18. Ogle and Prangen (1953) showed complete adaptation of fixation disparity after several hours to 2^{Δ} and 4^{Δ} of added vertical prism. Reprinted by permission of the publisher, from Ogle KN, Prangen A. Observations of vertical divergence and hyperphorias. Archives of Ophthalmology, 49:313–34. Copyright 1953, American Medical Association.

It is interesting to compare prism adaptation where the phoria returns to its original value with that observed in esotropic strabismus by Alpern and Hofstetter (1948). They observed a case of esotropia with anomalous binocular correspondence whose angle of strabismus (measured objectively by cover test) fully adapted to base-out prism worn for several hours. Interestingly, the perceived angle of diplopia or subjective angle of strabismus remained nearly zero (anomalous correspondence) before, during, and after adaptation to prism. This observation has also been reported by others (Mariani and Pasino, 1964; Hallden, 1952). These slow fusional responses to prisms observed in strabismus with anomalous correspondence have been called anomalous fusional movements (Bagolini, 1976). Circumstances similar to anomalous fusion may account for the constant subjective measures of the phoria and fixation disparity that occur with prism adaptation. Perhaps the objective phoria and fixation disparity are larger than subjective measures of these functions. If this were the case it would appear that complete adaptation had occurred by subjective measures, while it was still incomplete by objective measure. This interpretation assumes that normal binocular correspondence changes.

Evidence for such change comes from large differences in subjective and objective measures of ocular vergence where objective errors as large as 1 to 2 degrees can occur during single bifoveal fixation (Stewart, 1951; Fender and Julesz, 1967; Diner, 1978). Thus both perceptual and motor factors appear to contribute to the maintenance of a constant subjective angle of directionalization in both normal and anomalous correspondence. Normally, prism adaptation makes long-term adjustments in ocular alignment, however, in the short term, perceptual adaptations may occur to maintain single binocular vision if fast and slow fusional vergence do not completely align the eyes.

Maintenance of Hering's Law

Another function of prism adaptation is to maintain Hering's law of equal ocular movements (Hering 1942). Pathological, structural, and externally induced changes such as those that occur in noncomitant strabismus and in surgically corrected strabismus are compensated for by a spread of concomitance that restores Hering's law. The mechanism for these compensatory adjustments has been shown by Henson and Dharamashi (1982) to be vergence adaptation over limited motor fields or in specific directions of gaze ($\pm 20^0$). Similar direction-specific adaptations are instrumental in overcoming noncomitant phorias due to correction of anisometropia with spectacle lenses.

CLINICAL APPLICATIONS OF FIXATION DISPARITY

Chapter 15 by Sheedy and Saladin describes the use of forced duction fixation disparity curves for analysis of binocular disorders. These curves are used to evaluate prism adaptation. As described earlier in this chapter, fixation disparity is reciprocally related to prism adaptation such that clinical measures of fixation disparity can be used as an indicator of reduced or absent prism adaptation. Portions of the forced duction curves that have the lowest slope and that are closest to the horizontal axis represent the prism stimulus range resulting in the fastest and most complete prism adaptation, respectively. These observations can be used to interpret the significance of three diagnostic criteria from the forced duction fixation disparity curves that are used to diagnose and treat tonic disorders of binocular vision.

Associated Phoria

Two general criteria have been adopted for the prescription of prism based on measures of fixation disparity. The most commonly used method does not measure the magnitude of fixation disparity, but instead determines the amount of prism that will reduce fixation disparity to zero. The nulling or neutralization of fixation disparity with prism was referred to by Ogle and associates (1967) as the associated phoria, as opposed to the dissociated phoria measured under monocular viewing conditions. The associated phoria represents the amount of fusional vergence that has not been replaced by prism adaptation. Prism adaptation is mainly responsible for differences between the associated and dissociated measurements. Usually the associated phoria is less than the dissociated phoria (Ogle et al., 1967).

Paradoxical Fixation Disparity

Occasionally the two phorias are opposite in sign. For example, an intermittent exotrope with normal binocular correspondence can manifest esofixation disparity following orthoptic exercises. The paradoxical fixation disparity results from an overcompensation of fusional convergence by prism adaptation. Excessive adaptation produces a convergence error that is corrected during binocular viewing conditions by fusional divergence. The fusional divergence effort is associated with a purposeful esofixation disparity that prevents the decay of fusional divergence innervation. The effect of orthoptics is to increase the amplitude (Vaegan, 1979) and rate (North and Henson, 1981) of prism adaptation. Paradoxical fixation disparity resulting from orthoptics should be considered as a positive sign that will decrease when orthoptic exercises are discontinued.

The development of prism adaptation following orthoptics may reduce the associated phoria; however, fixation disparity in these postorthoptic cases may still be abnormally large (Schor, 1980a). Figure 14.19 illustrates measures of prism adaptation in three patients with occasional convergent strabismus. As indicated by the measures of vergence amplitude following occlusions of one eye, these patients showed a remarkable ability to adapt to divergent prism. This adaptation appears to be the mechanism developed by the orthoptic exercises from which patients learned to overcome their esotropia. Measures of forced duction fixation disparity curves in these same patients (Figure 14.20) show large amounts of fixation disparity in response to divergence prism even though adaptation was strong in that direction. Thus other factors in addition to prism adaptation influence the magnitude of fixation disparity.

Suppression

Sensory factors such as central suppression in strabismus can influence both prism adaptation and fixation disparity by limiting the stimulus to vergence eye movements to the peripheral retina (Jampolsky, 1956).

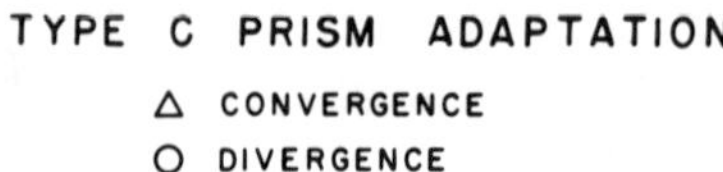

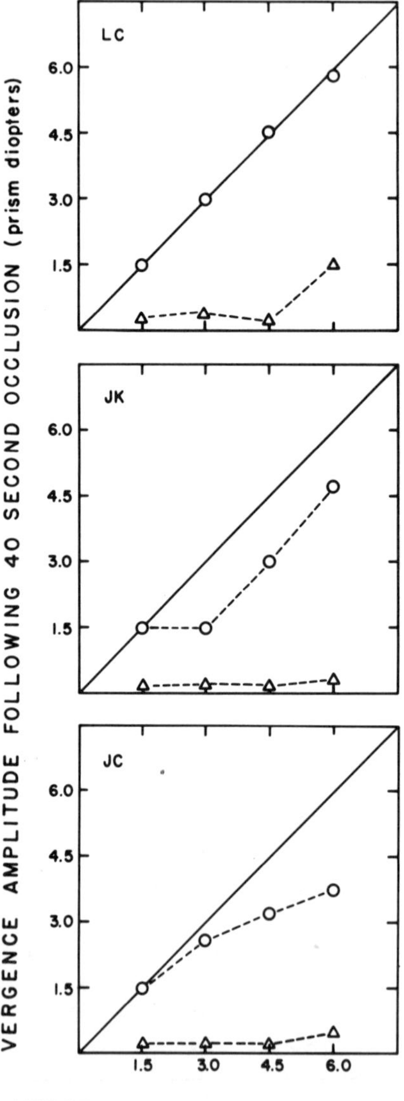

FIGURE 14.19. Adaptation to base-in prism by three subjects with occasional convergent strabismus. Reprinted by permission of the publisher, from Schor CM. The influence of rapid prism adaptation upon fixation disparity. Vision Research, 1979.

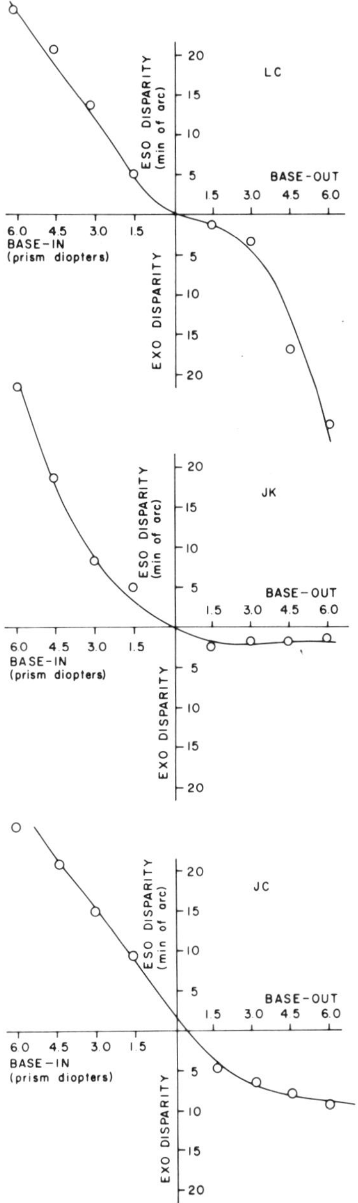

FIGURE 14.20. Prism-induced fixation disparity curves for three subjects with occasional convergent strabismus. Reprinted by permission of the publisher, from Schor CM. The influence of rapid prism adaptation upon fixation disparity. Vision Research, 1979.

As illustrated by Ogle and co-workers (1967) in Figure 14.6, fixation disparity resulting from a given prism stimulus is much greater when measured with a 6° rather than with a 0.75° fusion lock. Similarly, Carter (1964) has shown that prism adaptation is much more rapid and complete when conducted with central than with peripheral fusion locks. Clinical tests of the associated phoria take this into account by providing both central and peripheral fusion locks (Mallett, 1974). Central locks ensure that measured fixation disparity will be reduced to the same degree that it achieves in a normal environment. Removal of the central fusion stimulus would increase the fixation disparity and make the associated phoria easier to measure, however, it might also result in overcorrection of the usual associated phoria. In cases of binocular dysfunction associated with central suppression, clinical tests still provide peripheral fusion stimuli similar to those available in ordinary viewing conditions. Central suppression in strabismus may continue to cause increased fixation disparity even after orthoptic exercises have improved the rate and amplitude of prism adaptation (Schor, 1980a).

Motor Control Factors

Motor factors, such as the gain or response amplification of fusional vergence, have also been shown to influence the amplitude of fixation disparity (Schor, 1979b), which is considered to be a stimulus used to replenish the decaying innervation for fusional vergence. The gain of the fusional vergence control system will determine how large a stimulus is necessary to compensate for the decaying innervation. Normally the gain of disparity vergence ranges between 3 and 5.5 (Rashbass and Westheimer, 1961); however the gain is reduced by 40% in abnormal binocular vision (Grisham, 1980). Thus given the same amount of prism adaptation and the same decay of fusional vergence, a patient who has binocular dysfunction with reduced gain for vergence control will have a greater fixation disparity than a person who has a normal fusional vergence gain. Correction or reduction of the unusually large fixation disparity found in postorthoptic patients is only recommended if there are associated symptoms of asthenopia. Fixation disparity by itself does not suggest a binocular anomaly in need of correction. Studies of normal asymptomatic subjects reveal fixation disparity associated with either orthophoria or heterophoria (Palmer and von Noordon, 1978; Jampolsky et al., 1957). Symptoms of asthenopia appear to be related to abnormally low prism adaptation (Carter, 1965). If differences between measures of the associated phoria and dissociated phoria result primarily from prism adaptation, these two measures of the phoria are expected to have a higher correlation in symptomatic than asymptomatic patients. Similarly, fixation disparity and the associated phoria may be valid measures of binocular stress induced by the dissociated phoria for persons who are symptomatic. Since the associated phoria takes into account the effects of prism adaptation it also provides a more valid criterion for prescribing prism than the graphical technique, which computes a prescription based on measures of the dissociated phoria. Prism adaptation can be incorporated into graphical analysis, however, by plotting the associated rather than dissociated measures of the phoria within the zone of clear single binocular vision.

Center of Symmetry

The second major criterion for prescribing prism is based on the shape of the forced duction fixation disparity curve. A diagnostic feature of the curve is its flattest central region or the point at which the second derivative becomes zero. Ogle and colleagues (1967) refer to this inflection point as the center of symmetry (CS) (Figure 14.21). Prism is prescribed to shift the center of symmetry to the Y axis of the forced duction fixation disparity plot (Sheedy, 1980). As described earlier, the shape of the curve is determined primarily by prism adaptation (Schor, 1979a). The amplitude of fixation disparity is reduced by prism adaptation and the center of symmetry occurs where prism adaptation occurs most rapidly in response to changes in fusional vergence.

The flat region of the forced duction fixation disparity curve can be measured rapidly with the prism duction range over which fixation disparity remains zero (Godio and Rutstein, 1980). The test is conducted with a standard clinical device such as the Mallett unit and it is similar to tests of vergence ranges for the zone of clear single binocular vision. Usually the center of symmetry does not coincide with zero fixation disparity (the X axis intercept and associated phoria) because most patients prefer to adapt to a non-zero phoria and non-zero fixation disparity. This phenomenon was described earlier under functions of prism adaptation and phorization. Usually the associated phoria is greater than the center of symmetry so that prescriptions based on the latter criterion are usually less than those based on the former (Sheedy, 1980). Comparison of prism prescriptions based on the center of symmetry and the associated phoria indicate that the center of symmetry is the more successful criterion (Sheedy, 1980). Since prism adaptation is maximum and presumably most rapid at the center of symmetry, prescriptions based on this criterion optimize the response of prism adaptation to convergence and divergence fusional movements.

The slope of the center of symmetry also has some diagnostic value (Sheedy, 1980). Steep forced duction fixation disparity curves indicate

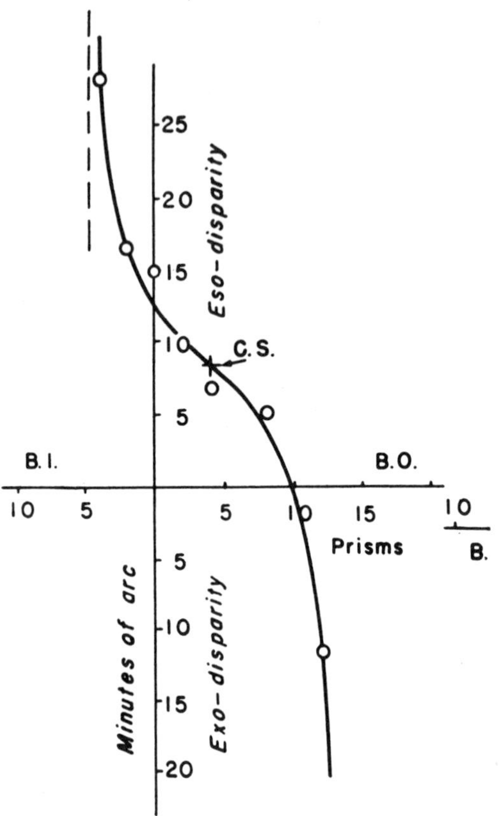

FIGURE 14.21. The center of symmetry (CS), found at the flattest central region of the forced duction fixation disparity curve, usually occurs at a smaller prism value than the point at which the forced duction curve crosses the X axis (associated phoria).

that the adaptive response to fusional vergence is abnormally slow and small. Orthoptic exercises will increase the rate (North and Henson, 1981) and amplitude (Vaegan, 1979) of prism adaptation and cause a flattening or reduced slope of the curves (Sheedy, 1980). Following orthoptics, prism is prescribed based on the lateral displacement of the center of symmetry from the Y axis. For patients with steep curves that do not flatten with orthoptics, prism prescriptions are recommended either on the basis of the associated or dissociated phoria criterion, since these two measures are very similar in these patients who lack prism adaptation.

Taken together, measures of the associated phoria and center of symmetry of forced duction fixation disparity curves give a complete analysis of tonic disturbance of the vergence adaptation process as well as the gain or internal amplification properties of the fusional vergence system. There have also been attempts in the past to use fixation disparity as a means of examining interactions between accommodation and convergence (Ogle et al., 1967). Measures of the *AC/A* ratio computed from equivalent amounts of fixation disparity produced by lenses and prisms, (Figure 14.22) do not correlate with the traditional open-loop measures of the *AC/A* ratio (Hebbard, 1960). Accommodative vergence is greater under binocular (closed-loop) viewing conditions than it is when the vergence loop is opened by occluding one eye (Hebbard, 1960). This discrepancy results from the operation of convergence accommodation, which has the effect of increasing the *AC/A* ratio under binocular viewing conditions (Schor and Narayan, 1982). This increase should cause the associated phoria to be greater than the dissociated phoria, however, the converse is usually found. As discussed in the following section, the increased interaction between accommodation and convergence under binocular viewing conditions is relieved by prism adaptation. The stimulus to convergence accommodation is reduced in 15 to 30 seconds as prism adaptation replaces fusional vergence innervation. Fixation disparity does not reveal transient stress on motor fusion caused by *CA/C* interactions because fixation disparity only measures sustained steady-state effects (Schor, 1980a), which remain after the occurrence of prism adaptation. A graphical method has been developed to predict both transient and sustained interactions between accommodation and convergence under binocular viewing conditions (Schor and Narayan, 1982).

ACCOMMODATIVE VERGENCE, VERGENCE ACCOMMODATION, AND FIXATION DISPARITY

Based on the Maddox (1886) classification of vergence, accommodation stimulated by spherical opthalmic lenses is expected to alter fixation disparity in a manner predicted by the accommodation convergence synkinesis. Accommodative convergence stimulated by ophthalmic lenses causes an increase in esophoria, which is corrected during binocular fixation by the fast and slow fusional vergence systems described in the preceding section of this chapter. Thus the increased demand on fusional vergence caused by accommodation can be equated to a specific amount of prism vergence by means of the *AC/A* ratio. An example of the influence of ophthalmic lenses on fixation disparity is shown in Figure 14.23. Minus power spheres stimulate accommodation and result in esofixation disparity, whereas plus powers relax accommodation and result in exofixation disparity. Forced duction fixation disparity curves have been obtained while accommodation was stimulated by ophthalmic lenses. The effect was to displace the fixation disparity curve laterally in the base-out direction with minus powers and in the base-in direction with plus

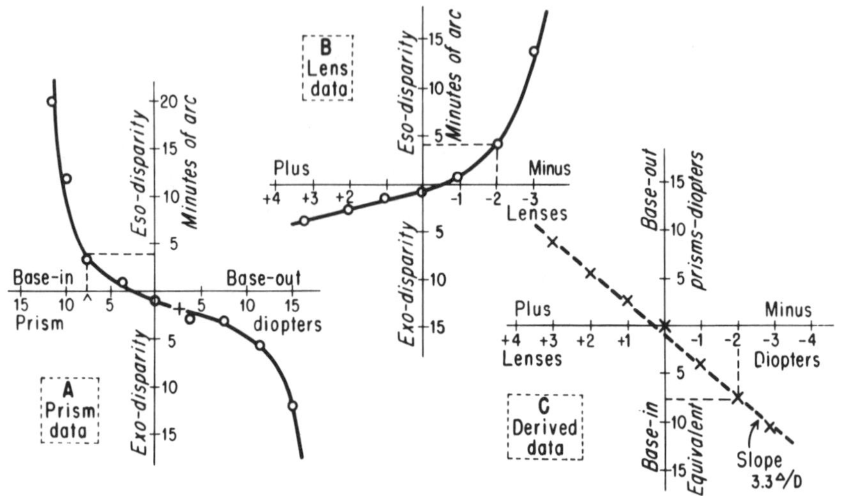

FIGURE 14.22. Graphical representation of fixation disparity as a function of prism vergence (A) and accommodative vergence (B). Derived data (C) show the relationship between change in stimulus to accommodation (lenses) and equivalent prismatic deviation. Reprinted by permission of the publisher, from Ogle KN, Prangen A. Observations of vertical divergence and hyperphorias. Archives of Ophthalmology, 49:313–34. Copyright 1953, American Medical Association.

powers. Thus minus powers resulted in an overall increase in esofixation disparity and plus powers caused an overall increase in exofixation disparity (Figure 14.23) (Hebbard, 1960; Ogle et al., 1967).

Martens and Ogle (1959) derived a measure of the *AC/A* ratio from fixation disparity plotted as a function of accommodation and fusional vergence stimulus amplitude (Figure 14.22). They plotted values of lens power and prism vergence that resulted in the same amount of fixation disparity as shown in Figure 14.22. The plot resulted in a straight line whose slope they believed measured the *AC/A* ratio under associated (binocular) viewing conditions. Comparisons reveal that the associated measure of the *AC/A* is almost always greater than the dissociated measure of the *AC/A* derived from changes of the phoria caused by monocular stimulation of accommodation. The two measures are poorly correlated (Martens and Ogle, 1959; Hebbard, 1960). In addition, the associated *AC/A* can be nonlinear while the dissociated measure is linear and different values of the associated *AC/A* are found depending on the method of derivation (Hebbard, 1960). Ogle and colleagues (1967) account for the differences in the two measures of the *AC/A* from differences in the accommodative response under monocular and binocular viewing conditions. This is an unlikely explanation since in some cases the accommodative response would have to double during binocular viewing conditions to account for the difference.

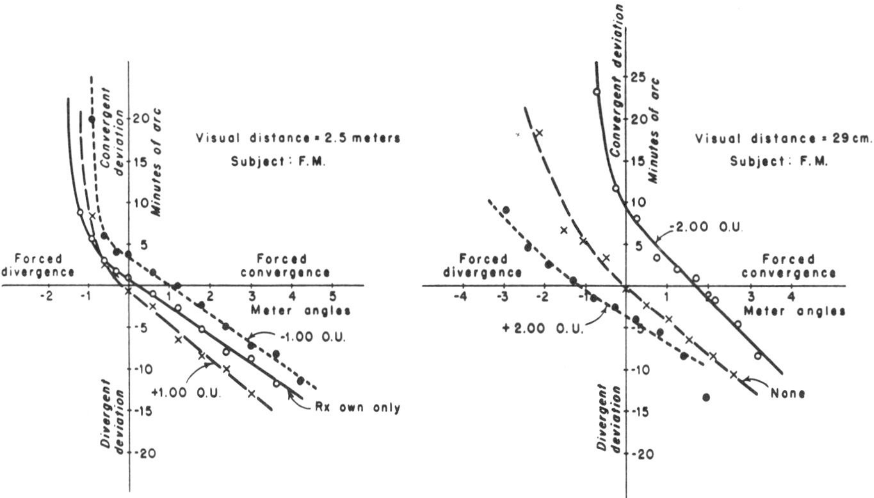

FIGURE 14.23. Effect of spherical lenses on forced duction fixation disparity curves for two viewing distances. Reprinted by permission of the publisher, from Ogle KN, Mussey F, Prangen A. Fixation disparity and the fusional processes in binocular single vision. American Journal of Ophthalmology, 1949.

Convergence Accommodation

Recently, Semmlow and Hung (1979) have shown that another variable, convergence accommodation, may account for differences in interactions between accommodation and convergence during monocular and binocular viewing conditions. The associated *AC/A* ratio reported by Ogle, Martens, and Dyer (1967) is derived from measures of fixation disparity. Semmlow and Hung compared forced duction fixation disparity curves measured with a pin-hole pupil (accommodation open-loop) and with normal pupils (accommodation closed-loop). They observed that fixation disparity was reduced by one-half when the accommodation loop was opened using the pin-hole pupil. They conclude that during closed-loop conditions forced convergence produced a change in accommodation by way of convergence accommodation. This change resulted in blur that was corrected for by optical reflex accommodation. The correction of blur also altered accommodative convergence in a way that increased the demand on fusional vergence and the magnitude of the resulting fixation disparity. For example, with forced convergence there is usually an exo-fixation disparity. The convergence effort stimulates accommodation by means of convergence accommodation, causing an excessive accommodative response. This error is corrected by reducing the output of the controller of optical reflex accommodation. The reduction in accommodative effort also reduces accommodative convergence, which in turn increases the phoria in the divergent direction. The increase in exophoria increases the amount of exofixation disparity that resulted from the high prism stimulus to convergence. Opening the accommodative servoloop with the pin-hole eliminated the correction of focus error caused by convergence accommodation and as a result reduces the amount of exofixation disparity caused by prism stimuli for convergence. Thus interactions between accommodation and convergence are complicated by convergence accommodation during binocular viewing conditions. This additional interaction will cause both lenses and prisms to have a greater effect on fixation disparity than if the convergence accommodation interaction did not exist.

These interpretations suggest that a pure *AC/A* ratio cannot be derived from fixation disparity as originally proposed by Martens and Ogle (1959). The relationship they derived may be more useful in determining equivalent lens and prism values for the correction of oculomotor imbalance, since their ratio is based on the mutual interactions between

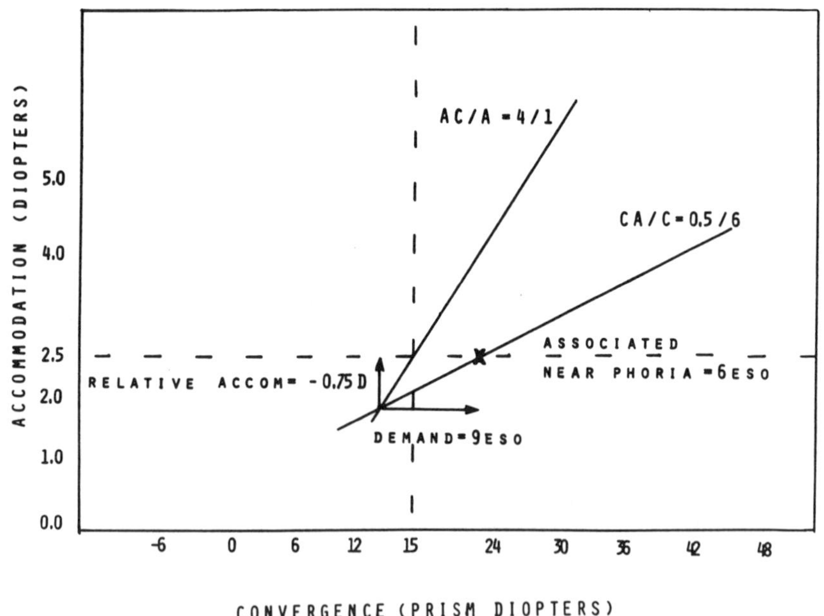

FIGURE 14.24. A The *CA/C* line is drawn through the associated phoria and the *AC/A* line is drawn through the convergence accommodation reference representing the near test distance. The *AC/A* and *CA/C* lines intersect at a point indicating the demand on accommodation (0.75 D) and convergence (9^{Δ}) necessary to correct or overcome an associated phoria of 6 eso for a person with a normal (0.5 D/6^{Δ}) *CA/C* ratio and a normal (4/1) *AC/A* ratio. B The *AC/A* and *CA/C* lines

accommodation and convergence that only occur during binocular viewing conditions.

Graphical Analysis of AC/A and CA/C Interactions.

A new graphical method for analyzing mutual interactions between accommodation and convergence is illustrated in Figure 14.24 (Schor and Narayan, 1982). Convergence is represented on the X axis and accommodation on the Y axis. The intercept of the two dotted lines indicates the accommodative and convergence stimuli presented by a fixation target at a 40-cm viewing distance. The near associated phoria (X) is plotted in reference to this intercept. Unlike classical graphical analysis (Hofstetter, 1945), the *AC/A* line is drawn through this near point reference rather than through the phoria point. The *CA/C* ratio is determined by a gradient method that uses either Tait's method of measuring the accommodative lag or the binocular cross-cylinder (Schor and Narayan, 1982). The *CA/C*

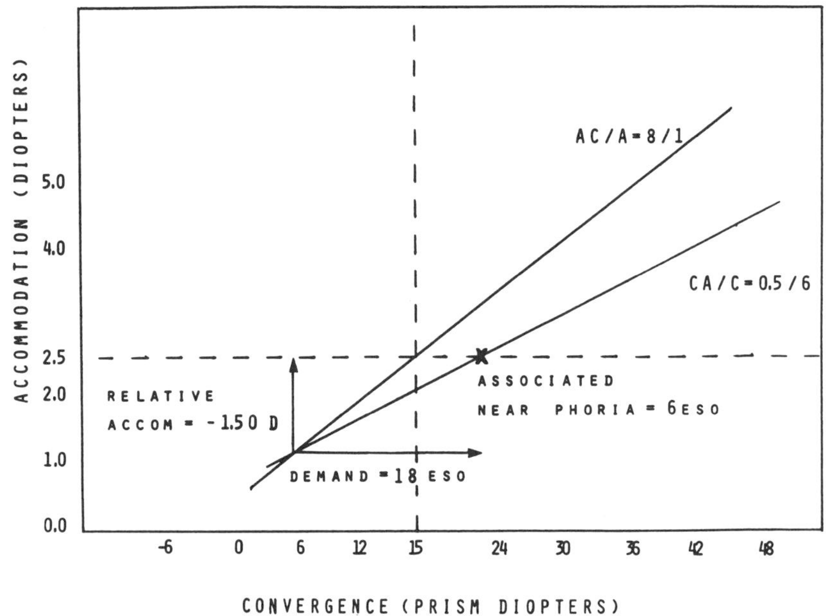

intersect at a point indicating the demand on accommodation (1.5 D) and convergence (18^{Δ}) necessary to correct or overcome an associated phoria of 6 eso for a person with a normal (0.50/6) *CA/C* ratio and a high (8/1) *AC/A* ratio. The demand on accommodation and convergence controllers will become very large as the slope of the *AC/A* and *CA/C* become parallel. Note that the reciprocal of the *AC/A* is plotted.

line is drawn through the associated phoria and indicates the amount that accommodation is altered when the eyes adjust their vergence posture from the associated phoria to the reference intercept. In the example shown in Figure 14.24 the near associated phoria is 6 Base-out. The patient has a *CA/C* ratio of $0.5D/6^{\Delta}$ such that 6^{Δ} of divergence to the near reference intercept would cause a -0.50^{Δ}D error of accommodation. Correction of the error by the accommodative system would stimulate accommodative convergence and result in recurrence of esophoria.

The additional amount of esophoria in this example would be 2^{Δ} for the *AC/A* ratio of $4^{\Delta}/1$. To avoid this error a negative vergence effort is needed that is greater than the associated phoria so that when the resulting error of accommodation is corrected, accommodative convergence will align the eyes at a vergence angle equal to the near reference intercept. The amount of fusional vergence and additional accommodation that is necessary for binocular alignment is indicated by the intersection of the *CA/C* line with the *AC/A* line drawn through the near reference point. The horizontal and vertical vectors from the intersection point to the associated phoria indicate the horizontal demand on convergence and additional adjustments of accommodation, respectively. In this example the associated phoria of 6 eso is corrected by a divergence effort equivalent to 9^{Δ} and an increase in accommodation of 0.75 D over the demand of the near viewing distance (2.5 D). This is a small difference because the slopes of the *AC/A* and *CA/C* are very different. If, however, the *AC/A* were abnormally high, such as $8^{\Delta}/1$ D as in a previous example, its slopes would be closer to that of the *CA/C* line. Figure 14.24 illustrates this graphically for a patient with the same *CA/C* ratio and with a normal *AC/A* ratio of 8/1. In this example the same accommodative error is caused by divergence of 6^{Δ}, but more esophoria is reinstated by the higher *AC/A* when the accommodative error is corrected. Consequently, the 6^{Δ}-associated esophoria is corrected with 18^{Δ} fusional divergence and a 1.50^{Δ}D increase in accommodative response. Without considering the *CA/C* ratio these two patients would appear to have the same demand fusional divergence when clearly they differ by a factor of two.

Prism Adaptation Reduces Convergence Accommodation

These proposed interactions are transient since they only occur during the first 15 to 30 seconds of a convergence or accommodative response. They do not occur during prolonged or sustained responses due to the operation of prism adaptation. Owens and Leibowitz (1980) have demonstrated that prism adaptation has no influence on the dark focus of accommodation. This suggests that prism adaptation occurs later in the feed-forward path of vergence system than convergence accommodation.

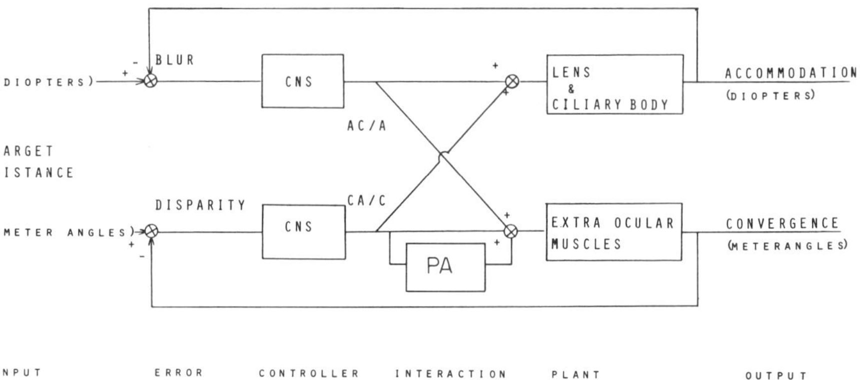

FIGURE 14.25. Systems block diagram illustrating the mutual interactions and feed-forward cross-links between the accommodative (*top*) and convergence (*bottom*) motor control systems. Tonic vergence (*PA*) occurs after the *CA/C* cross-link in the feed-forward path of the convergence system, since prism adaptation has no effect on the dark focus of accommodation. As prism adaptation (*PA*) relieves the CNS controller for fusional vergence, convergence accommodation is also relieved and its exaggeration of the *AC/A* ratio is eliminated. Thus excessive accommodative convergence interactions are transient since they are reduced within 15 to 30 seconds by prism adaptation.

As illustrated in Figure 14.25, the innervation from the fusional vergence controller marked *CNS* can influence the accommodative response through the *CA/C* cross-link, but the innervation for adaptive vergence marked *PA* cannot. As adaptive vergence innervation replaces fusional vergence innervation there is a reduction in the amount of convergence accommodation influencing the accommodative response. Thus for patients with normal prism adaptation, convergence accommodation only poses a transient problem prior to adaptive vergence. These patients have symptoms of transient blurred or double vision on changing viewing distance after working at a fixed distance for prolonged periods of time. For those patients with reduced or no prism adaptation, convergence accommodation presents a problem for both transient and sustained vergence responses.

THERAPY OF TRANSIENT AND SUSTAINED DISORDERS

Orthoptics

Different treatment options are recommended for accommodative vergence disorders associated with and without the ability to adapt to prism.

Transient disorders associated with normal prism adaptation would respond well to orthoptic exercises that train rapid and large fast fusional vergence responses to brief step presentations of lenses and prisms. Adaptation is indicated by differences between the associated and dissociated phorias. Their adaptive processes will respond to these trained fast fusional movements and relieve the excessive demands on convergence and accommodation caused by convergence accommodation. Patients who show reduced prism adaptation in conjunction with abnormal convergence accommodative interactions should receive orthoptic exercises to train both the rapid fusional and adaptive vergence processes (Vaegan, 1979). In cases where prism adaptation cannot be trained, several optical corrections can be considered.

Optical Correction with Lenses and Prisms

The simplest correction of accommodative vergence disorders is one that eliminates convergence accommodation so that the complex mutual interactions between accommodation and convergence will not occur (Schor and Narayan, 1982). In both of the examples illustrated in Figure 14.24 the error of accommodation caused by convergence accommodation and stimulated by the 6^{Δ} of fusional divergence used to correct the near associated phoria could be corrected with a +0.50 D add. Optical correction of this error shortcircuits the subsequent mutual interactions between convergence and accommodation that would normally occur. Note that the same plus add is used to eliminate convergence accommodative errors in two patients with markedly different *AC/A* ratios. The patients would also be corrected with 6^{Δ}BO prism, which would eliminate both fusional corrective movements and their effects on convergence accommodation. Thus correction of convergence accommodation errors with lenses or elimination of stimuli by full correction of the associated phoria with prism simplifies correction of binocular disorders by allowing the practitioner to ignore the complex mutual interactions resulting from the *AC/A* and *CA/C* cross-links. In cases where the associated phoria is large, it can be partially corrected and reduce the demands on convergence and accommodation to reasonable amounts. The effects of prescribed lenses and prisms are determined just as they are in standard graphical analysis, by moving the near reference point and the *AC/A* line to the left or right with base-in and base-out prism, respectively, and up and down with minus and plus lens additions, respectively. The demands on convergence and accommodation resulting from the remaining uncorrected portion of the associated phoria are computed with the graphical vector analysis described above.

Quantitative Predictions

Quantitative predictions of the demands placed on controllers of convergence (CD) and accommodation (AD) are derived below (Schor and Narayan, 1982).

Given

$$\text{Accommodative response } (AR) = AD + [CD \times (CA/C)] \qquad (k)$$

$$\text{Convergence response } (CR) = CD + [AD\,(AC/A)]. \qquad (l)$$

Where

AR = (1/viewing distance-depth of focus);
CR = (PD cm/viewing distance m) − (distance-associated phoria);

and AR and CR remain fixed for a given viewing distance since both accommodation and convergence feedback loops are closed.

Then by substitution

$$AD = \frac{AR - [CR \times (CA/C)]}{1 - (AC/A \times CA/C)} \qquad (m)$$

$$CD = \frac{CR - [AR \times (AC/A)]}{1 - (AC/A \times CA/C)}. \qquad (n)$$

Equations (m) and (n) predict that the response levels or demands on the accommodation and convergence controllers will always be greater than their stimuli predicted from target distance and the phoria. This is most evident when the AC/A and CA/C ratios are reciprocally related. Under these circumstances the denominators of equations (m) and (n) become zero, indicating that the interactions between accommodation and convergence will become unstable since the innervation required for their response will be infinitely large or reach saturation. The reciprocal relationship between the AC/A and CA/C is approximated whenever either ratio is abnormally high. The numerators of equations (m) and (n) are equal to the binocular cross-cylinder (accommodative phoria) (binoc cross-cyl) and the near convergence phoria, respectively. These are the open-loop responses of accommodation and convergence, respectively, while the other system (convergence or accommodation) is closed-loop. Hence these equations may be simplified to the following:

$$AD = \frac{\textit{binoc cross-cyl}}{1 - (AC/A \times CA/C)} \qquad (o)$$

$$CD = \frac{\textit{phoria at near}}{1 - (AC/A \times CA/C)}. \qquad (p)$$

The effects of added lenses and prism and an assumed depth of focus or lag of accommodation of 0.5 D on *AD* and *CD* are incorporated into the following equations:

$$AD = \frac{B\,X\,cyl - [(L + 0.5) + [\Delta(CA/C)]]}{1 - (AC/A \times CA/C)} \quad \text{(q)}$$

$$CD = \frac{Pn - [\Delta + [(L + 0.5)(AC/A)]]}{1 - (AC/A \times CA/C)} \quad \text{(r)}$$

where Δ = prism (+ = *BO*; − = *BI*);
Pn = near phoria (+ = eso; − = exo);
L = lens addition (+ = convex; − = concave).

Note that the accommodative and convergence demands can be calculated from one another using the tangent relationships of the *CA/C* and *AC/A*, shown in Figure 14.24, where

$$AD = [CD\,(CA/C)] + 2.5 - L; \quad \text{(s)}$$

$$AD = [(CD - Pn)/(AC/A] + 2.5 - L; \quad \text{(t)}$$

$$CD = (AD - 2.5 + L)/(CA/C); \quad \text{(u)}$$

$$CD = [(AD - 2.5 + L)\,(AC/A)] + Pn. \quad \text{(v)}$$

AD and *CD* are computed from equations (g) and (*h*) and *Pn* equals the near phoria. *L* equals any lens additions over the distance subjective. 2.5 − *L* is added to *AD* since the vertical vectors in Figure 14.24 only indicate the accommodative demand in addition to the reciprocal of the near working distance (1/0.4 m) − *L*. Thus *AD* computed from equations (*o*) and (*q*) is 2.5 D − *L* greater than the vectors graphed in Figure 14.24. *CD* will be positive for esophores and negative for exophores. *AD* will be positive for both esophores and exophores, however, *AD* will be negative for an exophore if the relative accommodation vector exceeds −2.50 D. In this case a negative accommodation beyond the far point would be required to see a target with clear single binocular vision at near.

Measurement of the *CA/C* Ratio

The application of the analysis described above requires the clinical measurement of the *CA/C* ratio. Based on principles similar to those used in the derivation of the gradient *AC/A* ratio, a gradient *CA/C* ratio can be determined at some near observation distance. The gradient *AC/A* which equals the change in convergence resulting from a unit change in accommodation is derived from the difference in two open loop convergence responses divided by the difference between their accommodative stimuli. This difference technique cancels all factors such as tonic and proximal convergence that are common to the two responses and reveals their difference; accommodative convergence. Similarly the difference in two measures of quasi open loop accommodative posture taken by binocular cross cylinder or dynamic skiametry divided by the difference in fusional convergence stimuli during these two measures yields a gradient measure of the *CA/C* ratio.

The accommodative loop is quasi opened during dynamic retinoscopy by beginning with a +3.50 D working lens that blurs the convergence stimulus at 40 cm by +1 D. Under blurred conditions the accommodative response is determined by the dark focus and any convergence accommodation. Retinoscopy is conducted using Tait's method (1928) in which the plus add is reduced until the retinoscopy reflex becomes a very fast against movement just outside of neutralization. The remaining plus equals the accommodative lag. Nott's method (1925) or the "observation behind fixation" is a similar measure of accommodative lag in which observation distance of the retinoscope is varied until a neutral reflex is observed. The modified estimate method or MEM (Weisz, 1980) is another retinoscopic method in which minus lenses of increasing amplitude are briefly placed before the plus add until a neutral reflex is observed. The MEM has the advantage of not influencing the patient's accommodative response. These methods of dynamic retinoscopy are conducted while the patient views a near target binocularly with and without 6 base in prism. The change in accommodative lag divided by the change in convergence stimulus yields the gradient *CA/C* ratio.

An alternative approach for determining the *CA/C* ratio utilizes the binocular cross cylinder test. This test is based upon the Mandelbaum effect (Owens, 1979) in which two superimposed stimuli to accommodation such as presented by the cross cylinder and grid pattern result in an accommodative response bias toward the patient's dark focus. Lenses are adjusted before the patient's eyes until the dark focus lies midway between the two focal planes of the cylindrical stimulus and the vertical and horizontal components of the grid pattern appear equally clear. The *CA/C* is determined by conducting the binocular cross cylinder with and without 6 base in prism. In all cases, base in prism is added since it results in less adaptation of the phoria than base out prism. The change in the test result divided by the change in the convergence stimulus yields the gradient *CA/C* ratio.

CLINICAL IMPLICATION

Forced duction fixation disparity curves of persons with disturbed binocular vision such as a large heterophoria accompanied by asthenopia reveal possible underlying disturbances that could cause these disorders. For example, Sheedy and Saladin (1978) have shown that curve type and slope at the Y intercept are the two most effective parameters for distinguishing between persons with symptomatic and asymptomatic binocular vision. Type I curves are associated with a lack of symptoms and the three remaining curve types are associated with symptomatic disorders. Curves that contain a flat central slope are more prevalent than those with steep slopes in persons who are asymptomatic. Both the curve type and central slope are determined primarily by prism adaptation. Thus we may interpret from clinical observations that prism adaptation is associated with asymptomatic binocular vision.

Sensory Disturbances

The lack of prism adaptation in symptomatic binocular vision as evidenced by steep forced duction curves may result from sensory disturbances. Carter (1964, 1965) found that rapid prism adaptation that characterized normal binocular vision only occurred with foveal fusion contours and did not occur if the eyes were dissociated by large amounts of prism. He also observed that adaptation to prism persisted many hours if binocular fusion was prevented, for example, by closing the eyes. Schor (1979b) observed that adaptation of the phoria was specific to disparity vergence and did not occur with monocularly stimulated accommodative vergence. These observations suggest that adaptation of the phoria to prism depends on binocular sensory fusion. Carter (1965) proposed that those persons who had reduced sensory fusion due to conditions such as uncorrected refractive error, anisometropia, central suppression, amblyopia, and aniseikonia did not have the ability to adapt to prism and as a result manifested large heterophorias and asthenopia. It is also possible that oculomotor disturbances such as a large heterophoria or strabismus could lead to some of these sensory disturbances.

Orthoptics and Curve Type

Two types of therapy used to correct asthenopia associated with unusual forced duction fixation disparity curves are the prescription of prism and orthoptics (ocular sensorimotor training). In the case of types II and III fixation disparity curves, prism is prescribed (Payne et al., 1974) to move the flat portion of the curve so that it is symmetric about the Y intercept. This therapy centers the operating range of prism adaptation about zero-prism stimulus or optimizes the range for normal viewing conditions. In cases where there is no flat region, orthoptics exercises are prescribed.

These have been found to reduce fixation disparity as evidenced by the reduced slope of the forced duction curves (Ogle et al. 1967; Arner et al., 1956; Sheedy, 1980; Hyde, 1979). Neither prism nor orthoptics is indicated for persons with the type IV curves who characteristically have extremely disturbed sensory fusion. Paradoxically, these persons show flat fixation disparity curves without the steep rise in slope prior to reaching the limits of fusion. It appears that they have slow fusional vergence or some form of prism adaptation, but lack fast fusional vergence as evidenced by their narrow operating range of forced vergence and lack of steep slope at the limits of this range.

Persons with occasional strabismus can also exhibit adaptation to prism (Alpern and Hofstetter, 1948; Schor, 1979, 1980) but lack fast disparity vergence eye movements. Interestingly, these strabismic patients do not always exhibit type IV curves. Figure 14.20 illustrates the steep slope of the forced duction fixation disparity curves from three occasional esotropes. The same subjects have marked prism adaptation (Figure 14.19). Factors interfering with sensory fusion such as central suppression may have been responsible for their marked elevation of fixation disparity. These observations illustrate that both fast and slow fusional vergence mechanisms are necessary for the operation of normal binocular vision. The importance of the slow fusional vergence mechanism is not always remembered, however, it was first recognized at the turn of the century by Hoffmann and Bielschowsky (1900), who stated ". . . the important factor concerning fusional movements is not the movement that leads to sensory fusion per se but the prolonged tonic fundamental innervation of the eye muscles that is adapted for the condition of single vision."

REFERENCES

Alpern MA. Types of movement. In: Davson H, ed. The eye. Vol. 3. New York: Academic Press, 1969:65–74.

Alpern M, Hofstetter HW. The effect of prism on esotropia. A case report. Am J Optom Arch Am Acad Optom 1948;25:80–91.

Ames A Jr, Glidden GH. Ocular measurements. Trans Sect Ophthalmol AMA. 1928;102–75.

Arner RS, Berger SI, Braverman G, Kaplan M. The clinical significance of the effect of vergence on fixation disparity—a preliminary investigation. Am J Optom Arch Am Acad Optom 1956;33:399–409.

Bagolini B. Part II. Sensorial-Motor Anomalies In Strabismus (anomalous movements). Doc Ophthalmol 1976;41:23–41.

Carter DB. Fixation disparity with and without foveal contours. Am J Optom Arch Am Acad Optom 1964;41:729–36.

Carter DB. Fixation disparity and heterophoria following prolonged wearing of prisms. Am J Optom Arch Am Acad Optom 1965;42:141–52.

Charnwood L. Retinal slip. Trans Int Optics Cong Br Opt Assoc Cond 1951;165–72.
Clark B. An eye movement study of stereoscopic vision. Am J Psychol 1936;48:82–97.
Crone RA. Diplopia. New York: American Elsevier, 1973.
Crone RA, Hardjowijoto S. What is normal binocular vision? Doc Ophthalmol 1979;47(1):163–99.
Diner D. Hysteresis in human binocular fusion: a second look. PhD dissertation California Institute of Technology, Pasadena, California 1978.
Ellerbrock VJ. Tonicity induced by fusional movements. Am J Optom Arch Am Acad Optom 1950;27:8–20.
Fender D, Julesz B. Extension of Panum's fusional area in binocularly stabilized vision. J Opt Soc Am 1967;57(6):819–30.
Flom MC. Some interesting eye movements obtained during the cover test. Am J Optom Physiol Opt 1958;35(2):69–71.
Godio L, Rutstein RP. The range of zero associated phoria in an asymptomatic clinical population. Am J Optom Physiol Opt 1980;58(6):445–50.
Grisham JD. The dynamics of fusional vergence eye movements in binocular dysfunction. Am J Optom Physiol Opt 1980;57(9):645–55.
Hallden U. Fusional phenomena in anomalous correspondence. Acta Ophthalmol 1952;(Suppl) 37.
Hebbard FW. Foveal fixation disparity measurements and their use in determining the relationship between accommodative convergence and accommodation Am J Optom Arch Am Acad Optom 1960;37:3–26.
Hebbard FW. Comparison of subjective and objective measurements of fixation disparity. J Opt Soc Am 1962;52:706–12.
Hebbard FW. Effects of blur on fixation disparity. Am J Optom Arch Am Acad Optom 1964;41:540–48.
Henson D, Dharamshi BG. Oculomotor adaptation to induced heterophoria and anisometropia. Invest Opthalmol 1982;21:234–40.
Henson DB, North R. Adaptation to prism-induced heterophoria. Am J Optom Physiol Opt 1980;57(3):129–37.
Hering E. Spatial sense and movements of the eye. Raddle CA, trans. Baltimore American Academy of Optometry, 1942.
Hirsch MJ, Alpern M, Schultz H. The variation of phoria with age. Am J Optom Arch Am Acad Optom 1948;25(11):535–41.
Hoffmann FB, Bielschowsky A. Uber dis der Willkue entzygenen Fusions—Bewegungen der Augen. Arch Ges Physiol 1900;80:1–40.
Hofstetter HW. The zone of clear single binocular vision. Am J Optom 1945;22(7):301–33.
Hyde I. Modification of fixation disparity by visual feedback. MS dissertation Pacific University, Forest Grove, Oregon, 1979.
Jampolsky, A. Esotropia and convergent fixation disparity. Am J Ophthalmol 1956;41:825–33.
Jampolsky A, Flom B, Freid A. Fixation disparity in relation to heterophoria. Am J Ophthalmol 1957;43:97–106.
Judd CH. Photographic records of convergence and divergence. Psychol Rev Monogr Suppl 1907;8:370–423.
Krishnan VV, Stark L. A heuristic model for the human vergence eye movement system. IEEE Trans 1977; BME-250:347–66.

Lau E. Neue Untersuchunger über das Tiefen—und Ebenensehen. Z Sinnesphysiologie 1921;53:1–35.

Lewin K, Sakuma K. Die Sehrichtung monokularer und binokularer Object bie Bewegung und das Zustandekommen des Tiefeneffektes. Psychol Fortschr 1924;6:298–357.

Ludvigh E, McKinnon P, Zartzeff L. Temporal course of the relaxation of binocular duction (fusion) movements. Arch Ophthalmol 1964;71:389–99.

Maddox EC. The clinical use of prism. 2d ed. Bristol England: John Wright & Sons, 1893:83.

Mallett RFJ. Fixation disparity—its genesis in relation to asthenopia. Ophthalmic Optician 1974;14:1159–68.

Mariani G, Pasino L. Variations in the angle of anomaly and fusional movements in cases of small-angle convergent strabismus with harmonious anomalous retinal correspondence. Br J Ophthalmol 1964;48:439–43.

Martens TG, Ogle KN. Observations on accommodative convergence: especially its nonlinear relationship. Am J Ophthalmol 1959;47(2):455–63.

McCullough RW. The fixation disparity-heterophoria relationship. J Am Optom Assoc 1978;49:369–72.

Mitchell AM, Ellerbrock VJ. Fixation disparity and the maintenance of fusion in the horizontal meridian. Am J Optom Arch Am Acad Optom 1955;32: 520–34.

Morgan MW Jr. The direction of visual lines when fusion is broken as in duction tests. Am J Optom Arch Am Acad Optom 1947;24:8–12.

North R, Henson DB. Adaptation to prism induced heterophoria in subjects with abnormal binocular vision or asthenopia. Am J Optom Physiol Opt 1981;58(9):746–52.

Nott, IS. Dynamic skiametry accommodation and convergence, Am J Physiol Opt 1925; 6:490–503.

Ogle KN. Fixation disparity. Am Orthopt J 1954;4(6):33–39.

Ogle KN. Researches in binocular vision. New York: Hafner, 1964:65.

Ogle KN, Prangen A. Observations of vertical divergences and hyperphorias. Arch Ophthalmol 1953;49:313–34.

Ogle KN, Avery DeH, Prangen A. Further considerations of fixation disparity and the binocular fusional process. Am J Ophthalmol 1951;34:57–72.

Ogle KN, Martens TG, Dyer JA. Oculomotor imbalance in binocular vision and fixation disparity. Philadelphia: Lea Febiger, 1967:108.

Ogle KN, Mussey F, Prangen AdeH. Fixation disparity and the fusional processes in binocular single vision. Am J Ophthalmol 1949;32:1069–87.

Owens DA. The Mandelbaum effect: evidence for an accommodative bias toward intermediate viewing distance. J Opt Soc Am 1979;69:646–52.

Owens DA, Leibowitz HW. Accommodation, convergence, and distance perception in low illumination. Am J Optom Physiol Opt 1980;57(9):540–50.

Palmer EA, von Noorden GK. The relationship between fixation disparity and heterophoria. Am J Ophthalmol 1978;86:172–75.

Panum PL. Physiologische Untersuchungen über das Sehen mit zwei Augen. Kiel: Schwerssche Buchhandlung, 1858.

Parks MS. The monofixation syndrome. Trans New Orleans Acad Ophthalmol 1971;121–53.

Payne CR, Grisham JD, Thomas KL. A clinical evaluation of fixation disparity. Am J Optom Physiol Opt 1974;51:88–90.

Rashbass C, Westheimer G. Disjunctive eye movements. J Physiol 1961; 159(2):339–60.

Richards W. Stereoblindness and fixation disparity. Abstract. Am J Optom Physiol Opt 1975;52(10):716.

Riggs LA, Niehl EW. Eye movements recorded during convergence and divergence. J. Opt Soc Am 1960;50(a):913–20.

Schor CM. The influence of rapid prism adaptation upon fixation disparity. Vision Res 1979a;19(7):757–65.

Schor CM. The relationship between fusional vergence eye movements and fixation disparity. Vision Res 1979b;19(12):1359–67.

Schor CM. Fixation disparity: a steady state error. Am J Optom 1980a;57(9):618–31.

Schor CM. Basic and clinical aspects of vergence eye movements: symposium discussion. Am J Optom 1980b;57(11):681–96.

Schor CM. The analysis of tonic and accommodative vergence disorders of binocular vision. Am J Optom Physiol Opt 1982a;58: in press.

Schor CM. Vergence eye movements: basic aspects. In: Lennerstraud, G, ed. Functional basis of ocular motility disorders. Stockholm: Pergamon Press, 1982b.

Schor CM, Narayan V. Graphical analysis of prism adaptation, convergence accommodation and accommodative convergence. Am J Optom Physiol Opt 1982;59:774–84.

Schor CM, Tyler CWT. Spatio-temporal properties of Panum's fusional area. Vision Res 1981;21:683–92.

Schubert G. Grundlagen der beidaugigen motorishen koordination P. flügers. Arch Ges Physiol 1943;247:279–91.

Semmlow JL, Hung G. Accommodative and fusional components of fixation disparity. Invest Ophthalmol 1979;18(10):1082–86.

Sheedy JE. Fixation disparity analysis of oculomotor imbalance. Am J Optom Physiol Opt 1980;57(9):632–39.

Sheedy JE, Saladin JJ. Association of symptoms with measures of oculomotor deficiencies. Am J Optom Physiol Opt 1978;55(10):670–76.

Stewart CR. A photographic investigation of lateral fusional movements of the eyes. PhD dissertation, Ohio State University, Columbus, 1951.

Tait EF. A quantitative system of dynamic retinoscopy. Trans Am Acad Optom, 1928;3:131–55.

Toates FM. Control theory in biology and experimental psychology. London:Hutchinson, 1975:169–73.

Tubis RA. An evaluation of vertical vergence tests on the basis of fixation disparity. Am J Optom Arch Am Acad Optom 1954;31:624–35.

Vaegan. Con and divergence show large and sustained improvement after short isometric exercise. Am J Optom Physiol Opt 1979;56(1):23–33.

Weisz, CL. The accommodative resting state. Rev of Optom 1980;7:60–70.

Woo G. The effect of exposure time on the foveal size of Panum's area. Vision Res 1974;14:473–80.

15 Validity of Diagnostic Criteria and Case Analysis in Binocular Vision Disorders

James E. Sheedy
J. James Saladin

The innervational pattern to the oculomotor system must be in balance so that a person can comfortably maintain bifixation of the object of regard. Individuals with an oculomotor imbalance may be able to maintain binocular vision, but do so with asthenopia, headache, blur, and/or intermittent diplopia. Asthenopia may be so severe after a prolonged visually intensive task that some avoid the task even when it is central to their occupations. The cost of oculomotor imbalances to the schoolchild may be even greater in that discomfort during near work (especially reading) may have long-term effects on educational development, career selection, and attitude. This chapter discusses the methods and criteria that are being used in differential diagnosis of horizontal oculomotor imbalances and suggests techniques that offer the promise of even greater diagnostic power.

PHORIA AND VERGENCE ANALYSIS

Clinical Measurement

The usual method of diagnosing horizontal oculomotor imbalances requires measuring heterophoria and vergence ranges, and takes into consideration the vergence demand point at several different fixation distances. Heterophoria is a tendency for deviation of the lines of sight from bifixation of the object of regard when fusion is eliminated. As such, it represents a rest position. It is commonly measured with the Von Graefe or Maddox rod subjective methods supplemented with the objective cover test. The magnitude of heterophoria varies with fixation distance (and therefore accommodative demand) if the AC/A ratio is not numerically equal to the patient's interpupillary distance. The amount of the heterophoria determines the fusional vergence needed to obtain bifixation. If either base-in or base-out prism is introduced under fused conditions, a negative or positive fusional vergence movement, respectively, must occur to reobtain the requisite alignment for fusion. As explained in Chapter 13 on Graphical Analysis, positive relative vergence is measured as the amount of base-out prism employed until a blur is noticed. Prism added until fusion is broken measures the positive and negative fusional vergences. It is common clinical practice for the prism amount to be reduced after diplopia is reported until the patient observes that the two diplopic images have become one. These three measurements are referred to as the blur, break, and recovery findings of the vergence measurement.

If the accommodative level is held fairly constant, the heterophoria measurement is easily repeatable within two or three prism diopters depending on the measuring method. Variability in the vergence amplitude measurements is greater. A difference of 10 prism diopters from one fusional vergence amplitude measurement to another is not unusual unless rigorous controls are applied. Not only do vergence ranges vary with the measurement method (prism bar or Risley prism), they also vary with the size and strength of the fusion stimulus, the attentiveness of the patient, the speed of prism change, and the immediate past history of vergence stimulation. With this variability in mind, one immediately sees that any criterion dependent on vergence ranges must be used according to some rather strict boundary conditions and instructions to the patient.

Normative Clinical Data

While the reader is referred to Borish (1970) and Chapter 13 for a complete description of the methods used for obtaining clinical data, a brief discussion of these methods is presented here with comments on analytical criteria. The methods can be divided into two general camps: those based on normative or expected values (an intersubject comparison), and those that compare various test results from a single patient (an intrasubject comparison). Examples of the first group include that proposed by Morgan (1944) and to a certain extent, the optometric extension program (OEP) analysis system (Lesser, 1974). Morgan's data are developed from the averages of over 800 prepresbyopic patients. The OEP table of expecteds was developed "by averaging the values found in thousands of cases" and a standardization process "from the clinical experience of practitioners" (Lesser, 1969). Morgan's and OEP data are presented in Table 15.1 together with similar data from Saladin and Sheedy (1979) that are based on a sample from a nonclinical population. Data from the three sources have a striking similarity considering the differences in construction of the studies. Saladin and Sheedy used conditions for heterophoria and vergence measurements, which were a compromise between those of Morgan (1944) and Sheard (1930). Measurements were made with the refractive correction in a phoropter, and the subject viewed a single column of 20/30 acuity letters. The heterophoria measurement was obtained by putting a 6^{Δ} vertical prism in front of one eye to obtain dissociation. The two images were aligned in the subject's visual space by varying a lateral Risley prism. Accommodative level was controlled by reminding the subject to keep the target clear, and one of the targets was flashed to minimize any subtle fusional effects. The vergences were measured by adding lateral prism slowly and equally to both eyes. Base-in vergences were measured before base-out. The amount of prism was recorded when the first sustained blur was detected (blur), and also when diplopia (break)

TABLE 15.1 Expected Values from OEP and Morgan Tables and Saladin-Sheedy Data

6 m	*OEP*	*Morgan*	*Saladin-Sheedy*
Phoria	0.5 exophoria	1 exophoria (2)	1 exophoria (3.5)
Positive vergences			
Blur	8	9 (4)	15 (7)
Break	19	19 (8)	28 (10)
Recovery	10	10 (4)	20 (11)
Negative vergences			
Break	9	7 (3)	8 (3)
Recovery	5	4 (2)	5 (3)
40 m			
Phoria	6 exophoria	3 exophoria (5)	0.5 exophoria (6)
Positive vergences			
Blur	15	17 (5)	22 (8)
Break	21	21 (6)	30 (12)
Recovery	15	11 (7)	23 (11)
Negative vergences			
Blur	14	13 (4)	14 (6)
Break	22	21 (4)	19 (7)
Recovery	18	13 (5)	13 (6)

Numbers in parentheses = standard deviation values.
All values are in prism diopters.

was noticed. The prism was slowly reduced until fusion (recovery) occurred with the subject trying to regain fusion.

Differences between Morgan's values and those of Saladin and Sheedy illustrate the difficulty in determining population norms. For example, Morgan's were mainly from a prepresbyopic clinical population. Saladin and Sheedy's were from a nonclinical, young adult (ages 20 to 30 years) population. Note the significant difference in positive vergence ranges. Ignoring any age differences, it would seem that a clinical population has smaller positive vergence ranges than does a nonclinical population. From which group is the positive vergence criterion to be chosen? Assuming that there is a relation between the positive relative vergence value and binocular efficiency and/or comfort, even the averages of a nonclinical (and visually healthy) population may not yield the best criterion value. Morgan's expecteds are always given with a range value, which, when taken into consideration, partly compensates for the difficulty just mentioned. Morgan provided a further compensation for this difficulty when he grouped the various clinical parameters that were best correlated with others in the group. For example, his group A consisted of negative relative vergence at distance, negative relative convergence and fusional reserve at near, positive relative accommodation, and amplitude of accommodation (Morgan, 1964). According to graphical analysis, this would be the top and the left (base-in) side of the zone. If all components of the group varied from an expected value in an appropriate direction, a reliable diagnosis could be made. Therefore Morgan's actual diagnostic criterion was not simply a series of numbers as listed in his Table of Expecteds, but a necessary agreement among subcriteria of correlated clinical parameters.

Clinical Analysis of Normative Data

From these concepts, several problems can be seen to develop when normative data gathered from a population are applied to a particular individual and used as criteria or indicators:

1. Population averages may not be the optimum value. As Morgan (1964) put it, "Averages tend to tell what a population is rather than telling what it should be."
2. There are differences in the averages for subpopulations. How many differences exist and how do we determine the subpopulations?
3. Some clinical data, particularly vergence ranges, have poor reliability even though the examiner uses the same conditions and patient instructions on which averages are based.

Analyses of graphically represented data provide the foremost examples of analytical systems that use criteria based on intrasubject data. Classical methods do not provide criteria for as many clinical parameters as do the OEP and Morgan's normative systems; therefore graphical analysis cannot be used as a complete substitute for either. Percival and Sheard give examples of classical criteria used in graphical analysis that depend on an intrasubject data comparison. Percival's (1928) is applied by measuring the positive and negative relative vergences, adding their absolute values, and determining the middle one-third of this vergence range. According to Percival, binocular comfort is to be expected when the demand point falls anywhere within this area or "zone of comfort."

Sheard's criterion (1930) can be stated as a requirement that the fusional reserve amount be twice the amount of the fusional demand. The fusional reserve is the relative vergence in the opposite direction from the heterophoria, and the fusional demand is the amount of heterophoria. For instance, a 6^{Δ} exophore should have at least 12^{Δ} of positive relative vergence at that fixation distance. The criterion was to be applied at several fixation distances. In actual practice, the application of Sheard's and Percival's criteria provide about the same results if the phoria falls in the middle of the vergence range. In a sense, both are based on a population norm just as Morgan's system and that of the OEP. Percival determined statistically that the middle one-third of the vergence range was a zone of comfort and Sheard similarly relied on clinical experience to determine that a 2:1 reserve:demand ratio was adequate.

FIXATION DISPARITY CRITERIA

Clinical Measurement of Fixation Disparity

In recent years, fixation disparity has been used to diagnose imbalances of the oculomotor system. Its chief advantage over phoria-vergence analysis is that the oculomotor system is examined under binocular and, presumably, more natural conditions. Fixation disparity is a small misalignment of the eyes under fused conditions from an exact bifixation of similar images onto corresponding points. The misalignment is on the order of a few minutes of arc. Such a small error is tolerated without diplopia because of the existence of Panum's areas. If a horizontal fixation disparity exists, the eyes will be slightly overdiverged or overconverged for the object of regard. In Figure 15.1 the eyes are overdiverged, and the lines of sight meet behind the plane of regard.

Figure 15.2 illustrates the Disparometer, a clinical instrument designed for measuring fixation disparity at a 40-cm viewing distance. The

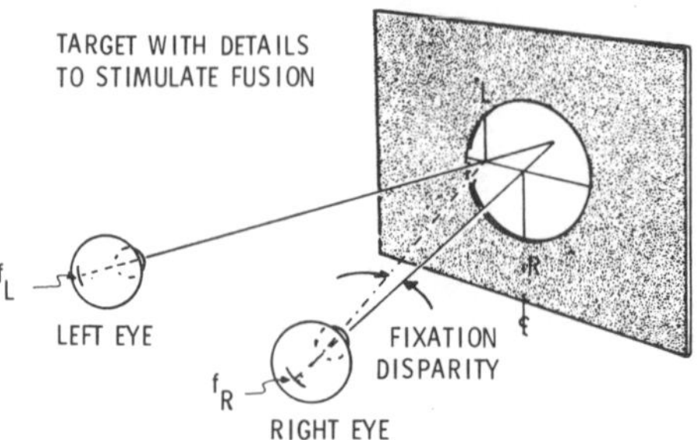

FIGURE 15.1. An illustration in perspective of an exofixation disparity. Note that the visual axes cross behind the plane of regard and that the nonius lines must have horizontal separation if they are to be imaged on the foveas. The fixation disparity angle is indicated by arrows. Adapted from Martens TG, Ogle KN. Observations in accommodative convergence, especially its nonlinear relationships. American Journal of Ophthamology, 1959. Reprinted by permission of the publisher.

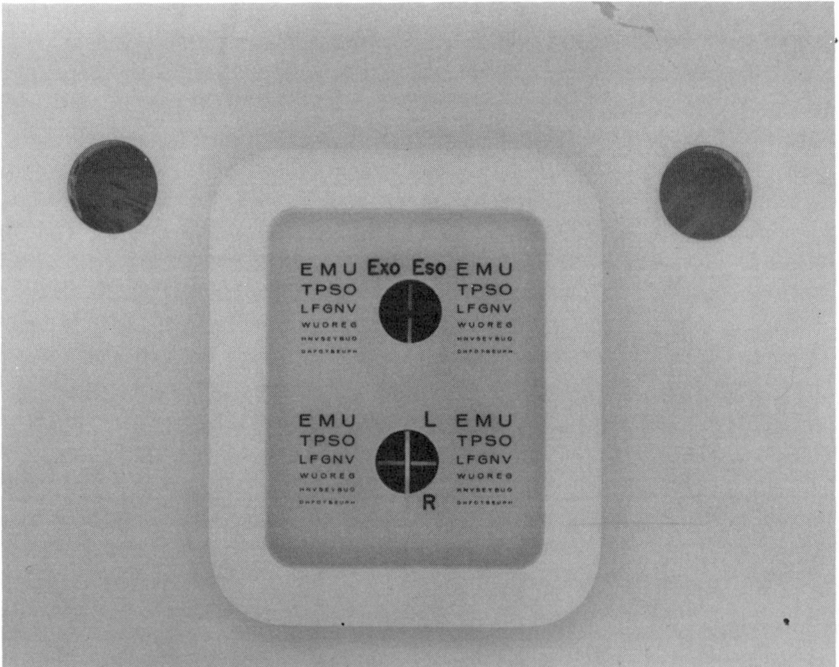

FIGURE 15.2. The Disparometer instrument for measuring fixation disparity at near distances. The subject is presented with different horizontal separations of the nonius lines until the two are seen vertically aligned. The fixation disparity amount can be read from a dial on the back. Note the small Snellen charts for use in stabilizing accommodation. (Vision Analysis, Box 14390, Columbus, OH 43214)

instrument has two binocularly seen circles, each of which subtends an angle of 1.5°. The upper stimulus is used to measure horizontal fixation disparity and the lower to measure vertical fixation disparity. Only horizontal fixation disparity is discussed here. Because nothing within the confines of the circle is seen by both eyes, the circle is the primary stimulus for fusion. The upper half of the circle is perpendicularly polarized with respect to the lower half. Each half-circle contains a polarized vertical line that can be seen by only one eye of the patient. Lateral misalignment of the two vertical lines is controlled by the examiner. If the vertical lines are aligned in real space but are seen as misaligned, a fixation disparity exists. Although the binocular system is using Panum's areas to maintain fusion, the oculocentric direction of each eye remains to be computed from the fovea. To measure the amount of fixation disparity, the lines are adjusted until the subject reports alignment in visual space. The physical horizontal misalignment that the two vertical lines subtend at the viewing distance is the angular measurement of fixation disparity. A horizontal midline through the circle is sometimes used to provide a vertical fusion lock. Accommodation is stabilized by instructing the patient to keep the visual acuity chart letters at the sides of the circle as clear as possible while the setting is being made.

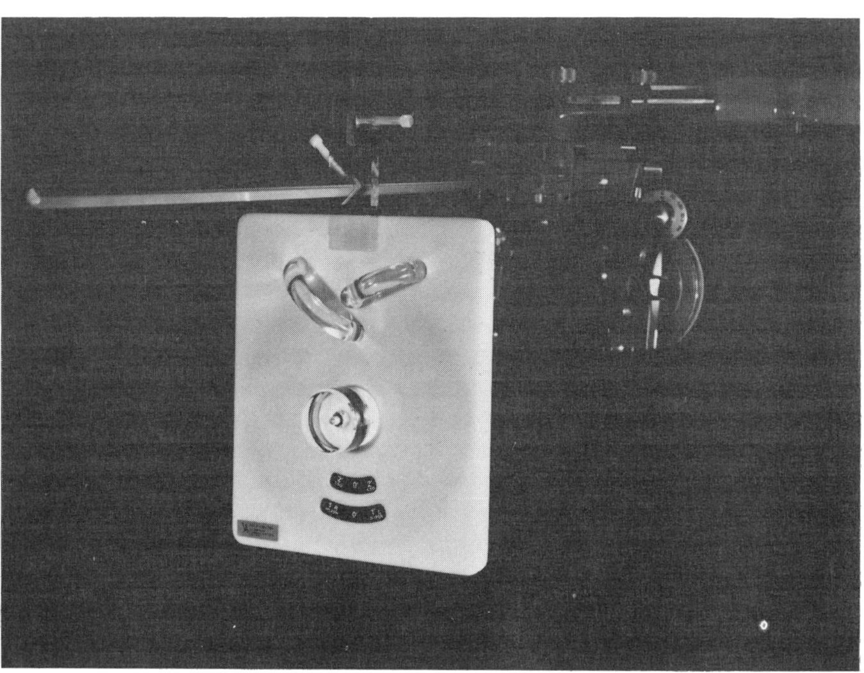

FIGURE 15.2. *(Continued)*

For a given accommodative stimulus level, the amount of fixation disparity can be manipulated by forcing vergence through the use of prisms. Figure 15.3 is a graphical representation of the relationship. On the horizontal axis the amount and base direction of the prism introduced before the eyes is indicated. Base-in is indicated to the left and base-out to the right. The corresponding fixation disparity angle is indicated on the vertical axis with esofixation (overconverged) disparity above the origin. Prism diopters are plotted on the horizontal axis and minutes of arc on the vertical axis. As indicated in the figure, base-out prism usually causes a relative exofixation disparity and base-in prism a relative esofixation disparity.

Analysis of Fixation Disparity Data

There are four descriptive characteristics of a fixation disparity curve (FDC) as shown in Figures 15.3 and 15.4. The first is curve type (shown in Figure 15.4). The second is the vertical axis intercept (Y intercept), which is a measure of the angular amount of fixation disparity with no induced prism stress. The third is the horizontal axis intercept (X intercept), which is the amount of prism needed to neutralize the fixation disparity to zero (associated phoria). The fourth point of interest is the

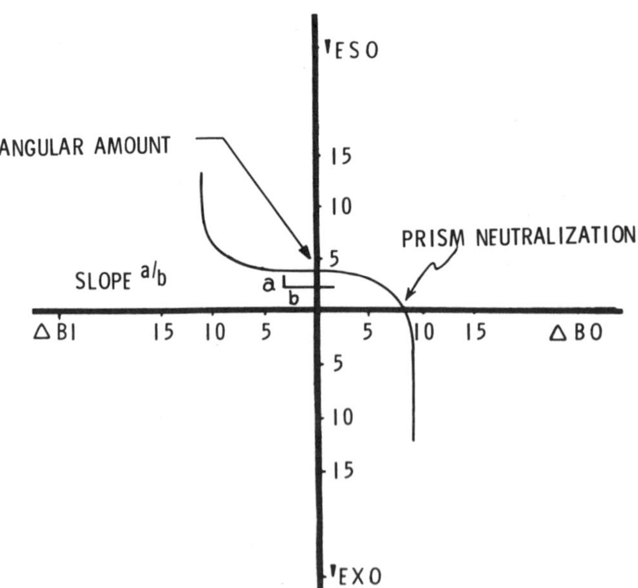

FIGURE 15.3. Slope, angular amount of fixation disparity, and amount of prism needed for neutralization of the fixation disparity are indicated.

slope of the curve as it crosses the vertical axis. Each characteristic could be used in the formulation of a criterion.

Ogle, Martens, and Dyer (1967) classified the curves according to shape. While this classification is not the only one and has some limitations, it is certainly the most widely referred to and is used in this chapter. The four curves are illustrated in the four sections of Figure 15.4. The most common (type I) is sigmoid-shaped and has a tendency for verticality on both ends. Type II curves lack the downward portion of the curve on the base-out side and type III lack the upward portion on the base-in side. A type IV curve is a sigmoid terminating in horizontal lines. The relative frequency of the curve types is given in Table 15.2 in which Saladin and Sheedy's (1979) data are compared to Ogle's. Type I curves are most frequent, followed by type II, type III, and type IV in that order. The differences among the data in the table are most likely due to the populations from which the samples were drawn. While Ogle, Martens, and Dyer (1967) reported that curve type can change with fixation distance, this conclusion needs to be verified. Additional studies are also needed on the effect of strength and size of fusion contours, accommodative state, and orthoptics on curve type.

The most widely used descriptive characteristic of fixation disparity is the horizontal axis intercept, which indicates prism amplitude that will neutralize fixation disparity. Ogle and associates (1967) called this point the associated phoria to distinguish it from the dissociated phoria described previously. The associated phoria is determined clinically with a Mallett unit (Mallett, 1964, 1966), Borish card (Borish, 1978), AO Vectograph, or Disparometer (Sheedy, 1980a). A successful variation of this neutralization technique based on Carter's (1965) work prescribes the least amount of prism that will neutralize fixation disparity for a 10-minute period. Excellent results have been obtained with this technique for correcting both vertical and horizontal imbalances. Carter maintains that if the fixation disparity cannot be neutralized with this technique,

TABLE 15.2 Relative Frequency of Curve Types

	Distance		*Near*	
Type	*Ogle, 1967 (%)*	*Saladin and Sheedy, 1979 (%)*	*Ogle, 1967 (%)*	*Saladin and Sheedy, 1979 (%)*
I	57.5	68.3	57.2	58.2
II	30.0	26.7	22.1	27.6
III	9.0	0	13.4	8.2
IV	3.4	5.0	4.9	7.2

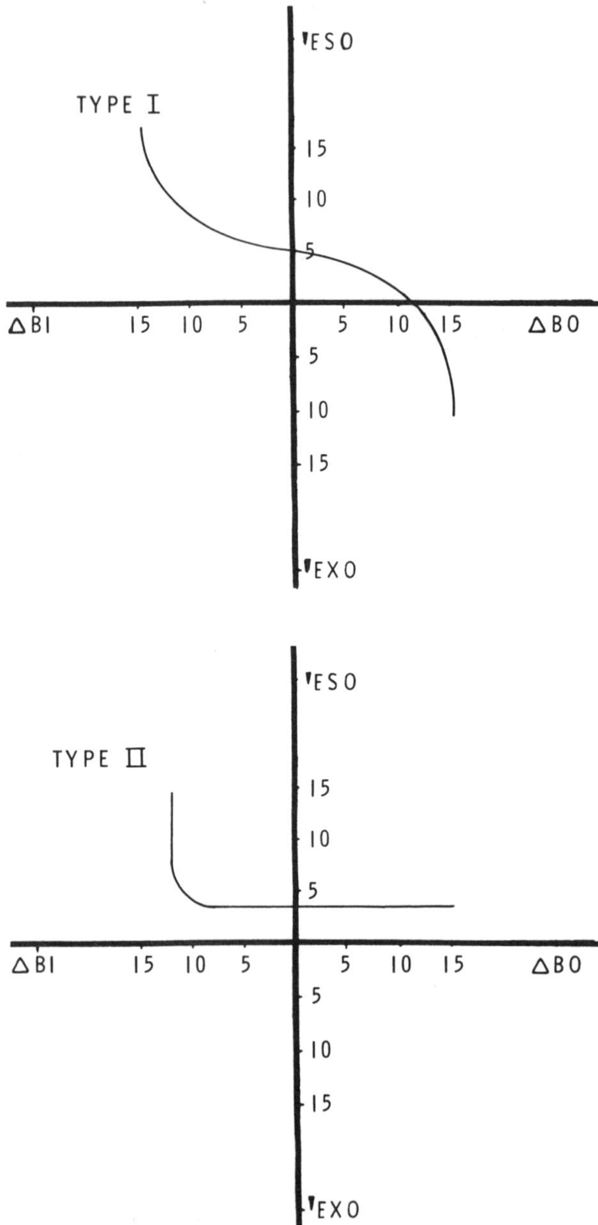

FIGURE 15.4. The four types of fixation disparity curves as described by Ogle et al., 1967. A Type I. B Type II. C Type III. D Type IV.

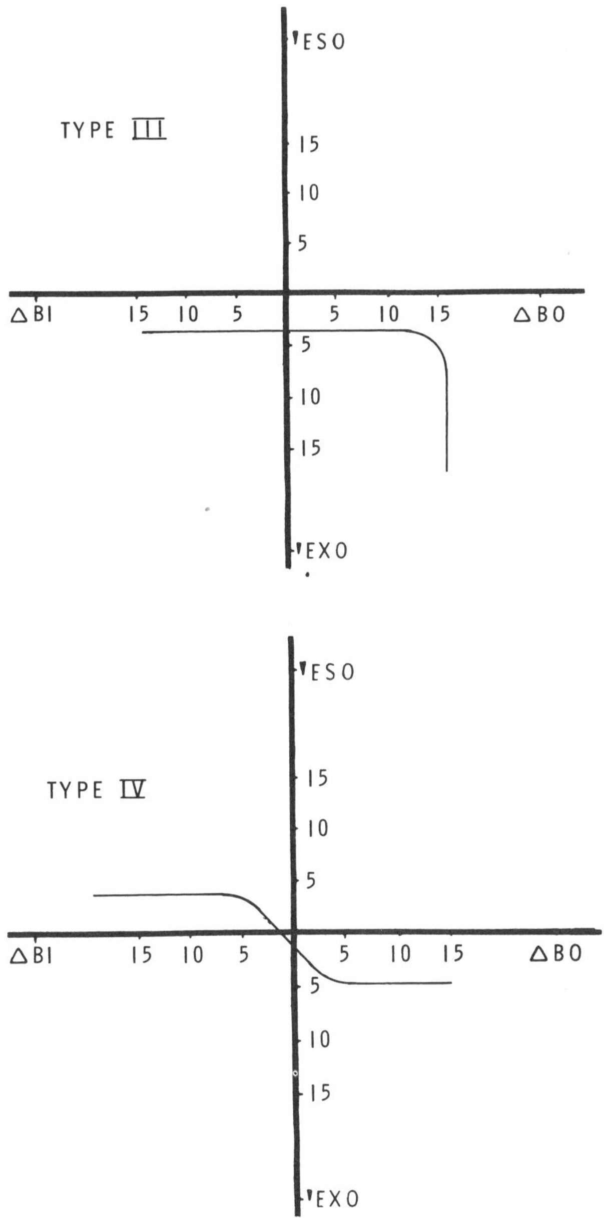

FIGURE 15.4. *(Continued)*

the patient's particular binocular system is very adaptable and probably will not profit by a prism prescription.

The Y axis intercept, or the angular amount of fixation disparity with no additional prism, shows promise of being of diagnostic use but its magnitude is more susceptible to variation than is the associated phoria. This leads to complication in its clinical application. For instance, the angular amount of fixation disparity is strongly dependent on the strength and size of the fusion contour. The greater the distance between the fusion contour and the fixation point, the greater will be the amount of fixation disparity. This relationship between size of fusion contour and the X axis intercept does not hold, however. Ogle and co-workers (1967) showed that as the fusion contour size increased the fixation disparity curve rotated about the X axis intercept. While there is some disagreement, it is our experience that this tentative conclusion is correct. Because of the stability of the X axis intercept, many practitioners who use the prism-to-neutralization method prefer to use a fixation disparity device without a central fusion lock. The prism needed for neutralization

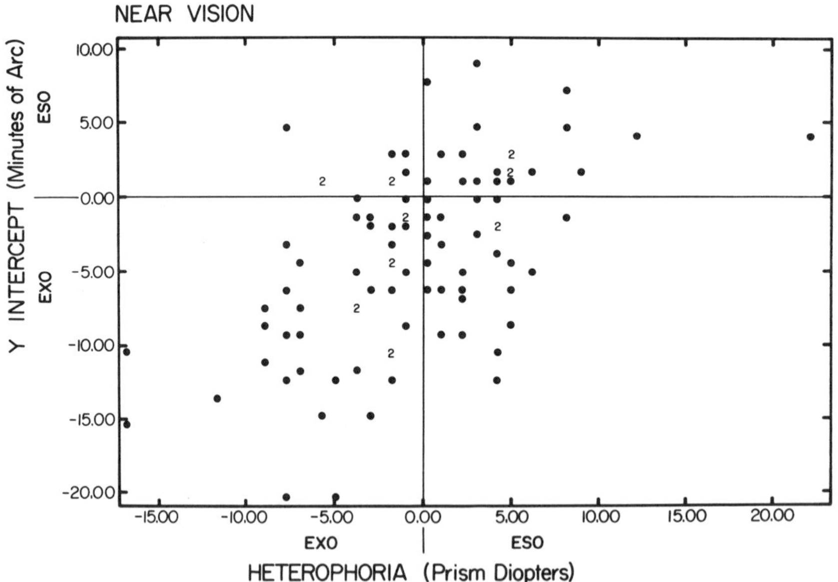

FIGURE 15.5. The amount and direction of heterophoria is plotted against the corresponding amount and direction of fixation disparity. Some 25% of the data points fall in quadrants 2 and 4, showing either esophoria with exofixation disparity or the reverse. These data were taken at a near (40 cm) testing distance. Reprinted by permission of the publisher, from Saladin JJ, Sheedy JE. Population study of fixation disparity, heterophoria, and vergence. American Journal of Optometry and Physiological Optics, 1978.

is the same with and without the central fusion lock, however, the patient's task is made easier by a greater apparent deviation of the two polarized nonius lines when they are absent.

The fourth point of interest on the fixation disparity curve is the slope (Figure 15.3). The steeper the slope, the less the binocular system is able to adapt to prism-induced stress without changing fixation disparity. We have defined the point on the horizontal axis indicating the habitual prism prescription (usually the origin) as the operating point. It is the slope of the curve at the operating point that may be of diagnostic importance. Variables that have an effect on slope include size and strength of fusion contour. The slope has a tendency to increase as the size of fusion contour grows and as its strength is lessened. The fusion contour can be strengthened by increasing contrast, sharpening borders, and to a certain extent, increasing the number of contours.

Relationship of Fixation Disparity and Phoria-Vergence

How closely related is the phoria-vergence relationship to fixation disparity? (See Figures 15.5 and 15.6.) If fixation disparity were due to the

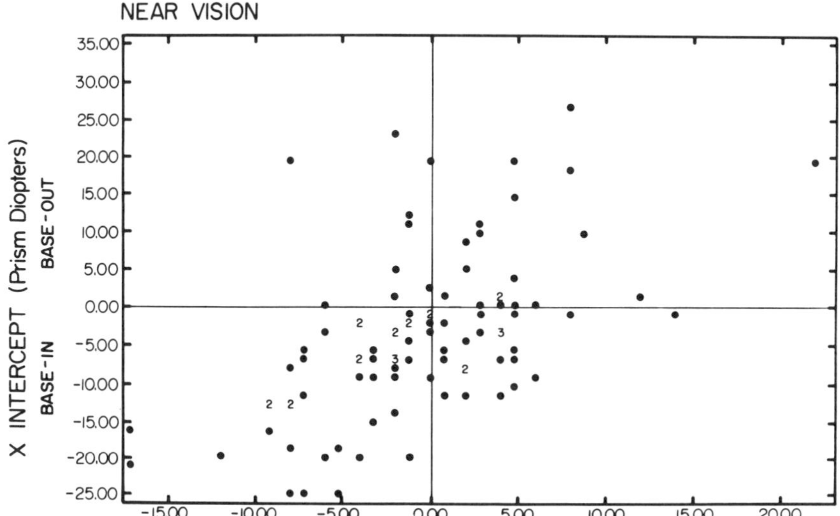

FIGURE 15.6. The amount and direction of heterophoria is plotted against the corresponding amount and direction of prism needed for neutralization of the fixation disparity. As in Figure 15.5, some 25% of the data points fall in quadrants 2 and 4. Reprinted by permission of the publisher, from Saladin JJ, Sheedy JE. Population study of fixation disparity, heterophoria, and vergence. American Journal of Optometry and Physiological Optics, 1978.

binocular system applying only a comfortable minimum of fusional vergence to overcome the phoria, one would expect that exophores would have an exofixation disparity and esophores an esofixation disparity. Figure 15.5 from Saladin and Sheedy (1979) shows that this is not true in at least 25% of the cases. One would also expect that an exophore would require base-in prism to more fully overcome the exofixation disparity and similarly, esophores would require base-out prism. Figure 15.6 shows that this is far from a general statement of truth. The explanation for fixation disparity must include more than the idea that it is a slight misalignment to conserve the neural effort involved in overcoming the heterophoria. A direct relationship between fixation disparity and phoria cannot be expected. As described in Chapter 14, fixation disparity is measured under binocular conditions, with an interchange occurring among accommodative convergence, convergence accommodation, and fusional vergence. A dissociated phoria measurement is made under nonfused conditions with binocular factors providing only a residual tonic effect. Fixation disparity and the phoria should be regarded as two somewhat dependent variables, but sufficiently independent to warrant both of their measurements for diagnosing horizontal oculomotor imbalances.

RELATIONSHIPS OF DIAGNOSTIC CRITERIA TO ASTHENOPIA

Symptoms

The most common manifestation of an oculomotor imbalance is asthenopia. The individual will complain of eye fatigue, intermittent diplopia, headaches, and/or inability to perform necessary visual tasks for an extended period of time. Symptoms will be associated with use of the eyes at the distance where the imbalance occurs; most frequently this is at the near working distance. The extent of symptoms will depend on both the severity of imbalance and on the individual's visual workload. Since elimination of symptoms is the goal of therapy, presence or absence of asthenopia has often been used as a criterion for evaluating the various clinical measures.

Arner and Colleagues Study

Arner and colleagues (1956) obtained an asthenopia measure on a group of 35 subjects by way of questionnaire and interview. They also measured the phoria, vergences, and fixation disparity curve (FDC) at a 2.5-meter test distance. The ordering of subjects according to degree of asthenopia was best correlated with the FDCs, which were ranked on the basis of (1) total length of curve, (2) slope of curve, (3) low amount of fixation disparity, and (4) symmetry of the curve around the point of demand. There was not a significant correlation between asthenopia ranking and rankings based on either Percival's or Sheard's criterion.

Sheedy and Saladin—First Study

Sheedy and Saladin (1977, 1978) studied the relationship between asthenopia and various clinical measures of oculomotor balance in two separate studies. In the first, 32 students were selected from a group of 50 on the basis of questionnaires and interviews to serve as an asymptomatic population; 28 patients from the orthoptics clinic at the Ohio State University were the symptomatic population. These patients had been referred to the clinic on the basis of an initial vision examination at which the diagnosis indicated an oculomotor imbalance with associated symptoms. Phorias, vergences, and FDC were measured on all 60 subjects.

Stepwise discriminant analysis (Klecka, 1975) was used to select the clinical test results (variables) that best indicated or predicted the proper segregation of the population into symptomatic and asymptomatic groups. The variables chosen were the phoria; blur, break, and recovery ranges; Percival's criterion; Sheard's criterion; vergence opposite the phoria; X intercept; Y intercept; and the slope of the FDC around 0 (the operating point). Stepwise discriminant analysis selected the variables one at a time in the order of their discriminability. After each was selected, the remaining variables were completely reanalyzed to assess which one was most discriminative *after* the previously selected ones were taken into account. This is similar to the approach a clinician uses in diagnosing a case; first, looking to the test result that is the best indicator of a problem, then looking at the result that best identifies problems the first test missed.

Table 15.3 lists the variables in the order in which they were selected in the first study (Sheedy and Saladin, 1977). The statistical analysis was performed on the entire population of 60 and also individually on the exophoric (n = 38) and esophoric (n = 19) segments of the population. Sheard's criterion was the best variable for the entire population and for the exophoric subjects, but was not selected for the esophores. For esophoric subjects the amount of deviation (phoria) was most discriminating. In each of the three categories the second variable chosen was fixation disparity. The slope of the FDC was the next best for the entire population and for the esophoric subjects. A steep slope was associated with the symptomatic population. For the exophoric subjects the second variable chosen was the Y intercept.

TABLE 15.3. The Order in which Clinical Values were Discriminative between Symptomatic Patients and Asymptomatic Students

All Subjects	*Exophores*	*Esophores*
Sheard's amount	Sheard's amount	Phoria
FDC slope	Y intercept	FDC slope
Vergence opposing phoria	X intercept	Recovery range
Recovery range	Vergence opposing phoria	Break range
Break range	Vergence recovery	Vergence opposing phoria
90% correct	89% correct	89% correct

Source: Sheedy and Saladin, 1977.

Sheedy and Saladin—Second Study

A second study (Sheedy and Saladin, 1978) was performed to substantiate the findings of the first and to institute additional experimental controls. A total of 103 optometry students served as subjects. A questionnaire evaluated frequency and severity of symptoms. Symptoms for known reasons other than oculomotor imbalance (e.g., contact lenses, allergies, etc.) were eliminated, creating an asymptomatic group of 44 and a symptomatic group of 33. This manner of obtaining the two populations, that is derived from a single homogeneous population, offered the advantage that the groups were not separated or selected on the basis of any previous analysis of clinical data. In the first study the symptomatic group was referred on the basis of an analysis of variables that were later statistically tested for discriminability. Also, at the time of referral, only phoria-vergence data were available, which would favor selection of those variables over FDC variables. The selection method in the second study is also advantageous since it resulted in symptomatic and asymptomatic groups that were similar in age and near vision workload requirements. A drawback, however, was that the severity of symptoms in the symptomatic group was not as great as in the first study, where symptoms were severe enough for subjects (patients) to seek professional care.

The variables used in the second study for stepwise discriminant analysis were slightly modified. Negative and positive blur, break, and recovery findings as well as the phoria were used. Sheard's and Percival's amounts were calculated based on the recovery and break findings as well as on the traditional blur findings. In addition to the FDC variables used in the first study, a variable that identified the type of FDC as type I or non-type I (II, III, or IV) was used. The results of the second study are presented in Table 15.4. Stepwise discriminant analysis was performed on the entire subject population, the exophoric and esophoric subpopulations, and the exofixation and esofixation disparity subpopulations.

TABLE 15.4. The Order in which Clinical Values were Discriminative between Symptomatic and Asymptomatic Students Derived from the Original Population

All Subjects	*Exophores*	*Esophores*	*Exofixation Disparity*	*Esofixation Disparity*
Sheard blur	Y intercept	Percival break	Sheard blur	FDC slope
FDC type	FDC type	Positive blur	FDC type	Percival recovery
FDC slope	Negative break	Negative break	FDC slope	X intercept
Negative blur	Phoria	Percival recovery	Negative blur	Percival break
Y intercept	Percival blur	FDC slope		
Positive blur		X intercept		
Phoria				
82% correct	92% correct	73% correct	76% correct	96% correct

Source: Sheedy and Saladin, 1978.

The results for the entire population were very similar to those of the first study. Sheard's criterion (the traditional one based on blur value) was the best discriminator. The FDC type, which was not used in the first study, was the second variable chosen. The non-type I curves was associated with the symptomatic group. The slope of the FDC was chosen third, having been chosen second in the first study.

The variables chosen for the exophoric and exofixation disparity groups were different from one another. The first variables chosen for the exofixation disparity group were identical to those for the entire population. As in the first study, Sheard's criterion followed by fixation disparity variables was discriminative for exodeviations. For the exophoric group the Y intercept and FDC type were the most discriminative values and Sheard's criterion did not appear as a discriminator. Sheard's criterion by itself was discriminative for the exophoric population at the 1% level of significance; but the discrimination provided by the Y intercept and FDC type explains the discrimination of Sheard's criterion so that it was not selected. The FDC type offered the most discrimination after the Y intercept, indicating that the information provided by these two variables was not redundant.

As in the first study, Sheard's criterion was not selected for esodeviations. Percival's criterion was selected; however, it was based on the break or recovery findings, which were also discriminative. The traditional Percival's criterion (1928) based on the blur findings was not selected as a major discriminative value in either study. The FDC slope was the best discriminator for the esofixation disparity group.

The percentage of the total population that was properly identified as symptomatic or asymptomatic was not quite as high in the second study as in the first (82% vs 90%). This was due to the subject selection method, which resulted in less severe symptoms in the second study. It is remarkable, however, that such highly successful percentages were obtained for the exophoric and esofixation disparity groups. Fixation disparity variables were the best discriminators for symptomatic and asymptomatic groups.

CLINICAL DIAGNOSIS

The Problem

There is no single measure that can be used to assess the patency of the oculomotor system. It is important to understand which of the clinical measures are most effective indicators of abnormality and how they may be used to complement one another for diagnostic purposes. Correlations with asthenopia show that those based on both fixation disparity curve and phoria-vergences are useful and that a diagnosis is strengthened when both types of measurements are made because they assess different aspects of the oculomotor system. The FDC is a measure of fine alignment of the system during binocular fusion and its reactions to induced stress. It is strongly influenced by the sensory fusional system. The phoria and vergence measurements are indications of the gross alignment and neuromuscular abilities of the system and are influenced strongly by the motor fusional system.

Fixation Disparity

It appears that the FDC type identifies a basic characteristic of the system and is the most diagnostic FDC parameter. Type I curves are most often associated with a lack of symptoms and the other types (II, III, and IV) with symptoms. Not all type I curves are normal, however, nor are all other curve types abnormal; but curve type is a primary indicator, and analysis of an FDC best begins here.

The slope of the FDC is the next aspect of an FDC to assess. Its value depends on which portion of the FDC is specified. The portion that is most important is where the patient is "operating," that is, around 0^{Δ} for the patient who is not wearing prism. As indicated by Schor in Chapter 14, a flat slope is most desirable. The slope value that best discriminates between symptomatic and asymptomatic patients is -0.96 minutes per $^{\Delta}$, or approximately -1.0 minutes per $^{\Delta}$ (Sheedy and Saladin, 1977) using the stimulus parameters shown in Figure 15.2. If prism diopters and minutes of arc are graphed equally, a slope of greater than 45° is poor. The clinical rule of thumb is that the fixation disparity in minutes should change less than the prism in prism diopters. The slope is more diagnostic for the esodeviations. Also, the critical value of the slope is flatter for esophoria than exophoria (-0.77 minutes per $^{\Delta}$ compared to -1.06 minutes per $^{\Delta}$), indicating that esophoria is less tolerant of a steep slope than is exophoria.

The Y intercept was also diagnostic, but more so for exodeviations than esodeviations. For exophores the criterion value that best discriminated between symptomatic and asymptomatic patients was 12.1′ exofixation disparity (Sheedy and Saladin, 1977). For esophores it was 0.2′ exofixation disparity, with esofixation disparity associated with the symptomatic group. This was an indication that any amount of esofixation disparity measured with the Disparometer may be suspect. The most common values are low amounts (less than 10′) of exofixation disparity. The associated phoria (X intercept) was not as diagnostically significant as the other FDC variables.

Stability is another aspect of fixation disparity that should be evaluated. Nearly all patients note small movements of the vernier lines with respect to one another. They are caused by small disjunctive eye movements. For most patients these movements do not seriously interfere with the measurement of fixation disparity. When encouraged to be critical, that is, forced to choose on the disparity presentations, most patients can reliably identify the amount of fixation disparity to within two minutes of arc. Excessive movement of the two lines indicates excessive eye movements and instability in the accommodative mechanism. These factors interfere with the patient's ability to assess which disparity presentation appears aligned. The amplitude of movement may be as high as 10′ or more as measured by finding the disparity presentations that bracket the range.

Phoria and Vergence

Sheard's and Percival's criteria provide the best means to analyze the phoria and vergences. The former, which states that the opposing blur vergence amount should be twice the phoria amount, is a powerful diagnostic aid—but only for exophoria. Implicit in Sheard's criterion is the concept that the opposing vergence overcomes the phoria. Hence the positive vergences overcome an exophoria. The positive vergences are an active process whereas the negative vergences are more passive. Esophoria should be analyzed with a revised Percival's criterion, which is that the positive break should not be more than twice the negative break. Meeting this criterion ensures that the patient operates in the middle one-third of the vergence range. The phoria is not even a part of this criterion and the criterion does not imply that vergence overcomes an esodeviation.

CLINICAL TREATMENT

A binocular imbalance needs to be treated if there are symptoms associated with use of the eyes that might result in poor visual performance or avoidance of use of the eyes (especially at near). Options for treatment are prism, lenses, vision training, or combinations thereof. The specific treatment for a given imbalance will depend on factors other than measurements of the oculomotor system. Motivation of the patient (especially for training), whether a refractive correction or contact lenses are worn, the amount and critical nature of visual use (especially at near), the binocular status at distance when prescribing for near, adaptability of the patient to a prism prescription, and patient history can all influence treatment. Analysis of clinical measurements, as presented below, must be tempered with these factors when treatment decisions are made.

Vision Therapy

Increasing the positive vergences with vision training will often reduce the symptoms of an exophore who has failed Sheard's criterion. Prism prescriptions are less effective than convergence training for these patients (Worrell et al., 1971). Percival's criterion (using the break findings) is diagnostically significant for esophoric imbalances. To meet this criterion, the negative vergences in esophoria must be increased either with ophthalmic aids or with vision training. Esophores are often prescribed prisms and lenses on the basis of FDC analysis. Lens prescriptions are also calculated on the basis of the AC/A ratio. Vision training is more difficult for an esophore than for an exophore. The negative vergences, which are a passive process, are best improved by strengthening sensory fusion, which allows the eyes to maintain sensory fusion for greater divergence levels. Strict adherence to this criterion would dictate that improving the positive vergences would be detrimental to an esophore. Increasing positive vergence ranges are usually the result of developed adaptation abilities, which can also transfer to adaptation and extension of the divergence prism range (see Chapter 14).

The primary effect of orthoptic training is to flatten the slope of the FDC. The slope of a steep type I curve, which is often found in conjunction with exophoria that fails Sheard's criterion, can be reduced. Gross motor training is indicated and may be followed by fine motor training in the form of jump vergences to reduce the slope of the curve where the patient is operating. The Y intercept may or may not change as the result of training. The slope of type II FDCs typically will not change; prism and/or lenses are usually the treatment of choice. The slope of type III FDCs can be reduced, but they are more difficult to alter than the slope of type I curves. We have had some success in reducing symptoms of patients with type IV FDCs. The type IV curve usually indicates binocular abnormality and it requires extensive sensory and gross convergence and divergence training. Type IV curves do not lend themselves to slope analysis since they are usually flat, yet associated with symptoms.

In some cases the amount of fixation disparity is unstable and the patient will show accommodative fluctuations during dynamic retinoscopy. Instability of the fixation disparity is associated with fluctuations of accommodative convergence. The fixation disparity is usually exodisparity in these cases, since the accommodative lag is often large. Accommodative training and/or plus lenses are the therapy of choice.

Lenses and Prisms

When prescribing from an FDC the goal is to enable the patient to operate on a portion of the curve that is relatively flat, and where the amount of the fixation disparity is stable (Sheedy, 1980b). The portion of FDC intersecting the Y axis where the patient is operating may be changed by prescribing prism or lenses. A plus lens in the form of reading glasses or a bifocal is indicated when there is esofixation disparity at near, especially if there is asthenopia or poor near performance such as is commonly observed in school children. In our first clinical study (Sheedy and Saladin, 1977) any amount of esofixation disparity in an esophore was associated with the symptomatic population. A plus lens addition can reduce or eliminate the esofixation disparity at near as described in Chapter 14. In cases of accommodative instability, where the amplitude of accommodation is fluctuating, the amount of the fixation disparity will also be fluctuating. Very often in these cases a plus lens addition will stabilize the accommodation and the amount of the fixation disparity.

Prism prescription is primarily based on analysis of the slope of the FDC. Many patients who are operating on a steep portion of the curve will have a flatter portion elsewhere. Enough prism should be prescribed to enable operation just inside this portion. If there is no flat portion of the curve, training is indicated to reduce the slope. If training is not possible or successful, prism should be prescribed to reduce the amount of fixation disparity. In some cases there may be a slight inflection in the curve, which indicates a center of symmetry (Ogle et al., 1967) and this may be used for a prescription. Reversal of the habitual fixation disparity is contraindicated so that the prism prescription should normally not exceed the X intercept (associated phoria). Prescription of prism will sometimes drastically improve the stability of the fixation disparity measurement (Y intercept). Increased stability may be used as a criterion for the amount to be prescribed. Some patients with large exophorias (even intermittent exotropia) will show a paradoxical esofixation disparity. In these cases the base-out prism prescription based on the FDC has been found to provide relief of symptoms (Sheedy, 1980b). A plus lens addition may also be considered for near distances. The FDC may be used to assess the effectivenes of tentative prism and near add prescriptions. The effects of prism and lens adds on FDC are described in Chapter 14.

SUMMARY

Armed with the measurements of the phoria, vergences, and fixation disparity, the clinician must assess whether asthenopia can be ascribed to a binocular imbalance. A clinically useful diagnostic method should yield reliable (repeatable) information that will be a direct measure of the binocular balance of the visual system under examination. Furthermore, the results should be analyzed in terms of an acceptance or rejection criterion. Some flexibility is necessary, however, since just as there is no sharply definable level between an inefficient and an efficient binocular system, there is no sharply defined criterion.

For any given patient the various criteria discussed here may agree or disagree. Disagreement need not suggest that one criterion is wrong and another right, rather that only certain aspects of the oculomotor system are not optimal and that the two criteria are not totally redundant. As an example, in a controlled study (Sheedy and Saladin, 1975) fixation disparity amplitudes predicted the lack of symptoms observed in presbyopes who disobeyed with impunity the conventional Sheard-Percival criteria of proper balance between the phoria and opposing vergence amplitudes. The lack of symptoms was explained by their flat fixation disparity curves. The original conclusion was that presbyopes had learned to substitute accommodative convergence innervation for positive vergence innervation; however, more recent evidence indicates that prism adaptation may be the explanation. This was a poignant demonstration that the phoria-vergence and fixation disparity criteria are indicators of different aspects of the oculomotor system. A complete analysis of any system would include analysis of both the phoria-vergence relationships and the various fixation disparity parameters.

REFERENCES

Arner RS, Berger SI, Braverman G, Kaplan M. The clinical significance of the effect of vergence on fixation disparity—a preliminary investigation. Am J Optom 1956;33:399–409.

Borish IM. Clinical refraction. Chicago: Professional Press, 1970.

Borish IM. The Borish nearpoint chart. J Am Optom Assoc 1978;49:41–44.

Carter DB. Fixation disparity and heterophoria following prolonged wearing of prisms. Am J Optom Arch Am Acad Optom 1965;42(3):141–52.

Klecka R. Discriminant analysis. In: Statistical package for the social sciences. 2nd ed. New York: McGraw-Hill, 1975.

Lesser SK. Optometric extension program postgraduate courses. Vol. 41. Series 18, no. 4. 13–15.

Lesser SK. Introduction to modern analytical optometry. Duncan, Okla.: Optometric Extension Program Foundation, Inc., 1974.

Mallett RFJ. The investigation of heterophoria at near and new fixation disparity technique. Optician 1964;148, No. 3844, 547–551.

Mallett RFJ. A fixation disparity test for distance use. Optician 1966;152, No. 3927, 1–3.

Martens TG, Ogle KN. Observations on accommodative convergence, especially its nonlinear relationships. Am J Ophthalmol 1959;47(1):455–62.

Morgan MW. The clinical aspects of accommodation and convergence. Am J Optom Arch Am Acad Optom 1944;21(8):301–13.

Morgan MW. The analysis of clinical data. Optom Weekly 1964;27–34; 23–25.

Ogle KN, Martens TG, Dyer JA. Oculomotor imbalance in binocular vision and fixation disparity. Philadelphia: Lea & Febiger, 1967.

Percival A. The prescribing of spectacles. Bristol, England: J. Wright & Sons, 1928.

Saladin JJ, Sheedy JE. A population study of relationships between fixation disparity, heterophorias and vergences. Am J Optom Physiol Opt 1978; 55(11):744–50.

Sheard C. Zones of ocular comfort. Am J Optom 1930;7(1):9–25.

Sheedy JE. Fixation disparity analysis of oculomotor balance. Am J Optom Physiol Opt 1980a;57(9):632–39.

Sheedy JE. Actual measurement of fixation disparity and its use in diagnosis and treatment. J Am Optom Assoc 1980b;51:1079–84.

Sheedy JE, Saladin JJ. Exophoria at near in presbyopia. Am J Optom Physiol Opt 1975;52(7):474–81.

Sheedy JE, Saladin JJ. Phoria, vergence, and fixation disparity in oculomotor problems. Am J Optom Physiol Opt 1977;54(7):474–78.

Sheedy JE, Saladin JJ. Association of symptoms with measures of oculomotor deficiencies. Am J Optom Physiol Opt 1978;55(10):670–76.

Worrell BE, Hirsch MJ, Morgan MW. An evaluation of prism prescribed by Sheard's criterion. Am J Optom 1971;48(5):373–76.

VI

DIAGNOSIS AND TREATMENT OF STRABISMUS

16

Kinematics of Normal and Strabismic Eyes

Ken Nakayama

Most contemporary investigators have measured eye rotations in only one direction, usually along the horizontal. In so doing, the very rapid movements of the eyes have been described with great precision, and significant classification of different types of movements has been possible: saccades, vergence, pursuit, and nystagmus (Robinson, 1968). In rarer instances, both horizontal and vertical movements have been considered, in which case the eye is treated as if it were a pointer (defined by the foveal axis). As such, two-dimensional descriptions of eye rotations specify the orientation of this pointer in space.

Much earlier, however, it was recognized that the eye can also make torsional movements about this pointer axis (Helmholtz, 1910). Therefore a full description of the rotary behavior of the eye also requires measurement of torsion. Far from being a formal exercise in completeness, consideration of all three degrees of freedom of eye rotation leads to some unique neurological conclusions regarding oculomotor organization. It may also provide an additional way of viewing the mechanics of eye musculature in health and disease.

Supported by NIH grants 5 R01 EY-01582, 5P30-EY-01186; and the Smith-Kettlewell Eye Research Foundation.

KINEMATIC LAWS OF EYE ROTATION

Although this subject can be explained simply, it can be confusing. Some of the difficulty stems from the need of previous writers to define the kinematic laws quantitatively, setting up a coordinate system based on a rigorously determined set of spherical angles. Although this is useful for empirical verification of these laws (see below), it is a poor way to introduce the subject. There is widespread lack of familiarity with three-dimensional spherical angle representations, and the choice of reference coordinates usually obscures the basic ideas.

Rather than describing eye kinematics with respect to a horizontal and vertical angular coordinate system as is usually done, this discussion begins intuitively and geometrically, without explicitly defining a coordinate system in any notational sense. A simple physical "ball and membrane" model of the eye is used (Nakayama, 1978). Figure 16.1 shows such a model positioned in the head of a supine observer gazing upward. The model consists of a spherical globe attached to a very tightly stretched elastic membrane carefully secured to the end of cylinder so that the membrane is equally taut in all directions. Because of the elastic quality

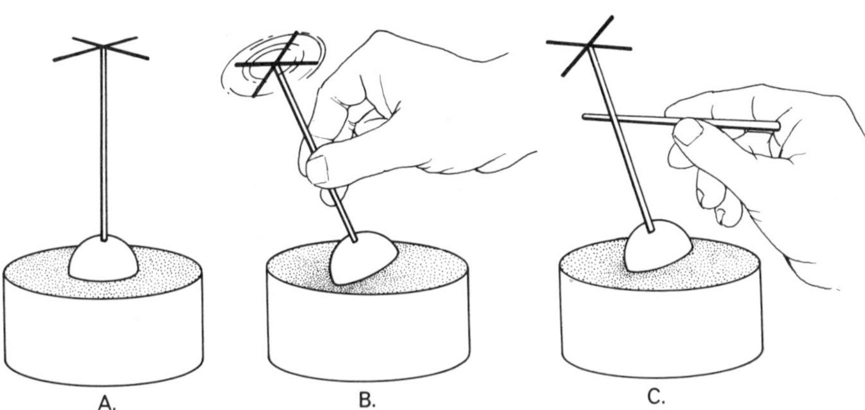

FIGURE 16.1. Ball and membrane model of the eye of a supine observer gazing upward. A Resting position of the "eye," when it is in the primary position. The foveal axis (see stalk) is perpendicular to the membrane and is oriented in the primary direction of regard. B Rotational displacement of the "eye" showing 3 degrees of rotational freedom; horizontal, vertical, and torsional rotations are possible. The stalk can be displaced as well as twisted between the fingers. C Rotational displacement of the "eye" having the capability of only 2 degrees of rotational freedom. Note that the smooth rod can displace the eye in only two dimensions. It has no control of the third dimension, torsion. This model obeys both Donders' law and Listing's law (see text).

of the membrane, there is a natural resting place for this eye model. Note the existence of a stalk attached to this globe. It represents the foveal axis and is perpendicular to the membrane. A cross is mounted on the end of the stalk to reveal the amount of twist of the globe around the axis. This position of rest is defined as the primary position, and the direction of the foveal axis, as represented by the stalk, corresponds to the primary direction of regard. The plane of this membrane when the model is at rest corresponds to Listing's plane for the eye. It is the frontoparallel plane passing through the center of the globe or sphere. The figure 16.1B depicts a situation in which the globe is rotated with three full degrees of rotational freedom. It can be rotated horizontally and vertically by displacing the stalk and torsionally by twisting the stalk between the fingers.

A third and most important case is shown in Figure 16.1c. Instead of moving the globe by grasping the stalk between the fingers, the fixation axis can be moved to any desired direction of gaze by pushing the foveal stalk with a smooth rod. In this case the model has sufficient rotational freedom to fixate any object, but it is limited to just two degrees of freedom, not three. The twist or torsion of the eye is no longer under external control because it cannot be twisted between the fingers. Its orientation is dictated by the elastic properties of the membrane, which ensures that it corresponds to the position having the lowest potential energy. Thus each direction of the foveal axis is associated with one and only one orientation of the globe.

What is essential to remember is that the behavior of this particular ball and membrane model is isomorphic with two of the most fundamental laws of human eye rotation: Donders' law and Listing's law. Donders' law states that for each gaze direction, that is, for each direction of the foveal axis in space, there is only one orientation of the globe in the orbit. Listing's law is much more specific, assigning the exact torsion of the eye in any gaze direction according to the model presented in Figure 16.1c.

This definition gives the most concise example of eye torsion and its relation to Listing's law. It says that the behavior of the eye (and of the model) shows a radial or axial symmetry, such that there is no net torsion of the eye with respect to an axial reference direction (the primary direction of regard). An equivalent and more common way to phrase Listing's law is to say that orientation of the eye can be predicted by assuming that the eye has made a geodesic (shortest path) rotation from the primary position to any other fixation position. The axis of this shortest path rotation is perpendicular to the intended direction of gaze, and thus lies in Listing's plane. For the case of the rubber membrane model, it means that the axis of the shortest path rotation lies in the plane of the membrane.

As with many other geometric and physical relations, the reason why the law can be stated with such simplicity is that we have a model that is couched in the proper coordinate representation to express Listing's law. Confusion has surrounded eye kinematics precisely because this most natural radial coordinate system has been neglected.

CONVENTIONAL COORDINATE REPRESENTATION OF LISTING'S LAW

To make actual kinematic measurements of the eye, it is often advantageous to use such nonradial angular coordinate systems. In particular, the angular coordinate systems that are usually chosen to describe eye rotation are based on the familiar concept of horizontal and vertical rotation. Two different systems, Fick and Helmholtz, specify rotations in this manner, although they are not identical (Alpern, 1969). For an appropriate model of the Fick system, consider a terrestrial telescope mounted on a set of two axes (Figure 16.2). The telescope can rotate horizontally about a vertical axis fixed to a stationary (earth-referenced) bearing and a vertical rotation can be made about a mobile horizontal axis. Thus any fixation direction can be specified in terms of two spherical angles.

In many ways, these two angles comprise a natural and suitable coordinate system that corresponds well with our sense of horizontal and vertical, and that is mechanically convenient for mounting the telescope. It can scan the visual field with ease and its gaze direction can be precisely specified by the two spherical angles (Θ, Φ) (Figure 16.2). The arrangement has one other advantage in that telescopic vertical always remains ori-

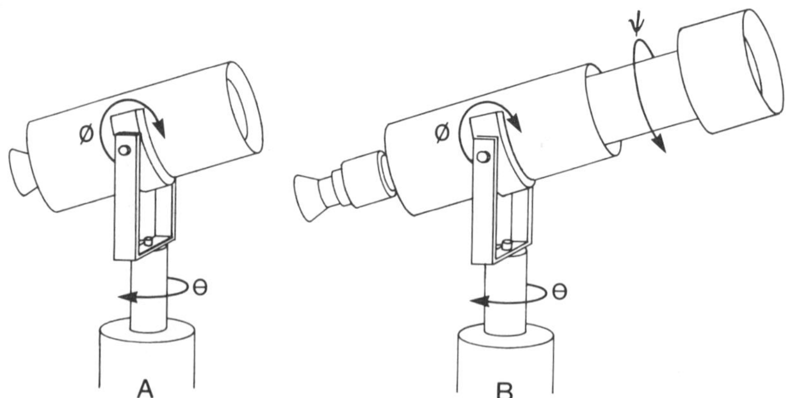

FIGURE 16.2. Fick coordinate system equivalent to a telescope model to describe the rotational behavior of the eye. A Description of a two-dimensional system that can be pointed to any desired direction of regard. It consists of freedom to rotate about a vertical axis, θ, and the freedom to rotate about a horizontal axis through an angle ϕ. B Same as in A with the addition of a third degree of rotational freedom. The telescope can also rotate about its optical axis by the angle ψ.

ented with respect to the environmental vertical. If we scanned the skyline of the city, for example, the vertical sides of any distant building would always line up with the vertical cross-hair in the telescope eyepiece. Although such a model is easy to understand, is easy to build, and has the property of preserving the parallel alignment of telescope and environmental verticals, it is very different from the behavior of the eye. It differs because it lacks the radial symmetry of Listing's law.

To describe adequately the radially symmetric rotational states of our normal eye fixations in this Fick system, we require an additional angular parameter, namely, a torsional one. The telescope needs to be twisted about its own axis (see Figure 16.2) according to the following equation:

$$\psi = \sin^{-1}\left(\frac{\sin\theta \sin\phi}{1 + \cos\theta \cos\phi}\right) \qquad (a)$$

where θ is the horizontal rotation, ϕ the vertical rotation, and ψ the required rotation to adjust the eye's orientation in accordance with Listing's law. This angle ψ is also called false torsion, as it is an apparent twist of the eye with respect to the vertical that needs to be "added" to make the eye conform to Listing's law. An extra parameter of this type is required for any coordinate representation of Listing's law that is not radially symmetric with respect to the primary direction of regard. As we can see from the ball and membrane model, however, no real torsion occurs as it moves from primary to oblique positions of gaze.

Empirical support for Listing's law comes from a number of measuring techniques. The simplest is to put a vertical afterimage on the retina when the eye is in the primary direction of regard, thus providing a visible indication of the "vertical" meridian of the eye as it makes different steady fixations on a target screen (Helmholtz, 1910; Hering, 1879). If the eye were to obey the telescope rule (as in Figure 16.2), such afterimages would always appear congruent with vertical lines on a target screen. This is because the longitude lines in Figure 16.3 project to vertical straight lines on a target screen. If the eye obeyed Listing's law, however, such afterimages should be tilted away from true vertical (Figure 16.3). If we were to project the afterimages on a normal planar surface they would be congruent to a family of hyperbolic arcs, as depicted in Figure 16.4 (Southall, 1961; Helmholtz, 1910).

IMPLICATIONS FOR NEUROMOTOR CONTROL

Listing's law has been stated. It holds under a wide variety of conditions, in particular when the observer is unconverged looking at distant targets and the head is erect (Nakayama, 1978). How is it maintained and why

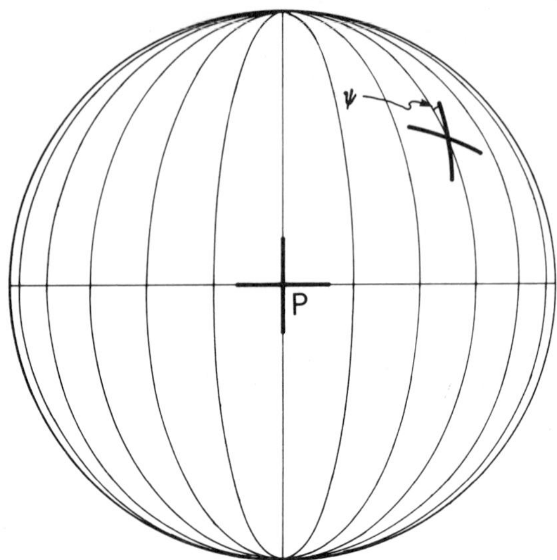

FIGURE 16.3. Representation of false torsion of the eye on a spherical field of fixation if the eye were to obey Listing's law. Vertical arcs represent longitude lines of the Fick system. They represent lines of constant horizontal angular displacement as well as as being congruent with vertical edges in the environment. Cross in the primary direction (represented by P) moves to a position in the upper right as a consequence of an eye movement in conformity with Listing's law. The vertical limb of the cross makes an angle of ψ with the true vertical in accordance with equation (a). This angle is defined as false torsion.

is it maintained? Is there a stiff rubber membrane in the orbit as described in Figure 16.1, mechanically obliging an adherence to Listing's law? A set of passive restraining tissues does exist in the orbit, comprised primarily of the stiff passive properties of each muscle and supplemented by nonmuscle tissue that surrounds the globe (Robinson, 1975). A partial cutaway drawing of some of the muscles and their attachments can be seen by looking ahead to Figure 16.11. Of importance is the arrangement of the muscles with respect to the primary direction of regard. The vertical rectus muscles pull back at an angle of 30° with respect to the primary direction. If Listing's law were to be explained by passive tissue elasticities, it would be very surprising if the primary axis of radial symmetry would lie in the primary direction of regard (see arrow). One might predict, for example, that the primary direction of regard would also be exodeviated by the same 30°, which it is not (Nakayama, 1978). Furthermore, there are oblique muscles that can provide the third degree of freedom, and thus there is really no obvious mechanical muscle constraint having sufficient stiffness to ensure Listing's law.

Some analogies might be useful at this point. Consider a soap bubble,

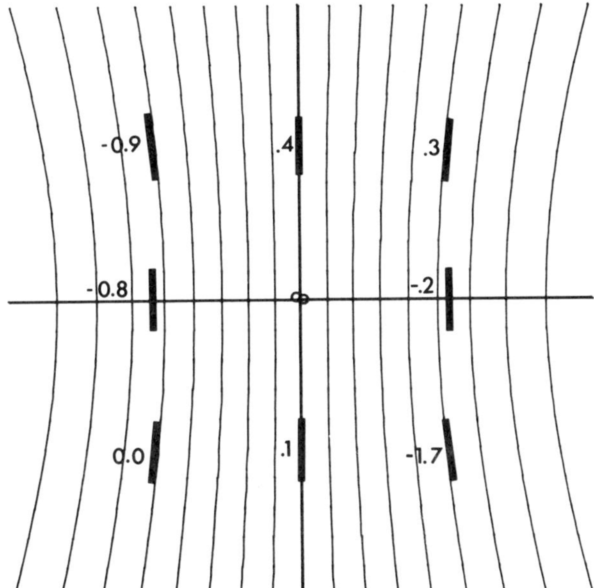

FIGURE 16.4. Experimental confirmation of Listing's law using afterimage alignment. If the law is correct, all afterimages should remain congruent to a family of hyperbolic arcs on a tangent screen. Such arcs are the central projection of vertical direction circles in the spherical field of fixation onto a frontoparallel planar surface (Helmholtz, 1910). Bold lines represent afterimage settings and accompanying numbers show the deviation from Listing's law in degrees. Eye screen distance is denoted by the horizontal line at the bottom of the figure. For more details, see text. From Nakayama K. A new technique to determine the primary position of the eye using Listing's law. American Journal of Optometry and Physiological Optics. Copyright 1978. Reprinted by permission.

a near perfect example of spherical symmetry. Few would ascribe this symmetry to a higher biological purpose, it is simply (though no less miraculously) the "solution" dictated by the classical physical principle of minimal surfaces. Likewise for the behavior of the ball and membrane model. It too has a symmetry (about an axis rather than a point) and this symmetry is the direct result of the constraining rubber membrane forces intrinsic to the model.

On the other hand think of a well-formed meatball. There is no intrinsic force in the meat to aggregate it into a spherical shape. What is required for it to exist is the "purpose" or "goal" of the maker, to ensure that the skillfull hand molds the meat into the desired symmetric form. The same holds for Listing's law. There is no intrinsic mechanical property of the muscles or the fascia in the orbit to dictate the observed radial symmetry seen for the rotational states of the human eye. As with the perfect meatball, it appears that the three-dimensional kinematic behavior of the eye can only be understood by looking beyond its immediate characteristics. One must invoke a higher biological purpose; its behavioral symmetry cannot be understood in terms of physics. Additional evidence to support this conclusion comes from deviations from Listing's law under specific conditions. It is violated with differing amounts of convergence (see below) as well as head tilt, it can be overcome with extensive voluntary effort (Balliet and Nakayama, 1978), and finally, it appears to break down in the state of sleep (Nakayama, 1975).

Because of these conclusions, it is argued elsewhere (Westheimer, 1973; Nakayama, 1975) that Listing's law is upheld by the central nervous system. Not only does it guarantee that the eye is pointed in the proper direction, it precisely apportions the flow of nerve impulses to the muscles so that Listing's law is also maintained. It is clear that many combinations of extraocular muscle innervation that would point the foveal axis in the desired direction are, as it were, forbidden. Only those states that simultaneously point the eye in the right direction and specify its torsional state are "permitted." Because there are essentially only two degrees of rotational freedom (as specified by Listing's law) and because various states of co-contracture during normal versional eye movements have not be observed (Robinson, 1970), the dimensionality of the six-muscle ocular system can be considered as only two, not six.

Several broad hypotheses can be proposed as to how this reduction of dimensionality could be accomplished. First, it should be clear that there must be a system formally equivalent to the model depicted in Figure 16.5, that is, there is a signal of orbital gaze direction expressed as a two-dimensional quantity, formally equivalent to two "command"

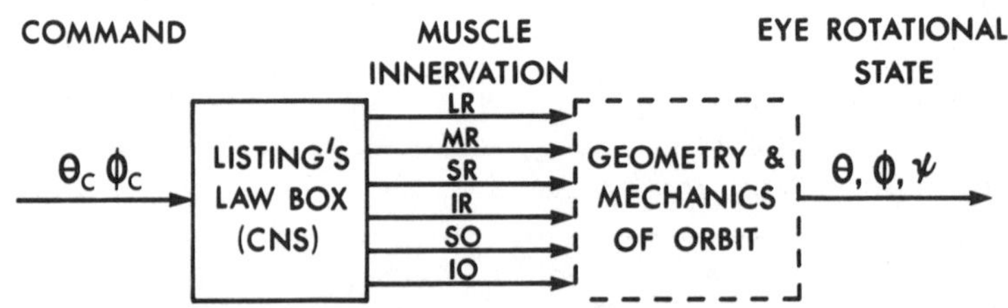

FIGURE 16.5. Block diagram showing that Listing's law is actively determined by the coordinated pattern of nerve impulses to the extraocular muscles. A two-dimensional command signal specifying two spherical angles θ_c, ϕ_c, provides input to the coordinating structure, Listing's law box. Thus in spite of the non-symmetric geometry and elasticities of the muscles and tissues, the torsion ψ is related to θ and ϕ by equation (*a*). Reprinted with permission from Basic Mechanisms in Ocular Motility and their Clinical Implications, G Lennerstrand, P Bach-y-Rita, eds., Nakayama K, Coordination of extraocular muscles, 1975, Pergamon Press, Ltd.

angles, θ_C, and ϕ_C. These commands go into a neural integrating network, Listing's law box, which then apportions the flow of impulses in such a way that the law is upheld, that is, that equation (*a*) is satisfied. Thus Listing's law is ultimately neurophysiological, and could be explicitly described as a set of synaptic weighting functions transforming a two-dimensional command signal to prescribed amounts of net excitation in the six separate motoneuron pools.

Why Listing's Law

This brings us to the more puzzling question of why, which might be best addressed by asking, how does the nervous system "know" that it is adhering to Listing's law? What feedback is given to the system to ensure this lawfulness? One alternative is that the nervous system is already prewired and precalibrated in its connectivity and strength of synaptic connections so that Listing's law is maintained without feedback. Thus the nervous system does not have to know it is regulating anything; it just happens to be preprogrammed. This seems unlikely because of the great change that occurs during development in the growth of the eye, muscles, and surrounding tissues. Small influences in early life could lead to larger imbalances later on. Furthermore, other open-loop aspects of the oculomotor system are known to be subject to parametric feedback (Ludvigh, 1952). For example, open-loop gains of the saccadic system (Optican and Robinson, 1980; Miller et al., 1980), as well as the vestibuloocular system (Melville Jones and Davies, 1976) can show very large shifts, specifically in terms of the open-loop gains of various subcomponents. Thus the problem of Listing's law becomes especially puzzling when considering the clear answer that has been received regarding the modifiability of saccades as well as the vestibuloocular reflex (VOR). In the case of saccades, there is a retinal position error signal that corrects the size of future saccades. For the VOR, retinal slip velocity can adjust its open-loop gain and phase. Such results suggest that a similar adjustment would be required to fine-tune Listing's law.

Three separable hypotheses have been advanced regarding the goal of Listing's law. The first is a motor hypothesis originally suggested by Helmholtz (1910). He asserted that Listing's law required the eye muscles to exert minimum energy. Such eye rotations require the muscles to do the least work in positions of eccentric gaze. Any other rotational state for a given fixation direction stretches the muscle or tissues beyond the minimum required. The assumptions are several. First is the question of whether eye movements obeying Listing's law actually require the least energy. As specified earlier, this is clearly the case for the rubber membrane model as depicted in Figure 16.1, but whether it holds for the eye is unproved. In fact the position of rest under neuromuscular paralysis changes with age, becoming progressively more divergent (DeGroot et al., 1976). No evidence as yet exists to suggest that the primary direction of regard (the axis of radial symmetry embodied in Listing's law) undergoes a concomitant divergence. In addition to this speculation, the argument assumes that the nervous system can also learn to accomplish the task of eye fixation at minimal energy cost and with great accuracy. It puts the nervous system in the position of performing an ergonometric analysis, measuring the work for each gaze direction and then calculating the rotational state that is associated with the least energy. Thus the hypothesis requires that Listing's law correspond to a set of minimum energy states and furthermore, that differences from the law are sufficiently great in terms of energy consumption that the nervous system can sense and act on them.

A second hypothesis, originally advanced by Hering (1868) and later considered by Westheimer and Blair (1972), is perhaps more ingenious. It is noted that eye movements made according to Listing's law preserve direction congruence for lines passing through the primary direction of regard. To get a modern flavor of this idea, think of a set of Hubel and Wiesel (1962) orientation-sensitive units in cortex. If any straight line is scanned so that it intersects the primary direction of regard, the relative dominance of orientation-tuned units best tuned for the orientation of the line when the eye is in the primary direction will also be the same set of units best tuned for gaze directions on the line in any other scanned portion (Figure 16.6). Thus straight lines will have the property of providing the same stimulation for a given orientation-tuned cell at any fixation along the straight line. In some fashion, therefore, the preponderant existence of straight lines could tune the oculomotor system's behavior so that it conforms to Listing's law.

This approach neglects the potential importance of straight lines that do not intersect the primary direction of regard. Consider the observer facing straight ahead and looking over to the right to scan a telephone pole. A vertically oriented Hubel and Wiesel unit would be optimally stimulated in the primary plane of regard (fixating at the object at eye level), but for points above and below this receptive field would be too extorted or intorted (see Figure 16.6). It might be supposed, however, that fixation of most straight lines of interest intersect the primary direction of regard as the observer can also turn his head for straight ahead frontal viewing. Consequently, off-axis fixations such as that depicted in Figure 16.6 could represent noise to be averaged out.

A third hypothesis suggests that Listing's law serves the cause of binocular vision by keeping the orientation of each eye the same in different directions of parallel gaze. This view suffers because other candidate laws are equally adaptive in this respect, for example, the telescope

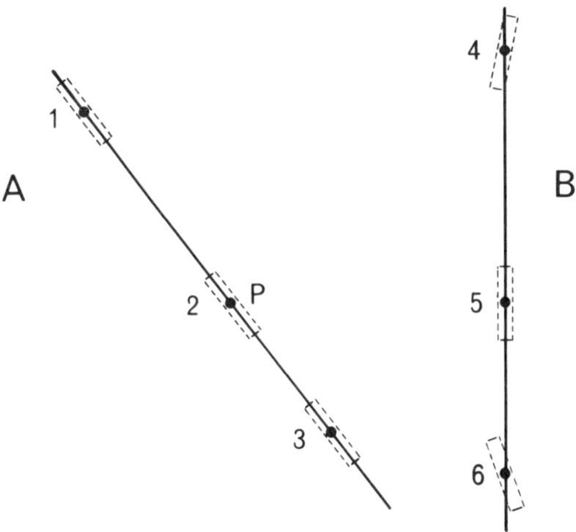

FIGURE 16.6. Preservation and lack of preservation of direction congruence as a consequence of eye rotations made in accordance with Listing's law. The primary direction of regard is designated by P and the sets of dashed rectangles associated with each line are the projection of foveal receptive fields were the eye to look at the various fixation positions (numbers 1-6). A For straight lines that have one point that passes through the primary direction of regard (this requires that the observer look directly at one point of the line), there will be a foveal receptive field orientation that will always line up with the line for other fixations. Thus at fixations 1, 2, and 3 the same class of cells with oriented receptive fields will receive optimal stimulation. B For eye fixations on lines not passing through the primary direction of regard, however, this property does not hold. Thus for fixations 4, 5, and 6 a given foveal receptive field (a vertically oriented one in this case) will not receive optimal stimulation at the different fixations along the line.

law as depicted in Figure 16.2. In this model the torsion of the eye with respect to the vertical would be identical for each direction of parallel gaze. An appropriate test of this binocular view might be to examine the eye kinematics of species having little or no binocular overlap, yet ones that make such large eye movements that adherence to Listing's law could be checked to a sufficient degree of precision. Animals such as the African chameleon may provide such an opportunity.

One might also consider the importance of Listing's law in maintaining binocular correspondence for nonparallel gaze. As it turns out there is some small advantage in this regard. (See below).

VERGENCE EYE MOVEMENTS

In general, versional eye movements obey Listing's law. Therefore as long as the foveal axes are roughly parallel, orientation of the vertical meridian of the eye can be predicted, as in equation (*a*). When the eyes are converged, however, the relation between gaze direction and eye torsion becomes altered, a finding that has been well recognized for more than a century (Hering, 1868).

As an example, consider the following experiment. An observer is placed in a bite apparatus and told to fixate a succession of points (F_1, F_2, F_3 as in Figure 16.7). In each fixation the gaze direction of the right eye is always the same, what varies is the direction of the left eye. This is the case of asymmetric vergence. The torsion of the right eye can be measured very accurately using a camera with telephoto lens as described by Balliet and Nakayama (1978) and this experiment can be repeated for several elevations of gaze. Figure 16.8 shows the change in torsion of the right eye as a function of the amount of asymmetric convergence for these different elevations. Clearly, for level and down gaze there is a large effect of convergence. Even though the right eye is looking in the same direction, the measured value of torsion progressively changes as the angle of convergence increases. This implies that the innervational pattern to a given eye for a given gaze direction will be different depending on the amount of convergence. Thus convergence eye rotations are clearly not mediated through the Listing's law integrating network (as in Figure 16.5), but must have some organization that bypasses this network.

There are several logical possibilities. In one case the vergence signal bypasses Listing's law box and directly innervates a single muscle pair, namely, the horizontal rectus system. This is the most simple conceptually and is in accord with the presumed importance of the horizontal rectus muscles in mediating vergence eye movements. Horizontal rectus muscles clearly must play a role in horizontal vergence movements and an attractive hypothesis is that they are directly innervated to produce vergence eye movements. It is also partially supported by the findings of Keller and Robinson (1971), who have shown that for a given horizontal gaze direction there is a particular discharge rate independent of whether the eye is engaged in versional or vergence movement. A second view is more complex, recognizing that Listing's law box must surely be bypassed

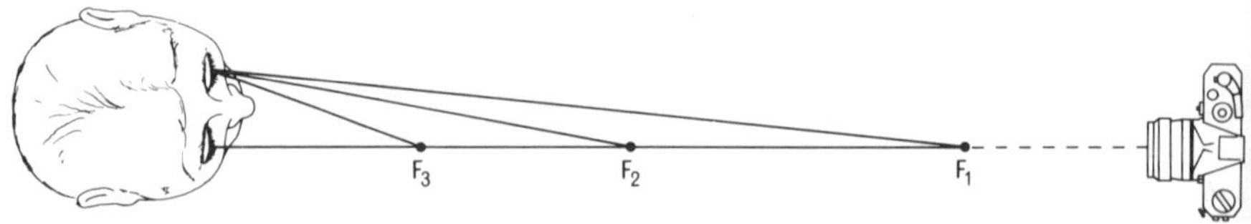

FIGURE 16.7. Schematic diagram of asymmetric convergence paradigm used to measure changes in eye torsion with differing amounts of convergence. Right eye is always in the same gaze direction regardless of the amount of convergence, whereas the left (unmeasured) eye changes fixation. Photographic measurement of torsion is thus confined to the right eye.

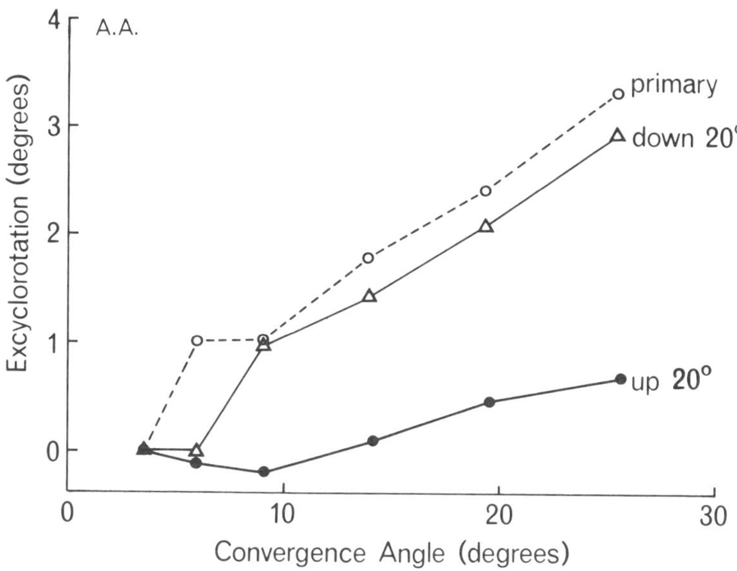

FIGURE 16.8. Torsion measured as a function of convergence for the differing elevations of gaze. Experimental apparatus as in Figure 16.7. Open circles represent level gaze, solid dots represent up gaze (20°), crosses represent down gaze (20°).

to produce the recognized deviations from Listing's Law, acknowledging that the separate contribution from the vergence system is likely to involve more than just the horizontal rectus system.

Experimental results and many other factors favor the second more complex alternative. First is the fact that excyclotorsion tends to increase with increased convergence, and this is especially prominent in horizontal gaze and in down gaze (as in Figure 16.8). From the geometry of the horizontal rectus muscles (they insert on the horizontal meridian of the eye and thus their axis vectors are vertical), one might expect that if there were torsional deviations from Listing's law they would be essentially opposite and of equal amplitude for fixations up versus down with respect to the primary plane of regard. Because the results show an asymmetric deviation from Listing's law, this view seems untenable. It appears that the vertical and the oblique muscles must play a role in vergence movement and furthermore, they must do so in a particular manner, ensuring a relative excyclorotation during convergence in down gaze and in level gaze, but not in up gaze. This participation of vertical and oblique muscles is also supported by some experiments on dark-reared kittens (Cynader, 1979). Such animals show prominent horizontal tropias after a period of dark-rearing during the critical period. Most important to note, however, is a large torsional deviation that accompanies this horizontal deviation.

As the animals recover from the strabismus, both the horizontal and torsional components disappear, demonstrating a strong link between tonic vergence and tonic cyclorotation under these experimental conditions. Both of these results suggest a new set of rules between muscle pairs must occur in vergence movements.

What can be said about vergence muscle coordination within an antagonistic pair? Keller and Robinson (1971) saw no deviation between the motoneuron rate versus position curve during vergence, but they did not measure the motoneuron discharge associated with vertical or oblique muscles. Human vergence appears to be accompanied by a measurable translation of the eye (Enright, 1980). It provides indirect evidence that during vergence various states of co-contracture within a muscle pair are possible, a clear violation of the Sherringtonian principle of reciprocal innervation. Simultaneous measurement of primate oculomotoneurons corresponding to antagonistic muscles during vergence and vergence might help settle the issue.

The functional question of why there should be a deviation from Listing's law in vergence has not received a satisfactory answer, although Hering's position (1868) that it must serve some aspect of binocular vision seems attractive. As one possible approach, consider the horopter in the vertical dimension, those points in space in binocular correspondence. Assuming a geometric model of retinal correspondence, the vertical horopter is a single vertical line through the fixation, at least for symmetric convergence in the horizontal plane (Helmholtz, 1910). In fact, however the empirical horopter is tilted backward and passes through the feet when a person is viewing targets at infinity (Helmholtz, 1910; Nakayama 1978; Nakayama et al., 1977), a view that has been collaborated with physiological recordings in cats and owls (Cooper and Pettigrew, 1979). The horopter tilt is a consequence of deviation from strict geometric correspondence between the two retinas, showing a physiological tilt of the vertical meridian in each eye. This very interesting point is discussed in greater detail in Chapter 7.

For parallel axes of the eye that are associated with viewing distant targets straight ahead and on the horizon the horopter line lies in the ground plane, a most convenient place for binocular vision to be optimal. With closer fixations in the primary plane of regard (assuming no violations of Listing's law), the horopter becomes oriented more and more close to the vertical (Figure 16.9).

Of interest is to see whether such torsional deviations from Listing's law might aid in keeping the vertical horopter line in a functionally appropriate orientation with the close viewing associated with convergence. To examine this issue, we note the factors that will determine orientation of the horopter line under these circumstances.

First is the physiological tilt of the vertical meridian of the eye (ψ_H

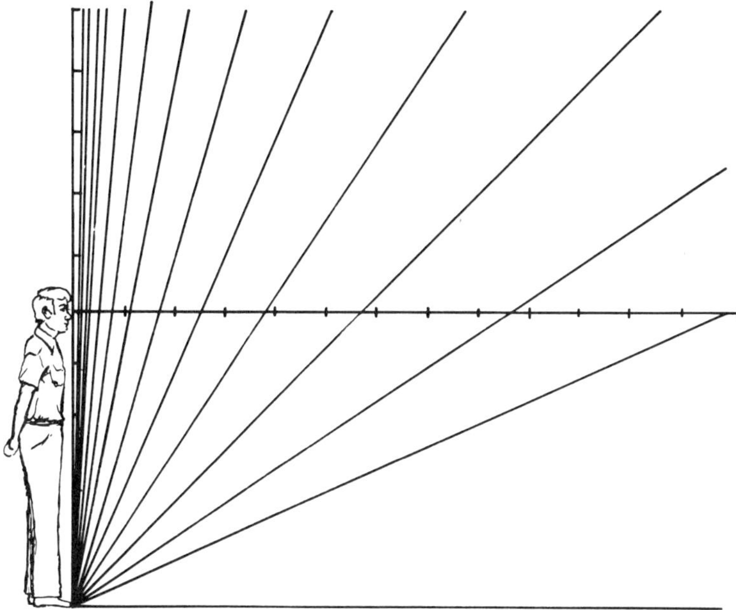

FIGURE 16.9. Position of the vertical horopter line for different distances of symmetric fixation in the horizontal plane of regard. Note that as fixation distance is decreased the horopter changes from a predominantly horizontal to a predominantly vertical orientation.

as originally hypothesized by Helmholtz and subsequently confirmed (Nakayama, 1977). Second is the torsion of the eye with respect to the environmental vertical. This eye movement contribution can be subdivided into two components: "false" torsion due to Listing's law in accordance with equation (*a*) (ψ_L), and torsion associated with convergence (ψ_C), which can be estimated from the data in Figure 16.8.

Figure 16.10 shows the orientation of the vertical horopter for three elevations of gaze, calculated from estimates of ψ_H, ψ_L, ψ_C. These are represented by the bold lines. In addition, the orientation of the horopter line without ψ_C (torsion changes due exclusively to convergence) is shown as the dashed line. From the figure it should be clear that a very slight advantage can be obtained by ψ_C as it tilts the horopter back by a small angle, at least in down gaze and level gaze. Inasmuch as the horopter line lies within a plane of best correspondence, this additional tilt at near distances may aid in the bincocular inspection of backwardly tilted surfaces. To the extent that such surfaces receive better illumination from overhead sources (presumably the sun or sky) especially in comparison to most vertical surfaces, they will be well placed to ensure optimal binocular stimulation. It must be admitted, however, that the effect is small.

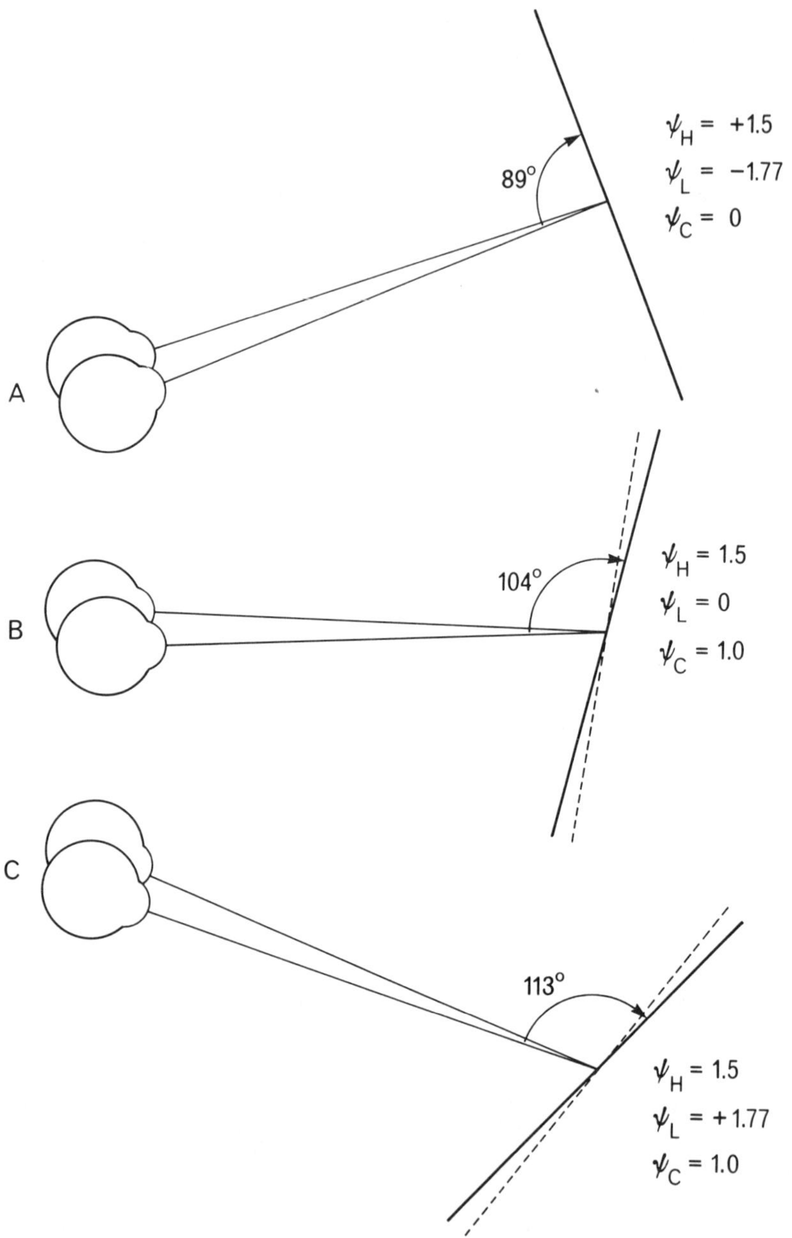

FIGURE 16.10. Orientation of the vertical horopter at a close viewing distance (19.3 cm) for three elevations of gaze: 20° elevation, level, and 20° depression. Bold solid lines in each case reflect the best estimate of the vertical horopter line orientation based on ψ_H (the physiological tilt of the vertical meridian as originally suggested by Helmholtz), ψ_L (eye extorsion introduced by Listing's law),

As the final note, it should be clear that the torsion associated with Listing's law during inward and downward gaze contributes an even greater tilt to the vertical horopter in the close viewing situation, much more so than the convergence-induced violation of Listing's law. Whether this is a cause or a byproduct of the law remains unanswered.

CLINICAL APPLICATIONS OF EYE KINEMATICS

Earlier sections of this chapter established the view that the relation between torsion and gaze direction was fixed by the nervous system. Thus whenever the eye is to make a saccade to a particular position in the orbit specifiable in terms of two angles, the brain allocates the innervation to the six muscles in a very stereotyped manner, ensuring that the third degree of freedom, torsion, is fixed.

The question to be considered is the degree to which this neurologic stereotypy can be used to assist in understanding disorders of the oculomotor system, especially those concerning the peripheral muscular pathology. At the outset, it must be noted that a similar type of reasoning based on neuronal stereotypy already exists as a cornerstone in the diagnosis of strabismus, namely, reliance on Hering's law of equal innervation. With Hering's law, the two eyes are assumed to be yoked neurologically and any changes in their conjugacy is attributed to peripheral factors, not to the possibility that Hering's law itself might be violated. Hering's law provides the scientific basis of the cover test, one of the most widely used tools in the diagnosis of strabismus.

Using analogous reasoning, one might also deduce pathological features of the peripheral oculomotor apparatus using Listing's law instead of Hering's law. One could assume that the neurologic machinery to maintain Listing's law is essentially intact at least over the short run and that any given deviation must be due to some form of mechanical abnormality of the oculomotor system. What is attractive is that such reasoning is based on the data from a single eye, and this could enable one more accurately to pin-point the abnormality especially in comparison to a test that simply compares the difference in rotation between the two eyes.

The variation with tropia as a function of gaze direction using the cover test, for example, can often localize the problem to four muscles; the four horizontal muscles for horizontal tropias or two pairs of oblique

---

and ψ_C (extorsion produced by convergence). Estimates of these parameters are set to the right of each condition. Dotted line represents tilt of the horopter without the extorsion produced by convergence. Numbers represent the angle of the horopter with respect to the line of sight. Note that it is larger in level and in down gaze.

and verticals for vertical deviations. Thus with a monocular test it may be possible to narrow the ambiguity by a factor of two. As yet the usefulness of this approach has still to be examined with a varied clinical population. It remains to be seen whether it will significantly add to our understanding of peripheral motor mechanisms associated with version or vergence, and as a separate issue, whether it will have peculiar advantages in the differential diagnosis of strabismus.

In this regard, it would seem that disorders involving vertical gaze would be most clarified through monocular kinematic analysis. In contrast to horizontal eye rotations, vertical eye rotations more obviously require the cooperation of several muscle groups, in particular, vertical rectus and oblique muscles. Figure 16.11 shows a cutaway view of the extraocular motor system with the axis of the vertical and oblique systems labeled. Each group acting independently will rotate the eye about an axis of rotation that is not in Listing's plane. The vertical rectus muscles will rotate the eye about an axis that makes an angle of 30° with Listing's

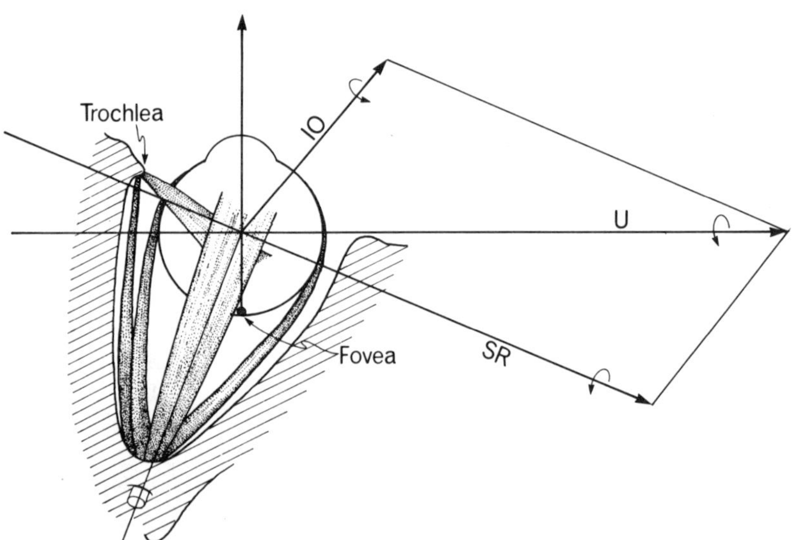

FIGURE 16.11. Partial schematic view of the extraocular muscle system showing that the action of the vertical and oblique muscles is far from being symmetrically arranged around the primary direction of regard. The action vector of the superior rectus muscle is denoted by $\hat{SR}$. Its direction represents the axis about which the eye would move if this muscle were activated alone and its length represents its relative torque for an infinitessimally small ocular elevation. $\hat{IO}$ represents the same for the inferior oblique muscle. Thus the vector sum of these torque vectors represents the resulting torque required for a vertical eye movement. This is labeled as the vector $\hat{U}$. Note that it must lie in Listing's plane so that the rotation is in accordance with Listing's law.

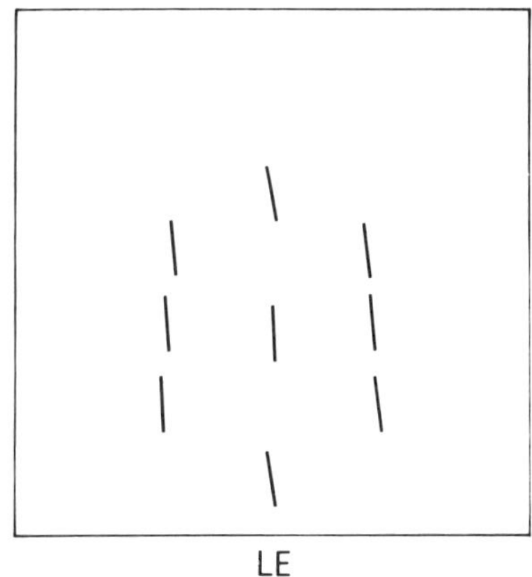

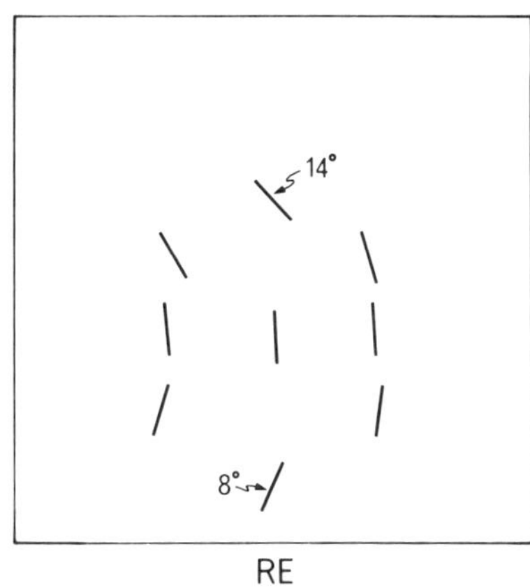

FIGURE 16.12. Normal and abnormal eye rotations. Torsional states of the eye (expressed as an angle that is three times the deviation from Listing's law) for different directions of gaze. Note that in the left eye there appears to be no marked deviation from Listing's law, whereas for the right eye there is a marked deviation. Right eye of this patient shows marked Brown's syndrome (see text).

plane and the oblique muscles will rotate the eye about an angle that deviates by about 51° in the opposite direction. From the geometry of the situation and knowledge of Listing's law one can deduce that each muscle group must contribute a certain rotational component (as depicted by the lengths of the rotational axis vectors) so that the resultant vector lies in Listing's plane. For example, in making a small elevation from the primary plane of regard it should require about twice as much torque from the superior rectus muscle as compared to the inferior oblique, otherwise vertical rotations from the primary direction of regard would not be in accordance with Listing's law. This can be most clearly seen by noting that only this ratio of torque vectors between the vertical and oblique systems can summate to give a resultant torque vector in Listing's plane (see Figure 16.11).

To give an example of how a monocular kinematic analysis might clarify a rather complex clinical case involving these muscles, following are data on one patient with Brown's syndrome. The patient has great difficulty in looking downward or upward. In particular, he had about 1 prism of right hypertropia in left, primary, and right gaze; 16 to 18 prisms of right hypertropia and 5 prisms of exotropia in up gaze; and 10 prisms of right hypotropia and 5 prisms of esotropia in down gaze. Independent evidence established that the cause of the motility disorder in the right eye was an adhesion of the superior oblique tendon in the trochlea, a side effect of nasal surgery.

Figure 16.12 shows a set of torsional measurements for different positions of gaze, obtained separately for each eye by measuring the orientation of a vertical afterimage at different locations on a tangent screen using a method described by Nakayama and Balliet (1977). The torsion is calculated as deviation from Listing's law and is represented by a line in each gaze position such that the torsional deviation is magnified by a factor of three. As expected, the normal left eye conforms to Listing's law. In contrast, there is a marked deviation for the right eye in the opposite direction in up gaze and down gaze.

To obtain a more intuitively satisfying spatial picture of this disordered set of torsional states, the orientation of the "equivalent" axis of rotation was calculated using an algorithm based on orthogonal matrices (Nakayama, 1974). This equivalent axis is the one about which the eye would rotate if it were to move directly to the measured fixation position with the measured amount of torsion. Thus it provides an analytical summary of how the eye can move from the primary position to any other measured rotational state by defining the axis of a shortest path rotation linking the two rotational states.

From the previous definition of Listing's law it should be clear that the axis vectors for all fixations of a normal eye should lie in Listing's

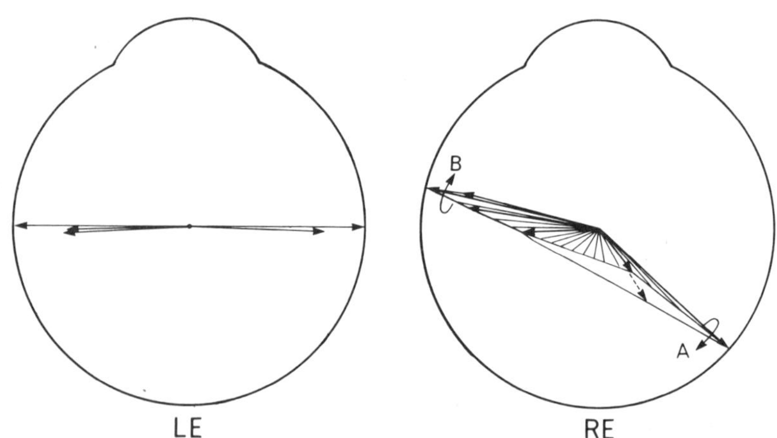

FIGURE 16.13. Top view of equivalent axes of rotation calculated for eye positions depicted in Figure 16.12. For each eye position away from the primary position (described in terms of three angles) it is possible to calculate an "equivalent axis of rotation" that will take the eye from the primary position to the measured fixation by the most direct rotation. If Listing's law is true, it is predicted that such axes will lie in Listing's plane, the frontoparallel plane passing through the center of rotation of the eye. It should be noted that such is the case for the normal left eye. For the right eye, however, such axes are clearly not in Listing's plane, deviating in the direction of the action of the vertical rectus system. As a comparison, note the similarity of the orientation of calculated axes of rotation and those of the vertical rectus system (as shown in Figure 16.11).

plane, that is the frontal parallel plane passing through the center of the eye. Figure 16.13 shows that this is definitely the case for the normal left eye and this congruence provides a nice confirmation of Listing's law.

For the right eye, however, the set of equivalent axis vectors is clearly outside Listing's plane. Note the orientation of arrows A and B, which describe the equivalent axes of rotation of pure up gaze and pure down gaze, respectively. They define an orientation that is very close to the axis of rotation of the vertical rectus muscles as shown in Figure 16.11.

Comparison of the measured equivalent axes and the known axes of the extraocular muscles, therefore, suggests an intelligible picture, one that does not immediately emerge from a consideration of the disordered torsional states as shown in Figure 16.12. The restriction at the trochlea prevents rotations in the axis of rotation of the oblique system, thereby leaving the rotation of the eye to be determined largely by the vertical rectus system. This can be seen by noting that the measured equivalent axes of rotation become tilted out of Listing's plane and are very close to those axes defined by the vertical rectus system.

The foregoing results offer a hypothesis that may be of some use in understanding complex muscle pathology. It suggests that if there is a restriction in any muscle system, in particular those movements requiring the cooperation of vertical and oblique muscles, the equivalent axis of rotation will shift out of Listing's plane toward the axis of rotation of the synergistic muscle system. Such a view if confirmed could conceivably aid in the diagnosis of vertical muscle disorders.

REFERENCES

Allen MJ. Dependence of cyclophoria on convergence, elevation and the system of axes. Am J Optom Arch Am Acad Optom 1954;31:297.

Alpern M. Kinematics of the eye. In: Davson H, ed. Vol. 3. New York: Academic Press, 1969.

Balliet R, Nakayama K. Training of voluntary torsion. Invest Ophthalmol Visual Sci 1978;17:303–14.

Cooper M, Pettigrew JD. A neurophysiological determination of the vertical horopter in the cat and owl. J Comp Neurol 1979;184:1–24.

Cynader M. Interocular alignment following visual deprivation in the cat. Invest Ophthalmol Visual Sci 1979;18:726–41.

De Groot J, Scott AB, Sindon A, Authier L. The human ocular anatomic position of rest; a quantitative study. In: Fells P, ed. Transactions of the Second Congress of the International Strabismological Association, Marseilles, May 1974. Marseilles: Diffusion Generale de Libraire, 1976:408–14.

Enright JT. Ocular translation and cyclotorsion due to changes in fixation distance. Vision Res 1980;20:595–601.

Helmholtz H. Treatise on physiological optics. Southall JPC, ed. New York: Dover, 1910.

Hering E. The theory of binocular vision (1868). Bridgeman B, Stark L, eds, trans. New York: Plenum Press, 1977.

Hering E. Der Raumsinn und die Bewegungen des Auges. In: Hermann L, ed. Handbook der Physiologie. Vol. 3. Leipzig: FCW Vogel, 1879:343–601.

Hubel DH, Wiesel TN. Receptive fields, binocular interaction and functional architecture in the cat's visual cortex. J Physiol 1962;160:106–54.

Keller EL, Robinson DA. Abducens unit behavior in the monkey during vergence eye movements. Vision Res 1971;12:369–82.

Ludvigh E. Control of ocular movements and visual interpretation of environment. Arch Ophthalmol 1952;48:442–48.

Melville Jones G, Davies P. Adaptation of cat vestibulo-ocular reflex to 200 days of optically reversed vision. Brain Res 1976;103:554–55.

Miller J, Anstis T, Templeton WB. Saccadic plasticity: parametric adaptive control by retinal feedback. J Exp Psychol Hum Percept Perform 1980;2:356–66.

Nakayama K. Photographic determination of the rotational state of the eye using matrices. Am J Optom Physiol Opt 1974;51:736–42.

Nakayama K. Coordination of extraocular muscles. In: Lennerstrand G, Bach-y-Rita P, eds. Basic Mechanisms in ocular motility and their clinical implications. New York: Pergamon Press, 1975:193–207.

Nakayama K. Geometrical and physiological aspects of depth perception. In: Benton S, ed. 3-D image processing. Society of Photo-Optical Instrumentation Engineers Proceedings, 1977:1–8.

Nakayama K. A new technique to determine the primary position of the eye using Listing's law. Am J Optom Physiol Opt 1978;55:331–36.

Nakayama K, Balliet R. Listing's law, eye position sense, and perception of the vertical. Vision Res 1977;17:453–57.

Nakayama K, Tyler CW, Appelman J. A new angle on the vertical horopter. Invest Ophthalmol 1977;(Suppl):82.

Optican LM, Robinson DA. Cerebellar dependent adaptive control of primate saccadic system. J Neurophysiol 1980;44:1058–76.

Robinson DA. The oculomotor control system: a review. Proc IEEE 1968; 56:1032–49.

Robinson DA. Oculomotor unit behavior in the monkey. J Neurophysiol 1970;33:393–404.

Robinson DA. A quantitative analysis of extraocular muscle coordination and squint. Invest Ophthalmol 1975;14:801.

Southall JPC. Introduction to physiological optics. New York: Dover 1961.

Westheimer G. Saccadic eye movements. In: Zikmund V, ed. The oculomotor system and brain function. Bratislava, Czechoslovakia: Publishing House of the Slovak Academy of Science, 1973.

Westheimer G, Blair S. Mapping the visual sensory onto the visual motor system. 1972;12:490–96.

17

Surgical Correction of Strabismus

Alan B. Scott

PURPOSE OF SURGERY

The first purpose of strabismus surgery is to aid function in one of the following categories:

1. Improvement of asthenopic or diplopic symptoms in phorias when prisms or exercises do not avail.
2. Restoration of binocular alignment in tropia acquired from injury or disease.
3. Development of binocular vision by providing alignment or by improving comitance.
4. Prevention of sensory abnormalities (suppression and anomalous correspondence) by surgery soon after onset of strabismus in children.
5. Correction of head turns and tilts in nystagmus and sometimes postively improving visual acuity.
6. Correction of head turns and tilts caused by extreme deviation of the fixing eye due to scar, paralysis, and so on.

The second general purpose is to improve cosmetic appearance. Both of

Supported in part by NIH grant EY-01186.

these purposes are addressed in the majority of strabismus operations; occasionally, purely functional or purely cosmetic considerations govern.

The surgical goals within this context are to achieve alignment in the primary position, to achieve or preserve concomitance (similar alignment in all gaze directions or distances of fixation), and to achieve stability of this result. These simple goals are often conflicting. For example, where binocular fusion is the primary goal, especially in childhood strabismus, a period of surgical overcorrection increases the rate of success, but at the cost of occasional instability requiring reoperation. Undercorrection leads to better stability of the strabismus, but with less frequent development of binocular fusion (Dunlap, 1971). Where binocular fusion is not expected to result (amblyopia or organic disease), most surgeons seek a position of slight esotropia as a more stable position than exact alignment in the primary position, thereby making secondary exotropia less common—stability at the cost of perfect alignment. Extensive weakening by recession of the lateral rectus in exotropia will cause a significant reduction in abduction amplitude, giving, however, stability at the cost of perfect concomitance. Some noncomitant strabismus patterns can be ameliorated by a simple operation on two muscles of one eye, but might require operation on five or six muscles for best correction of the noncomitance. In such a circumstance, simplicity and safety usually override perfection in the choice of procedure. Resolution of these conflicting goals constitutes one of the arts of strabismus surgery.

TIMING OF STRABISMUS SURGERY

Infantile Strabismus

When onset occurs before six months of age, most clinicians feel that there is some advantage in early surgery once the hereditary, general health, and neurologic aspects of the child are accurately assessed. Binocular cooperation is normally well underway by five or six months of age. Assuming normal eye structure and neurologic machinery, it follows that one should establish ocular alignment before this time; in any case as soon as possible. Irretrievable loss of cortical cell binocular responsiveness from experimental strabismus in young animals and the poor binocular fusional results of congenital esotropia corrected at late ages in humans are strong supports for early surgery.

Where inherent defects in the binocular machinery probably exist to limit prospects for binocular function (albinism or cerebral palsy or hereditary esotropia), surgical alignment can best be done later. For example, recently a mother, grandmother, and great grandmother, all with surgically straightened eyes but none with binocular fusion, came to the office with the latest generation, a four-month-old esotropic girl; not a stimulus to urgent operation for function.

Acquired Childhood Strabismus

A child up to age six years who had binocular fusion in infancy but later develops a manifest strabismus from any cause has an important backlog of fusion. It is truly urgent to correct this refractive error, any amblyopia, any major incomitance that had generated the strabismus, and to correct surgically any ocular misalignment that remains, if prisms are unable to accomplish this. Individuals of this kind have a high potential for restoration of normal or near normal binocular vision, which is often lost from six months or a year of conservative watching and waiting.

Acquired Adult Strabismus

Strabismus acquired in adulthood usually results from disease, injury, or breakdown of childhood strabismus. Following a trial of prisms and/or vergence amplitude training, cosmetic problems and symptomatic cases with potential for fusion should be operated on. In particular, paralysis of the sixth nerve without recovery after six months should be corrected before medial rectus contracture occurs to limit the ultimate motility result.

PHYSIOLOGY OF STRABISMUS SURGERY

The eye muscle system is complicated all out of proportion to the importance of strabismus as a health problem. At present, a long apprenticeship and experience with clinical cases is required to develop an understanding of when, how much, and what muscles to operate on. Empirical practice is being applied with the help of data systems, (Scott, 1975) and the physiological basis of strabismus surgery is now becoming known.

Mechanical Relationships

If eye muscles were stiff like ropes or cables, a 5-mm shortening of one muscle and a 5-mm lengthening of its antagonist would correct about 25° of strabismus. But such surgery actually provides about 10° of correction for an average operation in the usual strabismus range of 20 to 30 prism diopters. Furthermore, less effect is achieved from operating on paralyzed or weak muscles; greater effect is achieved from operating on stiff restrictive scars and on tight muscles. Understanding of the innervations, forces, and muscle actions involved with each such case is needed. Measurement of these force parameters and calculation of surgery is worthwhile and helpful in difficult cases (Collins et al., 1981).

Possible Training of Innervation

Strabismus surgery tightens or loosens muscles or moves the insertion to a new position, creating a different muscle plane. Do muscles adjust innervation to the task of the new position, learning to do something different? In adult humans and in monkeys, no evidence for innervation change was found; any apparent change in muscle effect is mechanical (Blodi and Van Allen, 1962; Metz and Scott, 1970).

About half of strabismus cases are concomitant, simple misalignments, with the eyes maintaining about the same angle of strabismus regardless of gaze direction or distance of fixation. The remainder are noncomitant with variation of strabismus angle depending on distance of fixation or gaze position. It is attractive to suppose that some innervational adaptability in infancy allows correction for the known variability of eye muscle anatomy in humans, but such noncomitant cases are evidence against adaptability.

Recession

If the insertion of a medial rectus muscle is detached and placed 5 mm posterior to the original, the tension on this muscle is reduced. In effect, the curve that describes the tension of the muscle in any horizontal gaze position has been displaced (Figure 17.1). The effect is greatest in the position of greatest action of the muscle, adduction; next is abduction, where the restriction effect of the medial rectus is significant; the least effect is in the primary position, where tensions are lowest. Surgeons are aware that in esotropia, recession of a restricting medial rectus muscle may have the greatest effect in the opposite (abduction) field of action, even more than into the field of action.

Resection

Resection operations shorten. The curve in Figure 17.1 is displaced upward along the length-tension lines. For an eye in esotropia, the lateral rectus muscle is usually thinner than the medial rectus muscle, which

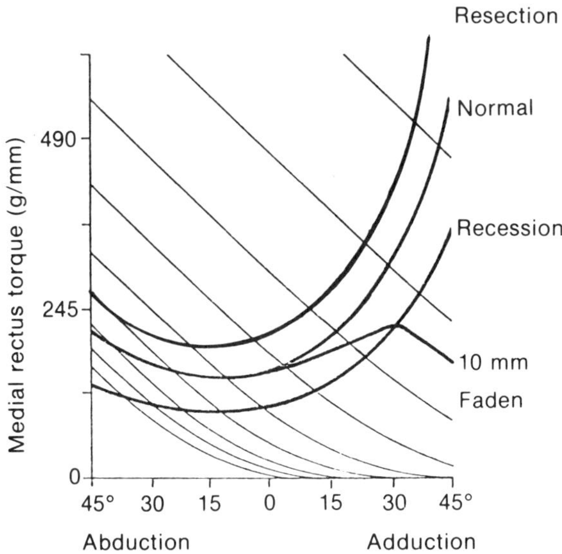

FIGURE 17.1. **Abscissa**, eye position. **Ordinate**, amount of torque (effective rotating force) on globe. Operations shift the muscle tension curve.

is stiffer and stronger. Thus it is no surprise that a 5-mm resection creates less angular change than a 5-mm recession. Large resections are often needed and actually remove muscle tissue. This increases muscle stiffness and reduces amplitude of eye movement.

Effect of the Antagonist

The agonist and antagonist together constitute a loop extending from the bony origin out to the eye (which acts as a pulley) and back again to the origin. Usually, operations are based on the assumption that the antagonist in this loop is intact and will normally take up the slack. If the antagonist lateral rectus is paralyzed, however, recession of the medial rectus to correct the estropia will have little effectiveness. If the antagonist is extra stiff and strong (as in endocrine exophthalmos), the effect of recession will be enhanced. Thus the status of the antagonist is important, and a concept of balancing of forces is necessary. Figures 17.2, 17.3, and 17.4 show some calculated muscle forces in normal, comitant strabismus and in lateral rectus paralysis (Garcia et al., 1976).

Arc of Contact

Muscle insertions are sometimes recessed to a position posterior to the point of tangency. Beisner (1941) has shown that change in alignment

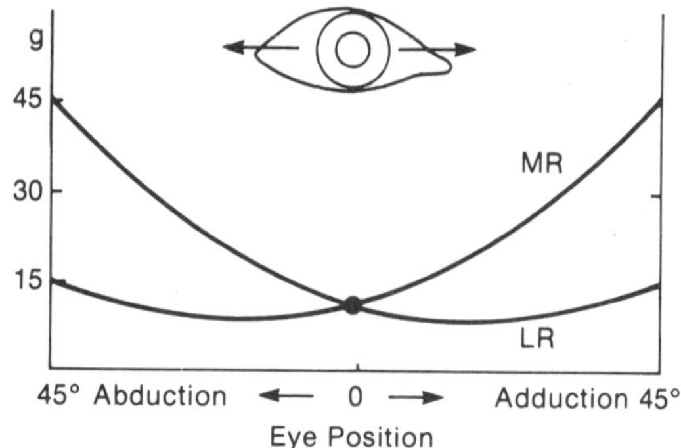

FIGURE 17.2. Tension of medial rectus (**MR**) is slightly higher than that of lateral rectus (**LR**). Balance for primary position is achieved by shift of innervation. **Abd**, abduction; **Add**, adduction. Adapted from Garcia H, Glanczspiegel R, Melek N, Ciancia AO. Forces in the oculomotor system. Archivos De Oftalmologia De Buenos Aires, 1976.

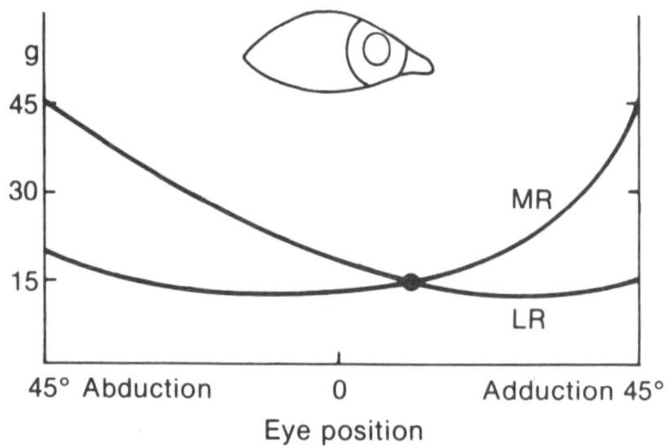

FIGURE 17.3. In concomitant esotropia, tension curves are displaced horizontally. **MR**, medial rectus; **LR**, lateral rectus; **Abd**, abduction; **Add**, adduction. Adapted from Garcia H, Glanczspiegel R, Melek N, Ciancia AO. Forces in the oculomotor system. Archivos De Oftalmologia De Buenos Aires, 1976.

near the primary position from such recessions is due to length-tension changes (Figure 17.5). There is progressive loss of effective lever arm with rotation after such large recession. Such an effect can be deliberately created by suturing the muscle to the globe without recession (the Faden operation of Cuppers (1976). This weakens rotation into the field of action, but not in the primary position (Figure 17.6), and is useful to limit eye rotation in nystagmus and in overactive muscles.

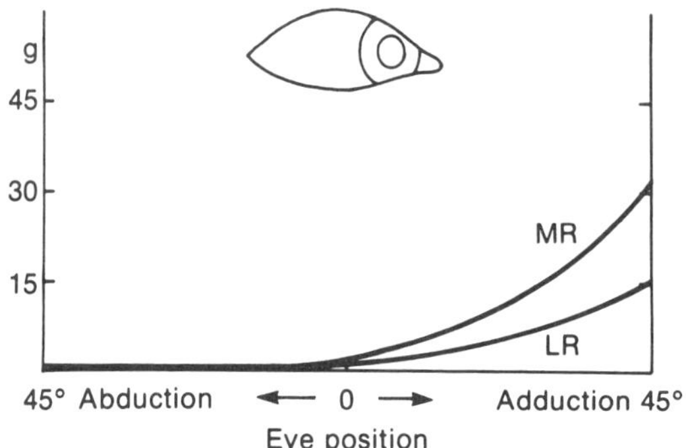

FIGURE 17.4. In lateral rectus (**LR**) paralysis, tension of both muscles is reduced in all gaze positions because lateral rectus does not keep medial rectus (**MR**) stretched. **Abd**, abduction, **Add**, adduction. Adapted from Garcia H, Glanczspiegel R, Melek N, Ciancia AO. Forces in the oculomotor system. Archivos De Oftalmologia De Buenos Aires, 1976.

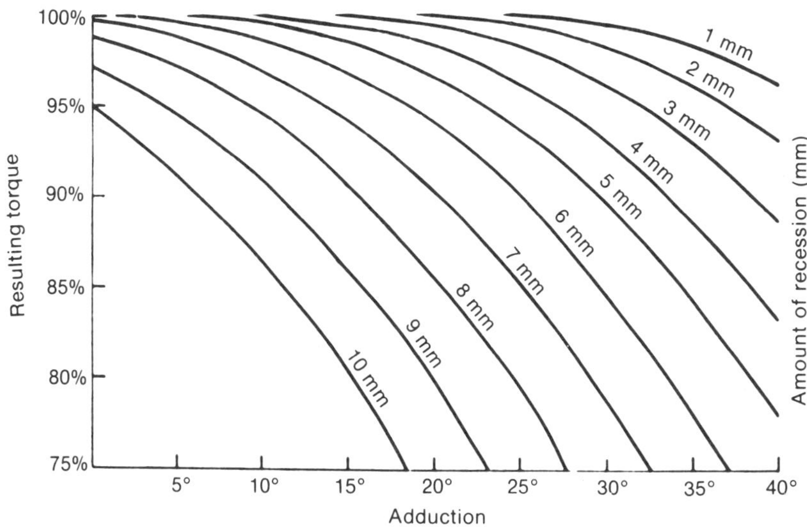

FIGURE 17.5. Curves show what happens when medial rectus muscle insertion is 1, 2, to 10 mm posterior to usual insertion. For example, a 7-mm recession puts muscle at tangency point; reduction of torque then occurs with adduction due to loss of level arm. Even so, the eye can rotate 30° before torque is reduced to 80% of normal. Adapted from Beisner DH. Reduction of ocular torque by medical rectus recession. Archives of Ophthalmology, 85:13–17. Copyright 1977, American Medical Association. Reprinted by permission of the publisher.

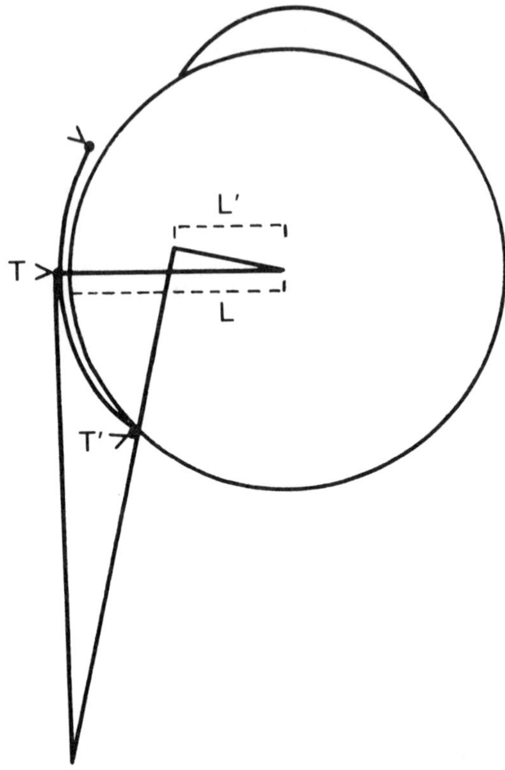

FIGURE 17.6. If muscle is sutured at **T**, then lever arm is **L**. Rotation of **T** to **T'** occurs with adduction, reducing effect of lever arm to **L'**.

Transposition Operations

If both the medial and the lateral rectus muscle insertions are moved to the area of the superior rectus insertion they will have a vertical torque also, instead of a purely horizontal one. This operation corrects from 12° to 15° of vertical strabismus, shifting 5 to 6 grams of horizontal force from each muscle to create supraduction. This is a small fraction of the 50-gram force created by the agonist muscle during lateral gaze; therefore the operation creates very little decrease in the amplitude of horizontal gaze movement. The two muscles are at normal length or close to it; thus horizontal alignment is unchanged, and the unchanged reciprocal innervation for horizontal gaze works well. These muscle insertions can also be transposed inferiorly; recession or resection can be done at the same time to correct horizontal strabismus.

When vertical rectus muscle insertions are transposed in a horizontal direction a lesser angular correction is usually seen. This is a consequence of the vertical muscles being smaller in cross-sectional area.

Bilateral Elevation or Depression of Muscle Insertions

If both lateral rectus muscle insertions were surgically moved upward, during up gaze they would be moved posteriorly and the tension in the muscle would be slacked off, reducing abduction. (Figure 17.7) This would be good for correcting the common V-pattern strabismus that has relative exotropia in up gaze. Downward surgical movement of lateral rectus insertions improves an A pattern (reversed effects for medial recti, of course).

Elevation of Medial Rectus and Depression of Lateral Rectus Insertion

There is no net effect on horizontal or vertical alignment in the primary position because one muscle is elevated as much as the other is depressed. Also, since muscle origins are far posterior, moving insertions does not

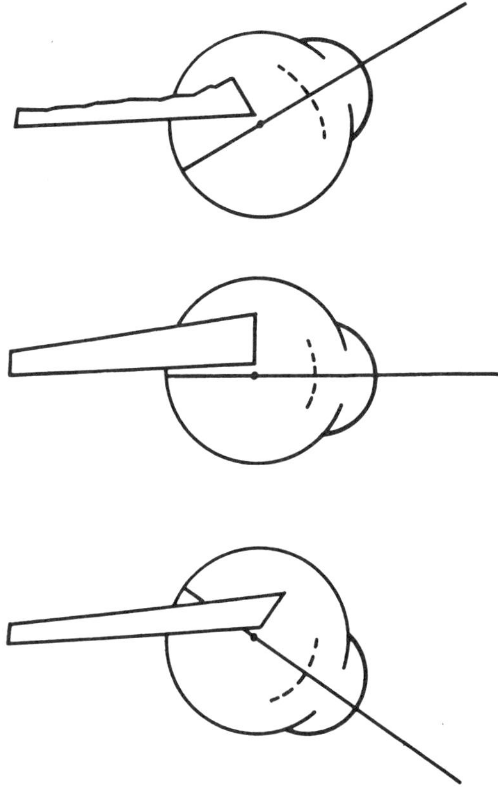

FIGURE 17.7. Medial rectus insertion recessed and elevated. Supraduction (at top) reduces length about 3 mm, reducing tension from 12 g to 6 g; infraduction (at bottom) tightens muscle about 3 mm, increasing tension from 12 g to 18 g.

create much change in the angle the muscle makes with the visual axis; a minimal torsional effect results. With upward gaze the medial rectus muscle tension will be diminished and the eye will thus tend to abduct; the lateral rectus in upward gaze will be tightened, further increasing abduction (Figure 17.8). With downward gaze the reverse occurs. This maneuver is helpful where the eyes tend to be more esotropic in upward gaze or more exotropic in downward gaze (the A pattern). The reverse, depression of the medial rectus and elevation of the lateral rectus insertion, is effective where the esotropia tends to increase in down gaze and exotropia tends to increase in up gaze (the V pattern).

Oblique Muscle Transpositions

It is possible to alter the insertion position of oblique muscle points to tighten or loosen them or to move them anteriorly or posteriorly in the orbit. Figure 17.9 and Table 17.1 show the effect of a number of placements of the superior oblique muscle insertions. In general, the more anterior it is, the less vertical infraduction effect and the less abduction effect; indeed, as one moves further forward this muscle becomes an adductor and an elevator. A similar analysis fits the inferior oblique, and Elliott and Nankin (1981) have shown in a clinical series that one can progressively weaken elevation in abduction as well as adduction by moving the inferior oblique insertion progressively anteriorly. With modern computers a rational mechanical analysis of these and many other maneuvers previously involving laborious calculation is now possible (France and Burbank, 1979). By careful accumulation of clinical data, helped by accurate modeling, clinical prediction is improving.

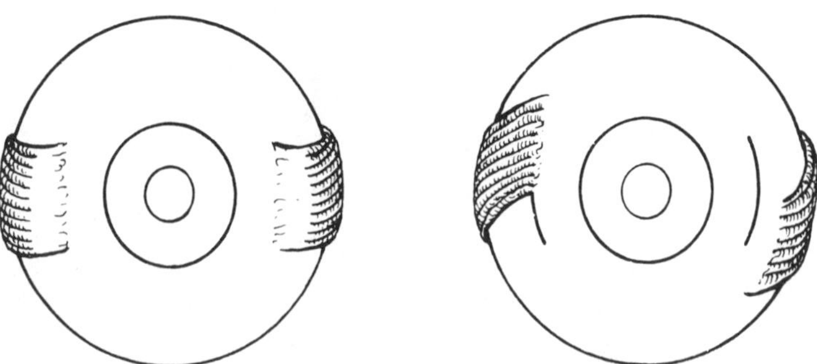

FIGURE 17.8. **Left**, Unoperated horizontal rectus muscles, right eye. **Right**, Elevation of left medial rectus insertion and depression (and recession) of lateral rectus insertion for A pattern. Adapted from Metz H, Schwartz L. The treatment of A and V patterns by monocular surgery. Archives of Ophthalmology, 55:252. Copyright 1977, American Medical Association. Reprinted by permission of the publisher.

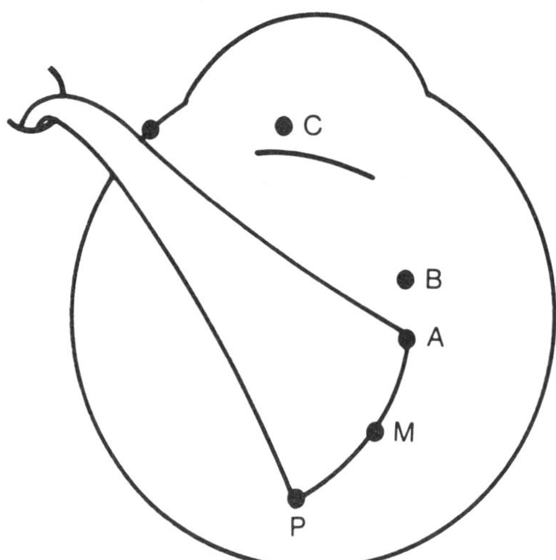

FIGURE 17.9. Insertion points are posterior (**P**), middle (**M**), and anterior (**A**) ends of normal insertion, a point 4 mm posterior to lateral end of superior rectus (**B**), and a point 2 mm anterior to medial end of superior rectus (**C**).

Special Techniques

The reintroduction and improvement of adjusting techniques made possible by new suture materials (Jampolsky, 1979) has increased the accuracy of surgery and reduced the need for reoperations by allowing fine-tuning of the muscle positions on the eye in the immediate postoperative period.

Stay-sutures (Callahan, 1961) to hold the eye in position for healing are akin to an orthopedic cast. These are crucial to stable results in some cases.

TABLE 17.1. Points of Insertion of Oblique Muscle and Degree of Effect

	*Effect (%) in primary position**		
Insertion†	*Horizontal*	*Vertical*	*Torsional*
Posterior (P)	23	47	30
Middle (M)	2	32	66
Anterior (A)	−4	11	86
Posterior to lateral end of superior rectus (B)	−3	12	85
Anterior to lateral end of superior rectus (C)	−62	−13	25

* Plus values, abduction, infraduction, intorsion; negative values, adduction, supraduction, extorsion. Effect is percent of rotation force around the three rotational axes.

† Points of insertion correspond to those in Figure 17.9.

COMPLICATIONS

The risks of strabismus surgery are now reduced by medical knowledge and technological improvement to a level where they are fully acceptable when significant cosmetic or functional improvement can be expected. About 70% to 80% reaches its goal in one operation (Cooper and Leyman, 1976; Helveston et al., 1978) and physical discomfort to the patient is usually modest. Psychological trauma to children should be virtually nonexistent when the experience is carried out in a concerned environment.

Nevertheless, general anesthesia and eye surgery are serious. An anesthetic accident still occurs once in several thousand cases despite skilled anesthesiologists, recovery room personnel, and monitoring devices. The incidence of visual loss from hemorrhage, infection, or surgical injury is not reported; 8 or 10 such cases in the 60,000 operations done annually in the United States is a reasonable estimate.

ALTERNATIVES

One can always do nothing. Mayan Indians thought esotropia a mark of beauty, and many people adapt to their appearance without a thought for the need of cosmetic repair. Similarly, some individuals with acquired strabismus become adapted to the presence of diplopia so that it no longer bothers them. In children, where functional binocular vision may be gained, thus stabilizing the deviation and preventing amblyopia, and where delay may reduce the chance of developing binocular vision, it is difficult to justify withholding treatment to align the eyes. In all other cases strabismus surgery is elective.

Glasses, contact lenses, and miotic eye drops are the first choice in accommodative esotropias. Minus lenses (−2.00, −3.00) in mild intermittent exotropia are useful as a measure to increase convergence.

Exercises to increase vergence amplitude are helpful when binocular vision already exists. Antisuppression exercises are commonly disappointing and if fusion is not attained, increase the incidence of late diplopia (Boyd et al., 1966).

Prisms reduce the fusional vergence need and may gain or regain fusion. With Fresnel prisms much larger strabismus angles can be so handled than with regular prisms.

For cosmetic purposes in small-angle esotropias, three or four prism diopters, base-out over the fixing eye and base-in over the esotropic eye can improve appearance. Injections of Oculinum, a long-acting myoneural-blocking agent derived from botulinum toxin into the overacting extraocular muscle to weaken it for two to four weeks is followed by permanent stretching of the injected muscle and shortening of the antagonist intact muscle with permanent alignment changes. While still experimental (120 cases), this technique has been spectacularly successful, with follow-up over three years and with no systemic complications. Such chemical recession is already the author's treatment of choice in small comitant deviations, in cases where extensive surgery has created much scar tissue without restriction, and in special situations in which health of the eye itself might be jeopardized by strabismus surgery. The injected eye is relatively immobile during a portion of the treatment. This results in esotropia with a gaze to one side and exotropia with a gaze to the other side. This visual experience seems to erase the suppression and anomalous retinal correspondence (ARC) associated with the deviation, with fusion resulting in several unexpected cases.

REFERENCES

Beisner DH. Reduction of ocular torque by medial rectus recession. Arch Ophthalmol 1971;85:13–17.

Blodi FC, Van Allen MW. Electromyography in intermittent exotropia; recordings before, during, and after corrective operation. Doc Ophthalmol 1962;16:21.

Boyd TAS, Ridgway CR, Budd GE. Childhood strabismus as a cause of persistent diplopia in adolescents and adults. Can J Ophthalmol 1966;1:199–205.

Callahan A. The arrangement of the conjunctiva in surgery for oculomotor paralysis and strabismus. Arch Ophthalmol 1961;66:241.

Collins CC, Carlson MR, Scott AB, Jampolsky A. Extraocular muscle forces in normal human subjects. Invest Ophthalmol 1981.

Cooper EL, Leyman IA. The management of intermittent exotropia. In: Moore S, Mein J, Stockbridge L, Orthoptics, past, present, future. New York: Stratton, 1976:563.

Cuppers C. The so-called Faden operation. In: Fells P, ed. Second Congress of the International Strabismological Association. Marseilles: Diffusion Gen. de Librairie 1976:394.

Dunlap EA. Overcorrection in horizontal strabismus surgery. Symposium on Strabismus, Transactions of the New Orleans Academy of Ophthalmology, 1971.

Elliott RL, Nankin SJ. Anterior transposition of the inferior oblique. J Pediatr Ophthalmol 1981;8(3):35–38.

France TD, Burbank DP. Clinical applications of a computer-assisted eye model. Ophthalmology 1979;86:1407–12.

Garcia H, Glanczspiegel R, Melek N, Ciancia AO. Forces in the oculomotor system. Arch Ophthalmol B. Aires, 1976;51:299.

Helveston EM, Patterson JH, Ellis FD, Weber JC. Enbloc recession of the medial recti for concomitant esotropia. Symposium on Strabismus, Transactions of the New Orleans Academy of Ophthalmology, 1978.

Jampolsky A. Current techniques of adjustable strabismus surgery. Am J Ophthalmol 1979;88:406–18.

Martin FJ et al., Factors influencing the surgical results of divergent strabismus.

In: Mein J, Moore S, eds. Orthoptics, research and practice. Transactions of the Fourth International Orthoptic Congress. London: Kimpton, 1981:182.

Metz H, Scott AB. Innervational plasticity of the oculomotor system. Arch Ophthalmol 1970;84:86–91.

Romano PE. Pediatric ophthalmic mythology. Postgrad Med 1975;58:146–50.

Scott AB. Botulinum toxin injection into extraocular muscles as an alternative to strabismus surgery. Ophthalmology 1980;87:1044–49.

Scott AB. Planning inferior oblique muscle surgery. In: Reinecke R, ed. Strabismus. Proceedings of the Third Meeting of the International Strabismological Association. May 10–12, 1978, Kyoto, Japan. New York: Grune and Stratton, pp 347–54.

Scott AB, Mash AJ, Jampolsky A. Quantitative guide-lines for exotropia surgery. Ophthal 1975;14:428–36.

Shea SF, Fox R, Aslin RN, Dumais ST. Stereopsis in human infants. Invest Ophthal & Vis Sci 1980;19:1400–4.

Taylor DM. Is congenital esotropia functionally curable? Trans Am Ophthalmol Soc 1972;70:529–76.

18

Strabismus Diagnosis and Prognosis

Nathan Flax

CLASSIFICATION

Under normal circumstances, vergence movements maintain eye position so that there is foveal bifixation, with the visual axis deviating from the point of regard within the limits of fixation disparity—30 minutes of arc or less. This rather precise positioning in individuals with normal binocular vision is mediated by a number of different vergence control mechanisms that have been classified by Maddox (1893) as tonic, accommodative, fusional, and proximal (Morgan, 1980). The net result of all the stimuli to vergence produces the precise motor response necessary to achieve bifoveal fixation, facilitating normal sensory integration of the two eyes.

In a substantial segment of the population there is failure to achieve or sustain such bifoveal alignment, resulting in the condition of strabismus (squint, tropia, or heterotropia). The incidence is most frequently reported as 2% to 3% of the population (Flom, 1963; Hugonnier and Hugonnier, 1969) but much higher figures are also given. The prevalence of strabismus is estimated in European studies at approximately 5.5% or 6% among six-year-olds (Graham, 1974). The National Center for Health Statistics of the United States Department of Health, Education, and Welfare gives an incidence of 6.7% among children ages 6 to 17 (Roberts, 1972, 1975).

At first glance, clinical management of strabismus would seem to be simple and straightforward. If the eyes are not properly aligned, isolate the factor responsible and select an appropriate approach to relieve the condition. Unfortunately, this is far easier said than done. Few aspects of eye care are as complex and difficult as is the treatment of strabismus. Although the condition has been identified from earliest times (Revell, 1971), its etiology is often not known and controversy surrounds its treatment.

Strabismus is classified in a number of different ways. The various schemata are often based on different models that overlap and occasionally contradict one another. Nonetheless, all are useful in that they shed some light on the condition, contributing to the diagnosis and, more important, point the way to appropriate management. Several different classification schemata are discussed, with comments on their utility in establishing a diagnosis. This chapter is not directed toward detailed procedures for all available clinical techniques but rather deals selectively with a few that are illustrative and useful for understanding the problems of diagnosis and management of the strabismic patient. Numerous texts give specific procedures (Griffin, 1976; Hugonnier and Hugonnier, 1969; Burian and von Noorden, 1980).

Depending on facial configuration, shape of the orbital fissure, width of the nose, separation of the eyes, angle kappa (the angle between the line of sight and the perpendicular to the cornea at the center of the pupil), and other anatomic characteristics, two patients with identical angles of deviation may appear to have very different conditions. Wide noses with prominent epicanthal folds tend to increase the appearance of esotropia or mask exotropia. Most pseudostrabismus is due to the very prominent epicanthal folds of infancy, which create the impression of turn by reducing the amount of visible nasal sclera, particularly on lateral gaze when the iris of one eye may be partially obscured. High positive-angle kappas can give rise to the appearance of exotropia in patients who are actually not strabismic. This author has encountered the situation where successful therapy for childhood esotropia has resulted in the need to reassure the parents who were then suspicious of a divergent strabismus. A high-angle kappa had initially minimized the appearance of the convergent strabismus. After successful treatment achieved bifoveal fixation, there was the illusion of a small exotropia. While appearance does not bear any relationship to functional outcome, it is perhaps the most important consideration in the initiation of treatment.

The most frequently used classifications for strabismus are based on motor alignment of the eyes. Distinction is made between unilateral strabismus, in which one eye continually deviates, and alternating strabismus. The prognosis for ultimate functional cure is approximately the same in both cases (Flom, 1963), but other characteristics of the condition do relate to this distinction. The likelihood of amblyopia is minimal in alternators. Furthermore, if there is alternate fixation at distance there is strong likelihood of approximately equal refractive states in the two eyes. If the alternation occurs as a function of fixation distance, with one eye being used at distance and the other at near, the probability of anisometropia is high.

Direction of deviation is the next most obvious classification. Esotropes, exotropes, and hypertropes show different characteristics with decidedly different prognosis. As a group, exotropes are easier to cure than esotropes but generalizations are very difficult because of the influences of other factors. A rather high percentage of exotropes are intermittent and in this group, nonsurgical functional cure rates are exceedingly high (Flax and Duckman, 1978). Esotropes tend to be constant and more difficult to treat functionally, particularly when anomalous retinal correspondence (ARC) is present (Flom, 1963). Hypertropia may involve a torsional component as well as elevation of an eye. In some instances, despite a small magnitude of deviation, functional results are difficult. Some vertical deviations can be compensated quite well with prism and show excellent results.

The angle of deviation is an important consideration, although not directly related to prognosis. There can be exceedingly high-angle esotropia with a large accommodative component, which can be well managed with convex lenses. Smaller angles of turn may be far more complex and resistant to treatment. Excellent results are achieved on intermittent exotropia of as much as 35 prism diopters, while poorer results sometimes occur in other patients who show anomalous retinal correspondence and constant esotropia of much smaller magnitude. Deviations of more than 35^{Δ} or less than 5^{Δ} tend to have a poorer functional prognosis (Flom, 1963).

An angle of turn that is constant in all directions of gaze is described as concomitant or comitant; an angle that varies as a function of the patient's direction of gaze is said to demonstrate lack of comitance or incomitance. Often incomitance is related to paralysis or paresis of one or more of the extraocular muscles, although anatomic abnormalities of the origin or insertion of a muscle, or of the orbital contents might also result in incomitance. In cases of paresis (or of hyperaction) of the extraocular muscles, the deficiency can be of the muscle itself or the innervation to the muscles. The classification of deviation by status of comitance does not give full insight into the condition. In some cases, such as a simple lateral rectus palsy, a patient may be left with perfectly intact binocular function in all fields of view except when the eyes move into the direction of action of the paralyzed muscle. The patient will be straight with bifoveal fixation on direct gaze but will demonstrate an increasing degree of esotropia when looking to the affected side. This condition may be a minimal handicap, since it is generally easy to compensate by turning the head or by suppressing vision of one eye on lateral gaze. Another patient with a similar involvement might not make a successful adaptation and consequently be bothered by intermittent diplopia. This patient may also suffer from asthenopia due to degradation of binocular function in the unaffected directions of gaze. Incomitance can take many forms and be of different degrees, ranging from inconsequential limitations of gaze on extreme version to significant limitation in or near primary gaze. Even minor muscle limitations can be disabling if they interfere with normal depression and convergence necessary for reading.

Still another diagnostic classification is the variability of turn angle. It is important to know if the angle of turn changes from one moment to the next and the conditions that precipitate change. It is not unusual for parents to report that a child's eyes appear straighter at the beginning of the day and more turned toward the end of the day or when the youngster is fatigued, ill, or emotionally upset. In other instances there is a variability in angle that does not relate to any specific time of day, state of fatigue, or particular task demand. A turn angle that varies as a function of detail of target or distance of fixation is suspicious of an accommodative component. Careful case history and repeated examination may be necessary to understand properly the fluctuations. One common circumstance that introduces variability is the distance of the fixation target. This change in motor status may be related to refractive considerations. This will be discussed later.

Strabismus can also be classified based on the frequency of deviation. A turn may be constant or intermittent. If intermittent, its occurrence may vary from occasional to frequent. It is generally not difficult to differentiate an intermittent from a constant strabismus at time of examination unless there is variability related to fatigue or time of day. Under such circumstance the patient might show a constant strabismus late in the day and an intermittent turn if examined earlier. Case history data are useful and important in making this distinction.

From a therapeutic point of view, frequency of turn is an exceedingly important consideration. It would seem to be unwise, for instance, to choose surgical interference, with its attendant risks, for a strabismic condition that appears only infrequently. Occasional turns have excellent functional prognosis with appropriate orthoptic therapy (Flom, 1963). The presence of any degree of intermittency improves the prognosis greatly as it implies some basis for normal function at least part of the time and a high probability of a functional neurosensory system. Careful and provocative testing is required to distinguish properly between a constant turn of variable angle and a true intermittent strabismus. Often, parental reports in this regard are misleading. It is possible for a child to be constantly strabismic, yet have an angle that varies from cosmetically acceptable to noticeable. This is often construed by parents as a shift from straight to turn. The prognostic implications are quite different when there is, in fact, bifoveal fixation at least part of the time as contrasted to a constant strabismus with an angle that reduces to cosmetically acceptable limits on occasion. In the latter case, intactness of neurosensory function cannot be assumed. When this author encounters such a situation and suspects that the parental report of straight eyes has actually been a response to a reduction in angle of deviation, the parents are brought into the examination routine and asked to assess eye position by their criteria so that the history can be properly interpreted.

Age of onset of strabismus is another important classification. It is highly desirable to ascertain whether it is congenital or acquired. Unfortunately, this is not always easily determined. It is generally accepted that congenital strabismus has a far more dismal prognosis insofar as functional binocularity is concerned, and it can also have a profound influence on amblyopia. Animal experiments point to critical periods very early in life that are vital to establishment and maintenance of the underlying neurology to permit clear central acuity. Animals deprived of form vision during the critical stages of neurologic development suffer irreparable loss of acuity together with demonstrable neural changes. Deprivation before and after a critical period produces functional deficits that are largely reversible with appropriate stimulation (Blakemore, 1974; Van Sluyters, 1978). Just exactly how to apply this research in humans is not fully clear. By consensus rather than experimental evidence it is usually assumed that humans have a somewhat longer and probably less critical "critical period" than do the animals studied. Most feel that acuity development in children is highly susceptible to deprivation up to the age of three or three and one half years. This has led to reconsideration of the role of early correction of refractive error (particularly astigmatism and anisometropia) in the interest of providing clear imagery during the sensitive period (Ikeda and Wright, 1975; Mitchell et al., 1973). Some difficulties in clinical management are not fully resolved. It would seem desirable fully to correct ametropia in very young children, however, refraction is not stable in infancy. Rapid changes in astigmatism, for instance, are normal in the first year or so of life (Atkinson et al., 1980; Mohindra et al., 1978).

Clinical decisions are not easy to make. Where there is high astigmia or high anisometropia, the need to provide clear focus on the retina almost seems to demand refractive correction. The question must be raised about the impact of high anisometropic correction on fusion due to problems of aniseikonia (image size) that may be created, and the introduction of variable prismatic stimulation to vergence. Is there the possibility that therapy to minimize the probability of amblyopia may have an adverse effect on fusion? The same question may be raised regarding the use of occlusion therapy in early strabismus. Not only does occluding an eye in a very young infant carry the risk of development of occlusion amblyopia in a previously sound eye (Burian, 1966; Ikeda and Wright, 1975; Thomas et al., 1979), the deprivation associated with early occlusion may in fact reduce the potential for later fusion. In animal experiments, reduction of the number of binocularly driven cortical cells as a function of occlusion during critical periods is well established (Blakemore, 1976; Hubel and Wiesel, 1965). Just how this relates to sensory fusion or motor control of the eyes in humans is speculative, but at very least it offers reason to be more cautious in the use of occlusion in infants. In general, it is accepted that congenital strabismics do not show a very hopeful prognosis for normal binocular function. Acquired strabismus of late onset generally has a good binocular function prognosis. Just where the transition line is remains to be established.

There are other important aspects of onset. Long-standing strabismus generally presents a different clinical picture than that of more recent onset. If its basis is a paretic ocular muscle, the specific offending muscle becomes far more difficult to detect with the passage of time. The motor deficiency tends to spread into other areas of gaze and becomes generalized (Burian and von Noorden, 1980). This is both good and bad. It complicates specific motor diagnosis but it may offer a more functionally useful motor system because a deviation that is consistent in all fields of gaze is easier to compensate by head-turning or use of a prism correction, and therefore may enhance the prognosis. Sensory concomitants of strabismus (which will be dealt with in some detail later in this chapter) such as diplopia, suppression, or anomalous retinal correspondence may change with the passage of time so that the functional status of a long-time strabismus may be quite different from one of recent onset. Sudden onset is highly suspicious of pathology, and must be investigated.

Another classification in diagnosis has to do with etiology. There are several potential causes of strabismus ranging from anatomic or mechanical interferences with eye movement because of congenital malformation or trauma, to functional or innervational abnormalities. It is desirable to ascertain etiology, although data in this regard are minimal and generally of questionable reliability. All too often investigation of the problem is done long after initial onset, making it difficult to establish clearly both time of onset and specific etiology.

The refractive state of the patient frequently relates to strabismus and becomes an important part of diagnosis. There are two different ways in which it relates to strabismus. One has to do with the direct influence of accommodative convergence on the alignment of the eyes. The other concerns influence of ametropia, particularly anisometropia, on sensory fusion processes. A frequent cause is uncorrected hyperopia, particularly in the presence of a high AC/A ratio. The accommodative effort necessary to compensate for the hyperopia induces so great an accommodative convergence response that the fusional vergence capability of the patient is overwhelmed, resulting in a loss of alignment. Typically, such strabismus develops fairly early in life, although later onset is possible. As a rule, accommodative esotropia is first noted at near, where the influence of accommodative convergence is greatest. In higher amounts of hyperopia (or in lower amounts with a high AC/A ratio) the squint may be present at all fixation distances. An important part of diagnostic evaluation involves ascertaining the influence of accommodation on the turn angle. The presence of a significant AC/A linkage in any strabismus, convergent or divergent, has a profound influence on therapeutic strategy and eventual outcome. A high ratio permits excellent leverage with use of lenses and should suggest caution when surgery is contemplated; the same high AC/A that may have precipitated a strabismus can be harnessed through lenses to assist in diverging the eyes. Failure to allow properly for an accommodative component can lead to postsurgical disaster. This writer has encountered patients with high AC/A ratios who were operated "successfully," only to have difficulty when it became necessary at a later date to correct existing hyperopia to alleviate asthenopia. Application of corrective lenses induced exotropia in a patient who had been esotropic before the surgery. Asthenopia and/or recurrence of the turn are generally avoidable consequences if the AC/A influence is appropriately planned for.

Refraction has an indirect influence on strabismus by virtue of its influence on the sensory processes of binocular vision. High astigmatism can cause amblyopia that degrades fusion. In an individual with high heterophoria this can become a factor in the manifestation of squint. Perhaps the most serious refractive interference to sensory fusion is that caused by anisometropia. Under normal circumstances it is assumed that the accommodative levels of the two eyes are the same and determined by the fixing eye. In uncorrected anisometropia it is not possible for the patient to maintain clear vision in each eye simultaneously (except possibly for special conditions of marked asymmetric convergence) (Rosenberg et al., 1953). If the eyes possess different degrees of hyperopia, the usual response is for the eye with the lower refractive state to set the binocular accommodative response, leaving the eye with the greater hyperopia continually blurred. This leads to amblyopia of the more ametropic eye, and in turn, produces confusion of clear and blurred images both appearing to be located in the same place, setting the stage for suppression. Suppression reduces the effectiveness of fusional vergence and contributes to squint. In myopic anisometropia, or when one eye is hyperopic and the other eye myopic, several possibilities exist depending on the degree of anisometropia. In milder cases the least myopic eye or the hyperopic eye may become dominant for distance and the more myopic eye dominant for near tasks. In such situations suppression is present although amblyopia is rare. If, however, the more myopic eye shows very high myopia, it may be suppressed at all distances with accompanying amblyopia. Exotropia and deep amblyopia of a highly myopic and anisometropic eye are not unusual.

Occasionally, strabismus may be due to deprivation because of early cataract or blindness in one eye. The latter condition traditionally has had a very poor prognosis but recent work with eye movement and biofeedback techniques offer the hope of straightening a blind eye (Goldrich, 1982; Hirons and Yolton, 1978).

There are two types of strabismus that involve a significant change in deviation. One is an exotropia that occurs past childhood or in old age following long-standing esotropia and the second is a postsurgical strabismus. Both have a guarded prognosis for functional binocularity.

There is one classification scheme for strabismus that is frequently used and with which this author disagrees. This is the use of the terms "latent" and "manifest" deviation. Some authors treat phoria and strabismus conditions as being essentially the same thing. They categorize by direction of deviation and differentiate between the two by classifying phoria as a latent strabismus and strabismus as opposed to manifest overt strabismus. This tends to minimize an exceedingly important distinction between them. Strabismus describes the condition whereby the two visual axes do not aim at a common point of regard when there is no artificial impediment to binocular vision. A phoria is an artificially produced circumstance in which fusional vergence cues are either not available or diplopic images are optically separated by so great an amount as to exceed any reasonable vergence capacity. Under these conditions the eyes deviate to a vergence position dictated by all of the Maddox innervations except fusion. In strabismus the eyes deviate despite the fact that the stimulus array contains cues that ordinarily permit a normal vergence mechanism to produce alignment. This is not to say that all strabismus is due to faulty fusional vergence, since there can be other considerations that preclude alignment. The important issue is that phorias and strabismus actually represent a significant change of state. Despite this, many authors lump the two together on the basis of the direction of deviation. Esodeviations and exodeviations are discussed and both phorias and strabismus included under one heading. Even surgical results are sometimes presented this way, a practice that this author feels is unwarranted and confusing (Burian and von Noorden, 1980).

ADAPTATIONS

Motor-based schemata are not sufficient to diagnose strabismus. Appropriate management requires understanding of the sensory aspects of the condition as well. As a consequence of the failure of a strabismic to align both eyes, the object of regard is imaged on the fovea of the fixing eye and some off-foveal point in the deviating eye. For the strabismic patient with normal retinal correspondence these two stimulated points do not give rise to the perception of common visual directions. This results in diplopia unless some compensatory mechanism is invoked. Suppression, the disappearance from consciousness of one image, is a frequent adaptive response to restore single vision. Suppression of a diplopically seen image does not involve the fovea of the deviated eye, but rather the off-foveal point in the eye that receives the same image as the fovea of the fixing eye.

Foveal suppression occurs for a different reason. Under normal circumstances the two foveas share a common subjective visual direction. Objects imaged on them are perceived as being located at the same place. In the absence of ocular alignment the two foveas carry images of different objects. Two different things would appear to occupy the same position in space. This "confusion" is a more disabling condition than is diplopia of a single object and hence there is suppression of data associated with the fovea of the deviated eye. The perception of two things in the same place is apparently so disturbing to overall function that it is a rare symptom. Patient reports of confusion are so infrequent as to indicate that suppression of the foveal image of the deviated eye probably occurs at the moment of turn. Even intermittent strabismics, who rather often experience diplopia, almost never report confusion. Diplopia can apparently be lived with more successfully and is more often reported. This author has encountered young patients with long-standing diplopia who never told anyone of it because they felt that "everyone saw that way." They reported a real-unreal distinction (McLaughlin, 1964) that permitted them to reach successfully for door knobs and the like. They used the preferred image for guiding movement and were surprisingly little bothered by the second "false" image. This is generally not the case in adult strabismics of recent onset who find it difficult or impossible to adapt to the diplopia.

Theoretical discussion of suppression makes it sound more constant an entity than it actually is. The suppression scotomas of the fovea and the off-foveal points discussed in the preceding paragraphs are not nearly as discrete as might be expected. In clinical testing suppression is most often an amorphous, continually shifting and changing phenomenon that is very much influenced by intensity of attention and variation in stimulus conditions. Brightness, color, size, and movement of stimulus have profound influence over what is suppressed and when. Suppressed objects can appear and disappear, wax and wane, as attention is directed to them, or their stimulus value changed by modification of the target or its surround. Merely changing ambient illumination or jiggling the target is often sufficient to overcome suppression and permit diplopia awareness. A small muscle light may be suppressed where a slightly larger bulb may be seen double. A red lens before the deviating eye can produce diplopia awareness and even the density of the red filter can influence suppression. Using a bell to add noise to the visual target or having the patient touch the target can reduce or eliminate suppression. Suppression by strabismics may also be a function of viewing distance, direction of gaze, refractive correction, and target detail. It is an elusive, variable, but often useful adaptation to strabismus.

Another sensory adaptation is anomalous retinal correspondence (ARC). While most frequently considered as a consequence, there is also the possibility that ARC can sometimes be the cause of deviation. This point of view has been offered, but most prevailing opinions are that anomalous correspondence follows rather than precedes deviation. In ARC the two foveas do not share common subjective visual directions. Rather, the fovea of one eye shares a common direction with an off-foveal point in the other eye. In harmonious ARC the corresponding retinal points are the fovea of the fixing eye and the point in the deviated eye that receives the same stimulus. This is a very utilitarian situation. There is no stimulus to diplopia. There could still be two areas of "clear" vision, one viewed by the fixing eye and one of some peripheral place where the fovea of the deviating eye happens to be pointed, but no confusion would exist since this clear image would be appreciated as peripheral to the point of regard (Brock, 1945; Cooper and Feldman, 1979).

Harmonious ARC would seem to be a most sensible adaptation to a motor deviation. The angle of anomaly, the angle between the subjective directionalization of the two foveas, is equal to the angle of turn and therefore the subjective angle of turn is zero. In effect the patient recalibrates sensory correspondence exactly to neutralize the angle of turn. Diplopia is avoided, both eyes can contribute to spatial judgments, and there may even be a bonus of a secondary area of clear vision in the field of view. Stereoacuity is reduced, but gross peripheral stereopsis is often demonstrated. Typically, a patient with harmonious ARC (HARC) is but little handicapped in normal environments. There is generally absence of asthenopia; there is no diplopia. Distance judgments are frequently quite accurate, particularly in a complex environment where decisions are not limited solely to disparity detection. Patients park automobiles in tight spaces successfully and this author has seen some who are highly skilled at hitting and catching a baseball.

While it is true that some patients with HARC (as well as many with monolateral strabismus and deep amblyopia) become remarkedly adept at using monocular distance and depth cues in normal environments, most also use binocular cues in daily life. This is easily demonstrated by occluding the deviated eye. In monolateral strabismus with suppression this maneuver has little impact on performance. In HARC cases, covering the turned eye degrades performance on the Brock stick-in-straw test

(Brock, 1956) in much the same way that it does for normals. This can sometimes be used as a diagnostic test for young patients incapable of response to more sophisticated tests. Noticeable degradation of spatial and depth judgment skills with turned eye covered is suggestive of HARC.

Harmonious ARC is a logical adaptive concomitant strabismus. Covariation of the angle of anomaly and the angle of deviation would seem to support this notion (Hallden, 1952). Presence of ARC while deviated and normal retinal correspondence (NRC) when aligned among intermittent strabismics (Cooper and Feldman, 1979) and the generally accepted clinical impression that among esotropes ARC is most likely to be demonstrated under circumstances closely relating to daily life and least likely to be manifested under circumstances remote from daily life are also consistent with this premise (Burian, 1951; Griffin, 1976; Burian and von Noorden, 1980). Unfortunately, like most things associated with strabismus, the problem of ARC is not always as cleanly dealt with as this discussion would imply. Not all patients show covariation. Of those who do, the covariation is not always precisely correlated to maintain mathematical equality of the objective angle of turn and the angle of anomaly (Kerr, 1969). Not all intermittent strabismics show the pattern of ARC while deviated and NRC while aligned. Not all ARC patients are harmonious.

Nonharmonious ARC (NHARC) presents a theoretical conundrum. There is an angle of anomaly other than zero but the angle of anomaly and angle of turn are not equal. This leaves the patient with a type of correspondence that is neither normal nor functional. Subjective and objective angles of turn do not agree but the functional advantage of this is not apparent. The patient with NHARC still has to suppress to avoid diplopia. Harmonious ARC is logical and useful; NHARC seems to have little purpose other than to complicate diagnosis and treatment. Several explanations are offered for the presence of NHARC. One is that the squint angle had been different at some prior time in the patient's life and that HARC developed as a compensation. Then something suddenly changed the angle of turn, leaving the patient with NHARC (Burian, 1945). This is plausible in some instances, particularly those in which surgical intervention has changed the angle of turn. A second explanation supposes that there is a gradual shift of NRC to HARC but that the adaptive process has not been sufficient to change the correspondence fully to match the squint angle (Ronne and Rindziunski, 1953). This author has great difficulty in accepting this line of reasoning. For such a process to occur there would have to be some positive reenforcement as the retinal correspondence shifted away from NRC toward HARC. No such reward exists since there is no patient benefit in terms of function in daily life from anything other than complete elimination of the subjective angle. Inbetween stages might actually be disadvantageous since they would shift a diplopic image (if there were no suppression) from the periphery toward the point of fixation, a situation that would seem to be more difficult to cope with than widely separated images.

There are several explanations offered for the physiological mechanisms whereby ARC is produced. Hallden (1952) proposed a sensory process in which retinal correspondence changes are independent of motor movements of the eyes. Morgan (1961) offers a theory of "registered" eye movements that produce change in retinal correspondence. These registered movements may be due to nonaccommodative vergence innervation. Kerr (1980) ascribes this to neurologically defective fusional vergence control. This might explain NHARC, since no purposeful adaptation is implied in this theory.

Another aspect of ARC that bears on diagnosis and management of strabismus is the variability of response in a single subject. It is possible for some patients to shift from normal to anomalous correspondence on the basis of a change in vergence angle or in various aspects of a stimulus array including size of target detail. Most fascinating is the condition wherein a patient exhibits ARC and NRC simultaneously. This phenomenon, called binocular triplopia, can sometimes be elicited in a major amblyoscope with first-degree targets placed at the objective angle. With flashing or oscillation of the targets and use of suggestion, it is sometimes possible for patients to view one of the targets in two different localizations simultaneously; one according to normal binocular projection and the other localized anomalously (Burian and von Noorden, 1980; Griffin, 1976). When this therapeutic procedure is used, the anomalous image fades from view; it does not shift position toward the normal image. This response pattern is not consistent with the hypotheses of a gradual shift of retinal correspondence from normal to anomalous.

Generally, ARC is felt to be a response to the misalignment of the eyes. The reverse situation cannot be dismissed completely, for if ARC was "wired in" then strabismus would result as a logical consequence. A patient with anatomically fixed ARC would seek strabismus in much the same way that normals seek alignment. Irregularities in retinal correspondence across the field of view are cited by Flom (1980) to explain some of the behaviors associated with strabismus. Regardless of whether or not ARC is the cause or effect of strabismus, its presence in any case other than intermittent exotropia complicates therapy. Congenital strabismics with consistent ARC on all tests almost always defy treatment to normalize correspondence.

In view of the complexities of both suppression and retinal correspondence, the diagnostic routine should include a variety of tests of each so as to ascertain the patient's sensory status over a range of different stimulus conditions. Each of the functions can and does change, in some instances, as a function of the particular test probe used (Burian and von

Noorden, 1980; Griffin, 1976). Another sensory aspect of strabismus has to do with the patient's fusion capability. Worth (1921) described three aspects of binocular integration that he labeled first, second, and third degrees. Some patients are capable of first-degree integration or simultaneous awareness of inputs of each eye in the absence of fuseable contours. Other patients can effect true sensory integration of second-degree targets, which requires coalescing of similar inputs from each eye into a single percept. Still others are capable of stereopsis (Worth's third-degree fusion). To probe these functions the test materials must either be presented at the crossing point of the visual axes in the case of esotropes or by use of optically dissociated stimuli along the line of sight of each eye. This latter technique can be accomplished by use of a Wheatstone or a Brewster stereoscope, or anaglyphs or vectograms.

As in so many other areas of strabismus work, some of the apparently obvious considerations do not necessarily pertain. It is erroneous, for instance, to think of simultaneous awareness, second-degree fusion (flat fusion), and third-degree fusion (stereopsis) as representing some sort of continuum in ascending order. This is not necessarily so. In a normal environment it is all but impossible to encounter first-degree stimulus conditions, and second-degree stimulus conditions are rare. There are almost always disparity cues available in real life situations. It requires careful manipulation of inputs to achieve first- or second-degree conditions. As a consequence, there are some strabismic patients who do better with third-degree fusion stimuli. Failure on a first-degree target does not preclude successful appreciation of a stereoscopic target. Diagnostic testing should include all three types of probes. Some strabismics, particularly intermittent exotropes, can at times maintain bifoveal alignment and demonstrate binocular integration more readily when presented with stereoscopic demands than when asked to deal with first-degree or second-degree stimuli (Flax, 1963; Goldrich, 1980).

Still another factor that must be checked is the capacity to make fusional vergence responses. If the patient is able to demonstrate second- or third-degree fusion either at a centration point in finite space where the visual axes cross or at the angle of deviation in a stereoscopic instrument, it is necessary to find out the patient's capacity to change the angle of deviation in response to a fusional vergence demand. This should be probed in both the converging and diverging directions from the angle of turn. Presence of a fusional vergence response, however slight, offers a favorable prognosis for ultimate binocular cure. In the case of an esotrope it is important to determine whether or not there is a centration range over which the eyes change vergence angle to achieve bifoveal fixation, regardless of how close to the patient this range might be. It is also useful to see if binocular alignment is triggered by a spatial manipulation task, such as placing a stick into a straw (which is held by the examiner in such a way that the task requires a depth judgment rather than aiming). This is sometimes the situation in near-point exotropes who do not converge just to look at a target but who will converge and bifoveally fixate when asked to make a spatial judgment that cannot be made accurately other than by use of either triangulation or stereoscopic data. The presence of such a positive response is a favorable indicator.

While motor and sensory factors are related, the linkage is not always consistent or predictable. Angle of turn does not necessarily correlate with magnitude or sensory impairment. Patients with small angle turns are not by definition more normal in function than those with larger angles of deviation. It is possible to find a patient with a large deviation who shows normal retinal correspondence, and another patient with a smaller turn angle with anomalous correspondence. Which is more normal? Does a patient with minimum motor deviation who is not capable of sensory fusion represent a greater or lesser departure from normal than another patient with a large angular deviation who can demonstrate a normal sensory relationship, including stereopsis, under appropriate stimulus conditions? It is even possible for an individual with strabismus to demonstrate more "normal" binocular function than does one with perfect alignment. For instance, one criterion of binocular vision is stereopsis. Yet there are nonstrabismics who have poor or no stereopsis (Movshon et al., 1972; Richards, 1969), while some with strabismus can demonstrate excellent stereoacuity so long as the disparity is presented in such a manner that the inputs are along the lines of sight of each eye.

There are situations in which patients who are strabismic may perform in a complex environment in a manner more efficient than others who do not have strabismus. For instance, in the condition variously labeled monofixational phoria (Parks, 1964), microtropia (Lang, 1968), or monofixational syndrome (Parks, 1969), there is misalignment of the visual axes in the order of 2 to 10 prism diopters with absence of bifoveal fixation, yet the patients will usually demonstrate fairly sophisticated functional binocularity. Such patients can show peripheral fusion (Burian, 1941) and stereopsis. They generally appear cosmetically straight and the turn is frequently not detected by the cover test, which is usually the most effective means of diagnosing the presence of strabismus. Patients with microtropia may fare better at daily tasks than nonstrabismics, who by virtue of a different type of binocular dysfunction, demonstrate frequent suppression or inadequate motor fusion ranges. Despite the fact that the eyes are straight in terms of motor function, the nonstrabismics may have asthenopia whereas the microtropics characteristically do not experience discomfort.

Some of the sensory concomitants of strabismus serve adaptive purposes. Harmonious ARC is functionally quite useful in normal environments. Suppression can eliminate diplopia or confusion and permit the strabismic patient to operate very well in daily life despite the absence of bifoveal fusion. Many people become quite adept at using so-called monocular cues to make spatial and depth judgments. Strabismic patients do not see a flat world; they see a three-dimensional world, although they are not always capable of normal stereopsis. At times the handicap can be small, there being poor correlation between degree of strabismically caused impairment in binocular function and difficulty in daily life. At times there may even be a negative correlation. Lesser degrees of binocular dysfunction may have greater impact on daily tasks than do greater dysfunctions. This writer has frequently encountered intermittent esotropes or moderate esophores who were asthenopic, in contrast to constant esotropes who have adapted successfully through suppression or ARC and showed minimal difficulty in normal activities. Intermittent strabismics would certainly have to be considered to have a higher degree of binocular function than constant strabismics, and yet this does not necessarily mean that the former are more comfortable or efficient. Using a grading scale based on the usual criteria of binocular vision, they would have to be rated as being better visually than their counterparts who show constant strabismus. Yet when faced with sustaining attention at reading they appear to be far more disabled than the constantly strabismic patient. This is an issue that has never been dealt with adequately in research studies and confounds the relationship between vision and academic performance (Flax, 1970; Spache, 1976).

Similarly, while the suppression amblyopia of strabismus certainly represents a serious visual deficiency, under ordinary circumstances it has less impact on daily function than might be anticipated. Suppression, by eliminating confusion or diplopia, may facilitate performance, particularly if the task can be accomplished without use of stereopsis cues. Suppression amblyopia degrades stereoacuity, but most tasks do not require fine stereopsis. The patient with amblyopia tends to have consistent (albeit reduced) binocular input, permitting reasonable performance, sometimes more so than a patient with a lesser degree of suppression who must deal with continually changing ocular inputs.

This author feels there is insufficient attention given to the relationship of the strabismic condition to performance. Most often the analysis of departure from clinical norms, emphasizing angle of turn or various aspects of binocular vision, pays scant attention to the impact of the ocular misalignment on the patient's ability to function out of the examination room. Treatment options are evaluated primarily in terms of the binocular measures and rarely consider overall performance, although this is actually more important than the binocular skills themselves.

TESTING

While it is not the intent of this chapter to discuss specific tests used in strabismus diagnosis, some comment is in order, particularly in view of the increased interest in early detection and diagnosis. In many instances the angle of turn is sufficiently large so that there is no question as to the presence of the condition. In other cases the turn angle may be small and the ocular and facial configurations such that strabismus is not readily apparent. With a cooperative patient the best single method to ascertain the presence of strabismus is the cover test. Successful application of this procedure requires that the patient be willing and able to maintain attention on a small target. Very young infants are captured by a bright and novel target presented at close distances and it is therefore possible to obtain satisfactory measurement at near, but it is exceedingly difficult to test at further distances. Older infants are particularly difficult to assess by cover tests, since it is not always possible to be sure that they are directing their attention as the examiner would like.

The presence of central fixation (or stable, consistent eccentric fixation) is another necessary condition for an accurate cover test. Demonstration of normal visual acuity can be taken as evidence of central fixation. Unfortunately, this is not always testable in infants and young children by usual clinical methods. When visual acuity can be measured, the presence of amblyopia should make the examiner suspicious of eccentric fixation. It is not an absolute indicator, however, since amblyopia can exist even with central fixation. There are several fairly refined procedures to ascertain the presence of eccentric fixation using entoptic phenomenona, such as the Haidinger brush or the Maxwell spot, which subjectively tag the directional locus of the fovea in space, but these require reasonably sophisticated patient responses (Ludlam, 1970). It is also possible to place the fovea under direct observation using a projection type ophthalmoscope that presents targets visible to both patient and examiner. This technique does not require the patient to describe a weakly perceived phenomenon such as a Maxwell spot or Haidinger brush, but does call for patient cooperation to the point of being able to participate actively (Burian and von Noorden, 1980). Infants will aim their eyes at a bright light such as presented with an ophthalmoscope but young children at times can be notoriously uncooperative. Certain at-risk populations, such as children with brain injury or cerebral palsy, who show high instances of strabismus and amblyopia are frequently unable to participate in this type of testing (Duckman, 1979; Harcourt, 1974). While larger degrees of eccentricity can be detected by observing the first Purkinje image of a muscle light, smaller degrees of eccentric fixation are all but impossible to detect with certainty in an uncooperative patient.

When the cover test cannot be applied it becomes necessary to rely on Purkinje image location to assess the presence and magnitude of strabismus. By means of a muscle light the location of the cornea reflection is noted in each eye under two-eyed viewing conditions. Asymmetry of the image location is assumed to be due to strabismus and the magnitude of asymmetry is a measure of the angle of the strabismus deviation. This Hirshberg method has been in use for many years. It is generally rather poorly specified so that converting the linear displacement of the corneal reflex to an angular measurement is fairly crude. For many years it was generally assumed that 1-mm displacement of reflected image represented 13 prism diopters of deviation (Morgan, 1963). Flom (1956) offered a formula that took into account the nonlinearity of the measurement, improving the accuracy of the Hirshberg test. Recently there have been several attempts systematically to compare Hirshberg estimates of squint angle to actual measurement of the deviation. This has produced a surprising result indicating that, on average, 1 mm displacement of the corneal light reflex equals approximately 22 prism diopters of angular deviation (Jones and Eskridge, 1970). Griffin and Boyer (1974) found that in individual patients 1 mm of corneal light reflex displacement varied from as little as 9.4 to as much as 68.2 prism diopters of deviation. In view of the enormous interest in early diagnosis and intervention it is ironic that so much of the clinical literature hinges on such crude measurements. Accurate determination of the existence and magnitude of small-angle strabismus in infants is based on fleeting observation and assumption of where the infant is in fact directing attention, and a crude method of interpreting the location of the corneal light reflex. Additionally, the use of a light as a stimulus does not afford good control over accommodative level.

There are many elegant tests for retinal correspondence and fusion (Griffin, 1976; Hugonnier and Hugonnier, 1969; Ludlam, 1970). Unfortunately, most are difficult if not impossible to use successfully with infants and young children. They all require subjective responses and a degree of cooperation not always present in preschoolers. In many cases the young child, highly suggestible and anxious to please the examiner, responds to other than visual cues when confronted with a confusing and demanding test circumstance. Use of objective tests such as visually evoked potentials (Amigo et al., 1978), elimination of ambiguity in testing by random-dot stereograms (Cooper and Feldman, 1978a; Reinecke and Simons, 1974), or behavior modification techniques (Cooper and Feldman, 1978b) all can serve to assist in permitting more accurate diagnosis of young children. Unfortunately, the number of procedures that have been developed thus far is relatively small and not all diagnostic areas can be tapped without reasonably sophisticated cooperation.

PROGNOSIS

The ultimate purpose of diagnosis is to arrive at a prognosis and a decision as to management. Many factors must be considered, of which perhaps the most important is cosmetic appearance. That this is so is attested to by the frequency of strabismus surgery as a therapeutic measure, despite the generally poor functional results. Multiple surgeries are frequent and reported functional cure rates vary widely, some as low as 10% (Ludlam, 1970). Burian and von Noorden (1980) report two series of congenital esotropes involving 100 patients in which 159 operations produced straight eyes, and the possibility of normal binocular function in only 7 patients.

Data regarding functional cures with surgery must be carefully analyzed since, in this author's opinion, most studies are seriously flawed either by inclusion of minimal success criteria or by nonidentification of criteria. Perhaps the most egregious deficiency is the use of success standards that were probably present in the patients *before* surgery. This is exemplified in a summary of 775 cases of operations for exodeviation (Burian and von Noorden, 1980). Inspection of the cited papers discloses such deficiencies as including intermittent exotropes who might have met the success criteria prior to operation (Burian and Spivey, 1965); using presence of stereopsis as a cure criterion in a sample comprised solely of intermittent exotropes (Pratt-Johnson et al., 1977), despite the fact that most intermittent exotropes show stereopsis when aligned (Cooper, 1977); treating half of the sample orthoptically in addition to surgery and accepting any degree of stereopsis as a functional result (Hardesty et al., 1978); ignoring near point function or alignment as criteria of satisfactory results while restricting the sample to patients who demonstrated fusion and stereopsis before surgery (Ballen, 1970); using alignment on cover test as an indication of binocular function with no tests for fusion or stereopsis (Windsor, 1971); or requiring fusion capability including stereopsis *before* operation, considering reduction of the deviation to within 10^{Δ} of straight as a success, and ignoring residual near deviations (Raab and Parks, 1969). The approximate 50% aggregate success really represents cosmetic improvement rather than functional cure.

Elimination of functional deficiencies in binocular vision, performance difficulties, and asthenopia should be considered in addition to cosmetic appearance. When feasible, this author considers orthoptics to be the preferred treatment (along with refractive correction and/or prisms). Inasmuch as the major emphasis in orthoptics is establishment of normal sensory fusion in order ultimately to effect alignment of the eyes, the approach is preferred to surgery. Unless surgery completely eliminates the strabismus it cannot be expected to have a significant impact on function. Even a slight residual misalignment of the eyes creates a situation that causes diplopia or requires functional adaptation by suppression or development of anomalous retinal correspondence. The adage "a miss is as good as a mile" must be kept in mind when relating functional outcomes with surgery. While it may infrequently result in normal retinal correspondence, this cannot be depended on (Burian and von Noorden, 1980). Thus it should be the back-up to orthoptics, not the other way around, since when feasible, orthoptics can produce more functional cures. Flax and Duckman (1978) reporting on 928 cases in 12 studies with well-stated, high-level success criteria, found 67% cure in orthoptics supervised by ophthalmologists and 86% cure when the orthoptic treatment was done by optometrists. Cosmetic surgery is always an option if functional results are not possible.

Optical limitations should be evaluated prior to undertaking therapy. For instance, if there is anisometropia, the introduction of possible anisophoria or aniseikonic difficulties must be considered. Hindrance to fusion may be caused by the variable prism induced by anisometropic spectacles. The cosmetic aspects of an anisometropic correction must also be considered. While contact lenses frequently are desirable, it must be established that the patient will tolerate them. In some instances it might be desirable to treat the strabismus by developing peripheral fusion to effect alignment and reasonably good binocular function without correcting the anisometropic refraction. In certain instances it is conceivable that full anisometropic correction may create more difficulties than benefits. Along the same line, the patient's potential fusional capabilities should be determined before undertaking treatment. In situations in which no fusion can be demonstrated under any circumstances during evaluation or, more particularly, in situations where horror fusionis is demonstrated, any therapeutic regimen should proceed very cautiously (Griffin, 1976). It is relatively easy to eliminate suppression; it is all but impossible to teach a patient to suppress. The best that can be done in situations of intractable diplopia is to use optical blur or occlusion in the hope of the patient developing suppression. This is not always successful. The possibility of asthenopia on conclusion of treatment should be considered if the optical and fusional factors indicate that at best, very tenuous or weak fusion might be achieved. The patient might best be treated in a manner not designed to introduce an uncomfortable situation. Thoughtless pursuit of a particular therapeutic objective at the expense of the patient's well-being is not desirable. For instance, one occasionally encounters a youngster who has been occluded for years in an attempt to improve an amblyopic eye, with total disregard of the effect of occlusion on the youngster's overall development. Methods of restraining a youngster from removing an eye patch are discussed (Hiles and Galket, 1974) with little concern about the effects on general performance and emotional well being of a child forced to function using a significantly amblyopic eye for an extended period of time with full knowledge that he or she possesses an eye that can see properly.

Heroic attempts to establish binocular alignment in cerebral palsied children may be ill advised. Many of these patients have great difficulty in successfully developing the usual functional adaptations that permit other strabismic children to perform. This author has encountered children with cerebral palsy who habitually fixated with the more amblyopic eye, turning what seemed to be the more functionally useful eye. Considering their multiple handicaps, including a high incidence of oculomotor dysfunction, one must carefully consider whether the surgical treatment of a strabismus is not possibly more harmful than beneficial, particularly in view of a very poor functional prognosis (Harcourt, 1974).

There are numerous factors that offer a favorable prognosis. Full and comitant motor capability is obviously an excellent prognostic sign. An accommodative component in esotropia or the ability to use accommodative convergence as a lever to affect alignment in an exotrope are highly desirable. Absence of anisometropia is also a favorable indicator. In an esotrope, the presence of normal retinal correspondence on all tests is a positive sign. Presence of ARC on any tests would tend to reduce the probabilities of a functional outcome but would not necessarily preclude success. In exotropia, anomalous retinal correspondence on certain tests can be ignored if the strabismus is intermittent. Many intermittent exotropias of the divergence excess type will show ARC when in deviated posture and normal retinal correspondence when aligned. From a practical standpoint this demonstration of ARC may be ignored, for as alignment is achieved the retinal correspondence takes care of itself through covariation. Constant exotropia, particularly if it is basic with large deviation at both distance and near, is usually more productively managed if the patients are likened to esotropes in determining prognosis. Intermittent exotropia has exceedingly high functional cure rate with orthoptics. The same cannot be said with certainty of constant basic exotropia. Demonstration of fusional capability, particularly fusional vergence capacity, is an excellent prognostic sign. In general, patients with fusional vergence, normal retinal correspondence, intact motor systems, and no optical problems should achieve functional cure. Depending on the angle of turn the cure may be effected with orthoptics alone, or in combination with surgery. In certain instances, surgery by itself may produce functional results.

Another important factor is the anticipated change in function in the normal environment. If daily function is better when the patient is binocular than when the patient is not, one can reasonably expect that treatment will proceed more efficiently. This is so because of heightened patient motivation and also by virtue of reenforcing effects of daily activity. The converse also exists. This author has encountered esotropic patients who had been responding quite well to orthoptics until such time as they began to develop a heavy interest in reading. At that particular stage in treatment they were ineffectively and uncomfortably binocular.

Since they could not function in a standard environment as binocular persons, they reverted to suppression and the turn angle increased. The heavy near point accommodative demands and the discomfort produced by fragile and unstable fusion was more disturbing than reverting to strabismus with deeper suppression. In many instances this situation is predictable and a change in the timing of therapy and possible convex lens prescription should be considered.

Planning the management of a strabismic problem must also include consideration of risk-benefit as well as cost-benefit factors. The former include the previously discussed possibility of the patient actually being worse after treatment than before. It is pointless to eliminate suppression unless there is the possibility of achieving alignment. It is unfair to offer surgery where there is high probability of diplopia or consecutive strabismus; anesthesia and health risks attendant to surgery must also be considered (Burian and von Noorden, 1980). Cost-benefit factors must be weighed not only in terms of money but of time and discomfort. The relationship between tangible benefits and the rigors of treatment must be considered. Persistent attempts to maintain acuity in an amblyopic eye in the absence of fusion may require almost constant therapy, which in itself reduces the patient's ability to function effectively.

It is essential that the decision include consideration of anticipated long-term consequences both without and with treatment. The question must be asked as to anticipated outcome if the condition is left untreated or if treatment is delayed until a later date. Frequently, parents are frightened into accepting surgery for strabismus for purposes of arresting or curing amblyopia before a child reaches age six or seven. This is not warranted for several reasons. Unless there is restoration of bifoveal fixation with full binocular function, the patient still has to suppress the fovea of the deviating eye. In most instances, amblyopia does not respond directly to surgical intervention. Furthermore, while there is good reason to institute amblyopia treatment procedures, such as refractive correction and stimulation of a turned eye, at as early an age as is possible, this does not mean that amblyopia cannot be treated at later dates. The age at which amblyopia develops is a more important factor in prognosis than the age at which active therapy is begun, particularly after the first few years of life. It may be more prudent to wait until the child is sufficiently mature, to assure more effective diagnosis and cooperation. Amblyopia treatment begun after age six is no less effective than that begun before this age (Birnbaum et al., 1977; Flom, 1970).

The anticipated results of treatment must be evaluated not only for their immediate impact but also for the long-term effects. Surgery for a strabismus is generally contraindicated when there is a strong accommodative component in the form of hyperopia that will almost certainly have to be corrected later in life. As long-term consequences are evaluated, it becomes apparent that compromise therapies may often be desirable. Given a poor prognosis for functional success, cosmetic surgery is certainly warranted. Partial functional results may also be a realistic objective of treatment. So long as the end result is cosmetically satisfactory and functionally useful it is sometimes appropriate to aim for peripheral fusion with stereopsis, leaving residual amblyopia and lack of bifoveal binocular function. Converting a large-angle turn to a stable and functionally useful mini-squint is not a failure but rather a resounding success from the patient's point of view. Naturally, it would be desirable to achieve full bifoveal alignment, full acuity, and central stereopsis but this is not always a practical goal. Similarly, there are instances in which control rather than cure should be the immediate objective. In the case of amblyopia where binocularity cannot be achieved, it is useful to improve the acuity of the amblyopic eye with intensive patching, pleoptics, and orthoptics just to establish a base-line capability in that eye. This has the very practical advantage of ensuring against blindness in case of injury to the normal eye and provides an enormous psychological benefit to the patient who no longer has one "blind eye." Then it might be well to permit the acuity to fall in that eye with occasional treatment to perk up the acuity rather than attempting constantly to maintain acuity against an impossible circumstance. Acuity will not be maintained unless full functional binocularity is achieved or the patient is made to alternate. Not all patients, for a variety of reasons, can become alternators.

Finally, it is important that strabismus be considered a disorder of a person. While some of the factors to be considered in diagnosis and prognosis reside in the eyes or the oculomotor system, the most important consideration should be the responses and behaviors of a person rather than of a pair of eyes. A humanistic assessment of the behaviors and problems of strabismus is required to provide maximal benefit. The therapeutic thrust should be to permit each and every patient to achieve the greatest improvement in ocular and overall performance as a consequence of appropriate diagnosis and management of the strabismus condition.

REFERENCES

Amigo G, Fiorentini A, Pirchio M, Spinelli D. Binocular vision tested with visually evoked potentials. Invest Ophthalmol 1978;17(9):910–15.

Atkinson J, Braddick O, French J. Infant astigmatism: its disappearance with age. Vision Res 1980;20:891–93.

Ballen PH. Surgical treatment of intermittent exotropia. J Pediatr Ophthalmol 1970;7:55.

Birnbaum MH, Koslowe K, Sanet R. Success in amblyopia therapy as a function of age: a literature survey. Am J Optom 1979;54(5):269–75.

Blakemore C. Maturation and modification in the developing visual system. In: Held R, Liebowitz HW, Tauber HL, eds. Handbook of Sensory Physiology. Vol. 8. Springer-Verlag, 1974:Berlin, New York: 377–436.
Blakemore C. The conditions required for the maintainence of binocularity in the kitten's visual cortex. J Physiol 1976;261:423–44.
Brock F. Binocular vision in strabismus. Optom Weekly 1945;36(3):67–68;179–180.
Brock F. Visual training. Part III. Optom Weekly 1956;2011–2148.
Burian HM. Fusional movements in permanent strabismus. A study of the rule of central and peripheral retinal regions in the act of binocular vision in squint. Arch Ophthalmol 1941;26:626.
Burian HM. Sensorial retinal relationship in concomitant strabismus. Trans Am Ophthalmol Soc 1945;81:373.
Burian HM. Anomalous retinal correspondence, its essence and its significance in prognosis and treatment. Am J Ophthalmol 1951;34:237–53.
Burian HM. Occlusion amblyopia and the development of eccentric fixation in occluded eyes. Am J Ophthalmol 1966;62:853.
Burian HM, Spivey BE. The surgical management of exodeviations. Am J Ophthalmol 1965;59:603.
Burian HM, von Noorden GK. Binocular vision ocular motility, theory and management of strabismus. 2nd ed. St. Louis: CV Mosby, 1980.
Cooper J. Intermittent exotropia of the divergence excess type. J Am Opt Assoc 1977;48(10):1261–73.
Cooper J, Feldman J. Operant conditioning and assessment of stereopsis in young children. Am J Optom 1978a;55(8):532–44.
Cooper J, Feldman J. Random-dot-stereogram performance by strabismic, amblyopic, and ocular-pathology patients in an operant discrimination task. Am J Optom 1978b;55(9):599–609.
Cooper J, Feldman J. Panoramic viewing, visual acuity of deviating eye, and anomalous retinal correspondence in the intermittent exotrope of the divergence excess type. Am J Optom 1979;56(7):422–29.
Duckman R. The incidence of visual anomalies in a population of cerebral palsied children. J Am Opt Assoc 1979;50(9):1013–16.
Flax N. The optometric treatment of intermittent divergent strabismus. Eastern Seaboard Vision Training Conference, Washington, D.C. January, 1963.
Flax N. Training intermittent exotropes. San Jose Vision Training Seminar, August, 1968.
Flax N. Problems in relating visual function to reading disorder. Am J Optom 1970;47(5):369–70.
Flax N, Duckman R. Orthoptic treatment of strabismus. J Am Opt Assoc 1978;49(9):1353–61.
Flom MC. A minimum strabismus examination. J Am Opt Assoc 1956;27(11):643.
Flom MC. Treatment of binocular anomalies of vision, in Vision of Children. In: Hirsch MJ, Wick RE, eds. Philadelphia: Chilton Book Co., 1963:197–211.
Flom MC. Early experience in the development of visual coordination. In: Young FA, Lindsley DB, eds. Early experience and visual information processing in perceptual and reading disorders. Washington, D.C., National Academy of Sciences, 1970:291–99.

Flom MC. Corresponding and disparate retinal points in normal and anomolous correspondence. Am J Optom 1980;57(9):656–65.

Goldrich SG. Optometric therapy of divergence excess strabismus. Am J Optom 1980;57(1):7–14.

Goldrich SG. Oculomotor biofeedback therapy for exotropia. Am J Optom 1982;59(4):306–17.

Graham PA. Epidemiology of strabismus. Br J Ophthalmol 1974;58(3):224–31.

Griffin JR. Binocular anomalies—procedures for vision therapy. Chicago: Professional Press, 1976.

Griffin JR, Boyer FM. Strabismus measurement with the Hirschberg test. Opt Weekly 1974;65(32):34.

Hallden U. Fusional phenomena in anomalous correspondence. Acta Ophthalmol 1952;37:(Suppl)1–93.

Harcourt B. Strabismus affecting children with multiple handicaps. Br J Ophthalmol 1974;58:272–80.

Hardesty HH, Boynton JR, Keenan JP. Treatment of intermittent exotropia. Arch Ophthalmol 1978;96:268.

Hiles DA, Galket RJ. Plaster cast arm restraints and amblyopia therapy. J Pediatr Ophthalmol 1974;11(3):151–52.

Hirons R, Yolton RL. Biofeedback treatment of strabismus: case studies. J Am Opt Assoc 1978;49(8):875–82.

Hubel DH, Wiesel T. Binocular interaction in striate cortex of kittens reared with artificial squint. J Neurophysiol 1965;28:1041–59.

Hugonnier R, Hugonnier SC. Strabismus, heterophoria, ocular motor paralysis. Troutman SV, trans. St. Louis: CV Mosby, 1969.

Ikeda H, Wright MJ. A possible neurophysiological basis for amblyopia. Br. Orthop J 1975;32:2013.

Jones R, Eskridge JB. The Hirschberg test—a re-evaluation. Am J Optom 1970;47(2):105–44.

Kerr K. Vergence-induced correspondence changes in anomalous retinal correspondence. University microfilms, Ann Arbor, Mich., 1969.

Kerr K. Accommodative and fusional vergence in anomalous correspondence. Am J Optom 1980;57(9):676–80.

Lang J. Evaluation in small angle strabismus or microtropia. Arruga M, ed. International Strabismus Symposium. Basel, New York: S. Karger, 1968:219.

Ludlam WM. Strabismus definition. In: Borish IM, ed. Clinical refraction. 3rd ed. Chicago: Professional Press, 1970.

Maddox EE. The clinical use of prisms and the decentering of lenses. 2nd ed. Bristol, England: John Wright & Sons, 1893.

McLaughlin SC. Visual perception in strabismus and amblyopia. Psych Monogr General and Applied 1964;78(12):1–23.

Mitchell DE, Freeman RD, Millodot M, Haegerstrom G. Meridional amblyopia: evidence for modification of the human visual system by early visual experience. Vision Res 1973;13:535–58.

Mohindra I, Held R, Gwiazda J, Brill S. Astigmatism in infants. Science 1978;202:329–31.

Morgan MW. Anomalous correspondence interpreted as a motor phenomenon. Am J Optom 1961;38(3):131–48.

Morgan MW. Anomalies of binocular vision. In: Hirsch MJ, Wick RE, eds. Vision of children. Philadelphia: Chilton Book Co., 1963:178–79.

Morgan MW. The Maddox classification of vergence eye movements. Am J Optom 1980;57(9):537–39.

Movshon JA, Chambers BEI, Blakemore C. Stereopsis and interocular transfer. Perception 1972;1:483–90.

Parks MM. Second thoughts about the pathophysiology of monofixational phoria. Am Orthoptic J 1964;14:159.

Parks MM. The monofixational syndrome. Trans Am Ophthalmol Soc 1969;67:609.

Pratt-Johnson JA, Barlow JM, Tilson G. Early surgery for intermittent exotropia. Am J Ophthalmol 1977;84:689.

Raab EL, Parks MM. Recession of the lateral recti. Arch Ophthalmol 1969;82:203.

Reinecke RD, Simons K. A new stereoscopic test for amblyopia screening. Am J Ophthalmol 1974;78(4):714–21.

Revell MJ. Strabismus, a history of orthoptic techniques. London: Barrie & Jenkins, 1971:1–6.

Richards W. Stereopsis and stereoblindness. Exp Brain Res 1969;10:380–88.

Roberts J. Eye examination findings among children. Vital Health Statistics 1972;11:115.

Roberts J. Eye examination findings among youth 12–17 years. Vital Health Statistics 1975;11:155.

Ronne G, Rindziunski E. The pathogenesis of anomalous correspondence. Acta Ophthalmol 1953;31:347.

Rosenberg R, Flax N, Brodsky R, Abelman S. Accommodative levels under conditions of asymmetric convergence. Am J Optom 1953;30(5):244–54.

Spache GD. Investigating the issues of reading disability. Boston: Allyn & Bacon, 1976;47.

Thomas J, Mohindra I, Held R. Strabismic amblyopia in infants. Am J Optom 1979;56(3):197–201.

Van Sluyters RC. Recovery from monocular stimulus deprivation amblyopia in the kitten. Ophthalmology 1978;85:478–88.

Windsor CE. Surgery, fusion, and accommodative convergence in exotropia. J Pediatr Ophthalmol 1971;8:166.

Worth C. Squint—its causes, pathology and treatment. Philadelphia: C Blakiston's Son, 1921.

19

Treatment of Binocular Dysfunctions

J. David Grisham

Treatment of vergence disorders in nonstrabismic patients is considerably easier and more effective than in cases of manifest strabismus or deep amblyopia. Muscle surgery is rarely indicated for patients who have basic sensory and motor fusion skills. Rather, some combination of spectacle prism, added lens power, and vergence training is usually sufficient to relieve both signs and symptoms. These minor disorders of vergence eye position and binocular vision are frequently associated with symptoms of eye strain, headaches, intermittent blurred and double vision, and early fatigue with sustained critical viewing. Strabismic patients rarely complain of any visual discomfort or inefficiency except when the squint is intermittent or recently acquired. It is more often the physiological minor disorders of binocular coordination that result in patient distress and performance limitations.

At our clinic approximately one in seven patients seeking services has a binocular dysfunction, physiological in nature, that interferes with daily tasks in some way. The reported prevalence of strabismus ranges from 2% to 4% in the general population (Hugonnier and Hugonnier, 1969); however, this condition receives a disproportionately large share of interest in the clinical literature. The emphasis of this chapter is on the treatment of binocular insufficiencies of various types: heterophoria, fusional vergence, and accommodative insufficiencies. The management techniques and principles are applicable at many points in treating the entire spectrum. Also, they fall in the realm of general clinical practice and have wide application.

Some of the principles guiding nonsurgical treatment of strabismus and amblyopia are presented, but no single chapter could adequately review the multitude of techniques, conditions, and often conflicting opinions regarding patient management. Consequently, this presentation deals with only the most common conditions and represents a particular point of view in favor at our clinic.

CHARACTERISTICS OF A VERGENCE DYSFUNCTION

Traditionally, a vergence dysfunction has been identified by comparing the measured parameters of the zone of clear single binocular vision to clinical standards for the general population. Morgan's table of clinical data is the most widely accepted standard (Table 19.1). If vergence, heterophoria, or accommodative range data for distance or near viewing fall outside of the low tail of the first standard deviation for the general population, the patient is suspected of having deficient binocular coordination. Discomfort or inefficiency can result depending on how the patient uses the eyes. In the light of a thorough history that includes discussion of symptoms, uses of critical vision, medical conditions, and medications, it must be determined that the identified binocular deficiency represents a practical problem for the patient. If so, there is a variety of treatment options.

One difficulty in applying Morgan's norms is the many sources of nonphysiological variation in the clinical measurement of the zone of

TABLE 19.1. Clinically significant data.

Test	*Clinical Data*
Heterophoria (6 m)	Esophoria $\geq 2^{\Delta}$; exophoria $\geq 3^{\Delta}$
Convergence ranges (6 m)	$\leq$ 5/11/6 blur/break/recovery
Divergence ranges (6 m)	$\leq$ 4/2 break/recovery
Heterophoria (40 cm)	Esophoria $\geq 2^{\Delta}$; exophoria $\geq 8^{\Delta}$
Convergence ranges (40 cm)	$\leq$ 12/15/4 blur/break/recovery
Divergence ranges (40 cm)	$\leq$ 9/17/8 blur/break/recovery
Relative accommodation (positive)	≤ -1.12 D
Relative accommodation (negative)	$\leq +1.50$ D

Clinical values falling outside the first standard deviation of the general population may indicate a binocular vision dysfunction.

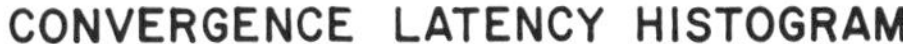

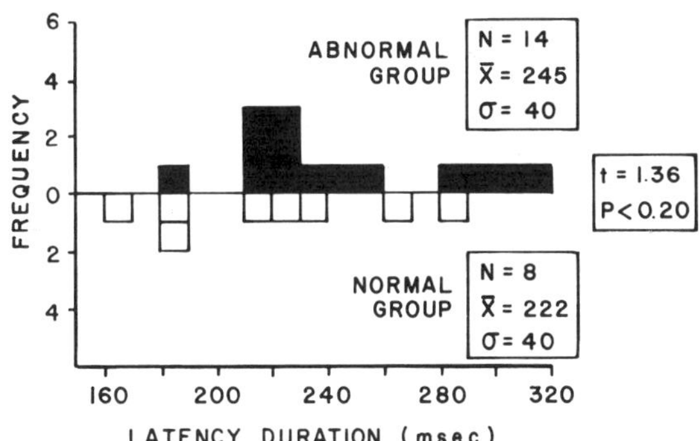

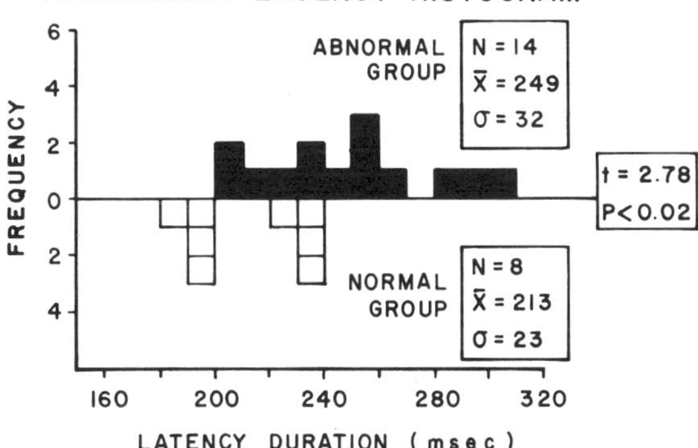

FIGURE 19.1. Fusional Vergence Latency Histograms. The mean group latency for subjects showing clinically abnormal vergence responses was significantly different from the mean latency of normal subjects only for responses in the divergent direction (student t test). Reprinted by permission of the publisher, from Grisham JD. The dynamics of fusional vergence eye movements in binocular dysfunction. American Journal of Optometry and Physiological Optics, 1980. (See textual explanation on page 609.)

clear single binocular vision. Test results are markedly influenced by such procedural factors as speed and smoothness of prism power induction (using Risley prisms), amount of contour in the fixation target, and phrasing of instructions (i.e., "Tell me when the target doubles," as opposed to "Try to keep the target single"). As with all subjective techniques, a patient's attention or arousal level can influence the test end points, as can other intangible factors such as tolerance of discomfort and precision of observation.

A fusional vergence dysfunction can also be defined in terms of objectively measured dynamic components of vergence response. This technique has generally verified the clinically established categories of vergence dysfunction (Grisham, 1980a). Two subject groups were designated by Grisham as either normal or abnormal on the basis of their clinically determined vergence and heterophoria data and Morgan's norms. The question was asked, "Can these groups be differentiated on the basis of certain objectively measured properties of fusional vergence response?" Divergence step latency, step convergence and divergence velocity, vergence step tracking rate, and percentage completion of step responses all discriminated between the clinical groups. These are shown

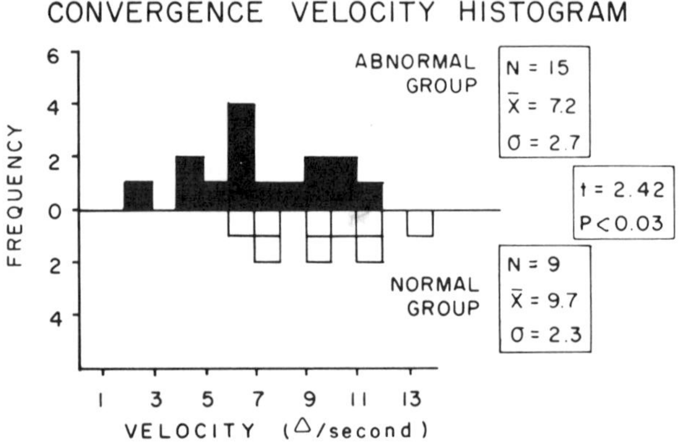

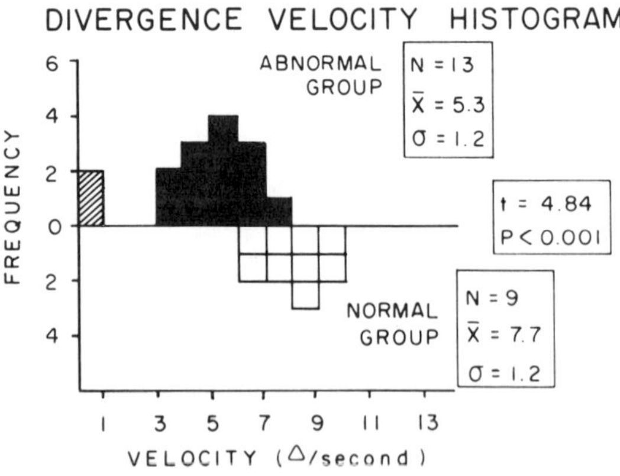

FIGURE 19.2. Fusional Vergence Velocity Histograms. The mean group velocity for subjects showing clinically abnormal vergence responses was significantly slower than the mean velocity of normal subjects for responses in both convergent and divergent directions. Reprinted by permission of the publisher, from Grisham JD. The dynamics of fusional vergence eye movements in binocular dysfunction. American Journal of Optometry and Physiological Optics, 1980.

in order of discriminating power, from weak to strong in Figures 19.1, 19.2, and 19.3.

Three general categories of vergence dysfunction were identified through analysis of fusional vergence dynamics of subjects in a clinically abnormal group ($N = 15$). One category of disorder was characterized by deficiencies in horizontal fusional vergence responses in the absence of abnormalities of tonic or accommodative vergence. That is, there was no significant heterophoria at distance or near fixation. These subjects exhibited deficits in response latency, velocity, or percentage of completed

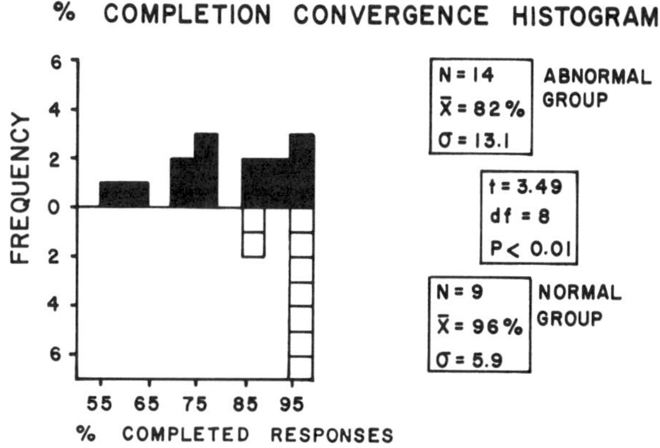

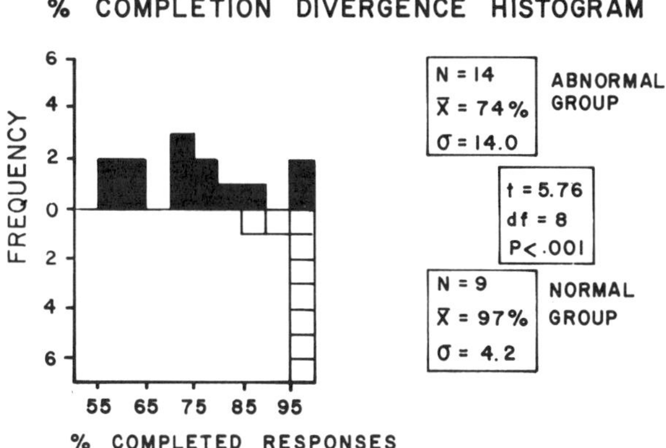

FIGURE 19.3. Percentage of Completed Response Histograms. Subjects in the clinically abnormal group completed fewer convergent and divergent step responses on average than subjects having clinically normal vergence at a high level of statistical significance. Reprinted by permission of the publisher, from Grisham JD. The dynamics of fusional vergence eye movements in binocular dysfunction. American Journal of Optometry and Physiological Optics, 1980.

responses in one or both horizontal directions. A second class of disorder was distinguished by unusually large heterophorias at either distance or near fixation as judged by Morgan's expected values, but the response characteristics of fusional vergence appeared normal. A third category was identified in which subjects showed large heterophorias and abnormalities in response dynamics. These functional classes parallel clinically established categories of vergence dysfunction (convergence or divergence excess and insufficiency) and confirm in a rigorous manner the clinician's analytical framework using graphical analysis.

CLINICAL ASSESSMENT OF VERGENCE FACILITY

Most clinicians are familiar with the standard techniques for assessing the functional status of the vergence system and binocular sensory fusion: cover test at distance and near, Risley prism vergence ranges, fixation disparity, test for central suppression, relative accommodation, near point of convergence, and the like. All of these procedures have been used for many years in the differential diagnosis of binocular vision dysfunctions. Except for the cover test and near point of convergence, most are subjective techniques, which is a common disadvantage. The patient indicates the end point of the procedure. This limits the assessment of vergence to only those patients who can make adequate subjective observations, and automatically eliminates infants, young children, and many handicapped individuals. It is often useful to make an objective assessment of fusional vergence function. Most clinicians do not have access to an infrared eye monitor for precise determination of latency, velocity, accuracy, and fatigue response characteristics. Clinical assessment can be made by direct observation of a patient's vergence response to a small-increment prism placed before the eyes, known as the reflex fusion test. It is similar to the four-prism diopter base-out test used in strabismus diagnosis, except both convergence and divergence functions are evaluated with respect to the dynamic components of response latency, velocity, accuracy, and fatigue. These observations comprise an evaluation of vergence "facility" in contrast to vergence "range of response," which stands as the traditional graphical analysis approach.

Observations made with the reflex fusion test are qualitative rather than quantitative, but they are objective. The clinician can learn from experience what observations suggest deficiencies in vergence function. Some guidelines for performing the test include asking patients to fixate a small detailed target at approximately 40 cm and instructing them to keep the target clear, refraining from any reference to single or double vision. The goal is to have patients accommodate accurately at the target plane and to avoid the influence of conscious control of vergence eye position while the characteristics of reflex disparity vergence are being tested. A small-increment loose prism, preferably six prism diopters, is introduced into the line of sight of either eye and the resulting vergence response to this asymmetric vergence stimulus is carefully evaluated. Interpatient variation in response to this simple procedure is wide, which gives the test its discriminating value. There is also some variation of response on repetition, which is worthwhile noting. Observations provide a sense of accuracy of response and rate of fatigue to repeated vergence steps. Both factors reflect the functional integrity of the disparity vergence system.

Vergence latency is assessed by observing the amplitude of version movement prior to vergence movement. The version and vergence systems appear to be functionally independent (Rashbass and Westheimer, 1961). If the vergence system is slow to respond, a sizable version movement can be seen since the version latency is approximately the same span as a normal vergence latency. The conjugate version movement is easily assessed by watching the prism-free eye. If latencies for both systems are approximately equal there will be little or no version movement of the eye without the prism. If there is more than two prism diopters of version before that eye changes direction to complete the vergence movement, one might suspect a slowly responding vergence system. It should be pointed out that disparity vergence latency is the same for equal increment steps along the vergence range for a particular vergence direction (Grisham, 1980a). The latency does not significantly change if prism is introduced at the patient's phoria position or close to the limits of fusional vergence response.

The clinician must determine which eye makes the largest disjunctive movement after the initial version and then evaluate the vergence velocity component. Experience with the technique serves as a guide in designating a slow, moderate, or fast response. We have found that with a little practice one can make accurate discriminating judgments regarding vergence facility. Patients showing slow reflex fusion responses often have restricted vergence ranges by Risley prisms. Grisham (1980a) found an inverse correlation of −0.70 between the total step vergence response time (latency and velocity) and a measure of range of step vergence responses. This relationship supports the use of the reflex fusion test as a valid indicator.

The direction and amplitude of heterophoria is included in the interpretation of the reflex fusion response. Step vergence velocity depends on the starting vergence position and decreases the further one samples from the phoria position. If a patient has a large exophoria, the expected reflex fusion response may be slow in the base-out direction (convergence) and fast in the base-in (divergence) direction. A slow reflex response in the convergence direction by a patient with a small to moderate exophoria would indicate poor vergence facility. Patients with slow step velocities in one vergence direction also tend to be slow for steps in the opposite direction, although there is wide variation in this regard.

CHANGING VERGENCE DYNAMICS WITH ORTHOPTICS

Besides being an objective indicator of vergence function, measurement of vergence dynamics provides a rigorous evaluation of the effects of various therapy techniques. The clinical literature has many reports of

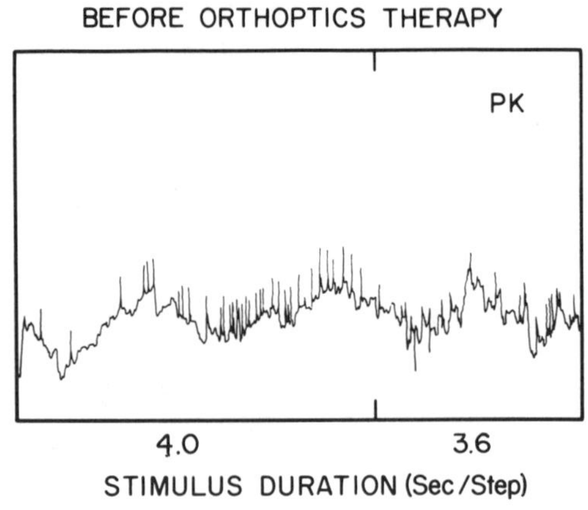

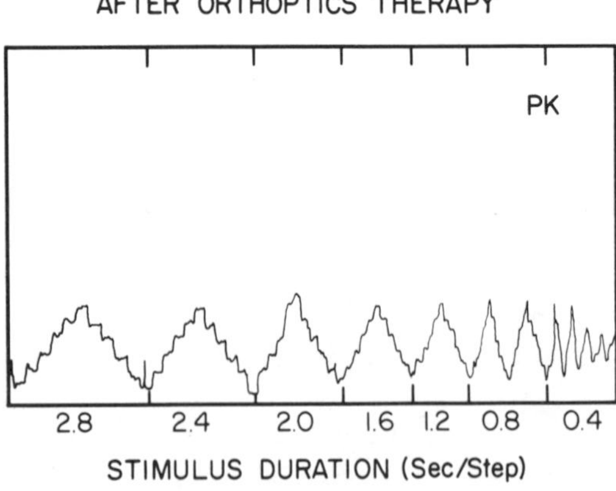

FIGURE 19.4. Step Vergence Tracking Recording Before and After Orthoptics. Prior to orthoptics therapy subject P.K. could not adequately track a step vergence staircase stimulus changing at the rate of 4 seconds per step. After 8 weeks of home orthoptics P.K. successfully tracks steps changing at the rate of 0.8 seconds per step. (Chan CL, Grisham JD, 1975)

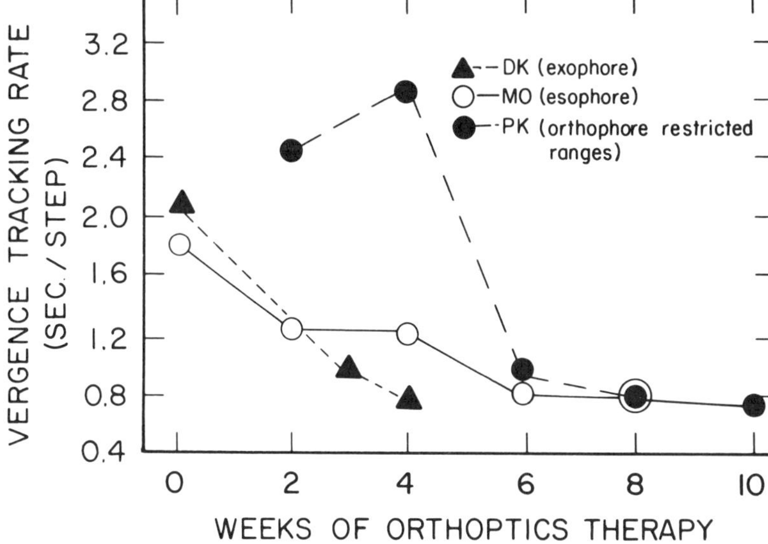

FIGURE 19.5. Changes in Vergence Tracking Rate with Orthoptics. Three subjects having clinical binocular deficiencies show significantly faster vergence tracking rates to a step staircase vergence stimulus as orthoptics therapy proceeds over several weeks. Three measures of tracking rate prior to therapy did not show significant differences in each case. (Chan CL, Grisham JD, 1975)

successful orthoptics treatment of various binocular vision and motility anomalies, but doubts remain regarding their validity since most studies have used subjective methods to determine a diagnosis and results of therapy. Even though the literature has many examples of improving vergence function through orthoptics procedures (Flom, 1954; Wick, 1977; Cooper and Feldman, 1980; Daum, 1982), changes in vergence function need to be studied in a more exact manner. Objective indicators such as vergence tracking rate provide a reliable means of showing the relative benefit of one technique over another (i.e., prism vs orthoptics, or step vergence techniques vs sliding vergence). Vergence tracking rate improves as a result of training in patients having minimal binocular dysfunctions and the change correlates with the increase in clinically measured vergence ranges (Chan and Grisham, 1975) (Figure 19.4). The step vergence tracking rate was determined for three patients diagnosed as having insufficient fusional vergence responses and complaining of asthenopia symptoms. To control for the effect of repeated testing, tracking rates were measured on three occasions prior to onset of orthoptic treatment. No significant variation was noted. Figure 19.5 shows that all three patients

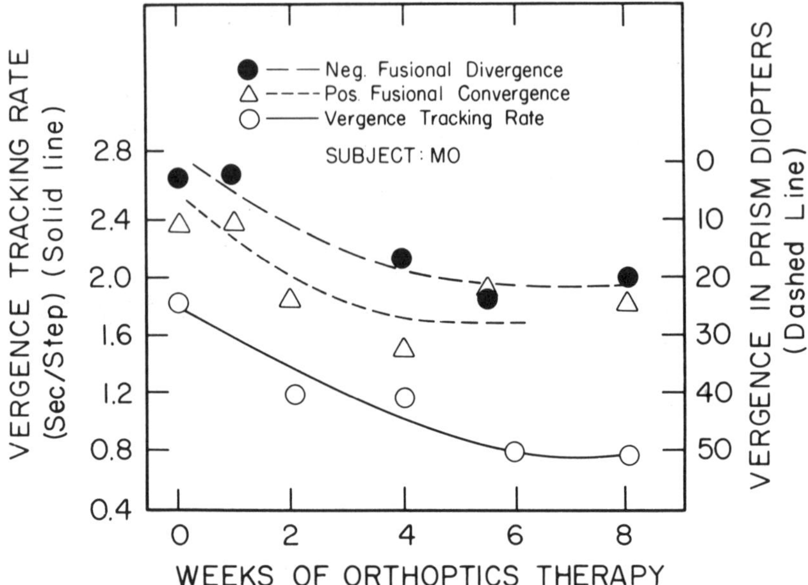

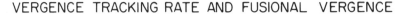

FIGURE 19.6. Changes in Vergence Tracking Rate and Fusional Vergence Ranges with Orthoptics. Subject M.O., an esophore at near, shows changes in the vergence tracking rate which appears to parallel an increase in convergence and divergence fusion ranges as measured with Risley prisms over the course of an orthoptics program. (Chan CL, Grisham JD, 1975)

showed normal tracking rates after four to eight weeks of vergence training at home for approximately 30 minutes per day. A normal rate is defined as successfully tracking a step vergence stimulus changing at the rate of one step per second or faster. In the case of one subject, an esophore at distance and near, increases in Risley prism vergence ranges paralleled changes in the vergence tracking rate over the course of orthoptic training (Figure 19.6).

PRINCIPLES OF CLINICAL TREATMENT

Numerous treatment options become available once it has been established that a dysfunction in vergence eye movements is not related to a systemic or ocular medical condition, to psychological factors, or to medication. In cases of heterophoria and vergence insufficiency, most clinicians prescribe one or more of the following therapy options: (1) prisms, (2) added lenses to alter the heterophoria through the *AC/A* ratio, and

(3) a variety of orthoptic exercises for establishing a higher quality of responses to sensory and motor fusion stimuli. It is assumed here that any significant refractive error has been corrected.

Prescription of Prism

Of all the criteria proposed for determining the amount of prism to prescribe, Sheard's criterion and the fixation disparity prism neutralization (associated phoria) remain the two most widely applied (Sheedy and Saladin, 1977). Both are derived from the relationship between habitual heterophoria for a given fixation distance and amplitude of the compensating vergence. Sheard's criterion, which was empirically determined, declares that the compensating vergence reserve (first sustained blur using Risley prisms) should be at least twice the heterophoria amplitude. If a patient's clinical data fail to satisfy this criterion and the history indicates present or impending symptoms, a prism can be prescribed using the following formula (Borish, 1970):

$$\textit{Sheard prism} = \frac{2(\textit{phoria}) - \textit{compensating vergence}}{3}. \qquad (a)$$

This represents the minimum amount of prism necessary for a patient's clinical data to satisfy Sheard's criterion. For example, if the near point heterophoria is 8^{Δ} exophoria and the compensating vergence (base-out prism to blur point) measures 10^{Δ} base-out, the Sheard prism would be:

$$\frac{2(8) - 10}{3} = 2^{\Delta} \textit{ base-in}. \qquad (b)$$

The associated phoria can be determined using commercially available instruments such as the Bernell unit, Mallett unit, or American Optical Vectographic slides. The patient wears polaroid glasses and judges the vertical and horizontal alignment of two fiducials, each seen monocularly, in a binocular viewing field. Prisms are placed before the eyes to neutralize any misalignment. The smallest amount of prism required to neutralize the disparity can be prescribed if the patient suffers from symptoms of binocular origin and shows other signs of binocular vision dysfunction (Ogle et al., 1967). Clinicians should avoid prescribing prism for any patient whose fixation disparity is independent of other signs and symptoms. Having a small fixation disparity is a normal physiological state for many people (Schor, 1980).

Frequently, patients can indicate the need for a prism prescription by their immediate subjective impression while the prism is held in place, for example, if the print appears clearer or if the eyes feel more comfortable with the prism than without it. The prism base is reversed and the response noted again. Reversing the prism is a control test for the Hawthorne effect where any change is considered an improvement. A prism prescription is indicated when the patient prefers the prism base that is consistent with the heterophoria or direction of fixation disparity in comparison to reversed prism or no prism.

When prescribing spectacle prism a number of optical factors should be considered that will promote proper and rapid spatial adaptation. Generally, large eye sizes should be avoided since the variation in prism thickness results in a spatially distorted image. When prism is base-down the floor appears concave and objects look taller than life. Significant base-up prism generates a convex field distortion as if one were standing on top of a hill (Michaels, 1975).

Prism distortion can be minimized in most prescriptions by steepening the lens base curves to +9.00 diopters or adding +3.00 diopters over stock, whichever is least. The adjusted base curve will not minimize other optical aberrations so that in some cases this adjustment is contraindicated. Adjusted base curves are appropriate for higher prism powers of 3^{Δ} or more per lens.

Prism is generally divided between the eyes to reduce distortions and to balance the weight of the spectacles. An exception is for vertical prism. When prescribing lenses, base-down prism should be avoided or minimized because magnification differences will be greatest in down gaze at the reading angle. Fresnel prism base-up is contraindicated due to a "venetian blind" reflection, where light from above is reflected off the prism bases into the eyes.

Prism adaptation can be expected to occur in several types of patients for whom prism glasses would be inappropriate. The following usually show considerable adaptation: (1) strabismic cases having anomalous retinal correspondence, (2) heterophoric cases where the fixation disparity-forced vergence curve terminates in suppression or diplopia before neutralization occurs, and (3) patients exhibiting a fixation disparity but all other indicators of binocular vision function are normal (Carter, 1980). People having normal binocular vision usually adapt to prism.

Added Lens Therapy

Spectacles or contact lenses can play a twofold role in the management of some binocular vision disorders. They generate clear retinal images that facilitate sensory fusion and they can establish a proper balance between accommodation and convergence, making motor fusion easier. If there is a moderate to high *AC/A* ratio, added spherical lens power beyond that needed for clear imagery can result in improved eye alignment. This of course applies only to patients who show adequate accommodation or to those whose accommodative responses can be sufficiently trained. The practice of prescribing add lenses is well known in the management of strabismics, particularly with accommodative esotropes and divergence excess exotropes. The approach is equally useful for patients with heterophoria with moderate to high *AC/A* ratios.

The question arises, How much added lens power is necessary for proper motor alignment of the eyes? Several methods are available for this computation. For example, consider a divergence excess exotrope, age 12, who while wearing glasses has 18^{Δ} of intermittent exotropia at 6 meters and an 8^{Δ} exophoria at 40 cm. The interpupillary distance measures 60 mm. He complains about reading eye strain and his parents report seeing one of his eyes turning out in the evenings. One method to determine the added lens power would be to calculate the *AC/A* ratio and prescribe lenses that would align the eyes at far and near viewing distances.

$$AC/A = PD\,(\text{cm}) + \frac{near\ deviation(^{\Delta}) - far\ deviation\ (^{\Delta})}{near\ focus\ (\text{D}) - far\ focus\ (\text{D})} \qquad (c)$$

exo: −; eso: +.

Example:

$$AC/A = 6 + \frac{-8^{\Delta} - (-18^{\Delta})}{2.5\ \text{D} - 0} = 6 + 4 = 10^{\Delta}/1\ \text{D}. \qquad (d)$$

Added lenses for distance = −1.75 D (18^{Δ} exo @ D requires −1.75 D add).

Added lenses for near = +1.00 D (if −1.75 D add is given overall, the near phoria changes from 8^{Δ} exo to 10^{Δ} eso, so a +1.00 bifocal is required for near).

The calculated added lenses provide a theoretical estimate, which is a starting point. An empirical prescription is refined with cover test measurements of the distance and near deviations using a variety of added lenses to align the visual axes. Other criteria than eye alignment might serve just as well or better. Added lens power that would bring the eyes into sufficient alignment to satisfy Morgan's norms or Sheard's criterion, or to neutralize the fixation disparity could also be used. It is preferable to prescribe the least amount of added power needed.

A confirmation test of the added lenses can be performed by evaluating the speed of fusional recovery. This is similar to the reflex fusion test discussed earlier. For example, in the case of divergence excess we calculated that a −1.75-D add for distance viewing would be adequate to bring the eyes into alignment. The patient is asked to fixate a distance target while wearing the tentative add in a trial frame or clip-overs. Either eye is occluded with a cover paddle and the patient is engaged in conversation to prevent a conscious vergence movement once the cover is removed. The eye under cover deviates to its dissociated or phoric position. The occluder is casually removed while the patient is speaking and one can judge the immediacy and velocity of the reflex fusion recovery to binocular alignment. If the response is immediate and fast, that amount of added lens power is likely to control the patient's deviation. The least amount of power that results in the maximum vergence response is found. This technique is particularly useful in divergence excess cases, which regress easily and tend to relapse into intermittent exotropia at distance. Most younger patients can adjust to as much as −3.50 diopters of added minus-lens power, if accommodative facility training is prescribed prior to or concurrent with the adaptation period to new lenses.

A significant shift toward myopia has not occurred in our patients wearing added minus lenses, but patients should be monitored for refractive changes as well as for control of deviation over the course of time. The amount of plus add that patients can accept is primarily related to their habitual near working distance. Most must form new near working habits if they are asked to wear a +3.00-diopter or greater add.

Orthoptics

Orthoptic training is often relied on for heterophoric patients to help maintain binocular alignment. Surgery is rarely necessary in the management of even occasional strabismus. In most cases of minimal binocular dysfunction essentially three interrelated processes are trained: sensory fusion, disparity vergence, and accommodation. The basic approach used to enhance sensory fusion and stereopsis is elimination of any suppression. The most effective orthoptics instruments are generally free-space devices that promote the transfer of learned skills to normal viewing conditions and, more important, which have suppression controls for each eye in the target design. The size of the suppression controls should be chosen to match the skill level of the patient. If suppression is deep and extensive, peripheral stimuli larger than 5° in angular extent are appropriate. If the suppression is light and foveal, large stimuli are of little value. In this case monocular details in the binocular field (i.e., suppression controls) should be foveal in extent (less than 1°) to provide some challenge for the patient during attempts to maintain them in the field. When suppression occurs, the clue to the suppressing eye will be perceived to disappear completely or to fade in and out of view. Usually the nondominant eye will manifest suppression, but a monocular control for each eye should be provided since suppression can and often does alternate between the dominant and nonpreferred eyes.

The following steps are involved in antisuppression training that is fundamental to orthoptics:

1. The size of suppression controls should be appropriate for the level of suppression. The suppression indicators should remain in perception most of the time, about 90%, but should also disappear occasionally.
2. When suppression does occur, some temporal stimulus to activate the suppression eye is introduced, for example, rapid blinking, flashing of lights, increasing illumination relative to the suppressing eye, target movement in the suppressed eye's field, and enlarging the target by moving closer.
3. As the control reappears, the patient actively focuses attention on maintaining the control in perception (called mental effort) for 10 seconds or some other specified time before proceeding to the next step. If the suppression control cannot be maintained after reasonable effort, a larger one is chosen to work with.
4. When the suppression clue is maintained for a criterion time, the vergence demand of the targets is increased (e.g., using Risley or loose prisms, sliding vergence targets or altering the fixation distance) and again suppression is monitored. Vergence training is stopped when suppression occurs, and the vergence stimulus is reduced. The suppression clue will reappear.
5. This process is continued until a normal range of fusional vergence, as judged by Morgan's norms or another criterion, is successfully achieved over which there is no suppression.
6. New targets having smaller suppression controls are introduced until the patient demonstrates normal vergence ranges with foveal size suppression clues (less than 1°).

One general principle is to establish sensory fusion prior to training motor fusion (Flom, 1954). Both can be enhanced simultaneously, but priority should be given to the sensory aspects as illustrated in antisuppression training. Motor fusion training itself can be accomplished with a variety of tasks, which should all be included in an orthoptics program.

Sliding Vergence

Fixation and accommodation are directed to the target plane. A disparity vergence stimulus is introduced slowly and smoothly (i.e., Risley prisms, variable vectograms or anaglyphs, amblyoscope, or mirror stereoscope). This is the most widely used technique. Blur, break, and recovery points are increased through repetition and concentration.

Near-Far Tracking

The stimulus is moved smoothly toward and away from the patient. This requires both accurate accommodative and vergence tracking. The patient's goal is to track without momentary double vision or blur from distance fixation to the near point of convergence. A well-known example is the pencil push-up but many free-space targets can be used in this manner (e.g., eccentric circles or vectograms).

Step Vergence

The patient fixates and clearly focuses a target at a fixed distance. A vergence stimulus is introduced in a discrete step, either large or small, by inserting a loose prism before one eye. As soon as the patient fuses and clears the image the prism is removed and refusion is required. The procedure is usually timed for a specified number of cycles and the goal is to increase the step vergence rate. This task is best suited to improve the velocity of the reflex fusion response. Many orthoptics targets have vergence steps incorporated in their design (e.g., most vectograms, anaglyphs, and stereograms) so that a loose prism is not always required.

Near-Far Jumps

In this procedure the patient alternates fixation between targets at different distances. Accommodation and vergence stimuli change together in discrete jumps. The jump duction exercise is a common example. Binocular lens flippers can be used as a variation on this procedure. Jumps or flips are timed and the patient endeavors to increase the rate while continuing an accurate accommodative and convergence response. This technique helps to integrate fusional vergence and accommodative responses and build flexibility in their relationships.

Liu and co-workers (1979) demonstrated that accommodative dynamics, latency, and velocity could be improved with standard orthoptics in patients diagnosed as having accommodative insufficiency. Both clinical data and dynamic optometer recordings confirmed the training effort, although persistence of improvement following completion of the exercises has not yet been investigated. Accommodative insufficiency is commonly associated with vergence deficiency, exophoria, uncorrected myopia, and latent hyperopia. If insufficient focusing responses are identified, accommodative facility training is the initial step recommended in an orthoptics program.

Once the diagnosis has been established, the patient and parents, if appropriate, are given a full description of the condition and its consequences in lay terms. This consultation should make reference to the following points: (1) a complete diagnostic statement, (2) cause of the condition, if known, (3) the consequences if the choice is not to treat, (4) prognosis using all therapy options, and (5) therapy alternatives and their practicality.

When considering an orthoptics program, a number of other issues should be raised. Will an in-office or a home-based program be required? Can the patient commit at least 30 minutes each day for exercises during the anticipated duration of the program? A specific time each day should be set aside when the exercises can be done. How long is the program expected to take and what will it cost? It is preferable to overestimate the length of the program by a few weeks rather than underestimate it. This avoids the unforeseen disappointment of slow progress. Some clinicians recommend a month-to-month commitment where progress and prognosis are reviewed regularly with the patient.

Our clinic prefers to use daily home-based training programs augmented by weekly or biweekly clinic visits. Thirty minutes per day of home training can be broken into two or three short periods distributed conveniently into the patient's schedule. Three exercises are given each week and the patient must demonstrate ability to perform each exercise correctly before terminating the weekly office visit. Printed instructions describing each technique are provided for review at home and a daily report sheet is completed by the patient and returned with each office visit.

Orthoptics patients need to be informed that training exercises will initially exacerbate symptoms. Eye strain, visual fatigue, and headaches are expected to some degree. Rest or mild analgesics usually make the symptoms tolerable. These symptoms usually decrease considerably by the third week of training.

At each office progress visit, the following steps occur:

1. The patient's symptoms and progress with the exercises are reviewed. Emotional support and encouragement are offered to offset the challenge of the program.
2. The patient demonstrates skill and technique doing the previous week's exercises. This affords the clinician an opportunity to offer helpful suggestions and to correct errors in performance.
3. Several standard tests of binocular function are performed to establish the currect diagnosis and to modify the program accordingly. Standard tests include the cover test, fixation disparity neutralization, vergence ranges, accommodative facility, central suppression, and stereopsis. Only appropriate tests for a specific patient need to be monitored regularly.
4. At least one new exercise is included in the weekly assignment of three for the sake of variety if not for functional considerations. As mentioned earlier, the patient must demonstrate the technique correctly

before it is assigned. Specific goals for each exercise are discussed. The goals should neither be too difficult nor too easy to achieve.

Treatment is not always required for cases of binocular insufficiency. There are some cases in which it is advisable simply to reassure the patients, educate them regarding their condition, and advise them to alter the way in which they use their critical vision, for example, taking frequent breaks while reading or avoiding sustained critical viewing in the evening when they are usually tired. This would apply to people for whom glasses and orthoptics are unacceptable or marginally required.

Management of Binocular Insufficiencies

Binocular insufficiencies are minor impairments of binocular vision resulting in asthenopic symptoms, deficient visual performance, or avoidance behavior to prevent onset of symptoms. Conditions include accommodative insufficiency or infacility, large heterophorias at distance or near fixation, convergence insufficiency, fusional vergence deficiencies, and subtle sensory fusion anomalies such as central suppression and reduced stereopsis. These disorders often appear concurrently and are interrelated, but they also may occur in isolation. Some binocular disturbances that are not classed as insufficiencies include manifest strabismus, anomalous retinal correspondence, amblyopia, and nystagmus.

Conditions categorized as binocular insufficiencies may be secondary to a host of precipitating diseases, drugs, and conditions, a partial list of which follows:

1. Blurred or reduced vision
2. Latent hyperopia
3. Aniseikonia
4. Oculomotor paresis
5. Neurologic disorders: cerebral palsy, multiple sclerosis, or myasthenia gravis
6. Endocrine imbalances: diabetes, thyroid
7. Most infectious diseases
8. Certain drugs: birth control pills, steroids, most tranquilizers
9. Systemic toxins: heavy metals, alcohol, etc.
10. Anemia
11. Poor diet
12. General fatigue
13. Visual fatigue
14. Pregnancy
15. Psychogenic stress

All these possible causes should be screened in the history and examination. A primary cause needs to be dealt with prior to or in coordination with any optical or exercise therapy designed to correct the binocular insufficiency. If pathological, drug, and optical factors have been dismissed as possible causes, the etiology can be presumed to be physiological, that is, developmentally immature responses, untrained responses, biological variation, excessive vision requirements, or fatigue. These physiological types have an excellent prognosis for improved function and remission of symptoms.

Accommodative Insufficiency

Signs

A nonpresbyopic accommodative deficiency is indicated by an abnormal reduction of accommodative amplitude. In some cases the near point of accommodation may be seen to regress with repeated measurement (four or five repetitions). Other signs include the report of alternate blurring and clearing while testing the accommodative amplitude or relative accommodation, a low negative and/or positive relative accommodation, and reduced monocular flipper rate.

The monocular flipper norms established at our clinic use the low tail of the first standard deviation as a reference point. For adults, an accommodative deficiency is suspected if the patient takes longer than 90 seconds to complete 20 cycles (40 flips) using ±1.50-diopter lens flippers at 40 cm (Table 19.2). For children grades 4 through 8, a disorder is suspected if 10 cycles of ±2.00-diopter lenses takes longer than 75 seconds while viewing targets at 33 cm with maintained visual attention (Pope et al., 1981).

The flipper test is performed by asking the patient to report "clear" each time a 20/25 print stimulus at near comes into focus through the alternating lenses. The examiner switches the flippers and maintains the correct testing distance. It is often useful to instruct children the meaning of "blurred" and "clear" vision at the beginning of the training period.

TABLE 19.2. Monocular accommodative flipper norms

Subjects	*Mean*	*SD*	*Clinically Significant*
Adults (optometry students) 20 cycles: ±1.50 D flippers @ 40 cm	64 sec	29 sec	> 90 sec
Children (grades 4–8) 10 cycles: ±2.00 D flippers @ 33 cm	52 sec	24 sec	> 75 sec

These monocular flipper norms can be used to compare a particular patient's accommodative skills with population expecteds. (Pope RS, Wong ID, Mah M, 1981)

Two refractive conditions associated with accommodative insufficiency in school-age children that can easily escape detection are latent hyperopia and pseudomyopia. If there is evidence of an accommodative spasm, such as a significant difference between retinoscopy and subjective refraction, a cycloplegic refraction should be performed. This is particularly true for the child who also has difficulty in learning to read. Eames (1937), Young (1963), and many other investigators find a higher prevalence of significant hyperopia in reading-disabled children compared with those who are achieving normally.

Symptoms

Patients may complain of discomfort, intermittent blur, headaches over the eyes, and a burning or a pulling sensation associated with near point activities. These sensations might occur after only a few minutes of reading. One frequent symptom is distance blur for a minute or more after a session of reading. Near point activity has induced a temporary spasm of accommodation.

Treatment

Eye strain due to accommodative insufficiency from any etiology can usually be relieved with a pair of reading glasses or bifocals. The most frequently prescribed added lenses for near range from +1.00 diopter to +1.75 diopters. Base-in prism can be incorporated if there is a significant exophoria induced through the add. Frequently, a patient is given a pair of loaner glasses to take home to wear for a trial period. Thus the effect of reading glasses can be assessed before the final correction is prescribed.

Home orthoptics training to correct a physiological accommodative deficiency usually takes about five weeks of 30-minute daily sessions (Figure 19.7). Symptoms of visual discomfort increase initially with training but by the third week of the program they are usually alleviated. Exercises frequently prescribed include: (1) pencil push-ups emphasizing clarity and working for increased amplitude of accommodation and accuracy of response (complete at least five sets of 20 cycles each day); (2) jump focus with alternate fixation and focus as rapidly as possible between two targets, one distant and the other close to the near point of accommodation; recording the time it takes to complete 20 cycles and trying to improve that time with practice (do at least five sets daily); and (3) monocular and binocular accommodative rock using ±1.00-D flippers initially and then increasing the amount up to ±2.00 diopters in subsequent weeks (complete a minimum of five sets of 20 cycles daily and record the best daily time for 20 cycles).

If the reading glasses and orthoptics do not bring symptomatic relief and improvement of skills within five weeks, the patient is screened again

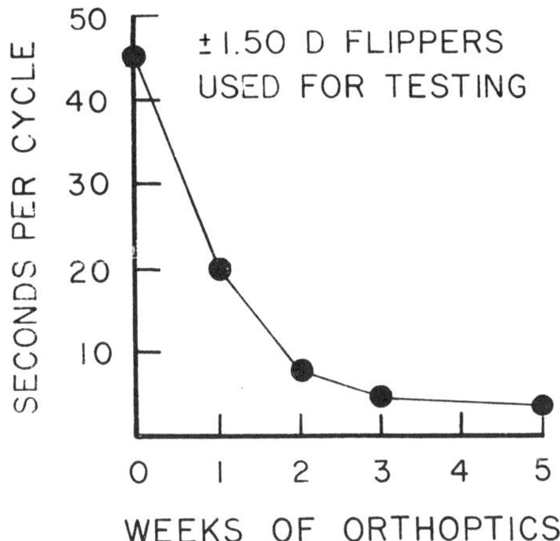

FIGURE 19.7. Change is Lens Flipper Rate with Orthoptics. Patient N.S., age 30, female. DX: Accom. Insufficiency. Accommodative flipper rate improves dramatically in first three weeks of home training (30 min/day), then levels out at a normal level of performance. Changes confirmed by dynamic optometry recordings (Grisham JD, 1978) (Lui J, et al., 1979).

for medical, drug, or psychological causes for the deficiency and referred to the appropriate professional.

Heterophoria and Convergence Insufficiency

Signs

The alternate cover test stands as the single most diagnostic test for large heterophorias at distance or near fixation. Occluding one eye for several minutes will manifest a latent component of the angle of deviation. Fusional and accommodative convergence may not relax immediately on testing and their persistence may mask a large tonic deviation. Comitance in the various fields of gaze should also be checked by a quick alternate cover test, particularly in down gaze where most near point activities take place. Heterophorias that fall outside Morgan's norms (Table 19.1) may present a problem. Other indicators include a fixation disparity that is neutralized by one or more prism diopters and a near point of convergence greater than 10 cm from the nose that regresses on repeated measures. A large exophoria at the reading distance is often associated with a low near point of convergence; however, reduced convergence may also be associated with near esophoria. Excessive demands on the fusional vergence system are often mirrored by deficiencies in sensory fusion. Depressed stereopsis and central suppression may be revealed by foveal size suppression controls.

Symptoms

Many asthenopic symptoms are associated with large heterophorias and convergence insufficiency such as intermittent blurring and doubling of print, eyestrain, tearing, and injection. Esophoric patients tend to report more severe symptoms such as eyestrain and frontal headaches than exophores with the same angle of deviation. Exophores typically complain of sleepiness or visual fatigue associated with concentrated visual tasks. Even a small degree of hyperphoria, 1^{Δ} or 2^{Δ}, can cause eyestrain and nausea. There is a large range of severity and individual differences in symptoms related to a heterophoria condition. For example, some patients with 10^{Δ} and more of hyperphoria can be completely symptom free and otherwise have normal binocular vision.

Treatment

If a high *AC/A* ratio is present, spectacle adds can be used very effectively. In cases of divergence excess exophoria and exotropia (large exodeviation at distance), a minus add can be prescribed overall to reduce the distance exophoria to within normal limits. It may also be necessary to incorporate a plus add bifocal to neutralize any near point esophoria induced by the minus add (see Added Lens Therapy section earlier in this chapter). With cases of convergence excess (large esodeviation at near), the prescription of an appropriate plus add bifocal reduces the esodeviation by relaxing the demand on accommodation for near work. Added plus lenses in reading glasses or bifocals is our preferred treatment opinion in esodeviation cases having a high to moderate *AC/A* ratio.

Spectacle prism is used effectively in cases where a significant heterophoria exists at both far and near fixation distances (i.e., moderate *AC/A* with a tonic vergence disorder). Prisms may also benefit patients having either a high or low *AC/A* ratio, but their prescription should be made with caution. A prism designed for use at a particular fixation distance may be entirely inappropriate for viewing at other distances and may therefore be rejected. In these cases glasses should be designed for a specific use and fixation distance.

Presbyopic exophores may benefit from prism prescribed for their reading distance. Some of these patients exhibit large exophorias at near while wearing their bifocals and experience visual fatigue when reading. Sabado and Louie (1974) examined 12 such patients who were given two pairs of glasses to wear on alternate weeks. One pair had sufficient base-in prism overall to neutralize the near point exofixation disparity. The other glasses had the same correction and frame but had no prism. After a trial wearing period, the patients were asked to choose one pair for their constant wear and return the other. Ten chose the prism glasses. The base-in prisms had induced a significant esophoria at distance for two patients who preferred glasses without prism. Clinicians should be aware of the possible benefits a prism prescription can have for presbyopic patients suffering from reading fatigue. Consideration of binocular vision for this group has often been neglected. In many cases, a little base-in prism in the reading glasses goes a long way to provide visual comfort and efficiency.

Prism prescriptions are recommended for large hyperphorias or smaller hyperdeviations that may accompany a lateral deviation. Clinicians usually prescribe sufficient prism completely to neutralize the hyperdeviation or the amount indicated by the neutralization of fixation disparity. A distinction should be made between vertical deviations under fused and unfused conditions. The vertical deviation may only occur under dissociated conditions manifest during the alternate cover test or Maddox-rod test. One method of making this distinction is to test for a vertical component with the alternate cover test after the horizontal component has been reduced using accommodative convergence stimulated by added lenses. If the vertical deviation disappears it is considered secondary and insignificant.

Orthoptics procedures are usually effective in treating significant lateral heterophorias and intermittent strabismus if the exercises are performed correctly and consistently. Most patients with exophoria and convergence insufficiency can achieve relief from binocular symptoms and show maximum training results in six to eight weeks of home-based orthoptics (30 minutes per day). Esophores typically take longer (8 to 10 weeks) and regress faster after training is discontinued. For this reason, esodeviations should initially receive maximum optical correction (added lenses and prisms) rather than orthoptics. If symptoms and signs of a dysfunction persist, visual training is indicated. Some patients are not disposed to structuring their life to accommodate an orthoptics program, and other therapy options should be offered them.

Fusional Vergence Deficiency

Signs

The traditional method of assessing vergence function is by measuring the vergence ranges (blur, break, and recovery points) using Risley prisms and comparing these results with various criteria, basically, Morgan's, Sheard's, and Percival's (Table 19.1). Another method is to test for a fixation disparity and investigate the fixation disparity-forced vergence curve. Curves having steeper slopes tend to be associated with vergence disorders (Sheedy and Saladin, 1977). Observing the speed of the reflex fusion response is still another way to evaluate vergence function (Grisham, 1980a). Clinicians also examine sensory fusion indicators such as reduced stereopsis and foveal suppression, which may underlie deficient vergence responses. A vergence dysfunction may occur without significant heterophoria, although they are often associated. Some patients have phorias within normal limits yet they have a restricted or narrow zone of clear single binocular vision (i.e., a tight motor zone) and fatigue rapidly with any sustained critical use of their eyes. The narrow zone is frequently associated with a sensory disturbance of binocular vision (Flom, 1954).

One way differentially to diagnose an accommodative infacility from a vergence dysfunction is to compare a patient's binocular ±lens flipper rate to the monocular flipper response. If the monocular rate proves to be within normal limits but the binocular rate is comparatively decreased, one can assume that vergence responses limited the binocular performance. Alternatively, if both monocular and binocular rates fall outside of normal limits and the patient was cooperative, accommodative facility may be the limiting factor or perhaps there is some combined deficiency of accommodation and convergence. The binocular rate is rarely faster than the monocular rate unless there has been some training effect or change in the patient's response criterion or attention.

Symptoms

The symptoms of fusional vergence deficiency are the same as those found with a large heterophoria. Often a minimal binocular dysfunction results from an inadequate relationship between the opposing forces of the heterophoria position and the compensating fusional vergence mechanism as indicated by fixation disparity and Sheard's and Percival's criteria. Symptoms are also inextricably tied to this relationship.

Treatment

Fusional vergence is a readily trainable visual skill (Flom, 1954; Chan and Grisham, 1975) (Figures 19.4 and 19.5). If there is a narrow motor zone or poor reflex fusion response (eyestrain) and if the patient is cooperative, orthoptics is the treatment of choice (Flom, 1954). The home training program (30 minutes per day) rarely takes longer than six weeks for maximum effect and learned skills usually do not quickly regress.

Common exercises given to patients include: (1) pencil push-ups emphasizing singleness, minimum of five sets of 20 push-ups daily; (2) jump ductions building speed of alternation, minimum of five sets of 20 cycles; and (3) loose prism steps increasing speed of reflex fusion response, with a minimum of five sets of 20 cycles for base-in and base-out prisms.

NONSURGICAL MANAGEMENT OF COMITANT STRABISMUS AND ASSOCIATED CONDITIONS

Cosmetic and functional therapeutic approaches to manifest strabismus depend on its etiology, associated conditions, and the patient's attitude regarding his squint. There is no single type of therapy that is best. Patching techniques, orthoptics, and surgery all have the potential to improve or degrade the quality of binocular vision. A good prognosis for functional correction is the best insurance that therapy will be beneficial. The most important factors that determine a favorable prognosis include an intermittent deviation, normal retinal correspondence, comitance, high-quality sensory fusion (stereopsis and no suppression), and motor fusion. Factors that predispose to poor functional prognosis include (1) a constant squint of long duration, (2) anomalous retinal correspondence that does not covary, (3) a noncomitant or variable deviation, (4) nystagmus, (5) moderate to deep amblyopia, and (6) deep suppression. Ideally, therapy should be initiated during early childhood when strabismus develops, so that the sensory consequences of eye misalignment (i.e., amblyopia, anomalous correspondence, and suppression) do not become well established.

The choice of a particular treatment option (i.e., surgery vs orthoptics or prisms vs added lens power) depends somewhat on the clinician's training and experience. There have been relatively few clinical trials that compare the effectiveness of various treatment options. In a literature review of 12 studies, Flax (1968) compared the relative merits of orthoptics and surgery in the treatment of squint. For the types of strabismus that were corrected, the orthoptics approach proved to be superior in providing functional and cosmetic results; however, the question remains as to similarity of case populations that were compared. Surgery is often the treatment of choice for the large and constant deviations, whereas orthoptics is more successful with smaller and intermittent squints. Comprehensive collaborative studies of alternative therapy approaches are urgently needed to establish relative effectiveness of various treatments and to define the patients who benefit most from a particular procedure. In our clinic patients with a favorable prognosis are encouraged to undergo orthoptics therapy, and if little progress is made surgical correction is recommended.

Optical Management

Frequently, correction of a small refractive error in either eye substantially improves the control of an intermittent squint. Similar sharply focused retinal images enhance the quality of sensory fusion and stereopsis, reduce suppression, and provide a strong stimulus to reflex fusional vergence (Flom, 1963). Even cases of constant strabismus, particularly in young children, may resolve themselves following correction of the ametropia (Mohindra, 1977). An accurate refraction is the first order of business in all types of binocular dysfunctions, including strabismus.

As in the treatment of binocular insufficiencies, glasses can serve not only to correct refractive error, but also to promote motor alignment of the eyes and establish better binocular integration. For most esotropes, full correction of manifest hyperopia is essential and any latent hyperopia should be revealed by cycloplegia. Besides a cycloplegic, several dry refractive techniques can be used to relax a spasm of accommodation. For example, the sudden-blur technique yields a hyperopic correction that usually can be tolerated by the patient after a short period of adjustment. The technique is performed after completing the standard subjective refraction. Additional plus is then added, about +0.50 diopters, to blur the 20/20 Snellen line slightly. Retinoscopy lenses (usually +1.50 diopters) are inserted under binocular viewing conditions for approximately 30 seconds. This blurs out the acuity line and should relax a portion of the latent hyperopia. When the retinoscopy lenses are extracted, the patient is asked if the line of print appeared crystal clear, even for a few seconds. If the answer is affirmative, another +0.25-diopter step is introduced to blur slightly the best acuity line again. The technique is repeated as long as the acuity line appears to be clear when retinoscopy lenses are removed. The prescribed hyperopic correction is the last amount of plus lens power that provided clear imagery; however, the prescription may not correspond exactly to the total latent hyperopia. This refractive technique usually does not result in "fogging" glasses, which should be avoided. Blurring distance objects degrades binocular vision and may be rejected by a child. A plus add bifocal can also be prescribed to promote the relaxation of an accommodative spasm while not reducing distance acuity.

If the horizontal angle of convergent strabismus is not too large (greater than 40^{Δ}), bifoveal alignment can be achieved by prescribing added plus lenses. When an esotrope focuses on distance objects there is a relative constant position in space, called the centration point, where the two visual axes cross. Of course, if the patient accommodates for a target placed at the centration point, the nondominant eye is converged additionally by the synkinesis of the AC/A ratio. The amount of added plus lens that would theoretically move the far point to coincidence with the centration point while accommodation is fully relaxed is calculated from the following formula (Flom, 1963):

$$\textit{plus add}(D) = \frac{\textit{angle of strabismus at distance } (^{\Delta})}{\textit{interpupillary distance } (\text{cm})} \qquad \text{(E)}$$

For example, if a constant comitant 24^{Δ} esotrope at distance has a 60-mm interpupillary distance, the plus add needed to align the eyes would be

+4.00 D at a centration point of 25 cm. Note that this add works independent of the AC/A ratio since the near phoria is not considered. This theoretical add can be checked quickly by unilateral cover test using trial lenses and a detailed fixation target at 25 cm. Plus adds resulting in binocular alignment are prescribed in bifocal form in conjunction with fusion training. Active orthoptics training can begin in free space at the centration point. Esotropic patients having anomalous retinal correspondence or a basic lack of fusion usually do not achieve bifoveal alignment using the centration point add. These patients have a residual esodeviation as measured by the unilateral cover test at the centration point. No matter how much add is used, bifoveal fixation is not achieved. In these cases bifocals are inappropriate since they do not completely correct the angle of squint. For example, reduction of an esotropia at near fixation from 40^{Δ} to 20^{Δ} when the patient looks through the lower segment does not promote functional binocular vision.

The effect of minus add lenses on an exotropia, intermittent or constant, should always be considered. As discussed earlier, intermittent exotropia at distance associated with moderate to high AC/A ratios (divergence excess) can often benefit from a minus add addition to the refractive prescription. Minus adds may also be useful with constant exodeviations at all distances associated with normal or even low AC/A ratios. They can be used while the exotropic patient alternately focuses distant and a detailed near point target to ellicit a gross convergence response. We frequently observe large-angle constant exotropes (greater than 50^{Δ}) who can make gross convergence movement after a little practice and achieve momentary bifoveal fixation of a target placed close to their near point of accommodation. A rapid change in accommodative convergence appears to begin the convergence response, which is then completed by reflex fusional vergence. These catalytic fusional skills are used to train exotropes before employing other therapy approaches. Surgeons who are concerned about overcorrecting the exotropia usually prefer that gross convergence exercises not be given immediately prior to surgical correction.

Some clinicians recommend the use of plus adds for near viewing with the divergence excess intermittent exotrope (Cooper, 1977; Flax, 1968). These patients often fuse at near but squint when viewing distance objects. The bifocal results in a similar convergence demand at near and far. The plus add approach may actually train fusional vergence ranges since the add may increase the measured exophoria at near fixation, which in effect increases the demand on the fusional vergence system. As the patient continues to wear these training lenses there may be an improvement in the control of distance exodeviation.

Prescription of ophthalmic prism to correct neuromuscular misalignment of the eyes dates back to the nineteenth century. Application of ophthalmic correction has expanded dramatically with the advent of the wafer-thin Fresnel prism. In addition to correcting strabismus with an excellent prognosis, some clinicians also advocate the use of prisms in treating an abnormal binocular sensory state such as anomalous retinal correspondence (Bagolini, 1966; Maraini and Pasino, 1965). A prerequisite for this therapy is elimination of amblyopia. Prism that overcorrects the esotropia is prescribed initially. This excessive base-out prism results in a slight exotropia as measured by the unilateral cover test. If the esotropia reappears after some time then prism adaptation is indicated and the prism power is increased again to overcorrect the angle of esotropia. After the prism is worn one to two months it is reduced to neutralize the deviation and create "sensory orthophoria," which is believed to promote the development of normal retinal correspondence. This approach is controversial (von Noorden, 1980) and requires verification. It may prove to be of great value in the management of strabismus in infants and young children during the interval between the onset of squint and its correction with either surgery or orthoptics.

During orthoptics therapy of concomitant strabismus with normal correspondence and no amblyopia, glass or Fresnel prisms are prescribed to neutralize the deviation. Orthoptics techniques are then conducted in a free-space environment to improve sensory and motor fusion responses. One key principle of management is to prevent strabismus from appearing during a visual therapy program. Everything possible should be done optically using prisms and added lens power to align the eyes for all viewing distances. If this goal cannot be achieved, one eye should be occluded to prevent the patient from suppressing that eye and reinforcing abnormal binocular sensory adaptations. For example, if a divergence excess exotrope fuses at near but squints at distance even after minus adds have been prescribed, patching the top half of one spectacle may be necessary. Thus fusion is preserved at near and suppression is prevented at distance. Constant complete occlusion should be avoided in cases of heterophoria or intermittent strabismus (Swan, 1947). Occlusion in heterophoria for a portion of the day, or graded occlusion such as with a frosted lens allows for adequate stimulation to maintain binocular alignment while eliminating suppression and other sensory obstacles to binocular vision.

Amblyopia

When sight of one eye is obstructed during the first five years of life, any resulting decrease in visual acuity that remains after correction of refractive error is called amblyopia, meaning "dullness of vision." The receptive field organization of the retina, particularly the fovea, has a coarser structure in amblyopic eyes than is normal (Meur et al., 1968). Uncorrected anisometropia and constant squint during early childhood are the most common causes of visual form deprivation and binocular inhibition culminating in amblyopia of the deprived eye.

A major obstacle to effective management of amblyopia is the common misconception that it cannot be treated successfully after the age of six years. This concept has been challenged by Birnbaum, Koslowe, and Sanet (1977) who analyzed the results of 23 published studies that provided sufficient acuity and age information to permit comparison of the success rate of amblyopia therapy achieved in patients under age seven years and over (Table 19.3). They used two criteria for success: improvement of four or more lines in acuity and achievement of 20/30 acuity or better. The total sample size was over 1,000 amblyopes. There proved to be no significant difference in the success rate between the two age groups using either criterion.

Seventeen studies were further analyzed into four age categories: under 7 years, 7 to 10 years, 11 to 15 years, and 16 years and older. No real differences appeared except in those age 16 years and older, which showed a lower success rate only by the first criterion. There only seems to be a slight age factor related to success of therapy. This difference is not unexpected since many difficult cases that persist beyond childhood are included in the population of older amblyopes, whereas the less severe

TABLE 19.3. Success of amblyopia therapy as a function of age at treatment

		Under 7 yr		*7 yr and over*	
		No.	%	No.	%
Criterion A	Success	110	52.1	429	53.8
	Failure	101	47.9	369	46.2
	Totals	211	100	798	100
Criterion B	Success	121	36.3	263	33.0
	Failures	212	63.7	535	67.0
	Totals	333	100	798	100

Source: Birnbaum et al., 1977.

Combined results of amblyopia therapy from 23 studies, comparing results achieved by patients under 7 and 7 years and older. Results are analyzed separately for improvement in acuity of 4 lines or better (Criterion A) and for improvement to 20/30 or better (Criterion B). Differences in results for the 2 age groups are not statistically significant (chi-square test: $P > 0.05$). Reprinted by permission of the publisher, from Birnbaum MH, Koslowe K, Sanet R. Success in amblyopia therapy as a function of age: a literature survey. American Journal of Optometry and Physiological Optics, 1977.

cases are treated successfully at younger ages. The success rate in this older group was 41.9%, which indicates that amblyopes should not be deprived of the possible benefit of therapy solely on the basis of age.

In general, the earlier amblyopia therapy is initiated the faster visual acuity and monocular fixation improve (Parks and Friendly, 1966). Even though therapy with adults is often successful, early detection and treatment cannot be overstressed. Once a child enters school and is beyond the watchful eyes of the parents, compliance with patching and wearing glasses frequently falls off. Considering the prevalence of amblyopia and squint, about 2% and 4% respectively, all infants should undergo a thorough vision examination before the age of one year, particularly if there is a history of strabismus in the family. To screen adequately for visual defects that could lead to visual deprivation, a minimum of four procedures should be done: (1) a complete case and family history, (2) an objective measure of the refractive error (Mohindra, 1977), (3) distance and near point cover tests for oculomotor deviations, and (4) a thorough internal health examination of the eyes. When the family history reveals other family members who have strabismus or amblyopia it is prudent to examine the child again at or about age three years to guard against late onset of strabismus.

Amblyopia has both sensory and motor aspects that need attention during a therapy program. The sequence of treatment objectives is (1) to establish steady foveal monocular fixation, (2) to improve monocular acuity maximumly (a functional success is considered to be 20/40 Snellen line acuity or better), and (3) to eliminate suppression and promote binocular sensory fusion and stereopsis.

Since its introduction by de Buffon in 1743, patching the dominant eye has become the mainstay of therapy. Not only does occlusion force the use of the amblyopic eye, but it removes the inhibitory effect of the normal eye under binocular viewing conditions. The most effective type is a piece of adhesive gauze (elastoplast) that is applied directly over an eye. Patches that attach to glasses are easily discarded or avoided by enterprising children. Tincture of benzoin can be applied topically before occluding a child who has sensitive skin. A hypoallergenic patch such as Opticlude is also effective in these cases.

Inverse occlusion (patching the amblyopic eye) has been advocated by Bangerter (1960) and others in cases of eccentric fixation to avoid reinforcing the use of the eccentric point and to provide the patient the benefit of sight with the normal eye. This is most often used in conjunction with active daily visual training (localization and fixation control with the amblyopic eye). Von Noorden (1965) has compared the relative effectiveness of direct and inverse occlusion. Direct patching is most effective for young children under the age of six (VerLee and Iacobucci, 1967); however, visual requirements of school (and the workplace for adults) may necessitate the use of inverse occlusion for at least part of the day.

Direct occlusion can be expected to improve acuity in four to six weeks or sooner for preschoolers. If no improvement occurs or if the fixation remains eccentric, inverse occlusion, active orthoptics training, or pleoptics should be conducted. Therapy, including patching, should continue for about six weeks beyond the last measurable improvement in acuity before the patient is dismissed. Ideally, binocular alignment and sensory fusion should be established to maintain the improved acuity and fixation. This is not always possible, particularly in strabismic amblyopia.

If a squint remains after amblyopia therapy, the patient should be taught to alternate fixation habitually for different distances or fields of gaze. Otherwise, occasional patching of the dominant eye (about two to three days a month) will be required indefinitely to preserve the improved acuity. If binocular vision has been achieved, then simple antisuppression activities can be used periodically to prevent regression. Anaglyphic or polaroid television trainers and reading bars are particularly suited for this purpose.

In the 1940s Bangerter coined the term pleoptics, meaning full vision, to describe his methods of active therapy of amblyopia with eccentric fixation. A bleaching light is projected onto the fundus while the fovea is shielded with a disc. The macula is then intermittently stimulated with flashes of light that are intended to eliminate foveal inhibition and promote central fixation (Bangerter, 1955). Cüpper's method uses the same bleaching procedure as Bangerter to decrease the physiological superiority of the eccentric fixation position over the fovea. In Cüpper's process, a negative afterimage is generated that identifies for the patient the location of the fovea in the free-space environment. Using this foveal tag the patient learns to make rapid, accurate saccadic movements and maintain steady fixation of designated targets placed about the room. Unfortunately, generation of the foveal afterimage in the amblyopic eye requires expensive and elaborate instrumentation as well as pupil dilation for each session. These constraints limit the utility of Cüpper's method for the private practitioner. This application has been limited in recent years to the most intractable cases where the amblyopia is unusually profound, the eccentric fixation ingrained, and conventional methods have proved ineffective.

Most cases of amblyopia can be adequately managed with a combination of patching and fixation training procedures. Other foveal tags can be used independent of bleaching the eccentric point. For example, the afterimage transfer technique is practical for home training with cooperative children over the age of five (Caloroso, 1972). A line afterimage is generated using an electronic flash attachment for a camera that has been masked with a slit aperture. After the dominant eye is flashed, it is held closed by the patient to ensure a proper afterimage transfer to the fovea of the amblyopic eye (Wick, 1974a). A blinking light will intensify the transferred afterimage. The patient maintains the position of the foveal tag on a suprathreshold target while counting outloud as long as the tag remains on the target. Some specified time is set as a goal, for example, 30 seconds, before fixation is directed to a smaller and more demanding target. The speed and accuracy of fixation can be improved with a series of suprathreshold and threshold acuity targets placed about the room. The patient is encouraged to make quick saccades from one target to another in synchrony with the beat of a metronome or within a specified time period. A Haidinger brush or Maxwell spot can also be used effectively as a foveal tag while employing the same basic procedures. Any demanding tasks or games involving hand-eye coordination with or without the use of a foveal tag may have training value. Children and adults usually respond to training programs with enthusiasm when required to perform such tasks as playing TV-pong, stringing small beads, throwing darts, tracing pictures, connecting dot-to-dot patterns, and the like using only the amblyopic eye.

The history of amblyopia therapy is replete with techniques and instruments that initially burst onto the scene and generate considerable enthusiasm. With time and experience they often yield a measure of disappointment. The CAM therapy is the most recent example of this scenario. Based on exposing the amblyopic eye to rotating grating patterns of various spatial frequencies for short durations, it does not appear to offer any advantages over direct patching for short durations, as has been found recently by a number of controlled studies (see review by Schor et al., 1981). Many clinicians are losing their enthusiasm for this approach.

In contrast, considerable interest has recently surfaced surrounding another new therapy, the application of auditory biofeedback to training accurate fixational eye movements. Flom, Kirschen, and Bedell (1980) noted remarkably fast improvements in the fixation pattern and acuity of amblyopes using auditory biofeedback in an experiment designed to measure the distribution of acuity with eccentricity from the fovea in amblyopic eyes. This technique is currently used in our clinic for selected patients. Auditory biofeedback gives a patient information about where the eye is pointing and how steady it is. An unpleasant noise associated with errors of fixation provides an incentive to hold correct fixation on a target as quickly as possible. Oculomotor biofeedback holds many possible applications for improving orthoptics techniques. It is a new field of very active clinical investigation that remain to be tested by clinical trial.

When the amblyopic eye's acuity improves to about 20/60, orthoptics procedures are undertaken to restore binocular vision and eliminate anomalous retinal correspondence and suppression. If binocularity cannot be achieved, acuity and fixation patterns of the amblyopic eye are maximumly improved and the patient is given continued treatments that will maintain the results of monocular therapy.

Anomalous Retinal Correspondence

The presence of anomalous retinal correspondence (ARC) is a factor that significantly influences the prognosis for a functional cure of strabismus. In anomalous correspondence the two foveas do not have the same oculocentric directional value. If the foveas of a patient were stimulated simultaneously, this patient would perceive diplopia. This integrative projection anomaly occurs in developmental strabismus and preserves some degree of binocular vision. Most strabismic patients showing ARC have the harmonious type in which the dominant eye's fovea and a theoretical point, the image point, in the turned eye have the same visual direction under binocular conditions. Even though patients with ARC are strabismic, they do not experience double vision, and can have 100 seconds of stereopsis along with slow fusional vergence eye movements.

Investigators generally agree that ARC associated with a constant convergent squint has a poor functional prognosis but that it is not a serious factor in intermittent strabismus. As previously noted, when the intermittent squinters make fusional vergence movements to straighten their eyes, covariation occurs and correspondence shifts to bifoveal projection as the eyes reach alignment (Morgan, 1961; Kerr, 1968). Positive fusional vergence movements are relatively strong and trainable. Some constant exotropes can be taught to straighten their eyes and initiate covariation so that ARC is not always a major stumbling block to successful therapy of exotropia. It is usually a negative sign in esotropia since voluntary fusional divergence eye movements are extremely limited.

Flom Swing Technique

In 1968 Flom developed a technique using an amblyoscope to stimulate fusional divergence and covariation in small-angle constant esotropes showing ARC. This is now referred to as the Flom swing, or covariation technique. Our clinic's functional success rate with patients who qualify for the procedure is 30%, which is very high for this category of patient (Grisham, 1980b). Conventional ARC therapy (the Chavasse technique) is least effective for these small-angle esotropes. The covariation technique works quickly if it works at all—in 10 sessions or less. No home training or patching is required. Usually by the second or third session the outcome can be accurately predicted and patients not showing response can be dismissed from further therapy.

A third-degree target having stereoscopic stimuli and suppression controls (e.g., a slide picturing a swing that is seen in depth when fused) is placed at the patient's subjective angle as measured on an amblyoscope under conditions of dim room illumination. A bright, rapid alternate flash (8 Hz) helps to enhance the stereopsis and break through any suppression (Schor et al., 1975). The patient's task is to maintain fusion of the swing target as the amblyoscope arms are diverged very slowly, 1° to 2° per minute, through the entire angle of strabismus. If fusion is broken or suppression occurs the angle is reduced slightly so that the correct perception can again be achieved. After several treatments many small-angle esotropes can straighten their eyes with the amblyoscope. There is a feeling of eyestrain if this has been done correctly. The patient holds the sensation of eyestrain while moving out of the instrument into free space as the room illumination is slowly increased. If the technique is successful the eyes remain straight, covariation has resulted in normal correspondence, and the patient reports markedly improved stereopsis. When moving out of the instrument, some patients immediately lapse back into the strabismic position and the technique needs to be repeated numerous times to build control.

After therapy, patients are considered to be completely cured if they have an esophoria and nearly 40 seconds of stereoacuity. Some patients exhibit a small eso flick during the unilateral cover test (Alvarez, Grisham, 1979) and reduced but improved stereopsis. These results are considered a partial success. To qualify for treatment a patient should have an angle of deviation of 20^{Δ} or less, harmonious anomalous correspondence, concomitance, and corrected visual acuities of 20/40 or better in each eye. Wick (1974) has written a thorough description of the technique and presented a case report for illustration. We have also used it for constant exotropes having ARC and as an additional procedure to build fusional ranges in normally corresponding strabismic patients.

Most clinicians consider anomalous retinal correspondence to be a sensory adaptation, developed over time in response to an early childhood strabismus (von Noorden, 1980). This new sensory coordinate system for binocular visual direction uses the fovea of the dominant eye and the target point of the turned eye as the straight ahead reference points rather than combining information from the two foveas into a single visual direction as in normal retinal correspondence. The classical technique for retraining normal retinal correspondence (NRC) involves patching an eye to prevent reinforcement of the anomalous binocular correspondence and to stimulate the foveas intensely with targets viewed binocularly until normal bifoveal correspondence occurs. Specifically, a series of first-degree and second-degree fusion targets is rapidly flashed on an amblyoscope aligned to the objective angle of deviation. The patient initially sees the targets in different locations since the foveas do not correspond in directional value but eventually (often several months) the targets may appear fused. Patients frequently report an interesting transition response where the targets are seen simultaneously as fused and in different directions (binocular triplopia).

For a complete description of the Chavasse technique refer to Lyle and Wybar (1967) and Wick (1975). It requires a high level of patient cooperation and extensive training. Frequently the chance of success is too low to merit the required effort.

Sensory and Motor Fusion Orthoptics

The objectives of this therapy sequence are essentially the same as in treating binocular insufficiency—clear single comfortable binocular vision during all waking hours. Specifically, training should be directed toward normalizing the following functions: (1) monocular and binocular accommodative facility as indicated by the lens flipper test, (2) good monocular acuities tested under binocular conditions such as with a Turville slide, (3) a base-in and base-out range of prism vergence equal to or greater than Morgan's norms, (4) no foveal suppression over the range of prism vergence, (5) zero associated phoria at all normal fixation distances and fields of gaze, (6) high quality of reflex fusion responses to small increments of base-in and base-out prisms (4^{Δ} to 6^{Δ}), and (7) the maximum stereoacuity possible, preferably 40 seconds of arc or better. These functions should all be surveyed periodically during therapy to update the prognosis and modify training.

If bifoveal fixation and rudimentary sensory fusion have been achieved at some point in real space using a combination of prism glasses, adds, or an active fusional vergence response, and if visual acuity is at least 20/60 in each eye, orthoptics can proceed with a good prognosis for functional correction. These cases respond well to free-space techniques and home-based training. When a squint is present at all distances, despite attempts to correct it optically, the prognosis for functional correction is reduced and a substantial amount of work with clinical instruments becomes necessary.

We have found the following free-space techniques to be valuable for rapid correction of conditions with a good prognosis for functional correction of binocular vision.

Red Lens-Prism Technique

This free-space technique is used to break through deep suppression, obtain pathological diplopia, and establish basic sensory fusion. Since there is a chance of inducing intractable diplopia, care should be taken in selecting patients for this procedure. Preference should be given to those having normal retinal correspondence and a good prognosis for a complete functional cure of strabismus. A combined hand-held red lens and loose prism is placed before the suppressing eye. The prism power should equal the angle of deviation and the prism base should be consistent with the squint direction (i.e., base-out for esotropia). Suppression is reduced and diplopia is stimulated with a bright fixation light in a darkened room. The red lens-prism combination is rotated to introduce a large vertical separation of the images. The eyes are covered alternately to demonstrate for the patient the two separate images, one red, the other white. Under binocular conditions, the patient is encouraged to maintain both images in view as long as possible. If one image should disappear, it can be renewed with vigorous blinking. Pathological diplopia can also be stimulated by moving the suppressed image with a continuously rotating prism or by having the patient sit closer to the fixation light and increase the size of the retinal image displacements. When the patient learns to maintain vertical diplopia the prism is rotated into a horizontal position to elicit a sensory fusion response; this is indicated by the perception of a single fused pink light or white light surrounded by a red glow. After training stable sensory fusion, low-power loose prisms (2^{Δ} to 6^{Δ}) can be interposed to develop the quality of reflex motor fusional vergence responses. Increasing room illumination makes the task more difficult.

Physiological Diplopia (Brock String and Beads)

This traditional procedure is designed to eliminate suppression. It allows the patient to monitor the state of sensory fusion during training. One end of a string is tied to a distant object and the other end is held close to the patient's nose along the midline. A bead is placed on the string at a point where fusion is possible. For esotropes using an appropriate plus add, this is usually the centration point. Exotropes must align their eyes on the bead using voluntary fusional vergence. A second bead is positioned at approximately one foot in front of the first bead so that when one bead is bifixated the other appears double because it falls outside the singleness horopter.

The correct physiological diplopia response is indicated when the patient reports seeing the fixation bead as single, the other bead as double, and the string forming an image of an X with the fixation bead at the intersection. If one string, or a Y, is reported or both beads appear single under binocular viewing conditions, suppression is suspected. The anti-suppression techniques of rapid blinking, increasing illumination of the suppressed bead, or movement of the string can readily be applied. In cases of deep suppression, pen lights or candles flickering in a dimly illuminated room can be substituted for the beads. When a physiological diplopia response can be maintained easily, motor fusion tasks such as jump ductions, loose prism steps, or bead push-up and push-away can be introduced. The patient monitors sensory fusion using the string and beads as a check against suppression. As sensory and motor fusion skills develop, the beads are shifted to distances away from the centration point, which requires higher levels of vergence control.

Mirror Stereoscope-Cheiroscope

The Javal folding mirror stereoscope is a free-space instrument that places targets at 33 cm along the strabismic angle of deviation so that sensory and motor fusion responses can be trained readily. Suppression can be controlled by changing the target size and adjusting the relative illumination between the two eye fields. Fusional vergence stimuli can be introduced in several ways. If training is to be effective with this instrument the patient must demonstrate normal retinal correspondence.

A large variety of instruments and techniques can be used effectively at this stage of strabismus therapy. If there exists some point in real space where the patient exhibits basic sensory and motor fusion the case can often be treated much like a binocular insufficiency as reviewed earlier. In addition to the Javal folding mirror, a partial list of appropriate training instruments includes vectograms, television trainers, reading bars, eccentric circles, aperture rule trainers, and Brewster stereoscopes[1] (see Griffin, 1976 for complete review). Amblyoscope therapy is needed in only the most difficult cases having a guarded prognosis.

The primary function of eye muscle surgery is to change the muscles' mechanical advantage to correct the strabismus without impairing ocular motility. Noncosmetic squints and heterophoria rarely require surgery but a surgical consultation is advisable in cases of cosmetic squints, where functional prognosis is poor, and in noncomitant deviations, where comfortable single binocular vision has not been satisfactorily achieved through visual therapy. In such cases close cooperation with a skilled surgeon cannot be overemphasized.

Horizontal strabismus starts to become cosmetically conspicuous when the angle of deviation exceeds 15^{Δ} to 20^{Δ}, and in the case of vertical deviations about 10^{Δ}. In borderline cases spectacle-yoked prisms often improve cosmetic aspects. For example, unilateral constant esotropes may benefit from prism placed base-out before the dominant eye. The prism directs the visual axis toward the nose and the strabismic eye moves conjugately outward. Base-in prism placed before the strabismic eye displaces the image of the turned eye temporally and further improves the

[1] The largest distributors of orthoptics instruments are Bernell Corporation, 422 E. Monroe St., South Bend, IN 46601; and Keystone View, 2212 E. 12th St. Davenport, IA 52803.

patient's appearance. Yoked prisms of various powers should be tested empirically to determine the optimum amounts.

What constitutes a functional correction of a squint? Flom's criterion is frequently quoted as a standard in the literature (Borish, 1970). A complete functional cure has the following characteristics:

1. Clear, comfortable, single binocular vision must be present at all distances up to a normal near point of convergence.
2. Stereopsis and a normal range of motor fusion.
3. An occasional squint (not exceeding 1% of the time) may be present provided diplopia occurs when the eye turns.
4. Spectacle lenses incorporating up to 5^{Δ} of prism may be worn if necessary.

The almost-cured category differs from the above in that stereopsis is not required, a squint may be present up to 5% of the time, and large amounts of prism may be used to maintain comfortable binocular vision.

Using Flom's criterion Ludlam and Kleinman (1965) investigated the persistance of a strabismus cure using orthoptics therapy. They reexamined 81 cured patients three to seven years after dismissal from training and found that 89% qualified for one of the two cure categories. These authors observed that patients who initially fell into the almost-cured category after training tended either to become complete functional cures or to drop into a Flom failure category over the intervening years. This suggests that a high level of sensory and motor fusion skills must be achieved to maintain long-range functional binocularity. Simple instruments such as television trainers, reading bars, loose prisms, and vectograms are routinely dispensed to dismissed patients for weekly monitoring of foveal suppression and reflex fusional vergence. If a deficiency is discovered, a short binocular insufficiency training program again brings these physiological indicators up to the high criterion of binocular vision.

Applications of Biofeedback

Although the idea is not new, application of biofeedback techniques to training of ocular motility has been an active area of clinical research during the last few years. Letourneau (1976) pointed out that clinicians have always given feedback to patients undergoing orthoptics by indicating success or failure on a particular procedure. Correct behavior is reinforced verbally, which in turn builds the patient's motivation to succeed further. Biofeedback is fundamentally an efficient means of giving patients immediate information regarding their performance; thus errors can be corrected without much loss of time and motivation remains high.

Letourneau and Ludlam (1976) demonstrated some of these advantages in a case report involving a limitation of gaze. Their patient made no progress using standard orthoptics techniques, but with biofeedback a significant expansion of motility was achieved.

Some types of vergence cases respond to biofeedback orthoptics. Several investigators are exploring the usefulness of this application. Manny (1980) demonstrated a vergence training effect in three subjects having clinically normal binocular vision. Hirons and Yolton (1978) used auditory biofeedback as the exclusive treatment in three strabismic cases. An intermittent exotrope and a constant small-angle esotrope achieved alignment and nearly normal sensory and motor fusion functions. Two years later, without further training, the esotrope remained straight but the exotrope lapsed back into intermittent deviation. A third case, a large exotrope having a dense unilateral cataract, was remarkable in that the patient succeeded in reducing the angle of deviation by 10^{Δ} in eight weeks of daily therapy, although alignment was not achieved.

In a follow-up study Van Brocklin and associates (1981) matched seven pairs of strabismic patients and included auditory biofeedback techniques as part of the office visual therapy for one member of each pair while the other member received traditional orthoptics. In five of the seven pairs the biofeedback member achieved the training objectives faster than did the control, but biofeedback demonstrated no particular advantage in the remaining cases. Based on patient observations the authors suggested that biofeedback should be applied prior to traditional training in a concentrated block of time rather than integrated with it. As might be expected, biofeedback orthoptics appears to be more effective with intermittent strabismus compared to constant deviations (also see Goldrich, 1982).

Inverso and Larsen (1981) applied auditory biofeedback orthoptics to 12 well-documented strabismic patients. Five of seven intermittent exotropes achieved a Flom criterion cure with daily treatment sessions ranging from 6 to 20 weeks ($\bar{x}$ = 12 weeks). There were also four patients with constant squint and an intermittent esotrope who did not reach the Flom criterion, but some did show reduction in their angle of strabismus.

Another promising application has been in training accommodation (Cornsweet and Crane, 1973). Trachtman (1978) described an interesting case of a 30-year-old man showing a spasm of accommodation resulting in functional myopia. An infrared optometer was used to monitor the refractive state and that information was converted into an auditory signal and feedback to the patient over stereophones. With practice, the report indicates the patient reduced the myopia by 0.50 to 1.00 diopter.

Several other types of oculomotor training using biofeedback techniques are being investigated. There are reports of some success using it with amblyopes (Flom et al., 1980; Schor and Hallmark, 1978), in cases of nystagmus (Abadi et al., 1980; Ciuffreda et al., 1980; Ciuffreda et al., 1982), and ocular pursuits (Letourneau and Ludlam, 1976). This therapy option appears to be expanding as new applications are found and as data support its use with selected patients.

REFERENCES

Abadi RV, Carden D, Simpson J. A new treatment for congenital nystagmus. Br J Ophthalmol 1980;64:2–6.

Alvarez S, Grisham JD. Orthoptics for the elderly: a case of microtropia. Rev Optom 1979;116(5):37–38.

Bagolini B. Postsurgical treatment of convergent strabismus. Int Ophthalmol Clin 1966;6:633.

Bangerter A. Die okklusion in der pleoptik und orthoptik. Klin Monatsbl Augenheilkd 1960;136:305.

Birnbaum MH, Koslowe K, Sanet R. Success in amblyopia therapy as a function of age: a literature survey. Am J Optom Physiol Opt 1977;54(5):269–75.

Borish IM. Clinical refraction. 3rd ed. Chicago: Professional Press, 1970:910.

Caloroso E. After-image transfer: a therapeutic procedure for amblyopia. Am J Optom Physiol Opt 1972;49(1):65–69.

Carter DB. Parameters of fixation disparity. Am J Optom Physiol Opt 1980; 57(9):610–17.

Chan CL, Grisham JD. Objective verification of fusional vergence orthoptics. OD thesis, School of Optometry, University of California, Berkeley, 1975.

Ciuffreda K, Goldrich S, Neary C. Use of eye movement auditory biofeedback in the control of nystagmus. Am J Optom Physiol Opt 1982;59(5):396–409.

Ciuffreda, KJ, Goldrich S, Neary C. Auditory biofeedback as a potentially important new tool in the treatment of nystagmus. Am J Optom Assoc 1980;51(6):615–17.

Cooper J. Intermittent exotropia of the divergence excess type. Am J Optom Physiol Opt 1977;40(10):1261–73.

Cooper J, Feldman J. Operant conditioning of fusional convergence ranges using random dot stereograms. Am J Optom Physiol Opt 1980;57(4):205–13.

Cornsweet TN, Crane HD. Research note: training the visual accommodation system. Vision Res 1973;13:713–15.

Daum KM. The course and effect of vision training on the vergence system. Am J Optom Physiol Opt 1982;59(3):223–27.

Eames TH. A frequency study of physical handicaps in reading disability and unselected groups. J Educ Res 1937;29:1–5.

Flax N. Training intermittent exotropes. San Jose Vision Training Seminar, 1968.

Flom MC. The use of accommodative convergence relationship in prescribing orthoptics. Penn Optometrist 1954;14(3).

Flom MC. Treatment of binocular anomalies of vision. In: Hirsch MJ, Wick RE, eds. Vision of children. Philadelphia: Chilton Book Co., 1963:197–228.

Flom MC, Kirschen DG, Bedell HE. Control of unsteady eccentric fixation in amblyopic eyes by auditory feedback of eye position. Invest Ophthalmol Visual Sci 1980;17(11):1371–81.

Goldrich S. Oculomotor biofeedback therapy for exotropia. Am J Optom Physiol Opt 1982;59(4):306–17.

Griffin J. Binocular anomalies, procedures for vision therapy. Chicago: Professional Press, 1976.

Grisham JD. A short program for accommodative insufficiency. Rev Optom 1978;35.

Grisham JD. The dynamics of fusional vergence eye movements in binocular dysfunction. Am J Optom Physiol Opt 1980a;57(9):645–55.

Grisham JD. Treatment of small angle esotropes with anomalous correspondence. Paper presented to American Academy of Optometry, December, 1980b; Chicago.

Hirons R, Yolton RL. Biofeedback treatment of strabismus: case studies. J Am Opt Assoc 1978;49(8):875–82.

Hugonnier R, Hugonnier SC. Strabismus, heterophoria, ocular motor paralysis. St. Louis: CV Mosby, 1969:131.

Inverso M, Larsen T. Biofeedback-enhanced vision training for strabismus. OD thesis, Pacific University College of Optometry, Forest Grove, Oregon, 1981.

Kerr KE. Instability of anomalous retinal correspondence. J Am Optom Assoc 1968;39(12):1107–08.

Letourneau JE. Applications of biofeedback and behavior modification techniques in visual training. Am J Optom Physiol Opt 1976;53(4):187–90.

Letourneau JE, Ludlam WM. Biofeedback reinforcement in the training of limitation of gaze: a case report. Am J Optom Physiol Opt 1976;53(10):672–76.

Liu J et al. Objective assessment of accommodative orthoptics. I. Dynamic insufficiency. Am J Optom Physiol Opt 1979;56(5):285–94.

Ludlam W, Kleinman B. The long range results of orthoptic treatment of strabismus. Am J Optom Physiol Opt 1965;42(11):647–84.

Lyle K, Wybar K. Lyle and Jackson's practical orthoptics. In: The treatment of squint. 5th ed. Springfield, Ill.: Charles C Thomas, 1967:205–59.

Manny RE. Monocular vergence movements produced by external visual feedback. Am J Optom Physiol Opt 1980;57(4):236–44.

Maraini G, Pasino L. Development of normal binocular vision in early convergent strabismus after orthophoria. Br J Ophthalmol 1965;49:154.

Meur G, Payan M, Vola J. Determination Indirecte de la Dimension des Champs Receptifs Retiniens de l'amblyope au Moyen Grilles de Hermann. Bull Soc Belge Ophthalmal 1968;150:615.

Michaels DD. Visual optics and refraction. St. Louis: CV Mosby, 1975:75.

Mohindra I. A non-cycloplegic refraction technique for infants and young children. J Am Opt Assoc 1977;48(4):518–23.

Morgan MW. Anomalous correspondence interpreted as a motor phenomenon. Am J Optom Physiol Opt 1961;38(3):131–48.

Ogle KN, Martens T, Dyer J. Oculomotor imbalance in binocular vision and fixation disparity. Philadelphia: Lea & Febiger, 1967.

Parks MM, Friendly DS. Treatment of eccentric fixation in children under 4 years of age. Am J Ophthalmol 1966;61(3):395–99.

Pope RS, Wong JD, Mah M. Accommodative facility testing in children: norms and validation. OD thesis, School of Optometry, University of California, Berkeley, 1981.

Rashbass C, Westheimer G. Independence of conjunctive and disjunctive eye movements. J Physiol 1961;159(2):361–64.

Sabado F, Louie S. The prescription of prism in presbyopic exophoria. OD thesis, School of Optometry, University of California, Berkeley, 1974.

Schor CM. Fixation disparity, a steady state error. Am J Optom 1980;57(9):619–31.

Schor CM, Hallmark W. Slow control of eye position in strabismic amblyopia. Invest Ophthalmol Visual Sci 1978;77–81.

Schor CM, Terrell M, Peterson D. Contour interaction and temporal masking in strabismus amblyopia. Am J Optom 1975;53:217–23.

Schor CM, Gibson J, Hsu M, Mah M. The use of rotating gratings for the treatment of amblyopia: a clinical trial. Am J Optom Physiol Opt; (in press).

Sheedy JE, Saladin JJ. Phoria, vergence, and fixation disparity in oculomotor problems. Am J Optom Physiol Opt 1977;54(7):474–78.

Swan KC. Esotropia following occlusion. Arch Ophthalmol 1947;37(4):444–51.

Trachtman JN. Biofeedback of accommodation to reduce functional myopia: a case report. Am J Optom Physiol Opt 1978;55(6):400–406.

Van Brocklin M, Vasche T, Hirons R, Yolton R. Biofeedback enhanced strabismus therapy. J Am Opt Assoc 1981;52(9):731–36.

VerLee D, Iacobucci I. Pleoptics versus occlusion of the sound eye. Am J Ophthalmol 1967;63(2):244–50.

von Noorden G. Burian and von Noorden's binocular vision and ocular motility. 2nd ed. St. Louis: CV Mosby Co., 1980:430.

von Noorden GK. Occlusion therapy in amblyopia with eccentric fixation. Arch Ophthalmol 1965;73(6):776–81.

Wick B. Visual therapy for small angle esotropia. Am J Optom Physiol Opt 1974b;51(7):490–96.

Wick B. Forced illumination of anomalous retinal correspondence in constant exotropia: a case report. Am J Optom Physiol Opt 1975;52(1):58–62.

Wick B. Vision training for presbyopic nonstrabismic patients. Am J Optom Physiol Opt 1977;54(4):244–47.

Wick B. Anomalous after-image transfer—an analysis and suggested method of elimination. Am J Optom Physiol Opt 1974a;5(11):862–71.

Young FA. Reading, measure of intelligence, and refractive error. Am J Optom Physiol Opt 1963;40(5):257–64.

VII

NEUROLOGIC ASPECTS OF VERGENCE EYE MOVEMENTS

20

Neurophysiological Correlates of Vergence Eye Movements

Lawrence E. Mays

The human oculomotor system can be considered as five functionally distinct subsystems (Robinson, 1981). The vestibuloocular and optokinetic systems serve to stabilize the eyes by compensating for head movements. The saccadic system generates high-velocity eye movements that can be used to acquire visual targets, while the pursuit system is capable of tracking relatively low-velocity target motion. All of these systems generate conjugate eye movements. The vergence system controls disjunctive eye movements, permitting fixating targets at various distances or following a target moving in depth.

There is good evidence that the vergence system is relatively independent of conjugate eye movement control systems. Rashbass and Westheimer (1961a, 1961b) demonstrated that pursuit and vergence eye movements can occur simultaneously with complete temporal and directional independence. Furthermore, vergence eye movements are dissociable from conjugate horizontal eye movements in certain cases of neurologic disease or injury (Smith and Cogan, 1959; Hoyt and Daroff, 1971; Sharpe et al., 1975). One well-known example is the syndrome of internuclear ophthalmoplegia, in which adduction (nasalward eye movement) is impaired for attempted conjugate eye movements but not for convergence. These reports suggest that the neural circuits that underlie

This work was supported by National Eye Institute Research grants EY-01189 to DLS and EY-03463 to LEM and a core facility grant EY-03039.

the vergence system are distinct from those of other eye movement control systems.

In this chapter the neurophysiological basis of an independent vergence system is developed from the motor output of the system back as far as possible to its underlying sensory mechanisms. Four pieces of information are needed in this effort. First, the form of neuronal signals to extraocular muscles must be determined. This is important in understanding the way vergence signals are formed and combined with commands for conjugate movements. Second, the site must be found at which vergence and versional (conjugate) eye movement control signals are combined. Vergence and versional control mechanisms, although neurologically distinct, must share part of the oculomotor output apparatus. Recent evidence from a number of sources supports the argument that vergence and versional signals are combined at the motoneuron. The third essential piece of information concerns the form of the vergence control signal before it is combined with conjugate eye movement commands. Neuronal signals recorded from midbrain sites in monkeys are consistent with a predicted vergence signal. Finally, the source of binocular disparity signal that controls fusional vergence movements must be determined. A cortical system that appears to provide the appropriate sensory information for disparity-driven vergence movements is described.

Although the neural mechanisms underlying conjugate eye movements have been under intense investigation during the last decade, the vergence system has received relatively little attention from neurophysiologists. Consequently, relatively little is known about the neural circuits that underlie vergence eye movements. This chapter summarizes existing data on the neurophysiology of vergence eye movements, develops hypotheses to fill the gaps in our knowledge, and provides an overview of how this system might work.

INNERVATION OF EXTRAOCULAR MUSCLES

Signals transmitted to the extraocular muscles by motoneurons can best be understood by considering the properties of viscoelastic forces on the globe. Passive forces on the eye are such that the oculomotor plant is an overdamped mechanical system (Robinson, 1964). Thus the mechanical response to a sudden change in force is quite sluggish. If, for example, the eye is deviated from its initial position by application of an external force, the sudden release of the eye (a step change in force) will result in its slow return that may take several hundred msec to complete. The velocity of this passive movement is quite similar to that of vergence movements, suggesting that a vergence movement results from a step change in innervation level, unlike saccades, which require an initial application of excess force to produce rapid acceleration and high velocity (Robinson, 1964).

Single-unit recording studies in monkeys have verified that motoneurons produce the control signals predicted by the mechanical properties of the globe and characteristics of the eye movements (Robinson, 1970; Schiller, 1970). There is an essentially linear relationship between motoneuron firing rate and eye position. The firing rate increases as the eye is moved in the pulling direction of the muscle it innervates (the unit's "on direction"). Motoneuron activity can be characterized by the slope of the rate-position curve and by its intercept, which is the eye position at which the unit becomes active. Firing rate-position curves for two abducens motoneurons are shown in Figure 20.1 (Keller and Robinson, 1972). As this figure suggests, there are large variations among units in slope and intercept. Keller and Robinson reported that the slope of 67 abducens neurons ranged from 1.1 to 14.5 (spikes/sec) per degree with a mode of 3.5 (spikes/sec) per degree. The variability in firing rate for any given eye position was quite small, however. A typical standard deviation of unit activity was only about 5% of the mean discharge rate.

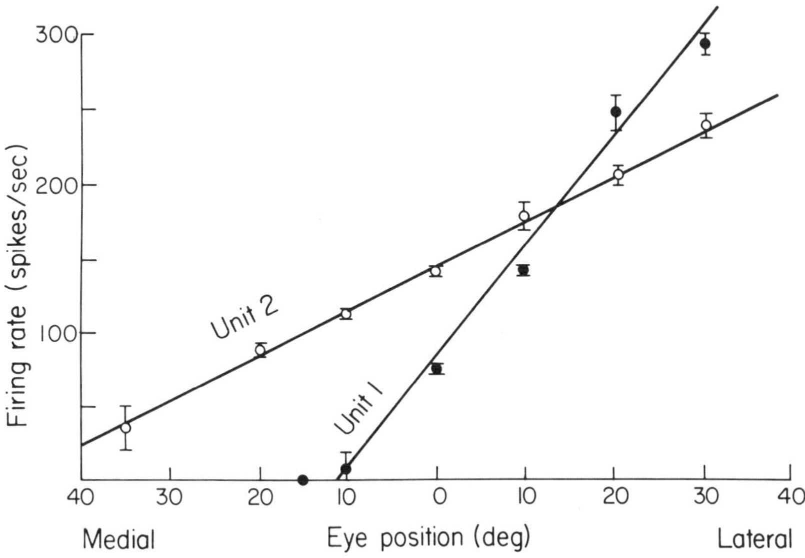

FIGURE 20.1. Firing rate-eye position curves for two lateral rectus motoneurons. The mean discharge rate was computed for several fixations at each position. Mean rates for unit 1 are shown by filled circles and rates for unit 2 by open circles. Standard deviations are given by the square brackets. Data were fit by straight lines of least square error. Reprinted with permission from Vision Research, 12, Keller EL, Robinson DA, Abducens unit behavior in the monkey during vergence movements, 1972, Pergamon Press, Ltd.

Motoneuron Activity During Saccades

For saccades in the on direction, each motoneuron provides a high-frequency burst of activity to accelerate the eye to saccadic velocities followed by a step increase in firing rate to hold the eye in the new position. An example of motoneuron activity during a saccade in the on direction is shown in Figure 20.2. The motoneuron is partially or totally inhibited during saccades in the off direction, and then resumes an impulse rate proportional to the new position. Changes in unit activity lead the saccade by about 6 to 10 msec. It is important to note that the combination of high-frequency pulse of activity and step change in rate are found within the same neuron. In this way a motoneuron can contribute both to phasic (rapid acceleration) and tonic (maintained position) components of the saccade. Because motoneurons may have a lower threshold eye position for phasic than tonic activity, more are active for the phasic than the tonic phase of most saccades.

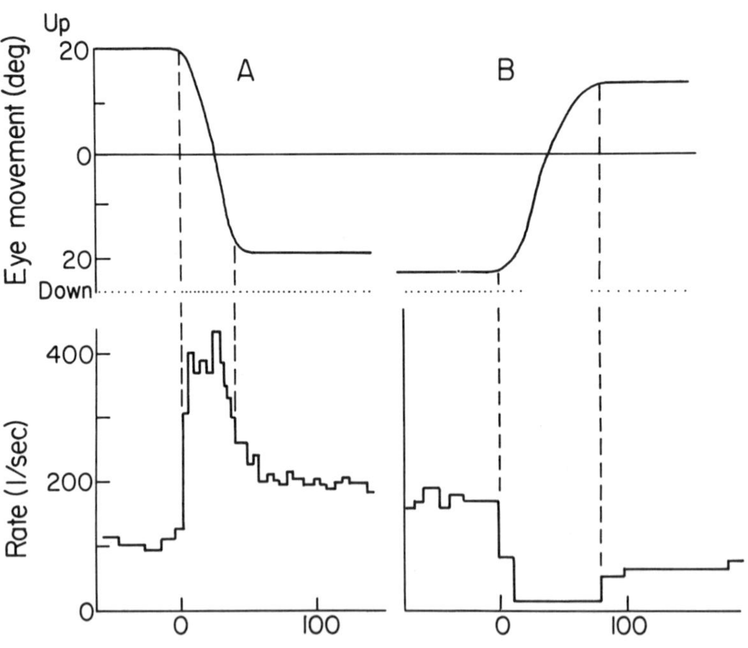

FIGURE 20.2. Instantaneous firing rate (reciprocal of interspike interval) of an oculomotor neuron during a saccade in its on direction (A) and its off direction (B). Reprinted by permission of the publisher, from Robinson DA. Oculomotor unit behavior in the monkey. Journal of Neurophysiology, 1970.

Motoneuron Activity During Vergence

Activity of medial and lateral rectus motoneurons has also been recorded during accommodative vergence movements (Keller and Robinson, 1972; Keller, 1973). In these experiments rhesus monkeys were trained to look at small illuminated targets at a distance of 17 cm or 2 m. The targets were usually aligned with the eye contralateral to the recording electrode. The other eye was covered and its position was measured accurately using the search coil technique (Fuchs and Robinson, 1966). A change in fixation from the far to the near target elicited an accommodative convergence movement of about four degrees in the eye ipsilateral to the recording electrode. All abducens neurons (presumably lateral rectus motoneurons) showed a decreased firing rate for convergence and an increased rate for divergence. Similarly, all medial rectus motoneurons displayed an increase in discharge frequency during convergence and a decrease during divergence. The pattern of neuronal discharge for vergence eye movements was a simple step change in unit activity. The activity of a medial rectus neuron during both convergence and divergence eye movements is shown in Figure 20.3. Unit activity is shown as instantaneous firing rate, or the reciprocal of interspike interval. The step change in motoneuron firing rate occurred for both abducens and medial rectus units and confirms the hypothesis that vergence movements result from a step change in innervation level.

In a quantitative analysis of motoneuron activity during accommodative vergence, Keller (1973) compared the firing rates of units for eye positions attained by vergence with the same positions attained by versional movements. For 13 of 15 abducens units and 13 of 13 medial rectus units, the differences were not statistically significant. Thus the control signals for pursuit, vergence, and saccadic eye movements have been perfectly combined at the level of, or prior to the motoneuron.

Functions of Muscle Fiber Types

Every motoneuron recorded by Keller participated in vergence, smooth pursuit, and saccadic eye movements. This is an important observation since it has been suggested that different muscle fiber types within extraocular muscle might subserve different eye movements (Alpern and Wolter, 1956; Jampel, 1967). Although six extraocular muscle fiber types can be distinguished on morphologic grounds (see Chiarandini and Davidowitz, 1979, for a review), muscle fibers can also be classified into "twitch" and "tonic" categories using criteria derived from observations on frog limb muscle (Peachey and Huxley, 1962). Twitch fibers are singly

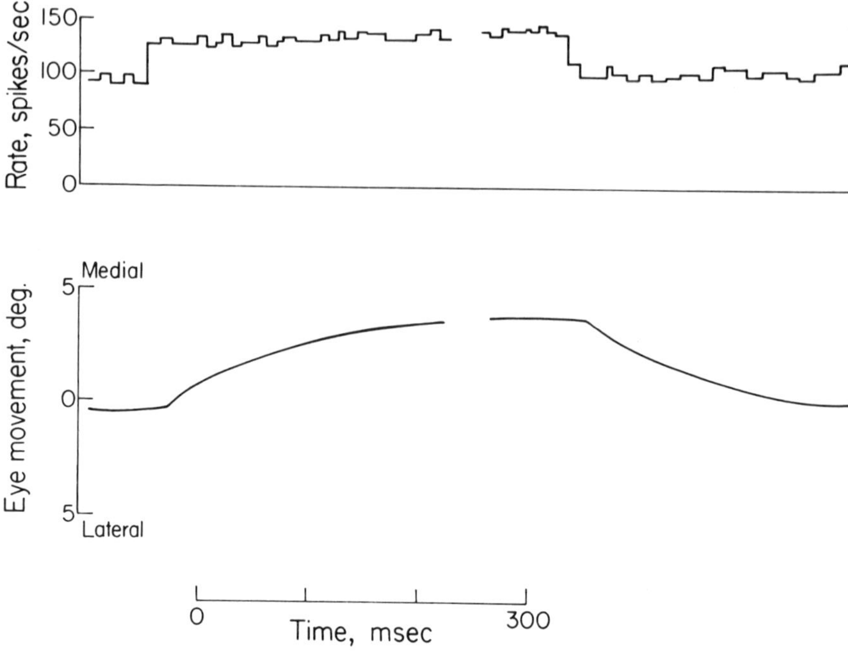

FIGURE 20.3. Instantaneous firing rate of an oculomotor neuron during a convergence movement (left lower trace) and a divergence movement (right lower trace). Reprinted with permission from Vision Research, 13, Keller EL, Accommodative vergence in the alert monkey, Motor unit analysis, 1973, Pergamon Press, Ltd.

innervated, can propagate action potentials, and appear to be less fatigue-resistant than tonic fibers. Tonic fibers are multiply innervated, typically do not conduct action potentials, and develop a graded sustained contraction when stimulated. Some multiply innervated fibers do conduct action potentials (slow twitch fibers), however.

Characterization of muscle fiber types as twitch and tonic had led to the hypothesis that tonic fibers are used for slow movements such as vergence, fixation, and pursuit, while twitch fibers are activated for saccades. This implies that the various muscle fiber types are innervated by different motoneurons that carry different command signals. The observation that each motoneuron participates in all types of eye movement and in fixation contradicts this hypothesis. Furthermore, Keller's finding that firing rates of motoneurons are indistinguishable for the same eye position achieved with or without vergence makes it highly unlikely that some as yet undiscovered motoneurons are primarily responsible for vergence movements. Recruitment of a population of "vergence motoneurons" would only serve to disrupt this precise firing rate-eye position relationship. Thus it is reasonable to conclude that all motoneurons, and hence all muscle fiber types, are involved in vergence as well as all versional movements. Nonetheless, the fact that motoneurons participate in all movements does not imply that all muscle fibers contribute equally to all components of the movement or fixation. Large differences between muscle fiber types in their response to the same innervation activity pattern would be expected from their morphologic and physiological characteristics.

COMBINING VERGENCE AND VERSIONAL SIGNALS

The best available evidence suggests that the motoneuron is indeed the site at which vergence and versional control signals are combined. The argument for this hypothesis is developed from our knowledge of supranuclear and internuclear conjugate eye movement control signals and the effects of lesions of the medial longitudinal fasciculus (MLF). A schematic representation of some of the neural circuits for horizontal eye movements can be seen in Figure 20.4. For simplicity, the vestibuloocular circuitry and some other connections have been omitted. All of the signals needed for horizontal conjugate eye movements are probably assembled in the paramedian pontine reticular formation (PPRF) adjacent to the abducens nucleus (VI). Lesions of the PPRF produce permanent deficits in horizontal conjugate eye movements toward the side of the lesion (Teng et al. 1958; Bender and Shanzer, 1964), and many neurons recorded in the PPRF have a discharge rate related to horizontal eye movements (Sparks and Travis, 1971; Cohen and Henn, 1972; Luschei and Fuchs, 1972; Keller, 1974). Medium-lead burst units in the PPRF (labeled B) discharge about 10 to 12 msec before saccades, just slightly before motoneurons. Nearly all medium-lead burst cells fire most vigorously for ipsilateral horizontal saccades. The PPRF also contains tonic cells (T), which have an impulse rate proportional to ipsilateral horizontal eye deviation. Together, these PPRF units appear to have the signals required by lateral and medial rectus motoneurons for both slow and quick conjugate eye movements, and PPRF neurons project directly to abducens neurons (Büttner-Ennever and Henn, 1976; Grantyn et al., 1980).

Abducens Internuclear Neurons

The abducens nucleus contains not only lateral rectus (L) motoneurons but also abducens internuclear (I) neurons (Graybiel and Hartwieg, 1974). Abducens internuclear neurons do not innervate extraocular muscles, but instead cross the midline at the level of the abducens nucleus and ascend in the MLF to the oculomotor (III) nucleus (Baker and Highstein, 1975;

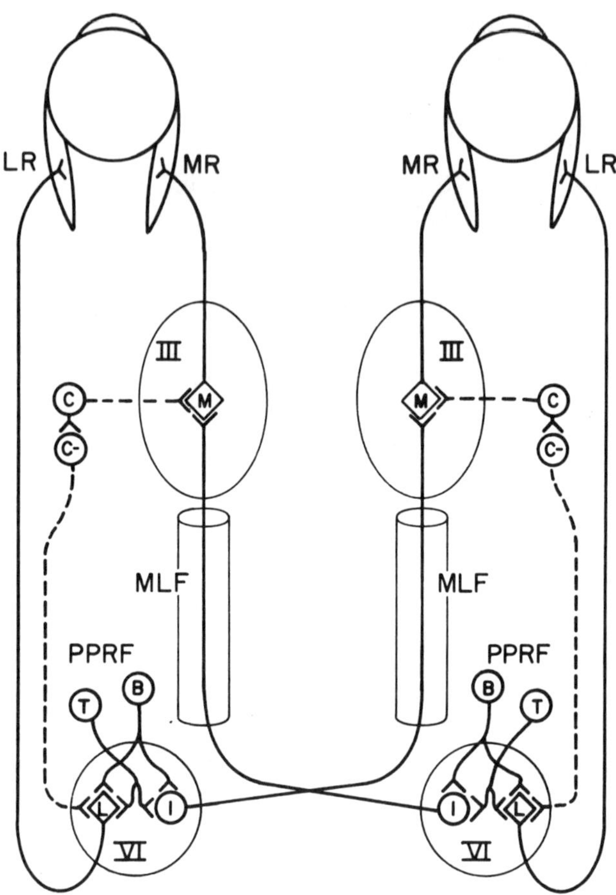

FIGURE 20.4. Schematic representation of some of the neural circuitry for the control of horizontal eye movements. The vestibuloocular circuitry and some other connections have been omitted. Lateral rectus and medial rectus muscles are designated as LR and MR. Horizontal burst neurons (B) and tonic eye position cells (T) in the paramedian pontine reticular formation (PPRF) have the signals required for all conjugate horizontal eye movements. These PPRF neurons probably provide similar input to both lateral rectus motoneurons (L) and internuclear neurons (I) in the abducens nucleus (VI). Abducens internuclear neurons cross the midline and ascend in the medial longitudinal fasciculus (MLF) to drive medial rectus motoneurons (M). A presumed convergence (C) input to medial rectus motoneurons is shown by dashed lines. A complementary convergence (C-) input to lateral rectus motoneurons is also assumed.

Highstein, 1977; Carpenter and Batton, 1980). These ascending fibers were thought to terminate in both the medial rectus and inferior rectus subdivisions of the oculomotor nucleus (Büttner-Ennever, 1977; Carpenter and Batton, 1980). Recent reexaminations of the location of motoneurons within the oculomotor nucleus revealed that some medial rectus motoneurons are found in the area considered to be the inferior rectus subdivision (Büttner-Ennever and Akert, 1981). Thus the medial rectus motoneurons are probably the sole target of abducens internuclear neurons.

In addition to this anatomic evidence, Highstein and Baker (1978) found that abducens internuclear neurons provide a powerful excitatory drive to contralateral medial rectus motoneurons (M). Very short latencies (0.5 to 0.8 msec) between stimulation of the abducens nucleus and the appearance of excitatory postsynaptic potentials (EPSPs) in medial rectus motoneurons suggest that this is a monosynaptic input. Abducens internuclear neurons appear to receive most of the same inputs as abducens motoneurons (Highstein, 1977) and their activity during conjugate eye movements is similar to that of abducens motoneurons (Delgado-Garcia et al., 1977). King, Lisberger, and Fuchs (1976) and Pola and Robinson (1978) recorded from fibers of the MLF between the abducens and oculomotor nuclei in awake monkeys. Nearly half (40%) of the fibers were classified as horizontal burst-tonic and most of the remainder were related to vertical eye or head movement. The majority of these horizontal burst-tonic fibers are probably axons of abducens internuclear neurons. The fibers have a discharge pattern that is indistinguishable from that of ipsilateral medial rectus motoneurons or contralateral abducens motoneurons for any conjugate eye movement. As Pola and Robinson state, abducens internuclear neurons are, in effect, surrogate medial rectus motoneurons. They convey all horizontal conjugate eye movement signals directly from the abducens nucleus to the contralateral medial rectus motoneurons, and so coordinate the action of lateral and medial rectus muscles.

Vergence and Abducens Internuclear Neurons

During vergence eye movements, however, medial rectus and lateral rectus motoneurons must not receive the same signals. Abducens internuclear neurons probably carry signals to medial rectus motoneurons for all horizontal eye movements except vergence. Evidence for this dissociation of control signals is found in cases in which the fibers of the MLF are damaged by injury or disease. The syndrome of internuclear ophthalmoplegia (INO) results from a lesion of the MLF between the abducens and oculomotor nuclei (Smith and Cogan, 1959). The condition is characterized by weakness or absence of ocular adduction for attempted conjugate gaze shifts and is presumed to be due to the interruption of abducens internuclear fibers (Highstein and Baker, 1978; Carpenter and Batton, 1980). Adduction for attempted convergence is spared in the INO syndrome. Carpenter and Strominger (1965) observed a similar syndrome as a result of experimentally induced electrolytic lesions of the MLF in monkeys. Thus the vergence control signal must arrive at the medial rectus motoneuron by way of a pathway other than the abducens internuclear input.

A direct test of the hypothesis that abducens internuclear neurons carry only versional control signals was attempted by Delgado-Garcia, Baker, and Highstein (1977). They reported that the activity of an identified abducens internuclear neuron was unaltered during disjunctive eye movements. Conjugate eye movements of similar amplitude were accompanied by impulse rate changes. It should be noted that this report was based on a small number of cells and that the eye movement records from the cat show unusually large asymmetric movements. Keller (personal communication) recorded from a small number of horizontal burst-tonic fibers in the MLF of monkeys trained on an accommodative vergence (Keller and Robinson, 1972) tracking task. He found no evidence that the activity of these fibers is modulated during vergence eye movements. This result supports the hypothesis that medial rectus motoneurons receive only conjugate signals by way of the abducens internuclear input. The obvious conclusion is that a vergence signal is added to this conjugate horizontal input at the medial rectus motoneuron. Since abducens internuclear neurons and abducens motoneurons have similar discharge patterns during conjugate eye movements and receive many of the same inputs, it is also reasonable to expect that versional and vergence signals are also mixed at the abducens motoneurons. The signal to abducens motoneurons must be opposite in sign to that sent to medial rectus motoneurons.

A plausible scheme by which a vergence signal might be added to the versional signal is shown in Figure 20.4. A presumed excitatory convergence (C) input mixes with the conjugate signal at the medial rectus motoneurons. A sign-inverting vergence signal (C-) is also sent to lateral rectus motoneurons. These presumed connections are drawn with dashed lines. A connection between convergence inputs on the two sides is not shown, but such a linkage is required to produce symmetric vergence inputs to the two eyes. Although the existence of a direct convergence input to medial rectus motoneurons has not been shown, there is reason to suspect that vergence signals may be found in the midbrain recticular formation near the oculomotor nucleus. Loss of convergence has been reported to result from lesions of the midbrain reticular formation (Nashold and Seaber, 1972). Convergence deficits are sometimes noted along with defects in vertical gaze in patients with midbrain lesions (Jacobs et al., 1973; Halmagyi et al., 1978).

VERGENCE SIGNAL

It is reasonable to assume that the vergence signal is the difference between abducens internuclear input and medial rectus motoneuron output. Therefore vergence input to the motoneurons is probably a frequency-coded signal in which the impulse rate is linearly proportional to the convergence angle. Because there is a linear relationship between motoneuron firing rate and eye position, the vergence controller needs no information about conjugate eye position. A given change in vergence input to the motoneuron would result in a fixed change in vergence angle without regard to absolute eye position. Thus the vergence input need provide only information about the degree of convergence. The addition of a signal linearly proportional to vergence angle at the level of the motoneuron to signals generated by conjugate systems would preserve the linear rate-position curve of the motoneuron. This hypothesis is also consistent with the observation of simple, linear addition of vergence and conjugate eye movements of similarly low velocities (Rashbass and Westheimer, 1961b; Miller et al., 1980).

Schiller (1970), recording from the area of the oculomotor nucleus in the rhesus monkey, found seven neurons that appeared to have an impulse rate proportional to the angle of convergence. Although the horizontal positions of the two eyes were not measured independently, these cells fired vigorously as a piece of food was moved toward the animal. The angle of approach (relative to the head) had no effect on the activity, and the firing rate did not show any clear relationship to conjugate eye position. Convergence of the eyes induced by prisms also resulted in a prolonged neuronal discharge. It appeared that the activity of these neurons was related to the angle between the eyes regardless of the direction of conjugate gaze, although some other component of the near response could not be ruled out. Schiller localized these cells near the caudal part of the oculomotor nucleus in the dorsolateral region. No convergence-related activity was observed in the midline area. Robinson (1970) also reported two cells in the oculomotor nucleus that appeared to be involved in the near response, but their activity was not studied further.

Recently, I began a systematic search for neural activity related to vergence in the midbrain of the monkey. Both the horizontal and vertical positions of the left and right eyes were measured using the electromagnetic search coil technique (Fuchs and Robinson, 1966). Monkeys were trained to look at small light-emitting diode (LED) targets for a water reward. One target array was positioned directly in front of the animal at a distance of 19 cm and another was placed at a distance of 83 cm. The LEDs were mounted in clear plexiglas so that the monkey could look through the near target array to see the far array. Each eye was carefully calibrated with these targets under monocular viewing conditions. By comparing this calibration to the monkey's eye positions during binocular viewing of the same targets, it was possible to verify that the eyes were properly aligned with the target and to reward the monkey for looking at it. Since the interpupillary distance of the monkey is about 2.8 cm, the convergence angles for the far and near targets were 1.9 degrees and 8.4 degrees, respectively. During the experiments the head was immobilized.

Preliminary data show that there are many midbrain neurons that have an impulse rate closely related to the angle of convergence. Figure 20.5 is a record from one of these cells during a single trial in which a

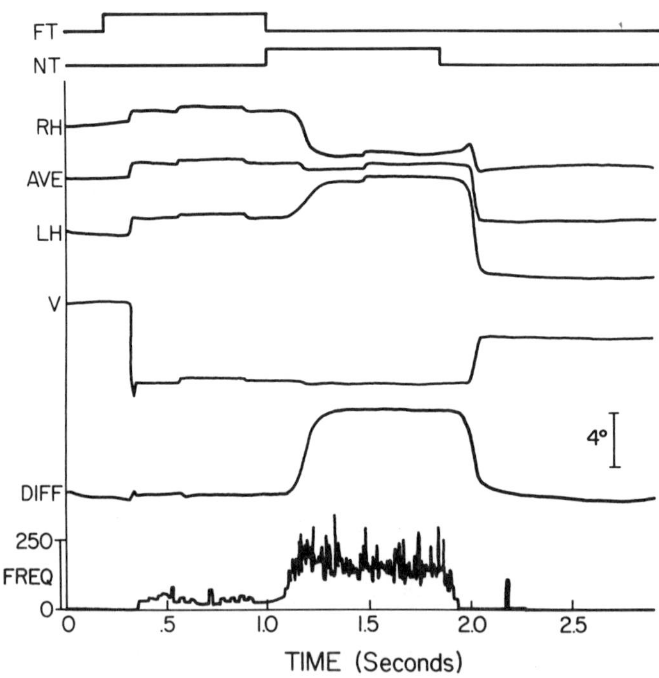

FIGURE 20.5. Instantaneous firing rate of a neuron related to the convergence angle of the eyes. Records of right horizontal (RH), left horizontal (LH), and vertical (V) eye positions are shown along with the average horizontal eye position (AVE). The difference between the left and right horizontal eye positions (DIFF) is a measure of the convergence angle. The presentations of a far target (FT, 83 cm distant) and a near target (NT, 19 cm) are shown at the top. Upward deflections represent rightward eye movements for RH, LH, and AVE; upward movement for V; and increased convergence for DIFF.

monkey was required to look to a far target (FT) and then to a near target (NT). Horizontal left and right (HL and HR) eye positions, the average (AVE) of horizontal left and right eye positions, and the difference (DIFF) between left and right horizontal eye positions are shown. Leftward horizontal movements are shown as downward deflections. Because the vertical positions of the eyes were identical, only one vertical eye position (V) signal is shown. The activity of the neuron is displayed as an instantaneous-frequency histogram (FREQ); AVE is a measure of conjugate horizontal gaze while DIFF shows the convergence angle between the two eyes. Prior to onset of the far target the monkey was free to look around the room. Just after the far target was turned on the monkey made a downward and rightward saccadic eye movement to look to it. The cell fired at a steady rate of about 50 spikes per second as the monkey looked at the far target. After 700 msec the far target was turned off and the near target was lighted. A nearly symmetric vergence movement was executed to look at the near target. The cell increased its firing rate to nearly 200 spikes per second just before this convergence movement and maintained that rate during fixation. When the near target was turned off the monkey was again free to look around the room and an abrupt decrease in unit activity preceded the divergence movement. Control trials showed that this cell's activity was not related to the position of either eye in the orbit. Rather, the firing rate was closely coupled to the convergence angle regardless of the direction of conjugate gaze. Cells of this type also showed increased activity during convergence elicited by monocular accommodative stimuli.

Tonic convergence cells could provide the signals required by medial rectus and lateral rectus motoneurons for convergence eye movements (see Figure 20.4). Some tonic divergence cells were also encountered in the same area of the midbrain and could provide a complementary input for divergence eye movements. Other cells fired only during the convergence movement (phasic convergence). All cells were recorded in the midbrain reticular formation lateral to the oculomotor complex. The location of a marking lesion at a representative recording site (R) is shown in Figure 20.6.

The activity of these cells is closely linked to vergence eye movements, but it is not yet possible to conclude that they drive motoneurons or even that they control vergence eye movements. The act of looking from a far to a near stimulus results in a near response (or triad) of convergence, accommodation, and pupillary constriction (Alpern et al., 1961). Thus the activity of these cells could also be linked to accommodation or pupillary constriction. The problem of identifying neural elements within the vergence system is difficult because of the complex interaction between accommodation and convergence. Semmlow and coworkers (Semmlow and Heerema, 1979; Hung and Semmlow, 1980) (also

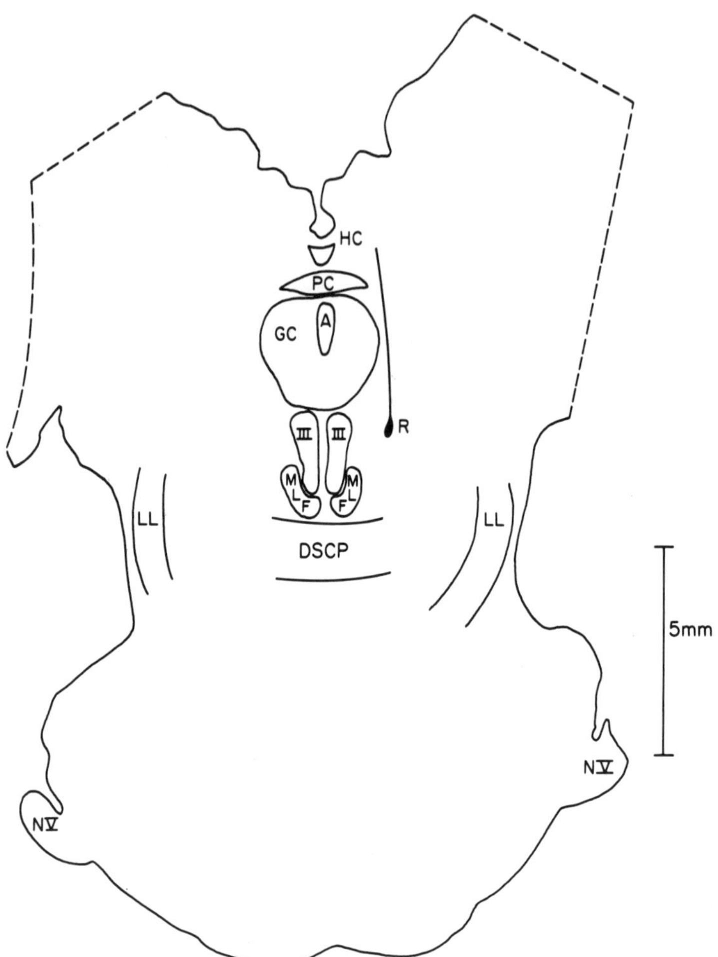

FIGURE 20.6. A drawing of a coronal section in the stereotoxic plane through the midbrain of a macaque showing a recording site (R) from which a convergence-related neuron was recorded. The electrode tract to R is also shown. HC = habenular commissure; PC = posterior commissure; CG = central gray; A = aqueduct; III = third nerve (oculomotor) nucleus; MLF = medial longitudinal fasciculus; LL = lateral lemniscus; DSCP = decussation of the superior cerebellar peduncle; and NV = fifth nerve.

see Chapter 7) have shown that levels of both accommodation and convergence are determined by the interaction of cross-coupled accommodation and vergence controllers. Vergence eye movements can be elicited by accommodative stimuli (accommodative convergence) and convergence induced by binocular disparity can also elicit accommodation (convergence accommodation). The neural mechanisms for these interactions are unknown.

CORTICAL PROCESSING OF BINOCULAR DISPARITY

Vergence eye movements can be elicited by binocular disparity or by retinal blur by way of the accommodation controller. Processing binocular retinal disparity information appears to be an important function of visual cortex. In the geniculo-striate pathway, signals from the two eyes are segregated until they reach primary visual cortex. Here the input is organized into ocular dominance columns and significant binocular interaction first occurs. Binocular disparity information is probably extracted at this level. Barlow, Blakemore, and Pettigrew (1967) found a number of neurons in the visual cortex of the cat that were sensitive to horizontal retinal disparities. More recently, Poggio and Fischer (1977) recorded from neurons in the visual cortex of alert monkeys trained to maintain fixation of a target light while an appropriate visual stimulus was moved in depth. The stimulus was a rectangle that could be suitably oriented in a cortical cell's receptive field. Many binocularly driven cells in visual cortex fired maximally when the visual stimulus was in the receptive field and at the same distance as the fixation point (tuned excitatory cells). Discharge rates decreased if the target was moved nearer or farther. Other cells fired most vigorously when the stimulus was either in front of or beyond the fixation plane (tuned inhibitory cells). In addition to these zero-disparity cells, other cells signaled that the target was nearer (near cells) or beyond (far cells) the fixation plane. The near and far cells were responsive to disparities of $\pm 1°$ or more, well beyond Panum's area. The vergence oculomotor system can also respond to large disparities (Westheimer and Mitchell, 1969). Poggio and Fischer suggested that near and far cells might be used to initiate vergence movements and that tuned excitatory cells could provide the feedback signal required to maintain fixation in depth.

Disparity Detectors

These observations provide neurophysiological support for an earlier hypothesis that there are three separate classes of detectors involved in wide-field stereopsis and the control of vergence. Using psychophysical tests in humans, Richards (1970) provided evidence that there were brain mechanisms to detect visual stimuli in the plane of fixation (zero binocular retinal disparity), in front of the fixation plane (crossed disparity), and beyond the fixation plane (uncrossed disparity). Individuals may lack one or more detectors, and the probability of this occurring in one hemisphere is about 0.30. Jones (1977) has shown that anomalous vergence responses are associated with these deficits in disparity detection. Binocular fusional vergence eye movements should be severely disrupted in individuals who lack all three detectors. The observed incidence of strabismus in the adult population is indeed quite close to the predicted percentage of the population expected to lack all three ($0.3 \times 0.3 \times 0.3 = 2.7\%$). That fusional vergence eye movements are absent in strabismics has recently been demonstrated by Kenyon, Ciuffreda, and Stark (1980), although they attributed a major portion of the deficit to suppression of input to one eye rather than to lack of disparity detectors.

Additional evidence of the importance of cortical areas for detecting binocular disparity and eliciting vergence movements is provided by Westheimer and Mitchell (1969). A human subject whose corpus callosum had been surgically sectioned for the control of epilepsy was tested for vergence eye movements. When a target moved from far to near in the peripheral visual field, the subject made a convergence eye movement to follow it. Since in this situation the images of the targets fell on the temporal retina of one eye and the nasal retina of the other, both retinal images reached the visual cortex on the same side of the brain. When the far target was viewed using the foveas, a target step from far to near along the midline caused the retinal images to shift to the temporal retina of each eye. Thus the retinal images for each eye were transmitted to separate cerebral hemispheres. In this situation the subject did not make a convergence eye movement. Similarly, a subject with a sectioned corpus callosum could not discriminate target depth induced by binocular disparity unless retinal signals were sent to the same hemisphere (Mitchell and Blakemore, 1970). These results suggest that the cortex is crucial for control of the vergence system by disparity cues.

Other Cortical Areas

Cortical areas other than the visual cortex have also been implicated in the control of vergence eye movements. Jampel (1960) reported that the near triad (convergence, miosis, and accommodation) could be elicited by stimulation of various sites in cortical areas 19 and 22 as well as the frontal lobe, including the frontal eye fields. These experiments, conducted on anesthetized monkeys, did not always yield consistent responses when the same sites were repeatedly stimulated. Robinson and Fuchs (1969) reported that electrical stimulation of the frontal eye fields of the alert, unanesthetized monkey yields short-latency, conjugate, contralateral saccades, and not vergence movements. Since low levels of anesthetic can change stimulation-induced saccades into slow or disjunctive eye movements (Robinson and Fuchs, 1969), some of Jampel's results may have been due to an interaction of electrical stimulation with anesthesia.

Recently, Sakata, Shibutani, and Kawano (1980) found that many visual fixation neurons of the posterior parietal cortex are sensitive to target depth. Neurons in area 7a were recorded in monkeys trained to look at a small visual target; at which time visual fixation units fired and increased their rate as the target was moved to a certain position in space. Many neurons fired more intensely when the fixation target was moved toward the animal, while others were activated by distant targets. Since neither convergence angle nor accommodation was measured, it is not possible to determine if these cells might control vergence or accommodation, or receive signals from these controllers.

CORTICOOCULOMOTOR PATHWAYS

The route by which a binocular retinal disparity signal might be transmitted from visual cortex to oculomotor areas is not known. Poggio and Fischer (1977) found that tuned excitatory cells were commonly encountered in layers V and VI of visual cortex, which project almost exclusively to the superior colliculus, pulvinar, and lateral geniculate nucleus (Lund et al., 1975). Near and far cells were usually encountered in the supragranular layers, which project to other areas of the cortex (Martinez-Millán and Holländer, 1975).

Although there is a strong anatomic projection to superior colliculus from visual cortex (Wilson and Toyne, 1970) and from the colliculus to oculomotor areas (Harting, 1977), there is no evidence implicating the superior colliculus in the control of vergence eye movements. It is known that many cells in the intermediate and deeper layers discharge prior to saccades of a particular vector (Wurtz and Goldberg, 1972), but the activity of superior colliculus neurons during vergence has not been investigated. Electrical stimulation of the colliculus produces short-latency saccades and not slow or disjunctive eye movements (Robinson, 1972; Mays and Sparks, 1980; and unpublished observations).

The pretectum is an area that may be involved in vergence eye movements or in some aspect of coordination of the near triad. Some cells in the pretectal region of the cat respond to stimuli moving toward or away from the animal (Straschill and Hoffmann, 1969). The response to movement in the sagittal plane does not depend on binocular vision since it can be produced by monocular visual stimulation. It should be noted that animals in this experiment were paralyzed and could not move their eyes.

The pretectal area has long been recognized as an important region for the control of the pupillary light reflex (Magoun and Ranson, 1935). In a recent examination of the connections of the pretectum, Benevento, Rezak, and Santos-Anderson (1977) concluded that the retina, superior colliculus, and cortex can only influence pupillary constriction and accommodation through their projections to pretectum. Thus coordination of the near triad may well involve pretectal nuclei, but there is as yet no direct evidence for a role for the area in ocular vergence.

OVERVIEW

Fusional vergence eye movements are controlled by binocular retinal disparity information. Neurons in the striate and prestriate cortex are capable of extracting disparity information that could initiate convergence or divergence eye movements (near and far cells). The range of disparities to which these cells respond is wider than that used in normal stereoscopic vision and may be comparable to the range to which vergence eye movements are made (Westheimer and Mitchell, 1969). Tuned excitatory cells could provide a feedback signal informing the vergence controller that the target is in the range of stereoscopic vision. Information about target disparities may be processed by other cortical areas, or may be sent directly to a vergence control mechanism in the midbrain. Since disparity information represents a desired change in vergence angle and not the desired vergence angle, a disparity error signal is probably integrated to produce a vergence signal. Phasic convergence cells, which have been recorded in the midbrain, may represent the input to this integrator and tonic convergence cells may be its output. The vergence signal is probably a frequency-coded impulse rate linearly proportional to the vergence angle. The best evidence suggests that it is combined in a simple, additive way, with versional signals at the motoneurons. The output of the motoneuron for any vergence movement is, in turn, a simple step change in impulse rate. It is very likely that the same motoneurons and hence the same muscle fibers are involved in all ocular movements regardless of whether they are slow or fast, disjunctive or conjugate. Not all muscle fiber types contribute equally to each type of movement, however, since muscle fibers vary in their response to neural input.

Relatively little is known about the neuronal mechanisms by which the fusional vergence system and the accommodation controller interact. Changes in accommodation caused by retinal blur can drive the vergence system, and vergence eye movements brought about by retinal disparity cues can change accommodation. Anatomic data suggest that the pretectum is a site at which this interaction might occur.

REFERENCES

Alpern M, Wolter JR. The relation of horizontal saccadic and vergence eye movements. Arch Ophthalmol 1956;56:685–90.

Alpern M, Mason GL, Jardinico RE. Vergence and accommodation. V. Pupil size changes associated with changes in accommodative vergence. Am J Ophthalmol 1961;52:762–67.

Baker R, Highstein SM. Physiological identification of interneurons and motoneurons in the abducens nucleus. Brain Res 1975;83:292–98.

Barlow HB, Blakemore C, Pettigrew JD. The neural mechanism of binocular depth discrimination. J Physiol (Lond) 1967;193:327–342.

Bender MB, Shanzer S. Oculomotor pathways defined by electric stimulation or lesions in the brainstem of monkey. In: Bender MB, ed. The oculomotor system. New York: Harper & Row, 1964:81–140.

Benevento LA, Rezak M, Santos-Anderson R. An autoradiographic study of the projections of the pretectum in the rhesus monkey (*Macaca mulatta*): evidence for sensorimotor links to the thalamus and oculomotor nuclei. Brain Res 1977;127:197–218.

Büttner-Ennever JA. Pathways from the pontine reticular formation to structures controlling horizontal and vertical eye movement in the monkey. In: Baker R, Berthoz A, eds. Control of gaze by brain stem neurons. New York: Elsevier, 1977:89–98.

Büttner-Ennever JA, Akert K. Medial rectus subgroups of the oculomotor nucleus and their abducens internuclear input in the monkey. J Comp Neurol 1981;197:17–27.

Büttner-Ennever JA, Henn V. An autoradiographic study of the pathways from the pontine reticular formation involved in horizontal eye movements. Brain Res 1976;108:155–64.

Carpenter MB, Batton RR III. Abducens internuclear neurons and their role in conjugate horizontal gaze. J Comp Neurol 1980;189:191–209.

Carpenter MB, Strominger NL. The medial longitudinal fasciculus and disturbances of conjugate horizontal eye movements in the monkey. J Comp Neurol 1965;125:41–66.

Chiarandini DJ, Davidowitz J. Structure and function of extraocular muscle fibers. In: Zadunaisky JA, Davson H, eds. Current topics in eye research. Vol. 1. New York: Academic Press, 1979:91–142.

Cohen B, Henn V. Unit activity in the pontine reticular formation associated with eye movements. Brain Res 1972;46:403–10.

Delgado-Garcia J, Baker R, Highstein SM. The activity of internuclear neurons identified within the abducens nucleus of the alert cat. In: Baker R, Berthoz A, eds. Control of gaze by brain stem neurons. New York: Elsevier, 1977:291–300.

Fuchs AF, Robinson DA. A method for measuring horizontal and vertical eye movement chronically in the monkey. J Appl Physiol 1966;21:1068–70.

Grantyn R, Baker R, Grantyn A. Morphological and physiological identification of excitatory pontine reticular neurons projecting to the cat abducens nucleus and spinal cord. Brain Res 1980;198:221–28.

Graybiel AM, Hartwieg EA. Some afferent connections of the oculomotor complex in the cat: an experimental study with tracer techniques. Brain Res 1974;81:543–51.

Halmagyi GM, Evans WA, Hallinan JM. Failure of downward gaze. Arch Neurol 1978;35:22–26.

Harting JK. Descending pathways from the superior colliculus: an autoradiographic analysis in the rhesus monkey. J Comp Neurol 1977;173:583–612.

Highstein SM. Abducens and oculomotor internuclear neurons: relation to gaze. In: Baker R, Berthoz A, eds. Control of gaze by brain stem neurons. New York: Elsevier, 1977:153–62.

Highstein SM, Baker R. Excitatory termination of abducens internuclear neurons on medial rectus motorneurons: relationship to syndrome of internuclear opthalmoplegia. J Neurophysiol 1978;41:1647–61.

Hoyt WF, Daroff RB. Supranuclear disorders of ocular control systems in man. In: Bach-y-Rita P, Collins CC, Hyde JE, eds. The control of eye movements. New York: Academic Press, 1971:175–235.

Hung GK, Semmlow JL. Static behavior of accommodation and vergence: computer simulation of an interactive dual-feedback system. IEEE Trans Biomed Eng 1980;BME-27:439–47.

Jacobs L, Anderson PJ, Bender MB. The lesions producing paralysis of downward but not upward gaze. Arch Neurol 1973;28:319–23.

Jampel RS. Convergence, divergence, pupillary reactions and accommodation of the eyes from faradic stimulation of macaque brain. J Comp Neurol 1960;115:371–400.

Jampel RS. Multiple motor systems in the extraocular muscles of man. Invest Ophthalmol 1967;6:288–93.

Jones R. Anomalies of disparity detection in the human visual system. J Physiol 1977;264:621–40.

Keller EL. Accommodative vergence in the alert monkey. Motor unit analysis. Vision Res 1973;13:1565–75.

Keller EL. Participation of medial pontine reticular formation in eye movement generation in the monkey. J Neurophysiol 1974;37:316–32.

Keller EL, Robinson DA. Abducens unit behavior in the monkey during vergence movements. Vision Res 1972;12:369–82.

Kenyon RV, Ciuffreda KJ, Stark L. Dynamic vergence eye movements in strabismus and amblyopia: symmetric vergence. Invest Ophthalmol Visual Sci 1980;19:60–74.

King WM, Lisberger SG, Fuchs AF. Responses of fibers in medial longitudinal fasciculus (MLF) of alert monkeys during horizontal and vertical conjugate eye movements evoked by vestibular or visual stimuli. J Neurophysiol 1976;39:1135–49.

Lund JS, Lund RD, Hendrickson AE. The origin of efferent pathways from the primary visual cortex, area 17, of the macaque monkey as shown by retrograde transport of horseradish peroxidase. J Comp Neurol 1975;164:287–304.

Luschei EA, Fuchs AF. Activity of brain stem neurons during eye movements of alert monkeys. J Neurophysiol 1972;35:445–61.

Magoun HW, Ranson SW. The central path of the light reflex. A study of the effect of lesions. Arch Ophthalmol 1935;13:791–811.

Martinez-Millán L, Holländer H. Cortico-cortical projections from striate cortex of the squirrel monkey (*Saimiri sciureus*). A radioautographic study. Brain Res 1975;83:405–17.

Mays LE, Sparks DL. Saccades are spatially, not retinocentrically, coded. Science 1980;208:1163–65.

Miller JM, Ono H, Steinbach M. Additivity of fusional vergence and pursuit eye movements. Vision Res 1980;20:43–47.

Mitchell DE, Blakemore C. Binocular depth perception and the corpus callosum. Vision Res 1970;10:49–54.

Nashold BS, Seaber JH. Defects of ocular motility after stereotactic midbrain lesions in man. Arch Ophthalmol 1972;88:245–48.

Peachey LD, Huxley AF. Structural identification of twitch and slow striated muscle fibers of the frog. J Cell Biol 1962;13:177–80.

Poggio GF, Fischer B. Binocular interaction and depth sensitivity in striate and prestriate cortex of behaving rhesus monkey. J Neurophysiol 1977;40: 1392–1405.

Pola J, Robinson DA. Oculomotor signals in medial longitudinal fasciculus of the monkey. J Neurophysiol 1978;41:245–59.

Rashbass C, Westheimer G. Disjunctive eye movements. J Physiol 1961a;159:339–60.

Rashbass C, Westheimer G. Independence of conjugate and disjunctive eye movements. J Physiol 1961b;159:361–64.

Richards W. Stereopsis and stereoblindness. Exp Brain Res 1970;10:380–88.

Robinson DA. The mechanics of human saccadic eye movement. J Physiol 1964;174:245–64.

Robinson DA. Oculomotor unit behavior in the monkey. J Neurophysiol 1970;33:393–404.

Robinson DA. Eye movements evoked by collicular stimulation in the alert monkey. Vision Res 1972;12:1795–1808.

Robinson DA. The use of control systems analysis in the neurophysiology of eye movements. Ann Rev Neurosci 1981;4:463–503.

Robinson DA, Fuchs AF. Eye movements evoked by stimulation of frontal eye fields. J Neurophysiol 1969;32:637–48.

Sakata H, Shibutani H, Kawano K. Spatial properties of visual fixation neurons in posterior parietal association cortex of the monkey. J Neurophysiol 1980;43:1654–72.

Schiller PH. The discharge characteristics of single units in the oculomotor and abducens nuclei of the unanesthetized monkey. Exp Brain Res 1970;10: 347–62.

Semmlow JL, Heerema D. The role of accommodative convergence at the limits of fusional vergence. Invest Ophthalmol Visual Sci 1979;18:970–76.

Sharpe JA, Silversides JL, Blair RDG. Familial paralysis of horizontal gaze. Neurology 1975;25:1035–40.

Smith JL, Cogan DG. Internuclear ophthalmoplegia. A review of 58 cases. Arch Ophthalmol 1959;61:687–94.

Sparks DL, Travis RP. Firing patterns of reticular formation neurons during horizontal eye movements. Brain Res 1971;33:477–81.

Straschill M, Hoffmann KP. Response characteristics of movement-detecting neurons in pretectal region of the cat. Exp Neurol 1969;25:165–76.

Teng P, Shanzer S, Bender MB. Effects of brain stem lesions on optokinetic nystagmus in monkeys. Neurology 1958;8:22–26.

Westheimer G, Mitchell DE. The sensory stimulus for disjunctive eye movements. Vision Res 1969;9:749–55.

Wilson ME, Toyne MJ. Retino-tectal and cortico-tectal projections in *Macaca mulatta*. Brain Res 1970;24:395–406.

Wurtz RH, Goldberg ME. Activity of superior colliculus in behaving monkey. III. Cells discharging before eye movements. J Neurophysiol 1972;35:575–86.

21

Clinical Dysfunction of the Vergence System

Gill Roper-Hall

Coordination of extraocular movements in humans is under the control of several distinct mechanisms, most of which subserve conjugate gaze. These include pursuit and saccadic movements, fixation, and the oculovestibular reflexes. The vergence mechanisms control disjugate (disjunctive) movements. While horizontal vergences comprise the major part of these movements, vertical vergences and cyclovergence movements also exist.

CONTROL AREAS

The final common pathway for all eye movements begins with the brainstem nuclei of the third, fourth, and sixth cranial nerves. The nervous impulses originate more centrally and are mediated through supranuclear control areas. The cortical centers, which subserve fixation, pursuit, and saccadic movement have been identified and for the most part are located in the frontal and parietooccipital motor cortex (Daroff and Hoyt, 1971; Burde, 1981; Roper-Hall, 1973). Certain brainstem centers including the superior colliculus, which may have a role in foveation, and the vestibular system, which is concerned with static gravitational and acceleration effects, may also serve as primary supranuclear control centers. Many other areas within the posterior fossa serve as subcenters or modulators, including the paramedian pontine reticular formation (PPRF), medial longitudinal fasciculus (MLF), and cerebellum.

Some eye movements, including vergences, can be controlled voluntarily as well as reflexly. Thus in addition to neurologic disorders that can affect the control areas, certain functional disorders can also influence eye movements.

Infranuclear and peripheral ocular motor problems do not produce vergence disorders or conjugate gaze problems although under certain conditions they can mimic them superficially. These peripheral conditions are easily differentiated by tests using forced ductions, intravenous injection of edrophonium chloride (Tensilon), doll's head maneuver or calorics, and Bell's phenomenon (Glaser, 1978).

VERGENCE SYSTEM

Vergence movements can be divided into convergence, divergence, vertical vergence, and cyclovergence. Horizontal vergences have the greatest amplitudes, with the excursion of convergence exceeding that of divergence. No specific centers for primary initiation of any of these movements have been determined, although it is known that lesions in the pretectal area of the midbrain rostral to the third nerve nucleus cause paralysis of convergence. Similarly, stereotactic stimulation in this area will produce convergence. This would suggest that there is a subcenter in the midbrain mediating convergence. Bilateral stimulation of the descending fibers from the frontal eye fields, as well as stimulation close to or in the midline of the rostral brainstem, also produces convergence, which indicates that supratentorial or central control is exercised over this region of the midbrain (Daroff and Hoyt, 1971; Jampel, 1960).

Components of the Vergence System

Convergence is an active process, and is synkinetically associated with accommodation and pupillary constriction in the near reflex. It is also associated with the binocular fusion mechanism, comprising the motor portion of the fusion reflex. Maddox divided convergence into four components: accommodative convergence comprises two-thirds of the total, and is produced to maintain bifoveal fixation on an object when a blurred image stimulates the accommodative mechanism. The remaining one-third consists of fusional, tonic, and proximal convergence (von Noorden, 1980). Fusional or relative convergence is synonymous with motor fusion, and is exerted to prevent an ocular deviation from becoming manifest. This applies to any heterophoria and to deviations induced by prismatic or haploscopic means, for example, when testing fusional amplitudes.

Tonic convergence is described as that convergence necessary to maintain the parallelism of the visual axes, preventing the eyes from reverting to a divergent position of rest. Proximal convergence is that which is induced by a sense of nearness. It is particularly responsible for the measurement artifacts when using haploscopic devices such as the synoptophore, which although set at optical infinity, induce a sense of nearness.

Divergence has been shown by electromyography to be an active process, and not just relaxation of convergence (Tamler and Jampolsky, 1967). No center for divergence has been identified, but lesions in the area of the sixth nerve nucleus can produce paralysis of divergence (Bielschowsky, 1943; Walsh and Hoyt, 1969a). Bilateral frontal stimulation can produce divergence (Pasik and Pasik, 1964). The divergence mechanism is closely linked with the fusional reflexes but it is not associated with accommodation. It is not under voluntary subjective control and therefore divergence dysfunction has been rarely linked to a functional problem (Lyle, 1954). A case of a patient who could voluntarily diverge his eyes has been reported, but this was most likely achieved by relaxation of a large exophoria rather than by active divergence (Walsh and Hoyt, 1969b).

Vertical and cyclovergences comprise a small part of the vergence system in humans. The extent to which the eyes can move disjugately in a vertical direction is a matter of a few degrees in individuals with no preexisting vertical muscle imbalance. Cyclovergence movements consisting of incyclovergence and excyclovergence are possible, although some authors dispute whether any motor fusional response exists. They suggest that all of the responses represent central psychosensory compensation (Kertesz and Jones, 1970; Kertesz, 1972, 1973; Sullivan and Kertesz, 1975; Krekling, 1973). Others state that in addition to the large central sensory response, a small motor cyclofusional portion also exists (Crone, 1971; Kertesz, 1971; Crone and Everhard-Halm, 1975). The ability to fuse cyclotorsional disparities varies considerably among normal individuals and according to the testing technique and size of target used (Crone, 1971). A small amount of incyclovergence is normally associated with any convergence movement. Large ranges of vertical and cyclovergence disjugate movements may be seen in patients with longstanding vertical or cyclovertical ocular deviations. These ranges can be extensive enough to control large ocular deviations with or without an associated compensatory head posture.

QUANTITATION OF VERGENCE ABILITY

Evaluation of the near point of convergence is an essential part of a routine eye examination, and should be tested although it need not necessarily be quantitated if the examination is normal in every other respect. Further investigation into accommodative or convergence function is indicated in any patient with ocular symptoms in the near position, a poor near point of convergence on initial screening, or a latent or intermittent exo-deviation, and in any case where a disturbance of the vergence system is suspected.

A thorough clinical examination of vergences includes quantitative measurement of the following parameters: near points of convergence and accommodation, ranges and amplitudes of accommodation, convergence, and divergence. If it is relevant, the amplitudes of vertical vergence and cyclovergence may be assessed.

The near point of convergence is measured in centimeters using an accommodative target. The most proximal point at which a single image can be seen is noted. The test should be repeated several times, and unless serial fatigue or improvement is noted an average reading may be taken. Diplopia may be noted subjectively at the breakpoint. The examiner should record which eye deviates at the near point.

The near point of accommodation is also measured in centimeters, and represents the point at which a clear image begins to blur. The target size should be recorded. Each eye is tested separately in a similar manner to that described for testing the near point of convergence.

It may be useful to know the ranges of accommodation or convergence in a particular patient. The range of either function is that distance between its nearest and farthest points, and is therefore also expressed in centimeters. The range is probably not relevant in a binocularly fixating emmetrope, as the far point is at optical infinity. In certain cases the far point of accommodation is closer than infinity, for example, in cases of accommodative spasm, and the measured range will be relatively small.

Amplitudes of accommodation are measured in spherical diopters (DS), and can be determined in a number of ways (Walsh and Hoyt, 1969a; Rubin, 1974; Roper-Hall, 1980). Amplitudes of convergence and divergence are generally measured in prism diopters ($^{\Delta}$). A prism bar or rotary prism is an ideal instrument for this test. Vergence amplitudes can also be measured in degrees using a haploscopic device such as a Synoptophore (Lyle and Wybar, 1967). Vertical vergences may be measured by either method. It is only possible to measure cyclovergences on instruments such as the Synoptophore or on experimental optical apparatus.

In all types of vergences the amplitude is determined by the extent over which a patient can maintain clear single vision, diplopia usually being appreciated at the breakpoint. The recovery point is also of clinical importance, the closer to the measured breakpoint that a patient can regain single vision being indicative of a strong binocular vergence mechanism. The farther a patient must retreat from the breakpoint before the images can be re-fused, the poorer the vergence amplitude (von Noorden, 1980;

Scobee, 1952). It is recorded as, for example, BO $30^{\Delta}/12^{\Delta}$, meaning that the patient can overcome increasing amounts of base-out prism by convergence until binocular fixation breaks at 30^{Δ}. The prisms are then decreased in strength until the diplopic images rejoin, in this case at 12^{Δ}, which indicates poor convergence ability.

RELATIONSHIP BETWEEN VERGENCE ABILITY AND FUSION

Fusion is a sensorimotor function in which an image perceived on the retina of one eye is able to be blended into one mental percept with the image falling on a corresponding area of retina in the other eye, and maintained over a measurable range. This necessitates relatively normal afferent input from each eye, normal cortical integration without suppression or adaptation, and a normal motor system that can direct the eyes into the position necessary to keep the images on the appropriate area of retina. This motor skill is provided by the vergence system, and is synkinetically linked with accommodation and pupil constriction in the near reflex.

Patients who have developed normal binocular vision in childhood can acquire fusional problems in later life. These problems are generally central, and can affect sensory or motor fusion. Sensory fusional problems are those in which the patient can make the necessary eye movements to align the two images but cannot blend or "lock" them. This condition usually results from severe closed head trauma (Pratt-Johnson, 1973; Pratt-Johnson and Tillson, 1979), but has also rarely been associated with diverse neurologic disorders such as migraine and brain tumor (Wade, 1960, 1965; Stanworth and Mein, 1971).

More commonly, acquired fusional disorders affect motor fusion. These patients are able to fuse or perceive stereoscopic detail when the images are aligned, but due to inadequacies in the vergence mechanism, the range over which fusion can be maintained is either reduced or absent. Disturbances to motor fusion can occur following severe closed head trauma and in certain neurologic and psychiatric conditions (Doden and Bunge, 1965; Diener, 1953), but in general these patients have no detectable illness.

The vergence system is generally unaffected in adult patients who develop diplopia from acquired nuclear or infranuclear neurologic causes. Sensory and motor fusion are usually intact. When all motor factors have been neutralized to realign the diplopic images, a normal fusion range can usually be demonstrated.

Asthenopic symptoms are common in patients with convergence insufficiency. The amplitudes of both convergence and divergence can be affected. There is usually no traumatic, neurologic, or functional basis to these symptoms, and the patients respond well to exercises designed to improve the near point of convergence and expand the fusion range. This apparent change in vergence ability is merely kinetic, the underlying system being normal. Patients with inherent fusional deficits (e.g., those with childhood strabismus) do not show significant improvement in the size of their fusion range in response to appropriately designed exercise programs.

CLINICAL DISORDERS AFFECTING VERGENCES

Neurologic disorders may disturb the control areas or pathways serving the ocular motor system, resulting in conjugate and disjugate gaze dysfunction. These disorders include vascular accidents, neoplastic growth, inflammatory and demyelinating processes, and degenerative diseases.

Lesions in the supranuclear areas or their pathways cause predominantly conjugate gaze difficulties but can affect convergence, particularly if the problem lies in or near the midline. Examples include Parkinson's disease and Huntington's chorea. Patients with progressive supranuclear palsy complain of difficulty reading or eating due to a conjugate paralysis of downgaze, rather than convergence weakness. In this disorder, associated neck rigidity adds further to the problem (Roper-Hall, 1973; Pfaffenbach et al., 1972).

Large lesions, particularly in the brainstem, are likely to produce complex neurologic findings. For an isolated ocular movement problem to occur, the lesions must be extremely discrete. Parinaud's syndrome (Walsh and Hoyt, 1969a) or the Sylvian aqueduct syndrome, the latter encompassing a broader range of clinical features than that originally described (Sanders and Bird, 1970), is caused by a lesion affecting the periaqueductal gray matter of the pretectum as well as the tegmental structures of the midbrain. The lesion may be caused by an intrinsic neoplasm or vascular accident or by an extrinsic pressure effect on the midbrain that results in raised intracranial pressure. A pinealoma is the most common cause. The syndrome generally includes defective vertical conjugate gaze, with saccadic function affected much earlier than pursuit and upgaze more greatly affected than downgaze, dissociation of the pupillary light/near reflex, and a poor response to a convergence stimulus (Walsh and Hoyt, 1969a). Convergence is often elicited in the extraordinary convergence retraction nystagmus seen on attempting to look up or make upward saccades (Smith et al., 1959). Nuclear lesions in the area of the third nerve complex affect convergence by their direct effect on medial rectus function.

Internuclear disturbances are produced by lesions involving the medial longitudinal fasciculus (MLF) and are commonly caused by microvascular accidents, postviral processes, or inflammatory or demyelinating disease. Bilateral internuclear ophthalmoplegia (INO) is most often produced by demyelinating disease (Walsh and Hoyt, 1969a), although occlusive cerebrovascular disease of the posterior circulation may also produce this entity, especially in an older age group (Gonyea, 1974). Classically INO is described as adduction weakness with abducting nystagmus in the fellow eye, but with convergence function spared. Rarely, a patient with a bilateral INO will demonstrate marked exotropia and the inability to adduct either eye or converge. Abducting nystagmus is generally absent (Daroff and Hoyt, 1971). The one-and-a-half syndrome as described by Fisher (1967) includes a horizontal gaze paresis to one side, and an INO to the other. This is produced by a lesion in the pons affecting the ipsilateral PPRF and MLF. The presence of the conjugate gaze paresis can mask involvement of the contralateral MLF. Underlying bilateral MLF involvement is likely when associated with impaired consciousness from basilar artery disease, as the reticular formation and MLFs share a common blood supply (Gonyea, 1974).

Infranuclear dysfunction can mimic a convergence problem because paralysis of a medial rectus or a depressor muscle will affect the final common pathway for gaze inward and downward and may mask normal convergence function, thus simulating a convergence weakness. Similarly, restrictive ocular muscle problems or myopathic conditions may prevent the intact vergence system from producing a smooth convergence movement, despite normal innervation. Peripheral muscle restrictions of this nature are common in such diverse entities as thyroid myopathy and orbital blowout fractures. These conditions show resistance when forced passive ductions are tested (Glaser, 1978).

Convergence weakness is often seen in systemic disorders when patients are debilitated or not fully alert, as it requires considerable voluntary effort and attention to converge. This is probably caused by a lack of supranuclear input or some nonspecific effect on the areas controlling convergence. Paresis of accommodation and convergence may be seen following viral illness, and does not always make a full spontaneous recovery. Organic causes for diminished accommodation are usually accompanied by associated convergence weakness, and rarely respond well to conventional orthoptic therapy or prisms. A carefully selected group of these patients does well with bilateral resection of the medial rectus muscles (von Noorden, 1976).

Systemic medications affecting the autonomic nervous system can disturb functions subserved by the parasympathetic and sympathetic nerve supply to the eye. These drugs can have both central and peripheral effects. Examples of such agents include tranquilizers such as diazepam (Valium) or chlordiazepoxide (Librium), which tend to weaken accommodation; parasympatholytic agents such as Lomotil, which contains atropine; and muscle relaxants (Norris, 1971). Alcohol and barbiturates also affect vergence function (von Noorden, 1980).

Since convergence is largely under voluntary control this part of the vergence system is susceptible to psychiatric disturbances and stress as well as malingering, a situation in which a patient has a particular need for secondary gain. Disturbances in the convergence mechanism can take any form, from complete paralysis of accommodation, convergence, or both, to a spasm of the near reflex at the opposite end of the spectrum in which the patient exhibits an esotropia, pupillary miosis, and accommodative spasm. Divergence, being an involuntary function, is not subject to the same type of derangement, although some authors believe this can occur (Lyle, 1954).

As mentioned earlier, trauma can cause organic paralysis of convergence and divergence as a sequela of severe closed head injury, although instances have been reported following whiplash injuries. In these cases there is apparent loss of motor fusion, occasionally accompanied by sensory fusional loss (Pratt-Johnson, 1973; Pratt-Johnson and Tillson, 1979; Wade, 1960, 1965; Stanworth and Mein, 1971; Doden and Bunge, 1965; Diener, 1953).

Patients with congenital or longstanding manifest strabismus frequently demonstrate inherently diminished fusional amplitudes. This results from the failure of development of binocular sensorimotor reflexes. If a new ocular, neurologic, or systemic problem occurs later in life, the preexisting fusional vergence disorder can be misleading. Similarly, longstanding previously asymptomatic heterophorias may decompensate, often fairly rapidly, producing asthenopic symptoms and presenting as an apparently acquired vergence problem.

DIFFERENTIAL DIAGNOSIS OF TRUE AND PSEUDOVERGENCE ANOMALIES

Patients with convergence anomalies will often complain of symptoms in the near position. Other conditions that can produce symptoms at near are those affecting downgaze because the normal position adopted for close work tasks is also slightly depressed (Roper-Hall, 1980). A-pattern exotropia or V-pattern esotropia, any infranuclear weakness affecting superior oblique or inferior rectus function unilaterally or bilaterally, and supranuclear disorders affecting saccadic or pursuit downgaze movement must be considered, as they all affect the ability to fixate in the reading position. Infranuclear involvement of one or both medial recti and certain cases of bilateral internuclear ophthalmoplegia can affect adduction and interfere with convergence.

Divergence paresis is manifested by the sudden onset of horizontal diplopia at distance. Inability to diverge the visual axes will produce a concomitant esodeviation that enlarges with increasing distance from the patient. Unilateral or bilateral weaknesses of the sixth nerve also demonstrate a relative esotropia for distance, but can be differentiated from divergence paresis by the presence of abduction limitation. The condition should also be differentiated from concomitant intermittent esotropia of the divergence weakness type often associated with increasing myopia, and from convergence spasm that presents as a variable esotropia with associated pupillary findings.

Infranuclear disorders can cause superior rectus or inferior oblique weaknesses that produce difficulties at distance, as can A-esotropia and V-exotropia. Restrictive ocular problems can produce symptoms in any position by preventing normal ocular motility and affecting ductions, versions, and the intact vergence system, and are generally differentiated from supranuclear entities by the presence of positive forced ductions.

CLASSIFICATION OF CLINICAL VERGENCE DYSFUNCTION

Disturbance of one of the vergence mechanisms is characterized by either an excess or insufficiency of effort expended for a necessary task. As accommodative and pupillary functions are closely linked with convergence activity, they should not be overlooked in disorders affecting horizontal vergences. Accommodative and pupillary dysfunctions are not normally associated with disturbances of divergence, vertical vergence, or cyclovergence.

Convergence Dysfunction

Insufficient Convergence

Convergence weakness is characterized by a remote near point of convergence associated with decreased fusional amplitudes with respect to the age and refractive error of the patient. Any degree of insufficiency can be seen from a mild condition producing only minimal asthenopic symptoms to a complete paralysis of convergence.

Paralysis or paresis of convergence is a supranuclear condition caused by such entities as cerebrovascular accidents, head trauma, or inflammatory or postviral illnesses. It is usually associated with a similar degree of accommodative dysfunction. Complete convergence paralysis causes exotropia of approximately 20 diopters in the near position, which becomes progressively less with increasing distance from the patient. The images may be fused at distance; however, a patient with preexisting exophoria in this position, previously controlled by positive relative convergence, may complain of diplopia due to a small manifest exotropia (Walsh and Hoyt, 1969a).

On examination no abnormality is seen in ductions or versions. An exotropia is demonstrable for near that measures the same in any gaze direction at one distance, regardless of the fixating eye. The deviation is maximal the closer the target is brought toward the patient. Crossed diplopia is noted subjectively in all near gaze positions. The pupils often react when attempts are made to respond to the near stimulus, but there are exceptions, particularly when the cause is functional (Walsh and Hoyt, 1969b).

Since the patient cannot make a convergence movement there is no point from which a near point can be assessed unless a prism is used to neutralize the deviation first. In complete paralysis there will still be no convergence ability demonstrable despite the neutralizing prism, as the convergence range, or motor fusion, is completely lost. These patients may also have inadequate divergence amplitudes. Sensory fusion and stereopsis are generally found to be normal when tested with the angle of deviation neutralized artificially, if the deficit affects motor fusion only. In certain cases, however, both motor and sensory fusion are involved (Pratt-Johnson and Tillson, 1979). When motor fusion is absent neither prisms nor surgery will be of benefit. Occlusion of one eye may be necessary, and if the accommodative mechanism is affected appropriate convex lenses may be needed.

In paresis of convergence, some ability to converge is maintained. Convergence paresis is seen as a stage in the recovery of a resolving convergence paralysis. Base-in prisms may be used at this stage if a sufficient range of convergence exists to keep the images fused for useful periods of time. Exercises to improve the near point and extend the convergence amplitudes may be helpful.

CASE REPORT MW. A 30-year-old pilot was injured in an airline crash. He sustained multiple injuries including severe concussion, a fractured mandible, facial lacerations including several near the left eye, and a peripheral seventh nerve palsy. Two days later an ophthalmologic examination was requested in the neurosurgical intensive care unit. Subcutaneous hematomata were present in both lids, and the patient preferred to keep both eyes closed. A small conjunctival laceration was found in the left eye. The pupils were approximately 3 mm and equal, reacting poorly (right worse than left) to light and accommodation. The ocular movements were grossly full. The patient was responsive to gross commands, but a full eye examination was not possible.

Eight days later the patient's mental status had improved dramatically and he complained of diplopia and poor vision. His glasses had been lost in the crash.

Bedside examination revealed a small exophoria at distance and a marked alternating exotropia at near. The ocular ductions and versions were full, but convergence ability was nil. A new myopic correction was prescribed with immediate improvement in visual acuity, but diplopia persisted in the near position. Regular bedside visits showed gradual daily improvement in his convergence problems. Although the patient was undergoing spontaneous resolution of his ocular problems, convergence exercises were given after he was able to fuse the exotropia. A full ophthalmologic examination 10 days later revealed some minor retinal damage, which was investigated and required no treatment. At this time the patient demonstrated normal fusion in all gaze positions and normal convergence ability, indicating that spontaneous recovery had occurred.

CASE REPORT JR. A 21-year-old male undergraduate student complained of blurred vision, intermittent horizontal diplopia, and pain in both eyes for nine months. The symptoms were exaggerated following a viral chest infection three months earlier. A slight left ptosis predated the onset of diplopia, and a neurologist diagnosed myasthenia gravis and began pyridostigmine (Mestinon) therapy. The patient also had a one-year history of a manic-depressive disorder and was taking the following daily medications when we first examined him: lithium carbonate, 1200 mg; chlordiazepoxide, (Librium) 25 to 75 mg; triclofose prn; pyridostigmine, 60 mg; and atropine, 1/125 g twice a day. His ocular symptoms were worse when tired, anxious, or depressed, or on maximal drug therapy.

On examination a moderate exophoria was noted greater at near than distance, and he read 20/25 OU with his myopic correction. Ocular movements were full and a 1-mm ptosis OS was noted. He converged to 15 cm with discomfort, and 8 to 10 cm with extreme effort. The near point of accommodation was between 10 and 14 cm OU, the image blurring and clearing with effort. The pupils were large (6 mm) but reacted appropriately to light and near stimuli.

A diagnosis of intermittent exotropia with associated convergence and accommodation insufficiency was made. The systemic medical problems and medications were considered to be a large contributing factor. Convergence therapy was attempted with limited success because frequent changes were prescribed in the dosages or types of drugs needed for his various illnesses. Several sessions were canceled because he was too sleepy or depressed to benefit from exercises, and on some occasions when the medications were discontinued or decreased, the near points of convergence and accommodation and his fusional amplitudes were absolutely normal. It was concluded that further convergence therapy would be inappropriate unless these other factors could be controlled. Plus 1.00 lenses were given for reading.

Convergence insufficiency is a nonneurologic concomitant condition unrelated to any organic cause. The condition can produce severe asthenopic symptoms and mimic convergence paralysis or paresis. The near point of convergence recedes, amplitudes of convergence are diminished, and the patients complain of eyestrain related to close work. Most of these patients recall that they were never able to converge voluntarily ("cross their eyes") in childhood. Onset is gradual, but symptoms are frequently associated with a change in occupation or a period in which intense study is necessary, placing a strain on the mechanism. The symptoms are common in students, bookkeepers, seamstresses, and many others who do detailed work. Similarly, some patients with convergence insufficiency are concurrently experiencing a period of stress, and the condition is sometimes seen in individuals who are also mildly depressed or neurotic. When the subjective symptoms exceed those that seem possible from the degree of the disorder, a functional component such as depression or malingering should be suspected.

With the exception of those with an associated accommodative insufficiency, patients respond extraordinarily well to orthoptic exercises designed to teach recognition of the breakpoint of diplopia and improve the convergence near point and fusional amplitudes (von Noorden, 1980). If therapy is discontinued at this stage the condition may recur. A future recurrence is unlikely if the patient is taught to exert positive and negative relative convergence using such therapeutic aids as stereograms and stereoscopes. Some therapists suggest that these exercises be practised on a regular basis indefinitely to ensure permanent relief of symptoms. The final stage in treatment is to teach voluntary convergence, that is, the ability to converge the eyes without the stimulus of a fixation target, as patients who have this ability will rarely develop future symptoms.

CASE REPORT DWK. A 24-year-old male graduate engineering student noted ocular fatigue for three years when doing graphs. Six months before our first examination he complained of increasing ocular discomfort after prolonged close work. At that time a neurologist noted decreased convergence and upgaze ability and the patient was admitted for a full neurologic evaluation to rule out myasthenia gravis or a possible Parinaud's syndrome caused by pinealoma. The findings were entirely negative for any pathology and he was referred for neuro-ophthalmologic examination. Visual acuity wearing his myopic correction was 20/15 OU. Cover testing revealed an exophoria of 12^{Δ} at near and 1^{Δ} at distance associated with a slight V pattern. The near point of convergence was 14 cm, to 6/7 cm with immense effort accompanied by head-shuddering from 10 cm. The near point of accommodation was normal for his age and refractive error. Ocular movements with the exception of convergence were normal as was the rest of the eye examination. Base-in fusional amplitudes were normal, being $6^{\Delta}/6^{\Delta}$ at distance and $18^{\Delta}/16^{\Delta}$ (his exophoria was 12^{Δ}) at near. Base-out amplitudes were $30^{\Delta}/25^{\Delta}$ at near, but with extreme discomfort he could achieve $40^{\Delta}/40^{\Delta}$ at both distance and near.

A diagnosis of exophoria with convergence insufficiency was made despite the relatively good near point and amplitudes of convergence. A course of five convergence treatments was given over the next four months. Large amplitudes were achieved without discomfort, and he could overcome 40^{Δ} of prism base-out by jump convergence at near and exhibit voluntary convergence without needing a fixation target. Exercises were discontinued for three months; at the return visit all findings were normal and the patient was still asymptomatic.

Excessive Convergence

The relationship between accommodative convergence and the amount of accommodation exerted is known as the AC/A ratio. When accommodation is excessive, or the ratio is high, more convergence is exerted than necessary to align the visual axes and overconvergence or esotropia results. This is usually seen as an acquired concomitant strabismus occurring in young children around three to four years of age. Two types of accommodative esotropia are recognized, the first having a normal AC/A ratio and the second a high ratio. In the first type a moderate degree of uncorrected hyperopia produces a blurred image. The patient can clear this by accommodating but is unable to exert negative relative convergence to maintain binocular vision, and the deviation becomes esotropic. This strabismus is said to be fully accommodative when it is completely eliminated by wearing the appropriate hyperopic correction, and partially accommodative if the deviation is reduced but not eliminated by the glasses.

The second condition, convergence-excess esotropia, is due to a high AC/A ratio. These patients have a small esophoria for distance, with an appropriate hyperopic correction if needed. The deviation becomes esotropic at near fixation because of the excessive convergence occurring where accommodation is maximal. A bifocal correction or anticholinesterase therapy are often used to alleviate the excessive convergence produced by accommodative effort. Surgical intervention is often necessary to obtain a binocular result.

CASE REPORT DG. The five-year-old son of an ophthalmologist was seen in evaluation of his convergence-excess accommodative esotropia. Two weeks before his second birthday his left eye turned in. He was examined and given a cycloplegic refraction the same day! A hyperopic correction was ordered but no occlusion therapy was found to be necessary. A course of miotic therapy and bifocals was given, and a 4.5 mm medial rectus recession and 7 mm lateral rectus resection of the left eye was performed. Postoperatively he continued to wear the bifocals.

On examination, his visual acuity was 20/20 OD and 20/15 OS, wearing

+5.50, +0.50 at axis 48° OD and +5.50, +0.50 at axis 140° OS. An esophoria of 3^{Δ} was measured with this correction at distance. A 5^{Δ} esophoria was measured becoming an 18^{Δ} intermittent esophoria through the top segment at near. The esotropia increased markedly without correction, becoming 45^{Δ} at near and 40^{Δ} at distance. A full fusion range without suppression was elicited and he demonstrated excellent stereoscopic responses. The bifocal add was reduced to +1.75 OU with no significant change in his examination.

Convergence spasm, or spasm of the near reflex is a form of excessive or inappropriate convergence, which is an acquired disorder. It is almost always functional. It often has its onset during periods of stress, for example, during final examinations in school or college. Rarely, it can be caused by inflammatory conditions and has been seen occasionally after head trauma (Walsh and Hoyt, 1969a). It is rare before puberty and is more common in females than males. The condition may present with subtle findings often coexisting with other ocular complaints, or manifest itself as a large esotropia with associated accommodative and pupillary findings.

The condition is generally intermittent and recurrent, and is characterized by variability of esodeviation, associated pseudomyopia due to inappropriate accommodation for distance, and pupillary constriction noted when the visual axes converge inappropriately. Near and far points of accommodation are also variable, and may be so close to each other at times during testing that the range is only a few centimeters. The near point of convergence may appear normal, but the patient cannot relax the visual axes very much beyond that point before becoming esotropic, so the range of convergence is usually small. Prism amplitudes show variable convergence ability, but divergence is usually poor and can be nil. Although this is a concomitant supranuclear condition, incomitant measurements may be noted on lateral gaze due to the variability of convergence effort during testing. This same effort may produce apparent limitation of abduction during ocular movement testing, thus simulating bilateral sixth nerve weakness (Walsh and Hoyt, 1969b). Convergence spasm should be carefully differentiated from the divergence weakness group of disorders and from any true unilateral or bilateral infranuclear abducens weakness.

Management of this condition can be difficult because of its functional nature. The condition may be superimposed on other unrelated ocular problems that may be causing anxiety, and sometimes when these are treated the spasm will clear spontaneously. Most patients can be taught to control the episodes once the nature of the problem has been explained to them. Patients are encouraged to interrupt their activities or remove themselves from the stressful situation when possible as soon as the symptoms begin, and relax for five to ten minutes or until symptoms abate. If the attacks cannot be broken by these means, a trial of weak cycloplegic agents is often helpful. Cases where stress, depression, or other psychiatric disturbances appear to be the underlying cause should be referred for competent specialist therapy.

CASE REPORT KC. A 26-year-old female graduate student noted the sudden onset of horizontal diplopia with blurring of vision after a strenuous day three years prior to our examination. The symptoms cleared gradually over the next few days. Further episodes occurred over the next three years, some as frequently as once a week, and some lasting 14 days. In the past three months the frequency, duration, and severity of her symptoms had increased and were exacerbated if she was upset or under stress. On examination the patient's visual acuity was 20/15 OU wearing −2.75 OD and −1.50 OS. A variable intermittent esotropia of approximately 4^{Δ} at near and 6^{Δ} at distance was measured. The ductions and versions were normal and the deviation remained the same to each side at the measured distance. A Hess chart showed variable but concomitant esodeviation without paresis.

The bifoveal near point of convergence was 6 cm, but the accommodative near point was variable from 12 to 16 cm. The pupils reacted normally during efforts to converge or accommodate at near but constricted inappropriately during distance testing. Base-out fusional amplitudes were excellent, being $40^{\Delta}/40^{\Delta}$ at near. Her base-in amplitudes were variable, from normal at times to poor during a spastic moment, being $8^{\Delta}/6^{\Delta}$ to $0^{\Delta}/1^{\Delta}$ at distance and $16^{\Delta}/14^{\Delta}$ to $2^{\Delta}/1^{\Delta}$ at near during the same examination. The rest of her ocular findings were normal. A diagnosis of spasm of the near reflex was made. Cycloplegic refraction confirmed that her myopic correction was appropriate, and a prescription for 1% cyclopentolate (Cyclogyl) three times a day was prescribed, with relief of symptoms five days later. A recurrence a few days later was again successfully alleviated by repeating the cycloplegic therapy for another week.

Convergence retraction nystagmus is another clinical entity in which inappropriate convergence is demonstrated during certain eye movements. This is caused by simultaneous co-contracture of all the ocular muscles in an attempt to make an upward eye movement rather than by a true convergence effort. This co-contracture explains the retraction seen in the repeated convergence movements. It is a characteristic finding in Parinaud's syndrome in which convergence ability to a near stimulus may be diminished or absent. This therefore is a supranuclear disturbance of convergence, as convergence movements can be elicited, although inappropriately, during attempted upward saccades. It is demonstrated most effectively with a downward-moving optokinetic tape (Walsh and Hoyt, 1969a; Smith et al., 1959).

Divergence Dysfunction

Insufficient Divergence

A form of longstanding nonaccommodative esodeviation exists that is classified as esotropia of the divergence weakness type. This is the converse of the convergence-excess type already described in that the esodeviation is generally small and fused for near, becoming larger and often manifest for distance fixation. The patient must exert negative relative fusional divergence if the deviation is to be controlled for distance. In patients of this type who are myopic, the deviation is increased when refractive correction is worn, particularly if there is an overcorrection. This distance deviation will often become manifest with the increasing myopia of early teenage years. The patient describes symptoms of uncrossed diplopia for distance, which is concomitant across the gaze field. These patients are treated easily with an appropriate base-out prism, which places the deviation within the range where divergence can be exerted. The prism can be incorporated into the spectacle correction if glasses are worn. If the myopic correction is significant, some of the prismatic effect may be achieved by decentration. If the prism required for fusion exceeds that which can be incorporated or worn without complaints about the weight or cosmesis, ocular muscle surgery may be indicated. Orthoptic exercises to expand the divergence range are rarely effective.

CASE REPORT AO. A nine-year-old boy complained of horizontal diplopia at distance for three months, at first intermittent, becoming constant. He had no complaints in the near position.

His uncorrected visual activity was $20/15^{-1}$ OU. An exophoria of 6^{Δ} was measured at 1/3 m, becoming a right esotropia of 10^{Δ} with diplopia at 1 m and 14^{Δ} at 6 m. His ocular movements were full, no incomitance was demonstrable on Synoptophore measurements, and a good fusion range with stereoscopic responses was elicited. Fusional amplitudes at near were $40^{\Delta}/35^{\Delta}$ base-out and $4^{\Delta}/4^{\Delta}$ base-in. At distance the deviation was neutralized first with 14^{Δ} base-in; base-out amplitudes were $11^{\Delta}/11^{\Delta}$ (from 14^{Δ} to 25^{Δ}), and base-in were $4^{\Delta}/4^{\Delta}$ (from 14^{Δ} to 10^{Δ}).

A diagnosis of concomitant decompensated esodeviation of the divergence weakness type was made. Five-diopter base-out prisms OU were ordered in plano lenses with immediate relief of diplopia. Orthoptic exercises to improve divergence amplitudes were unsuccessful and the patient could not be weaned from the prismatic correction. A 4.5 mm left medial rectus muscle recession and 3 mm left lateral rectus muscle resection was undertaken. Postoperative measurements showed a 2^{Δ} esophoria at near and an 8^{Δ} intermittent esotropia at distance. Wearing his original prism glasses for a few months stabilized the distance deviation until the patient reported that diplopia was no longer present at distance without his glasses.

Although his latent deviation could be dissociated easily in a clinical setting and his divergence amplitudes were still poor (1^{Δ} placed base-in immediately broke his fusion at distance), the patient was asymptomatic at home and in school, so the prisms were discontinued.

Divergence-insufficiency type esotropia should be differentiated from the supranuclear entity of divergence paralysis (Walsh and Hoyt, 1969a). This neurologic condition is characterized by a sudden onset of symptoms, the patient describing horizontal uncrossed diplopia for distance. Occasionally patients will describe a sudden onset of blurred vision, rather than diplopia. This is binocular blurring, and is a *forme fruste* of diplopia. It is alleviated with either eye covered or when the deviation is neutralized with prisms. This symptom is more common in supranuclear disturbances of ocular movement than from infranuclear causes (Roper-Hall and Burde, 1977).

On examination, no ocular version or duction weakness is found. Abduction in particular, is normal. There is an esodeviation that is small and usually fused if present at near, becoming an esotropia that increases in size with receding fixation. The deviation is concomitant, not changing in any direction at a specified distance. The amplitudes of divergence are diminished or absent at distance and near. Convergence and accommodative amplitudes are often normal, although a convergence insufficiency may accompany the condition, producing an exotropia within the range of single vision. The patient may have other associated neurologic signs or symptoms, but the condition can exist as an isolated neurologic entity. It is most often caused by a sudden microvascular or inflammatory event in the brainstem or following head trauma (Walsh and Hoyt, 1969a). It is also reported in association with raised intracranial pressure, aqueductal stenosis, and in certain cases of cerebellar tumor (Walsh and Hoyt, 1969b; Kirkham et al., 1972; Hogg and Schoenberg, 1979; Lippmann, 1944).

CASE REPORT TD. A 54-year-old woman noted the sudden onset of horizontal diplopia at distance, occurring a few weeks after a left maxillary sinus infection. Surgical exploration of the maxillary sinus revealed no pathology, and no association between the two conditions could be made. Her past ocular history included a branch retinal vein occlusion OS three years earlier. Medical evaluation at that time revealed no systemic disorders.

Ocular examination showed corrected visual acuity of 20/20 OD and $20/20^{-1}$ OS. An esotropia was present at distance and measured 25^{Δ} to 30^{Δ} in primary and lateral gazes; and was less in the near position. Ocular ductions were full, although at times on version testing a questionable underaction of the right moreso than the left lateral rectus was thought to be present. A Hess chart confirmed the concomitant nature of the condition and the absence of any abduction limitation.

A diagnosis was made of divergence paralysis on a presumed vascular basis. At this stage the patient's divergence amplitudes were nil, and she required the full neutralizing prism to eliminate the diplopia. As this was a high-power prism it was elected to occlude one lens of her bifocal spectacles. She was seen at monthly intervals for the next six months, during which time she made a steady and almost complete spontaneous recovery. On the second monthly visit the deviation became exophoric at near, and the esodeviation of 14^{Δ} at distance was fused with a 12^{Δ} base-out Fresnel prism on the top segment of her left lens. At each subsequent visit the deviation decreased and the strength of prism was reduced appropriately. At a final visit when the residual deviation was stable, a new manifest bifocal correction was given, with a 1^{Δ} base-out prism incorporated into the left lens, giving a full field of binocular single vision.

Divergence paresis describes the condition in which a patient retains some ability to diverge, but that is inadequate to maintain binocular control. It is a mild version of divergence paralysis and represents the same etiologic condition either as a less severe entity or perhaps, full paralysis in resolving stages. The totally concomitant esotropia with full abduction has been reported to display some incomitant features as it resolves, occasionally becoming a nuclear sixth nerve weakness (Bielschowsky, 1943; Walsh and Hoyt, 1969a). Divergence paralysis and paresis both have the same neurologic significance, and all patients with these findings should undergo thorough neurologic investigation. They respond well to temporary use of base-out Fresnel prisms.

Excessive Divergence

Excessive divergence at distance can produce an intermittent exotropia, called divergence-excess type. This exodeviation becomes progressively larger with increasing distance from the patient. It is believed that the condition develops slowly from an exophoria present in early childhood and becomes manifest, at first intermittently, by the preteens or early adulthood. Subjective symptoms may be minimal, as these young patients develop dense areas of suppression (Pratt-Johnson et al., 1981).

CASE REPORT RM. A three-year-old girl was examined after her mother and pediatrician noted her left eye turning out intermittently. No strabismus was detected at a routine ophthalmologic examination one year previously. Her uncorrected visual acuity was 20/20 OD and 20/20 OS. On prism measurements an exophoria of 6^{Δ} at near and a left exotropia of 20^{Δ} at distance were found. Plus 3.00 lenses to relax any accommodative effort at near did not alter the size of the deviation and a diagnosis of true divergence excess exotropia was made. An atropine cycloplegic refraction revealed hyperopia of +1.50 OD, +1.75 OS, but no glasses were ordered. Fundus examination was normal.

Seven millimeter bilateral lateral rectus recessions were carried out under general anesthesia. Immediately postoperatively a 5^{Δ} esophoria at near and 2^{Δ} left esotropia at distance were measured. Slight overcorrection is a desired surgical result. In the later postoperative period a gradual increase in her esodeviation necessitated a combined course of miotic therapy, plus lenses, and later, weak base-out prisms to correct the deviation. After this therapy was completed she maintained a small esophoria in all positions without refractive correction. Her acuity was 20/15 OU, she had a good fusion range without suppression, and she demonstrated gross stereoscopic responses.

Convergence and Divergence Dysfunction

Occasionally a patient simultaneously will lose the ability to converge and diverge. This condition is always acquired and organic. It represents a total loss of vergence ability, or motor fusion. The characteristics are those described for convergence paralysis, with the addition of diminished or absent divergence amplitudes.

Vertical Vergence Dysfunction

Insufficient Vertical Vergences

Strictly speaking, this is not a distinct entity but a normal situation that occurs with infranuclear paresis or paralysis of one of the vertically acting extraocular muscles. The normal amplitude of vertical vergence ability is a diopter or two at most in either direction. Hyperdeviation greater than one diopter therefore will produce symptomatic hyperphoria, or diplopia from hypertropia. Prismatic correction of the vertical diplopia caused by a recently acquired hypertropia therefore requires almost full neutralization of the deviation, and is only practical when the incomitance permits an adequate field of binocular single vision (Roper-Hall and Burde, 1979). This is unlike the situation in horizontal deviations in which often less than half the deviation need be corrected by prisms, the rest being controlled by the patient's horizontal fusional amplitudes.

CASE REPORT DHK. A 52-year-old man noted vertical diplopia following neurosurgical removal of a meningioma from the trigeminal nerve in the cerebellopontine cistern area. A diagnosis of trochlear nerve damage secondary to surgical manipulation was made. Ophthalmic examination was normal except for a typical right superior oblique palsy. A right hypertropia was present, measuring 10^{Δ} at distance and 14^{Δ} at near. The deviation increased in downgaze and head tilt to the right, and was maximal in left downgaze. Torsional testing revealed minimal excyclotorsion of the right eye only, in primary and downgaze. No deviation was measurable on upgaze and the patient intermittently depressed his chin to use this diplopia-free position. Almost the full neutralizing prism was necessary to permit binocular fusion as the patient had normal small vertical fusional amplitudes of one to two diopters. A 12^{Δ} Fresnel prism placed base-down on his right lens relieved the diplopia for distance and near, providing he depressed his chin to read.

The patient was seen four more times over the next seven months, during which time the hypertropia continued to improve and the prisms were reduced and then discontinued accordingly, as complete spontaneous recovery took place.

Skew deviation is another acquired clinical entity causing a sudden onset of hypertropia. There may be little or no deviation in primary gaze, but a hypertropia of any degree appears in lateral gaze to one or both sides. The deviation is often concomitant in lateral up and downgaze to one side, preventing one muscle from being isolated as an infranuclear paralysis. The deviation may be laterally incomitant or periodic. The condition is caused by a lesion in the posterior fossa, and may be associated with nystagmus or internuclear ophthalmoplegia (Walsh and Hoyt, 1969a, 1969b). The patient may notice binocular blurring rather than diplopia when the deviation is manifest (Roper-Hall and Burde, 1977).

CASE REPORT DK. An 18-year-old female noted the sudden onset of vertical diplopia four days earlier. She could obtain single vision by turning her face to the left.

Her visual acuity was 20/30-1 OD and 20/50 OS with her myopic correction. A moderate left hypertropia of 6^{Δ} associated with a small left exotropia was present in primary gaze, increasing in left gaze. The hyperdeviation did not alter in right or left head tilt, and measured the same in left upgaze as in left downgaze. The Hess chart confirmed the concomitant nature of the deviation and a diagnosis of skew deviation was made.

Ocular findings included gaze-paretic nystagmus in left gaze, a 2 mm ptosis OS, decreased corneal sensation OS, and an enlarged blind spot OS on visual field testing. These ocular symptoms were followed soon after by paresis of both lower extremities. She was hospitalized for neurologic evaluation and a probable diagnosis of multiple sclerosis was made. She was treated with intravenous steroid drip followed by subsequent clearing of all symptoms. Over the next five years recurrent episodes of lower extremity weakness with full remissions confirmed the diagnosis of multiple sclerosis.

Excessive Vertical Vergences

Any individual with a congenital or longstanding hyperdeviation capable of being fused intermittently has by definition a large vertical fusion range. Some patients with gradually developing hypertropias, such as seen in thyroid ocular myopathy, may also display expanded vertical vergence ability. This ability is an adaptation to an abnormal condition and requires a developmental period, usually in childhood. Assessment of the vertical fusional amplitudes is often helpful in differentiating preexisting from recently acquired neurologic disorders.

CASE REPORT MQ. A 16-year-old boy was evaluated for intermittent upward drifting of his right eye. His parents first noticed this at two years of age when he was tired. He had been delivered by forceps and sustained subsequent swelling of the right side of his face. Present symptoms included occasional vertical diplopia, but the main concern was poor cosmetic appearance when his eye deviated.

His uncorrected visual acuity was 20/15-2 OU. A noticeable head tilt to the right with variable chin elevation was present, with which a marked right hyperphoria of 20^{Δ} was measured at distance. This increased without the head posture to 30^{Δ} at distance and 35^{Δ} at near, although the deviation was easily dissociated to a right hypertropia. This means that the patient had large vertical fusional amplitudes of between 20^{Δ} and 30^{Δ}. It was associated with a 10^{Δ} exodeviation in all positions. The right hypertropia also increased in left gaze and when the head was tilted to the right. Ocular movements documented on the Hess chart showed a concomitant deviation due to spread of comitance, underaction of the superior oblique muscle, and corresponding overactions of the right inferior oblique and inferior rectus muscles. No obvious torsion was measured. The rest of the ocular examination was normal.

The patient underwent a right superior oblique tuck and right inferior oblique myectomy with complete relief of symptoms, including head tilt.

Dissociated vertical divergence (DVD) is an unusual clinical entity first described in detail by Bielschowsky (1943). It is a disjugate condition in which one eye at a time becomes elevated and extorted spontaneously, or when covered, returning to primary gaze when uncovered. This would suggest extraordinary powers of motor vertical vergence, because not only can one eye deviate markedly and apparently be controlled moments later, demonstrating a vertical amplitude of twenty or more diopters, but the other eye is capable of the same ability in the opposite fusional direction. These patients rarely demonstrate true sensory fusional responses, however.

Bielschowsky (1943) originally described a phenomenon present in DVD that could be elicited using a dark glass wedge. The Bielschowsky phenomenon is generally tested now using a bar of neutral filters of increasing density (von Noorden, 1977). This bar is placed before the fixating eye. The opposite eye is occluded, and elevates behind the cover as just described. The bar is moved before the fixating eye, beginning with the least dense filter. The covered eye is observed to move downward from its elevated position, often becoming hypotropic. The fixating eye meanwhile remains in the midline, looking through filters of increasing neutral density. This test is used to differentiate DVD from alternating hypertropia caused by paresis of vertically acting muscles, the latter generally being associated with marked overaction of the inferior oblique muscles.

Dissociated vertical divergence can be congenital or develop in early childhood, and may be associated with any type of baseline deviation (usually a small hypotropia). It is frequently accompanied by latent nystagmus (Mein and Johnson, 1981), and rarely produces symptoms apart from the cosmetic aspects of the intermittent hypertropia.

CASE REPORT SR. A 19-year-old female noted intermittent vertical diplopia for at least 10 years. Her mother recalled observing the daughter's left eye elevating noticeably on occasion in early childhood, but with spontaneous improvement. She had noticed the eye elevating again recently, and the patient also reported an increase in the frequency of diplopia.

Her uncorrected visual acuity was 20/15 OU. A 6^{Δ} left esotropia with a variable left hypotropia of 3^{Δ} to 8^{Δ} was present in primary gaze. A compensatory head posture consisting of chin elevation reduced the deviation, which could then be fused, to a 2^{Δ} esophoria with a 2^{Δ} right hyperphoria. On cross-cover dissociation in primary gaze the left hypotropia was gradually converted to moderate left hypertropia of approximately 15^{Δ}. As the left eye elevated behind the occluder it also extorted. The occluder was then transferred to cover the right eye and the left eye moved down and intorted, bobbing slightly below the midline before resuming fixation in primary gaze. The covered right eye meanwhile elevated and extorted similarly behind the cover, producing right hypertropia of approximately 18^{Δ}. These findings were consistent with DVD.

Ocular movements showed variable overaction of both inferior oblique muscles and some bilateral superior rectus muscle weakness. On diplopia testing, binocular responses were occasionally reported at near, but at all other times alternating suppression and not diplopia was elicited. A good fusion range and reasonable stereoscopic responses were demonstrable on Synoptophore examination, although only 200 arc-seconds of stereoacuity were obtained on the Titmus (fly) vectograph test, and no stereoscopic responses were elicited using the Titmus random-dot stereotest.

A diagnosis of left esotropia with left hypotropia and DVD was made. The deviation was associated with a gross form of normal fusion and stereopsis often masked by alternating suppression and occasionally dissociating to produce vertical diplopia. This degree of fusion is unusual in deviations associated with DVD, and in general the presence of suppression prevents symptoms. Reduction of her basic deviation using a 6^{Δ} prism base-down OD alleviated the diplopia and permitted the chin to be lowered while maintaining single vision.

Cyclovergence Dysfunction

Insufficient Cyclovergence

Similar to that situation found in insufficient vertical vergences, this condition occurs in any sudden onset of a cyclovertical deviation. The normal cyclofusional range is thought to be 5° to 6°, but the findings vary among different researchers (Kertesz and Jones, 1970; Crone, 1971; Kertesz, 1971; Linwong and Herman, 1971). Any patient with an acutely acquired defect without preexisting cyclodeviation will be unable to fuse images that become tilted beyond the normal range. This problem is seen most commonly in unilateral or bilateral superior oblique paralyses. These muscles are the primary intorters of the eye and have a major secondary vertical action in the adducted position. Patients with superior oblique muscle palsy will suffer more from the effects of a slanted or tilted image than from the vertical separation of diplopic images. Even if the images can be superimposed, for example with prisms, a large torsional disparity cannot be fused. In unilateral conditions the extorsion can often be reduced by a head tilt, bringing the images within a cyclofusional range. In bilateral conditions, tilting the head to one side merely exaggerates the extorsion present in the affected opposite eye. A patient may require occlusion of one eye, with a head tilt also in some cases, to overcome the monocular torsion. Others adopt a chin depression, which avoids both the bilateral excyclotorsion and V-pattern esotropia produced in the downgaze position by bilateral superior oblique paralyses. Neither exercises nor prisms can correct torsional difficulties, and surgery is usually indicated in cases that do not resolve spontaneously.

CASE REPORT JT. A 19-year-old male was first examined by us two months after he sustained bilateral superior oblique palsies from closed head trauma received in an automobile accident. He claimed torsional diplopia, now intermittent, in straight ahead gaze and worse in downgaze, accompanied by vertical diplopia in lateral gaze to each side. The symptoms had improved slightly since the injury, and the diplopia could now be alleviated by chin depression.

Corrected visual acuity was 20/15 OU. Asymmetric underaction of both superior oblique muscles, right worse than left, was noted and documented on the Hess chart. Prism measurements in primary gaze showed right hyperphoria of only 1^{Δ} associated with 1^{Δ} of esophoria at distance, and 2^{Δ} of exophoria at near. A 4^{Δ} right hypertropia was present in left gaze and increased to 8^{Δ} in right head tilt. The deviation became 2^{Δ} left hypertropia in right gaze increasing to 4^{Δ} in left head tilt. A V-pattern esodeviation was present. Double Maddox rods showed excyclotorsion of 10° OD and 0° OS on upgaze, 5° OD and 2° OS in primary gaze, and 15° OD and 12° OS on downgaze.

A combination of a small base-out prism and base-down prism OD permitted superimposition of diplopic images in the reading position, but binocular blurring was present. This disappeared when the images were fused using chin depression, so it was assumed to be caused by the bilateral excyclotorsion. No further recovery of the paralysis occurred. The patient declined any ocular surgery, preferring to adopt his head posture to read.

Excessive Cyclovergence

This is an abnormal situation and usually represents adaptation to a cyclovertical muscle weakness in one or both eyes. It does not always result in fusion, and is commonly seen in concomitant strabismus in which both horizontal and vertical deviations exist. Oblique muscle dysfunction is responsible for the marked torsional movements seen. The excyclotorsion seen as either eye dissociates and elevates in DVD is such an example of large cyclofusional ability, especially when binocular responses are demonstrable in primary gaze.

Another condition displaying an unusual disorder of cyclovergence is superior oblique myokymia. It is a relatively rare, frequently undiagnosed condition (Hoyt and Keane, 1970; Susac et al., 1973; Roper-Hall and Burde, 1978) characterized by brief recurring episodes during which the patient describes visual symptoms often accompanied by physical ocular sensations. Visual symptoms can consist of intermittent oscillopsia of the object of regard or of intermittent diplopia, either vertical or torsional. This subjective description of oscillopsia might easily be confused with the more common conjugate problem. The diplopic image may vibrate, jiggle, shimmer, or jump up and down. The rate of oscillation varies between patients. The ocular sensations are of the eye twitching, jumping, or moving, and a pulling or drawing sensation may accompany or precede an attack. The condition usually affects one eye only. If the affected eye is observed during one of these episodes, fine vertical or cyclotorsional jerks are seen. These subtle movements are maximal in the field of action of the superior oblique muscle, namely in the depressed adducted position or on tilting the head to the side of the affected eye. Ophthalmoscopic examination of the conjunctival vessels and fundus may enhance clinical findings. The patient is unable to overcome these episodes by any physical means, and prisms cannot alleviate an oscillating and intermittent condition. It has been reported that superior oblique myokymia responds to the use of systemic carbamazepine (Tegretol). (Susac et al., 1973).

CASE REPORT SH. A 39-year-old woman complained of sudden onset of intermittent diplopia four months earlier. The images separated vertically with a torsional element. The diplopic episodes lasted a few seconds and occurred as often as every few minutes. Her past medical history included infrequent migraine headaches and an automobile accident with loss of consciousness.

A small exophoria on cover testing was occasionally associated with a small left hyperphoria, but the ocular movements were full and binocular results were elicited on diplopia testing. The rest of the ophthalmic examination was entirely normal, including a Tensilon test, but the patient denied experiencing any symptoms. During the head tilt test a jerky cycloversional movement was noted, worse in the left eye, as the patient straightened her head. A few moments later she noted the spontaneous onset of symptoms and the first of several "attacks" was observed. A rapid intorsional jerking was apparent in the left eye when the eyes were fixating in right downgaze. The right eye was unaffected. Tilting her head to the left and regarding an object in right downgaze would precipitate an episode if the phenomenon was quiescent. This maneuver stimulates superior oblique contraction. The slight left hyperphoria present in the resting phase and representative of mild superior oblique weakness became a small left hypotropia secondary to superior oblique overaction or spasm, with underaction of the right inferior rectus muscle, its contralateral synergist, during an attack. Ophthalmoscopic examination showed torsional jerking of the fundus of the left eye, and a diagnosis of left superior oblique myokymia was made. One month later these episodes had diminished in frequency and subsequently ceased without recurrence.

Acquired Fusional Dysfunction

Clinically, it is not possible for a fusional range to be too large; thus all disorders affecting fusional performance are those of insufficient fusional ability. As already mentioned, fusion has sensory and motor components, the latter being served by the vergence system. Both components must function adequately for fusion to be achieved.

Any barrier developing in early childhood that prevents good alignment of the visual axes or clear vision in both eyes will result in poor motor and sensory fusional skills if left untreated. This fact is useful when differentiating this condition from acquired loss of fusion in adults. Adaptations such as suppression, residual amblyopia, or anomalous retinal correspondence, together with poor fusional amplitudes help to conclude that the condition is longstanding and of little neurologic significance. In patients with sudden loss of motor fusion due to trauma or other organic causes, none of these adaptations is found and they are generally able to fuse binocular images and appreciate stereopsis at the neutralized angle of deviation.

Occasional cases have been reported in which patients retain gross motor fusional ability to converge and diverge, but are unable to achieve a correctly superimposed or fused image. This represents central sensory loss of fusion and is rare and should be differentiated from more common peripheral causes such as aniseikonia or metamorphopsia. A grossly limited field of ocular movement or torsional misalignment of the image due to a restricted or paralyzed ocular muscle can also prevent fusion of superimposed images. Central loss of both sensory and motor fusion following trauma has been reported and is extremely rare (Pratt-Johnson and Tillson, 1979).

REFERENCES

Bielschowsky A. Lectures on motor anomalies. Hanover, N.H.: Dartmouth College Publications, 1943.

Burde, RM. Control of eye movements. In: Moses RA, ed. Adler's physiology of the eye. 7th ed. St. Louis: CV Mosby, 1981:122–65.

Crone RA. Human cyclofusional response. Vision Res. 1971;11:1357–58.

Crone RA, Everhard-Halm Y. Optically induced eye torsion. I. Fusional cyclovergence. Albrecht Von Graefes Arch Klin Exp Ophthalmol 1975;195:231–39.

Daroff RB, Hoyt WF. Supranuclear disorders of ocular control systems in man. In: Bach-y-Rita P, Collins CC, Hyde JE, eds. The control of eye movements. New York: Academic Press, 1971:175–235.

Diener F. Zur Kenntnis traumatischer Schädigungen der Naheinstellung und der fusion. Schweiz Arch Neurol Neurochir Psychiatr 1953;72:18–26.

Doden W, Bunge H. Fusionsstörungen nach Schädelhirntraumen. Klin Monatsbp Augenheilkd 1965;146:845–53.

Fisher CM. Some neuro-ophthalmological observations. J Neurol Neurosurg Psychiatr 1967;30:383–92.

Glaser JS. Neuro-ophthalmologic examination: general considerations and special techniques. In: Glaser JS, ed. Neuro-ophthalmology. Hagerstown, Md.: Harper & Row, 1978, 25–46.

Gonyea EF. Bilateral internuclear ophthalmoplegia. Association with occlusive cerebrovascular disease. Arch Neurol 1974;31:168–73.

Hogg JE, Schoenberg BS. Paralysis of divergence in an adult with aqueductal stenosis. Arch Neurol 1979;36:511–12.

Hoyt WF, Keane JR. Superior oblique myokymia. Arch Ophthalmol 1970;83:461–66.

Jampel RS. Convergence, divergence, pupillary reactions and accommodation of the eyes from faradic stimulation of the macaque brain. J Comp Neurol 1960;115:371–400.

Kertesz AE. More on cyclofusional response. Vision Res 1971;11:1359.

Kertesz AE. The effect of stimulus complexity on human cyclofusional response. Vision Res 1972;12:699–704.

Kertesz AE. Disparity detection within Panum's fusional areas. Vision Res 1973;13:1537–43.

Kertesz AE, Jones RW. Human cyclofusional response. Vision Res 1970;10:891–96.

Kirkham TH, Bird AC, Sanders, MD. Divergence paralysis with increased intracranial pressure: an electro-oculographic study. Br J Ophthalmol 1972; 56:776–82.

Krekling S. Comments on cyclofusional movements. Albrecht Von Graefes Arch Klin Exp Ophthalmol 1973;188:231–38.

Linwong M, Herman SJ. Cycloduction of the eyes with head tilt. Arch Ophthalmol 1971;85:570–73.

Lippmann O. Paralysis of divergence due to cerebellar tumor. Arch Ophthalmol 1944;31:299–301.

Lyle DJ. Divergence insufficiency. Arch Ophthalmol 1954;52:858–64.

Lyle TK, Wybar KC. Lyle and Jackson's practical orthoptics in the treatment of squint. 5th ed. London: HK Lewis, 1967:97–132.

Mein J, Johnson F. Dissociated vertical divergence and its association with nystagmus. In: Mein J, Moore S, eds. Orthoptics, research and practice. Transactions of the Fourth International Orthoptic Congress. London: Kimpton, 1981:14–16.

Norris H. The action of sedatives on brain stem oculomotor systems in man. Neuropharmacology 1971;10:181–91.

Pasik P, Pasik T. Oculomotor functions in monkeys with lesions of the cerebrum and the superior colliculi. In: Bender MB, ed. The oculomotor system. New York: Harper & Row, 1964:40–80.

Pfaffenbach DD, Layton DD, Kearns TP. Ocular manifestations in progressive supranuclear palsy. Am J Ophthalmol 1972;74:1179–84.

Pratt-Johnson JA. Central disruption of fusional amplitude. Br J Ophthalmol 1973;67:347–50.

Pratt-Johnson JA, Tillson G. Acquired central disruption of fusion amplitude. Ophthalmology 1979;86:2140–42.

Pratt-Johnson JA, Pop A, Tillson G. The complexities of suppression in intermittent exotropia. In: Mein J, Moore S, eds. Orthoptics, research and practice. Transactions of the Fourth International Orthoptic Congress. London: Kimpton, 1981:172–73.

Roper-Hall G. Disturbances of the supranuclear control of ocular movements. Br Orthopt J 1973;30:3–16.

Roper-Hall G. Ocular difficulties in the near gaze position. Am Orthopt J 1980;30:109–20.

Roper-Hall G, Burde RM. Sensorimotor adaptations in comitant strabismus. Am Orthopt J 1977;27:21–32.

Roper-Hall G, Burde RM. Superior oblique myokymia. Am Orthopt J 1978;28:58–63.

Rubin ML. Optics for clinicians. 2nd ed. Gainesville, Fla.: Triad Scientific Publishers, 1974:133–38.

Sanders MD, Bird AC. Supranuclear abnormalities of the vertical ocular motor system. Trans Ophthalmol Soc UK 1970;90:433–49.

Scobee RG. The oculorotary muscles. 2nd ed. St. Louis: CV Mosby, 1952:346.

Smith JL, Zieper I, Gay AJ, Cogan DG. Nystagmus retractorius. Arch Ophthalmol 1959;62:864–67.

Stanworth, A, Mein J. Loss of fusion after removal of cerebellar tumour. Br Orthopt J 1971;28:97–98.

Sullivan MJ, Kertesz AE. The nature of fusional effort in diplopic regions. Vision Res 1975;15:79–83.

Susac JO, Smith JL, Schatz NJ. Superior oblique myokymia. Arch Neurol 1973;29:432–34.

Tamler E, Jampolsky A. Is divergence active? An electromyographic study. Am J Ophthalmol 1967;63:452–59.

von Noorden GK. Resection of both medial rectus muscles in organic convergence insufficiency. Am J Ophthalmol 1976;81:223–26.

von Noorden GK. In: von Noorden—Maumenee's atlas of strabismus. 3rd ed. St. Louis: CV Mosby, 1977:156–59.

von Noorden GK. Burian—von Noorden's binocular vision and ocular motility: theory and management of strabismus. 2nd ed. St. Louis: CV Mosby, 1980.

Wade SL. Third nerve palsy with loss of fusion. Br Orthopt J 1960;17:114–15.

Wade SL. Loss of fusion following brain damage. Br Orthopt J 1965;22:81–83.

Walsh FB, Hoyt WF. Clinical neuro-ophthalmology. Vol 1. Baltimore: Williams & Wilkins, 1969a:237–39.

Walsh FB, Hoyt WF. Clinical neuro-ophthalmology. Vol. 3. Baltimore: Williams & Wilkins, 1969b:2534.

Supplementary Glossary of Control System Terminology*

George K. Hung
Kenneth J. Ciuffreda

attentuation — a decrease in gain.

automatic control system — a feedback control system whose goal is to reduce the difference between input and output to near zero.

band-pass filter — an element that passes midfrequencies of an input signal but attenuates the low and high frequencies.

bandwidth — the range of frequencies to which a system will respond; it is usually measured at the half-power points, which are the upper and lower frequencies at which the output power is reduced to one-half or the magnitude is reduced to $\frac{1}{\sqrt{2}}$ (= 0.707) of the mid frequency response.

bias — an offset; a bias introduced into the pathway

* This glossary is meant to supplement control system terms already discussed in the book. The intent is to familiarize non-engineers with engineering terminology. For those interested in a more comprehensive understanding of these terms and concepts, see the reference list at the end of this glossary.

Supported in part by NIH grants EY03709 and EY03541.

of a system which will result in a constant offset in system response level.

Bode plot — a semilog plot in which frequency of sinusoidal input is specified on the abscissa (logarithmic scale) and either response magnitude (in decibels) or phase (in degrees) is specified on the ordinate (linear scale); given a transfer function G(ω), where G is a complex function of frequency (ω) of the form $a + jb$, the Bode magnitude is plotted as $20 \log_{10} \sqrt{a^2 + b^2}$ versus ω, and the Bode phase is plotted as $\tan^{-1} \frac{b}{a}$ versus ω.

closed-loop gain — $\frac{G}{1 + GH}$, where G is the forward loop gain and H is the feedback gain of the system.

closed-loop system — a system in which all or part of the output is fed back to the input.

controller — an element in a feedback control system that corrects for a particular error between the output and input.

critically damped — in the response to a step input, it is the amount of damping just sufficient to prevent overshooting.

dampen — to reduce oscillation; this makes the response more sluggish.

deadspace — that portion of the operating range of a control element over which there is no change in output for a given input.

decibel (dB) — a unit used to express the magnitude of a transfer function G(ω), designated as $|G(\omega)|$, such that

$$|G(\omega)|_{dB} = 20 \log_{10} |G(\omega)| = 20 \log_{10} \left| \frac{\text{output}}{\text{input}} \right|;$$

for example, if at a certain frequency (ω) the magnitude $|G(\omega)| = 1/\sqrt{2}$ (=0.707), this magnitude expressed in decibels is $20 \log_{10} 1/\sqrt{2} = -3$ dB.

feedback — the process in which all or part of the output signal is fed back to the input.

first-order system — a system whose transfer function has the form $\frac{b}{s + a}$; the step response of such a system takes the form of an exponential.

gain — the ratio of output magnitude to input magnitude.

high-pass filter — an element that passes the high frequencies of an input signal but attenuates the low frequencies.

Laplace transform — a mathematical technique that converts an expression from the time domain to the complex frequency domain; subsequent computations can then be done using relatively simple algebraic procedures rather than more complex differential equations.

linear — a system that obeys the principle of superposition, so that if

$y_1(t)$ = the system response to $x_1(t)$

and

$y_2(t)$ = the system response to $x_2(t)$, then

$ay_1(t) + by_2(t)$ = the system response to $ax_1(t) + bx_2(t)$

low-pass filter — an element that passes low frequencies of an input signal but attenuates the high frequencies.

negative feedback — the process whereby all or part of the output is subtracted from the input to give the error signal driving the controller; it is a means of improving stability characteristics of the overall response.

open-loop gain — GH; see definition of closed-loop gain for symbols.

open-loop system — a system in which none of the output is fed back to the input.

overdamped — in the response to a step input, the amount of damping is in excess to prevent overshooting.

phase angle — describes the relationship of the output to the input at a particular frequency and can be thought of as the number of cycles the output

	either lags or leads the input (note 1 cycle $= 2\pi$ radians $= 360°$).
plant	the controlled physical component of a system; this is in contrast to the controlling component such as neural circuitry.
positive feedback	the process whereby all or part of the output is added to the input to give the error signal driving the controller; this results in system instability.
rise time	the time required for a system response to a step input to change from 10 to 90 percent of the final steady-state value.
saturation	the limit of an element's response beyond which the output will not change with additional input.
second-order system	a system whose transfer function contains S^2 as the highest power of s in the denominator for a 2nd order low-pass filter of the form $\frac{b^2}{S^2 + 2abs + b^2}$; the step input response may show overdamping, critical damping, or underdamping depending upon the damping ratio a.
settling time	for a step input, the time (approximately equal to 4 time constants) for the output to reach and remain within 2 percent of the final steady-state value.
step input	an input whose value is zero prior to some reference time and a different constant value after that time.
time constant	for a first-order system, the time for the (exponential) response to a step input to reach 63 percent of its final value.
time delay	the time between the application of an input and beginning of the response; latency.
transfer function	a mathematical expression that describes the input-output relationship of a control element or system.
underdamped	in the response to a step input, the amount of damping is insufficient to prevent overshooting.

REFERENCES

Bahill AT. Bioengineering: biomedical, medical and clinical engineering. Englewood Cliffs, N. J.: Prentice-Hall, 1981.
Bibbero RJ. Dictionary of automatic control. New York: Reinhold Pub., 1960.
Clason WE. Elsevier's dictionary of computers, automatic control, and data processing. New York: Elsevier, 1971.
Emanuel P, Leff E. Introduction to feedback control systems. New York: McGraw-Hill, 1979.
McFarland DJ. Feedback mechanisms in animal behavior. New York: Academic Press, 1971.
Milsum JH. Biological control systems analysis. New York: McGraw-Hill Book Co, 1966.
Sante DP. Automatic control system technology. Englewood Cliffs, N.J.: Prentice-Hall, 1980.
Stark L. Neurological control systems: studies in bioengineering. New York: Plenum Press, 1968.
Toates F. Control theory in biology and experimental psychology. London: Hutchinson Educational, 1975.

Name Index

Abadi, R.B., 644
Abel, A., 460
Abraham, S.V., 26, 27, 42, 146
Abrams, D., 440
Adler, F.H., 29, 30, 31, 32, 42, 55
Aguilonius, F., 199, 204, 207
Akert, K., 657
Albrecht, D.G., 271
Alexander, K.R., 85
Allen, M.J., 115, 416, 434
Alpern, M., 3, 9, 55, 76, 77, 78, 80, 82, 84, 86, 91, 101, 102, 118, 120, 122, 127, 129, 130, 131, 132, 138, 140, 142, 143, 144, 177, 178, 180, 303, 308, 310, 354, 376, 383, 388, 389, 390, 412, 418, 452, 461, 467, 488, 493, 513, 546, 653, 661
Alvarez, S., 638
Ames, A., Jr., 330, 465, 468, 469
Ames, A.A., 82
Amigo, G., 595
Anstis, S.M., 266
Apkarian, P.A., 228, 229, 230, 244
Arditi, A., 339
Arner, R.S., 513, 530
Asher, H., 83
Aslin, R.N., 41, 42, 45, 115
Atkinson, J., 583
Bach-y-Rita, P., 354, 550
Bagolini, B., 157, 493, 632
Bahill, A.T., 355, 383
Baker, A.G., 252
Baker, F.H., 163
Baker, R., 655, 657, 658
Ball, E.A.W., 102
Ballen, P.H., 596
Balliet, R., 550, 554, 562
Balsam, M.H., 430, 431, 432, 433
Bangerter, A., 634, 635
Barany, E.H., 231
Barlow, H.B., 218, 243, 310, 663
Batton, R.R., III, 657, 658
Becker, W., 384, 385
Bedell, H.E., 144, 145
Beisner, D.H., 569, 571
Bender, M.B., 655
Benevento, L.A., 666
Berens, C., 30, 31
Bevan, W., 232
Beverley, K.I., 261, 262, 263, 264
Bielschowsky, A., 58, 157, 330, 465, 513, 673, 688, 691, 692
Bird, A.C., 676
Birnbaum, M.H., 599, 633
Bishop, P.O., 218, 243, 315, 339
Björk, A., 29

Blake, R., 161, 231, 233
Blakemore, C., 239, 252, 256, 259, 260, 275, 276, 288, 583, 584, 664
Blodi, F.C., 385, 568
Bohman, C.E., 45
Boring, E.G., 46, 287
Borish, I.M., 77, 518, 525, 606, 642
Bour, L.J., 102, 112
Bourdy, C., 32, 33, 34, 35, 54
Boyd, T.A.S., 576
Boyer, F.M., 595
Braddick, O.L., 285
Bradford, R.T., 82
Brandt, T., 53
Brecher, G.A., 30, 31, 330
Breese, B.B., 233
Breinin, G.M., 26, 29, 129, 132, 133, 135, 140, 143, 385
Breitmeyer, B., 214
Brock, F.W., 143, 145, 147, 588, 589
Brodkey, J., 9, 115, 118
Brown, H.W., 154
Bunge, H., 675, 678
Burbank, D.P., 574
Burbeck, C.A., 275
Burde, R.M., 671, 687, 689, 690, 694
Burian, H.M., 29, 79, 81, 82, 87, 88, 89, 143, 157, 318, 329, 580, 584, 586, 589, 590, 592, 594, 596, 597, 599
Büttner-Evener, J.A., 5, 655, 657

Calaroso, E., 635
Callahan, A., 575
Campbell, F.W., 102, 105, 106, 144, 145, 147, 181, 227, 275, 278, 288
Campos, E.C., 55
Cantonnet, A., 89
Carpenter, M.B., 657, 658
Carpenter, R.H.S., 377, 389
Carter, D.B., 55, 56, 65, 469, 472, 475, 476, 477, 480, 484, 488, 492, 498, 512, 525, 616
Catellani, C.O., 55
Chan, C.L., 612, 613, 614, 628
Chang, J.J., 241, 274
Charman, W.N., 109, 110, 111, 147
Charnwood, L., 474
Check, R., 232
Chiarandini, D.J., 653
Chin, N.B., 129, 132, 133, 143
Ciuffreda, K.J., 7, 11, 80, 83, 114, 117, 120, 121, 126, 145, 146, 148, 149, 150, 151, 152, 164, 644
Clark, B., 467
Clark, M.R., 5, 106, 355, 376
Clatworthy, J.L., 284
Cline, D., 448
Cobb, W.A., 233
Cogan, D.G., 26, 43, 216, 657
Cohen, B., 655
Cohen, M.M., 140
Collewijn, H., 5, 376
Collins, C.C., 568
Collyer, S.C., 232
Colson, Z.W., 30, 31
Comerford, J.P., 395
Cook, G., 5, 183, 355, 358
Cooper, E.L., 576
Cooper, J., 88, 135, 154, 156, 588, 589, 595, 596, 613, 631
Cooper, M., 556
Cornell, E., 87, 89
Cornsweet, T.N., 643
Costenbader, F., 145
Crane, H.D., 101, 106, 376, 643
Craske, B., 60
Crawshaw, M., 60
Crone, R.A., 5, 11, 55, 180, 328, 332, 335, 468, 492, 673, 693
Cross, A.J., 404, 405, 406, 409
Cuppers, C., 570
Cynader, M., 263, 555

Daroff, R.B., 7, 671, 672, 677
Daum, K.M., 613
Davidowitz, J., 653
Davies, P., 551
Davis, C.J., 131
DeGroot, J., 552
Delgado-Garcia, J., 657, 658
Denieul, P., 106
Dharamashi, B.G., 494
Dickerson, R.E., 272
Diener, F., 675, 678
Diner, D., 224, 467, 494
Doden, W., 675, 678
Donders, F.C., 7, 129, 439, 443
Dove, H.W., 282
Drake, S., 230, 231
Duane, A., 129
Duckman, R., 581, 594, 597
Duke-Elder, S., 29, 30, 440
Dumais, S.T., 42
Dunlap, E.A., 566

Eames, T.H., 624
Easter, S.S., 7
Ebenholtz, S.M., 60, 64, 65, 66
Ellen, P., 3, 118, 120, 122, 376, 383, 389, 390
Ellerbrock, V.J., 55, 318, 326, 330, 331, 345, 346, 477, 481, 488
Elliot, R.L., 574
Emsley, H.H., 440
Enoch, J.M., 145

Enright, J.T., 556
Epstein, W., 84
Eskridge, J.B., 132, 133, 309, 595
Everhard-Halm, Y., 5, 11, 328, 332, 335, 673

Fankhauser, F., 145
Fechner, G.T., 297
Feinberg, I., 144
Feldman, J., 588, 589, 595, 613
Felton, T.B., 252
Fender, D., 223, 273, 318, 319, 326, 328, 383, 467, 494
Filliozat, J., 89
Fincham, E.F., 33, 34, 35, 38, 43, 45, 101, 102, 132, 147, 178, 179, 180, 181, 187, 190, 367, 419
Findley, J.M., 41
Fischer, B., 243, 253, 255, 663, 665
Fisher, C.M., 677
Flax, N., 581, 591, 593, 597, 629, 631
Flieringa, H.J., 418, 440, 460
Flom, M.C., 127, 129, 134, 135, 136, 137, 143, 144, 164, 440, 460, 467, 579, 580, 581, 582, 590, 595, 599, 613, 619, 628, 629, 630, 636, 642, 643
Foley, J.M., 47, 85, 246, 257, 264, 273, 284, 285, 286, 287, 309, 315
Forrest, E.B., 89
Fox, R., 231, 232, 233
France, T.D., 574
Franceschetti, A.T., 79, 81
Francis, E.L., 38, 39, 40, 54
Frey, K.J., 60
Friedman, R.B., 205
Friendly, D.S., 634
Frisby, J.P., 251, 253, 258, 284
Fry, G.A., 19, 126, 132, 133, 178, 202, 218, 308, 405, 406, 407, 419, 420, 421, 427, 428, 429, 430, 431, 432, 433, 440, 441, 451, 453, 461
Fuchs, A.F., 354, 382, 653, 655, 659, 664, 665
Fujii, K., 102

Galket, R.J., 597
Ganz, L., 269, 276, 278
Garcia, H., 569, 570, 571
Getz, D.J., 86
Gibson, H.W., 134
Gibson, J.J., 248, 278
Giles, G.H., 89
Givner, I., 143, 145, 147
Glaser, J.S., 672, 677
Glidden, G.H., 465, 468, 469
Godio, L., 499
Gogel, W.C., 47–48, 86, 286
Goldberg, M.E., 665
Goldrich, S.G., 586, 591, 643
Gonyea, E.F., 677
Gouras, P., 227
Graemiger, A., 146
Graham, N., 267
Graham, P.A., 579
Grant, V.W., 47
Grantyn, R., 655
Graybiel, A.M., 655
Green, D.G., 105, 145
Gregory, A.H., 145
Griffin, J.R., 580, 589, 590, 591, 595, 597, 641
Grisham, J.D., 498, 607, 608, 609, 611, 612, 613, 614, 625, 628, 238
Guber, D., 139
Guth, S.K., 429, 430
Guzzinati, G.C., 83

Haines, F., 440
Hallden, U., 157, 231, 467, 493, 589, 590
Hallmark, W., 643
Halmagyi, G.M., 659
Halveston, E.M., 576
Hamasaki, D., 129, 427
Hampshire, R., 158
Hampton, D.R., 329, 330, 346
Harcourt, B., 594, 598
Hardesty, H.H., 596
Hardjowijoto, S., 55, 468, 492
Harter, M.R., 227
Harting, J.K., 665
Hartweig, E.A., 655
Heath, G.G., 102, 134, 145, 461
Hebbard, F.W., 43, 466, 467, 474, 484, 501, 502
Hecht, S., 238
Heerema, D., 179, 180, 426, 661
Heineman, E.G., 85
Held, R., 64, 268
Helmholtz, H.L., 43, 206, 207, 210, 214, 217, 223, 231, 234, 375, 410, 433, 543, 546, 548, 549, 551, 556, 558
Hendley, 412
Henn, V., 655
Hennessy, R.T., 35, 43, 82, 112
Henry, G.H., 315
Henson, D.B., 55, 480, 494, 495, 500
Hering, E., 3, 7, 16, 118, 201, 205, 212, 217, 280, 297, 298, 373, 374, 375, 376, 377, 380, 391, 394, 395, 397, 404, 494, 548, 552, 554, 556
Herman, S.J., 693
Hermann, J.S., 118, 153
Hermans, T.G., 85
Heron, G., 109, 111
Hess, A., 354

Hess, C., 440
Hess, R.S., 144, 145, 147, 148
Highstein, S.M., 655, 657, 658
Hiles, D.A., 597
Hillebrand, F., 212
Hirons, R., 586, 643
Hirsch, M.J., 125, 126, 132, 239, 492
Hochberg, J., 84
Hoffmann, F.B., 58, 330, 465, 513
Hoffmann, K.P., 665
Hofstetter, H.W., 76, 78, 79, 80, 82, 91, 129, 134, 153, 403, 406, 417, 428, 433, 434, 439, 440, 442, 443, 451, 452, 453, 460, 461, 462, 467, 493, 513
Hogg, J.E., 687
Hokoda, S.C., 79, 80, 83, 150, 151
Holländer, H., 665
Hollins, M., 214
Holway, A.H., 287
Hooten, K., 5, 11, 335
Howard, H.J., 238
Howard, I.P., 376, 380, 389
Howe, L., 440
Howell, E.R., 144, 148
Hoyt, W.F., 671, 672, 673, 674, 676, 677, 680, 684, 686, 687, 688, 690, 694
Hsu, F.K., 7, 355
Hubel, D., 163, 218, 243, 246, 256, 257, 258, 552, 584
Hugonnier, R., 579, 580, 595, 605
Hugonnier, S.C., 579, 580, 595, 605
Hung, G.K., 92, 104, 106, 114, 148, 150, 180, 182, 183, 184, 185, 186, 187, 189, 192, 426, 469, 503, 661
Hurvich, L., 309, 373
Huxley, A.F., 653
Hyde, I., 513

Iacobucci, I., 634
Ikeda, H., 163, 583, 584
Inverso, M., 643
Ishak, I.G.H., 283
Ittleson, W.H., 82
Ivanoff, A., 32, 33, 34, 35, 54

Jackson, R.W., 42, 115
Jackson, S., 134, 135
Jacobs, L., 659
Jaeger, R., 184, 185
Jameson, D., 309
Jampel, R.S., 354, 412, 653, 664, 672
Jampolsky, A., 161, 466, 467, 468, 469, 470, 495, 498, 575, 673
Jobe, F.W., 131
Johnson, F., 692
Johnson, S.C., 273
Jones, R., 9, 253, 298, 300, 304, 305, 306, 310, 311, 312, 313, 315, 331, 335, 595, 664, 673, 693
Joshua, D.E., 218, 243
Judd, C.H., 465
Judge, S.J., 137
Julesz, B., 223, 234, 240, 243, 244, 245, 248, 249, 250, 251, 252, 256, 258, 259, 264, 269, 272, 273, 274, 275, 276, 277, 279, 281, 282, 318, 319, 326, 328, 467, 494
Jurgens, R., 384, 385

Kakizaki, S., 233
Kasai, T., 106
Kaufman, L., 47, 257, 339
Kaye, M.G., 236, 237, 251, 258, 282
Keane, J.R., 694
Keiner, E.C.J.F., 146
Keller, E.L., 119, 124, 303, 354, 554, 556, 651, 653, 654, 655, 658
Kelly, D.H., 275
Kelindorfer, J., 102
Kenyon, R.V., 7, 11, 115, 117, 120, 121, 122, 123, 124, 125, 154, 157, 158, 159, 160, 161, 162, 163, 309, 381, 390, 397, 664
Kerr, K.E., 9, 300, 304, 310, 311, 312, 589, 590, 637
Kertesz, A.E., 82, 218, 221, 319, 320, 321, 322, 323, 324, 325, 326, 328, 329, 330, 331, 332, 333, 334, 335, 336, 337, 339, 340, 341, 342, 343, 346, 347, 673, 693
King, W.M., 657
Kirkham, T.H., 687
Kirschen, D.G., 144, 148
Klecka, R., 531
Kleiner, K., 65
Kleinman, B., 642
Knoll, H.A., 77, 427
Koenderink, J.J., 259
Konishi, M., 244
Kowal, C.T., 230, 231
Kowler, E., 384
Krekling, S., 673
Kretschemer, S., 157
Krishnan, V.V., 5, 7, 9, 11, 101, 115, 117, 118, 119, 182, 183, 184, 186, 300, 308, 350, 352, 357, 359, 360, 362, 363, 364, 366, 477, 485, 486, 489

Lack, L.C., 231
Landolt, E., 439
Lang, J., 592
Langlands, N.M.S., 253
Larsen, J., 5
Larsen, T., 643

Larson, B.F., 142, 143
Lau, E., 465
Lawson, L.J., 82
LeGrand, Y., 44
Lehmkuhle, S.W., 161, 233
Leibowitz, H.W., 35, 36, 37, 38, 39, 43, 45, 46, 48, 49, 50, 53, 54, 60, 61, 62, 63, 66, 82, 85, 112, 506
Lennerstrand, G., 550
Lesser, S.K., 440, 441, 518, 519
Letourneau, J.E., 642, 643, 644
Levelt, W.J.M., 231, 232, 233
Levy, J., 33, 34–35
Levy, M., 78, 80
Lewin, K., 465
Leyman, I.A., 576
Lie, I., 47
Linksz, A., 221
Linwong, M., 693
Lippmann, O., 687
Lit, A., 283
Liu, J.S., 5, 11, 104, 106, 620, 625
Loomis, J.M., 248
Louie, S., 626
Luckiesh, M., 43, 429, 430
Ludlam, W.M., 594, 595, 642, 643, 644
Ludvigh, E., 468, 485, 486, 551
Luschei, E.S., 354, 655
Lund, J.S., 665
Lyle, K., 134, 135, 639, 673, 674, 678

McCready, D.W., 47
McCullough, R.W., 468
MacGillavry, T.H., 439, 443
MacKay, D., 256
McKee, S.P., 283
Mackensen, G., 148
McLaughlin, S.C., 587
Maddox, E.E., 15–18, 27–29, 30, 43, 55, 75, 92, 101, 118, 177, 180, 187, 298, 404, 406, 477, 501, 579
Maffei, L., 227, 278
Magoun, H.W., 666
Mallett, R.F.J., 467, 498, 525
Malmstrom, F.V., 83, 90
Manas, L., 78, 125, 126, 137
Mann, I., 26, 42
Mann, S.M., 146
Mannen, D.L., 89
Manny, R.E., 643
Marg, E.P., 9, 83, 427
Mariani, G., 157, 493, 632
Marr, D., 251, 258, 282, 283
Martens, T.G., 76, 79, 83, 89, 125, 128, 129, 178, 466, 502, 504, 522
Martinez-Milán, L., 665
Mayhew, J.E.W., 251, 258
Mays, L.E., 665
Mein, J., 675, 678, 692
Melville Jones, G., 551
Metz, H., 574
Meur, G., 632
Meyer, H., 199
Michaels, D.D., 616
Miles, F.A., 137
Miller, J., 258, 551
Miller, J.M., 323, 387, 388, 659
Miller, P.J., 7
Mintz, E.U., 238
Mitchell, A.M., 3, 157, 298, 300, 308, 350, 353, 388, 389, 481
Mitchell, D.E., 38, 40, 205, 252, 304, 306, 310, 311, 350, 353, 583, 663, 664, 666
Mitchell, R., 87
Mohindra, I., 583, 630, 634
Moldover, J., 29
More, 91
Morgan, M.W., Jr., 9, 11, 18, 19, 44, 55, 76, 77, 78, 80, 82, 86, 89, 91, 93, 101, 102, 104, 115, 126, 131, 134, 180, 182, 427, 477, 488, 518, 519, 520, 521, 579, 590, 595, 606, 625, 627, 637
Morris, C.W., 126
Moss, F.K., 44
Movshon, J.A., 592
Mueller, J., 101, 115, 118, 177
Murphy, B.J., 384
Myers, E., 7

Nadell, M., 91, 129
Nagel, A., 330, 332, 439, 440
Nakamizo, S., 388, 389, 393, 396
Nakayama, K., 214, 220, 248, 544, 548, 549, 550, 554, 556, 557, 562
Nankin, S.J., 574
Narayan, V., 501, 505, 508
Nashold, B.S., 658
Nelson, J.I., 244, 245, 251, 332
Neumaier, R.W., 143
Neumueller, J., 80
Niehl, E.W., 3, 5, 157, 158, 359, 383, 388, 389, 484, 485
Norcia, A.M., 252, 255, 275
Norris, H., 678
North, R., 55, 480, 495, 500
Nott, I.S., 511

Ogle, K.N., 38, 39, 76, 79, 81, 83, 87, 88, 89, 101, 102, 125, 128, 129, 132, 137, 138, 139, 178, 179, 202, 205, 208, 212, 213, 220, 221, 235, 238, 239, 240, 250, 253, 283, 299, 309, 310, 328, 330, 345, 346, 359, 466,

Ogle, K.N. (cont.)
467, 468, 469, 472, 473, 474, 475, 477, 480, 484, 486, 488, 489, 491, 492, 493, 498, 499, 501, 502, 503, 504, 513, 522, 525, 526, 527, 615
Olmstead, J.H.D., 182
O'Neill, W.D., 9
Ono, H., 85, 124, 379, 380, 381, 386, 387, 388, 389, 391, 392, 393, 394, 395, 396
Optican, L.M., 332, 551
Otto, J., 146, 147
Owens, D.A., 35, 36, 37, 38, 39, 40, 43, 45, 46, 48, 49, 50, 54, 60, 61, 62, 63, 65, 66, 85, 109, 111, 112, 506, 511

Pali, E., 379
Palmer, E.A., 468, 469, 498
Panum, P.L., 200, 201, 216, 217, 220, 221, 222, 224, 225, 226, 227, 234, 249, 250, 275, 465
Parks, M.M., 153, 592, 596, 634
Parks, M.N., 83
Parks, M.S., 467
Pasik, P., 673
Pasik, T., 673
Pasino, L., 157, 493, 632
Payne, C.R., 512
Peachey, L.D., 653
Peli, E., 395
Percival, E.A., 460, 461, 521, 531, 534, 536, 627, 628
Pereles, H., 439
Perry, N.W., 227
Perlmutter, A.L., 319, 320, 321, 322, 323, 324, 325, 326, 346
Peters, H.B., 131, 180
Pettigrew, J.D., 243, 244, 257, 262, 367, 556
Pfaffenbach, D.D., 676
Phillips, S.R., 9, 102, 107, 111, 112, 113, 144
Pickwell, L.D., 119, 158, 395, 396
Piggins, D., 216
Pilar, G., 354
Pitts, G., 443
Poggio, G.F., 243, 253, 255, 663, 665
Poggio, T., 251, 258, 282, 283
Pola, J., 656
Pope, R.S., 623
Post, R.B., 51, 53, 54, 66
Powell, W.H., 30, 31
Prangen, A., 467, 469, 474, 477, 484, 488, 491, 492, 493
Pratt, C.B., 77
Pratt-Johnson, J., 161, 596, 675, 678, 680, 688, 696
Prentice, C.F., 440
Pulliam, K., 270
Pye, D., 55

Quere, M.A., 158

Raab, E.L., 596
Radner, M., 278
Rady, A.A., 283
Raibert, M., 265
Ramachandran, V.S., 285
Randle, R.J., 83, 90
Ranson, S.W., 666
Rasche, F., 233
Rashbass, C., 5, 35, 125, 140, 157, 300, 303, 325, 346, 359, 363, 377, 384, 385, 407, 408, 425, 484, 485, 486, 498, 611, 649, 659
Regan, D., 261, 262, 263, 264
Reinecke, R.D., 595
Revell, M.J., 580
Richards, W., 47, 236, 237, 238, 246, 251, 258, 282, 284, 309, 315, 389, 481, 592, 663
Riggs, L.A., 3, 5, 157, 158, 359, 383, 388, 389, 484, 485
Rindziunski, E., 589
Ripps, H., 176, 187
Ritter, M., 85
Roberts, J., 579
Robinson, D.A., 118, 119, 303, 354, 355, 383, 384, 543, 549, 550, 551, 554, 556, 649, 650, 651, 652, 653, 657, 658, 659, 664, 665
Roelofs, C.O., 440
Roenne, G., 218
Rogers, B.J., 380
Rohler, R., 145
Ronne, G., 589
Roper-Hall, G., 671, 674, 676, 687, 689, 690, 694
Rosenberg, R., 102, 585
Rubie, C., 76
Rubin, M.L., 674
Rutstein, R.P., 499

Sabado, F., 626
Safra, D., 146, 147
Saida, S., 381, 386
Sakata, H., 665
Sakuma, K., 465
Saladin, J.J., 45, 79, 91, 104, 106, 512, 519, 520, 525, 528, 529, 530, 531, 532, 533, 535, 538, 539, 615, 628
Samson, C.R., 118, 153
Sanders, M.D., 676
Saye, A., 253, 284
Schapero, M., 129, 191
Schiller, P.H., 651, 659
Schlodtmann, W., 157
Schmiedt, W., 439
Schober, H., 44, 113

Schoenberg, B.S., 687
Schoessler, J.P., 157
Schor, C.M., 57–60, 68, 183, 186, 205, 224, 467, 468, 469, 474, 477, 479, 480, 481, 484, 485, 486, 487, 488, 495, 496, 497, 498, 499, 501, 505, 508, 512, 513, 615, 636, 638, 643
Schubert, G., 476, 492
Schulman, P., 78
Schumer, R.A., 252, 269, 273, 276, 278
Schwartz, L., 574
Scott, A.B., 203, 206, 219, 221, 222, 236, 254
Seaber, J.H., 658
Sears, M., 139
Semmlow, J.L., 9, 11, 92, 93, 104, 114, 117, 118, 119, 120, 122, 123, 124, 144, 148, 150, 163, 176, 178, 179, 180, 182, 183, 184, 185, 186, 187, 189, 193, 426, 469, 503, 661
Senders, J.W., 103
Shanzer, S., 655
Shapero, M., 78, 80, 91
Sheard, C., 404, 405, 406, 440, 460, 461, 519, 521, 531, 534, 536, 537, 615, 627, 628
Sheedy, J.E., 79, 91, 202, 218, 499, 500, 512, 513, 519, 520, 525, 528, 529, 530, 531, 532, 533, 535, 538, 539, 615, 628
Shirachi, D., 106
Shulman, P., 125
Sieback, R., 44
Silanpaa, V., 309
Simons, K., 595
Slater, A.M., 41
Smith, D.R., 88
Smith, J.L., 657, 676, 686
Southall, J.P.C., 549
Spache, G.D., 593
Sparks, D.L., 655, 665
Spekreijse, H., 227
Sperling, G., 251, 282
Spivey, B.E., 596
Stanworth, A., 675, 678
Stark, L., 5, 7, 9, 11, 27, 93, 102, 104, 106, 115, 117, 118, 120, 121, 125, 157, 175, 181, 182, 183, 184, 298, 302, 303, 324, 350, 352, 358, 359, 363, 477, 485, 486, 489
Steinbach, M.J., 380, 387
Steinman, R.M., 5, 376, 384
Stern, A., 80
Stewart, C.R., 350, 425, 426, 467, 494
Stoddard, K.B., 102
Straschill, M., 665
Stromeyer, C.F., III, 276
Strominger, N.L., 658
Sullivan, M.J., 333, 334, 335, 336, 337, 339, 340, 341, 342, 343, 673
Susac, J.O., 694, 695
Sutter, E.E., 260, 261
Sutton, P., 276
Swaine, W., 440
Swan, K.C., 632

Tait, E.F., 78, 83, 571
Takahashi, E., 137
Tam, W.J., 392, 394, 395
Tamler, E., 385, 673
Tanzman, I.J., 282
Templeton, W.B., 376, 389
Teng, P., 655
Thomas, J., 584
Thompson, D.A., 81, 182
Tietz, J.D., 47, 48
Tillson, G., 675, 678, 680, 696
Tinor, T., 117, 118, 144
Toates, F.M., 26, 29, 30, 101, 105, 177, 181, 184, 359, 381, 468
Tomlinson, A., 147, 191
Torok, N., 352
Toyne, M.J., 665
Trachtman, J.N., 643
Travers, T., 161
Travis, R.P., 655
Tremain, K.E., 163
Troelstra, A., 102, 119
Tubis, R.A., 469
Tucker, J., 110, 147
Tyler, C.W., 205, 216, 220, 221, 222, 224, 230, 234, 241, 245, 248, 252, 255, 256, 257, 258, 259, 260, 261, 264, 265, 267, 268, 269, 273, 275, 276, 277, 278, 281, 467, 474

Urist, M.J., 145

Vaegan, 55, 469, 495, 500, 508
Van Allen, M.W., 385, 568
Van Brocklin, M., 643
van der Hoeve, J., 418, 440, 460
van der Tweel, L.H., 233
van der Wildt, G.J., 106
van Doorn, A.J., 259
van Hoven, R.C., 418, 419, 420, 428
Van Sluyters, R.C., 583
Venkiteswaran, N., 118, 119, 120, 122, 123, 125, 178
Verhoeff, F.H., 202, 217, 330
VerLee, D., 634
Volkmann, A.W., 206
von der Heydt, R., 243, 244, 259, 261
von Hofsten, C., 60, 65
von Noorden, G.K., 29, 87, 143, 148, 154, 155, 157, 468, 469, 498, 580, 584, 586, 589, 590, 594, 596, 597, 599,

von Noorden, G.K. (cont.)
632, 634, 638, 672, 674, 677, 678, 682, 692

Wade, S.L., 675, 678
Wales, R., 232
Wallach, H., 60, 85
Walls, G.L., 43, 204
Walsh, F.B., 673, 674, 676, 680, 684, 686, 687, 688, 690
Walton, J., 45, 179, 180, 190
Watanabe, A., 9, 106, 116
Weaver, A.M., 412
Weber, R.B., 7
Wee, H.S., 161
Weil, M.P., 253
Weisz, C.L., 511
Westheimer, G., 3, 31, 32, 35, 83, 90, 102, 106, 125, 126, 128, 140, 141, 142, 157, 181, 184, 282, 283, 298, 300, 303, 304, 308, 310, 325, 346, 350, 353, 359, 363, 375, 377, 383, 384, 388, 389, 407, 408, 425, 440, 460, 484, 485, 486, 498, 550, 552, 611, 649, 659, 663, 664, 666
Wetzel, P., 179, 193
Weymouth, F.W., 239, 440
Wheatstone, C., 199
Whiteside, T.C.D., 112
Whiteside, T.D.M., 51
Wick, B., 613, 636, 638, 639
Wiesel, T.N., 163, 218, 243, 246, 256, 257, 258, 552, 584
Williams, R.A., 383
Wilmer, W.H., 30, 31
Wilson, D., 117
Wilson, M.E., 665
Windsor, C.E., 596
Winter, H.J.J., 199
Wist, E.R., 31, 32
Wolfe, J., 268
Wolfson, D.M., 66
Wolter, J.R., 303, 354, 653
Woo, G., 309
Woo, G.C.S., 223, 467
Wood, I.C.J., 147, 191
Woodburne, L.S., 238
Worrell, B.E., 537
Worth, C., 591
Wright, J.C., 331
Wright, M.J., 163, 583, 584
Wright, W.D., 283
Wurtz, R.H., 665
Wybar, K., 29, 30, 639, 674

Yamamoto, H., 115, 119
Yarbus, A.L., 383, 388, 389, 392
Yolton, 586, 643
Yoshida, T., 9, 106, 116
Young, F.A., 624
Young, L.R., 358

Zimmerman, A.A., 26
Zuber, B.L., 5, 125, 157, 182, 302, 303, 324, 358, 359, 363, 388
Zuckerman, C., 85

Subject Index

Abducens internuclear neurons, 655–656, 657–659
AC/A ratio, 115, 178, 404
  and added lens therapy, 616–617
  and age, 129–132, 403, 427–428
  and CA/C ratio, 180, 404, 509–510
  and convergence dysfunction, 683
  and disparity controller, 190–191
  in divergence excess exotropia, 88, 154
  in double parallelogram model, 451
  effects of drugs on, 140–143
  effects of orthoptics on, 132–138
  effects of surgery on, 139–140
  and fixation disparity, 501–504
  future studies on, 163, 164
  graphical analysis of, 505–506
  individual differences in, 433–434
  innateness of, 153
  linearity and nonlinearity of, 125, 128–129
  plasticity and critical period of, 132–133, 433
  and strabismus, 115, 134, 584–585
  twin studies of, 434
  variability of, 125, 132–133, 433
Accommodation
  and accommodative convergence, 17, 410–411, 416
  in amblyopia, 143–153
  biofeedback training for, 643
  and convergence, relation between, 7–11, 19, 99–195, 404–416, 443–462
  in darkness, 34, 36–38, 42
  dual process model of, 44–45
  effects of drugs on, 141, 142–143, 677
  effects of eccentricity on, 112–114
  effects of prism adaptation on, 61, 65
  effects of spatial frequency on, 107–112
  effects of surgery on, 140
  even-error stimulus, 102
  and fixation disparity, 501–502
  in graphical analysis, 439
  Maddox view of, 16–19
  measurement of, 43–45, 440
  models of, 44–45, 181
  monocular flipper test for, 623
  neural control of, 111, 132–133, 411–413
  normal, 101–114
  and pretectum, 666
  stimulus situation for, 389
  stimulus to, 449
  power-spectrum analysis of, 106
  systems analysis of, 106
  and tonic vergence, 42–46
  See also Near triad response
Accommodation amplitude, 106, 113

Accommodation amplitude (cont.)
and age, 129, 427
and amblyopia, 146, 150–151
in double parallelogram model, 451
and graphical analysis, 403, 439
testing of, 674
measurement of, 449
Accommodation bias, 102, 104, 110
Accommodation controller, 140, 142–143, 148, 175, 184, 509–510
Accommodation controller gain (ACG), 148–150, 192
Accommodation dynamics, 106, 111
Accommodation esotropia, 87, 683
Accommodation excess, 683
Accommodation feedback control system, 181, 184
Accommodation gain, 118, 144, 145
Accommodation insufficiency, 618, 620, 623–625
Accommodation lag, 505, 511, 105, 182
Accommodation latency, 106–107, 111, 126
Accommodation paresis, 677
Accommodation range, 674
Accommodation stimulus-response curve, 102, 111
Accommodation time constant, 106
Accommodative convergence, 16, 119–125, 672
in ambylopia, 143–145, 153–163
and accommodation, 17, 410–411, 416
and convergence accommodation, 415–416, 430–433, 501–506
disorders of, 507–511
and disparity vergence, 155–163, 308–309
early views of, 177–181
effect of drugs on, 140, 141
effect on phoria, 58
effect of surgery on, 140
and equal components proposition, 389, 390–391
and fixation disparity, 501–506
motoneuron activity during, 653
Maddox view of, 27
measurement of, 20, 153–155
neural mechanisms in, 132–133, 411–413
and night myopia, 45–46
nonlinearities of, 117
normal, 114–125
peak velocity: amplitude in, 115–117
and proximal vergence, 90–92, 128–129
and strabismus, 143–145, 153–163
and triad pupil response, 427
in vergence abnormalities, 11
in vergence system modeling, 93
Accommodative vergence control signal, 124
Accommodative vergence dynamics, 115
Accommodative vergence gain, 117–118, 144, 145
Accommodative vergence latency, 115
Acetylcholine, 142, 143
Adaptations, 48, 54–67, 183, 276, 586–593
Added lens therapy, 616–618
Additivity proposition, 381, 385–388, 396–397
Afferent pathways, in amblyopia, 148
African chameleon, 553
Aftereffects, 138, 233, 252, 276, 278–281
Afterimage alignment, 548–549, 562
Afterimage transfer technique, 635–636
Age
and AC/A ratio, 129–132, 164, 403, 427–428, 433–434
and amblyopia, 633–634
and strabismus, 566–567, 583–584
Alcohol
effect on AC/A ratio, 140
effect on vergence, 30–32, 140, 678
Amblyopia
accommodation in, 143–153
accommodative vergence in, 143–145, 153–163
and age, 633–634
animal studies of, 161–163
associated anomalies of, 143, 144–145
distance perception in, 86
fusional vergence in, 161
management of, 145, 146, 599, 632–637, 643
model applications to, 148–149, 191
organic and functional, 146–147
pathways in, 148
prevalence of, 143
saccadic latencies in, 148
and strabismus, 581, 583–584, 585–586, 593
surgery for, 565, 576
American Optical Vectographs, 525, 615
Amobarbital sodium, 141
Amphetamines, 31, 32, 140–142
Amytal sodium, 140
Anaglyphs, 591
Anatomic resting position, 26–27
Anesthesia, 26, 30, 664–665
Angle kappa, 580
Angle of direction, 581
Angle of turn, 582, 589, 592, 595, 598
Angular coordinate systems, 546–549
Animal studies, 161–163, 583, 584. *See also* Cat; Monkey
Anisometropia, 146

management and prognosis, 597–598
and strabismus, 581, 583, 585–586
Anomalous fusional movements, 493
Anomalous retinal correspondence (ARC), 144, 157, 492–494, 553
harmonious and nonharmonius, 588–590
management of, 577, 616, 637–644
prognosis of, 581, 598, 637–644
Anticholinesterase, 142, 143, 683
ARC. *See* Anomalous retinal correspondence
Arc centune, 440
Associated phoria, 179, 471, 494–495, 498–501, 615
and diagnosis, 524, 535, 531–536
Asthenopia, 512, 530–534
Astigmatism, 583
Asymmetric vergence, 3, 102, 158, 209–210, 221, 554
Asymmetric disparity presentations, 321–323, 339–341
Atropine, 341, 419, 678
Auditory biofeedback, 636
Autostereogram, 241

Ball and membrane model, 544–546, 548
Bandwidth limitation, 256–257, 269
Barbiturates, 30–32, 40, 140–142, 678
Base-in prism adaptation, 478–480, 484, 501
Base-in prism limit, 406–409, 452, 461
Base-out prism adaptation 480, 483, 501
Base-out prism limit, 406–409, 451, 461
Bernell unit, 615
Bichrome test, 448
Bielschowsky phenomenon, 692
Bifocal treatment, 87
Bifoveal fixation, 16–17
Binocular anomalies, 86–90, 93
Binocular correspondence, 492–494, 553
Binocular disorders
case analyses of, 401–540
management of, 536–538, 605–646, 622–623
validity of diagnostic criteria of, 517–540
Binocular mixture, 230–231
Binocular neurons, 218–220, 227–230
Binocular optical system, 351
Binocular triplopia, 590
Bioengineering models, 5
Biofeedback, 586, 636, 642–644
"Black box" modeling, 353–354, 358
Bleaching, 635
Blur, 176
and accommodation, 9, 102, 114
and accommodative vergence, 114–115
diagnostic value, 531–534
in graphical analysis, 447–448
and Jampel center, 413
measurement of, 518, 519
and Panum's area, 474
and vergence, 118, 176, 177, 180
Blur-break range, 403, 406–409, 421–424, 451–454, 461
Blur points, 406, 417
Bode diagram, 5
Borish card, 525
Brainstem, 676
Break, 447–448, 452–454, 518, 519, 531–534
Break points, 406
Brewster stereoscope, 591
Broca Pupillometer, 415–416
Brock stick-in-straw test, 588–589, 591–592
Brock string and beads technique, 640–641
Brown's syndrome, 561–562

CA/C ratio, 163, 501, 510–511
and AC/A ratio, 180, 505–506, 509–510
and disparity controller, 190–191
Campimeter, 424
Carbamazepine (Tegretol), 695
Cartesian coordinates, 439, 441
Cat, visual cortex of
disparity detectors in, 310
single-unit studies of, 259, 412, 663
Center of rotation, 442
Center of symmetry (CS), 499–501
Centrad, 440
Central nervous system, and Listing's law, 549–553
Central processor, 451
Cerebral palsy, 597–598
Chain reflex, 410, 416
Chameleon, 553
Chavasse technique, 639
Chlordiazepoxide (Librium), 677
Chromatic aberration, 102
Ciliary muscle tone, 146
Circle of equal convergence, 299
Circular vection, 53
Clear single binocular vision (CSBV), 178, 409, 426–427, 447, 451, 452, 460, 461, 606–607
Closed-loop accommodation, 106, 503–504
Closed-loop disparity vergence, 303–304, 323–324
Closed-loop response, 184, 359–360, 490, 509–511
Coincidence optometer, 146, 147
Color luminance, 231, 234–235

Comitance, 589, 592–593
  management and prognosis of, 581–582, 598, 629–632
  surgery for, 565, 577
Computer simulation, 181, 189–192, 349–350, 486–488
Confusion, 144, 587
Conjugate eye movement, 299–300, 377–381, 404
Constant accommodation, 389
Continuous control system, 301, 358–359
Contrast
  and accommodation, 102, 107, 111
  effect on Visual Evoked Potential (VEP), 229
Contrast sensitivity, 111, 147–148
Controller gains, 362, 365, 367
Controllers, 181–184, 359–367, 485–491. *See also specific types*
Control systems, 175, 301, 349–350, 369–371
Convergence
  and accommodation, 443–462
  disorders of, 679–686, 689
  and cyclorotation, 434
  in graphical analysis, 439
  lesions affecting, 676
  measurement of, 440, 444–447
  neural control of, 672
  in newborns, 41
  See also *Vergence*
Convergence accommodation, 9, 113–114, 177–181, 506–508
  and accommodative convergence, 415–416, 430–433, 501–506
  measurement of, 428–430
Convergence excess, 683–686
Convergence insufficiency, 87, 89, 625–627, 675–676, 679–683
Convergence paralysis, 679–680
Convergence paresis, 677, 679, 680
Convergence range, 674
Convergence retraction nystagmus, 685
Convergence spasm, 679, 684
Convergence weakness, 677
Coordinate system, 439, 441, 546–549
Corpus callosum, 664
Corresponding retinal points, 200, 202–204, 492–493, 553
  and fusion, 297
  and horopter, 556
  normal and anomalous, 157, 298
  testing of, 595
  training of, 638–639
  variations in, 466–467
Cortex
  cyclopean level in, 243
  disparity processing in, 253–254, 663–665
  hypercyclopean processing in, 275–279
  near triad processing by, 664
  orientation-sensitive units in, 552
  and receptive field size, 256
  single-unit studies of, 663
  stereoptic model of, 244–249
  See also Visual cortex
Cortical cells, reduction of, 163
Corticooculomotor pathways, 665–666
Cosmetic surgery, 596–597, 600
Counterphase gratings, 216
Course/fine disparity, 249, 251–253
Course guide of accommodation, 111
Cover test, 467–468, 559–563, 594, 625
Critical period, 133, 583–584
Cross-cylinder test, 429, 448, 505
Cross-link effectiveness, 189
Cüpper's method, 635
Cyclofusion, 220–221
Cyclofusional amplitude, 331, 333–334
Cyclofusional disparity vergence, 317, 330–348
Cyclofusional eye movements, 330–331, 332, 337, 411
Cyclofusional range, 693
Cyclofusional stimulation, 344–346
Cyclopean disparity, 249, 274–275, 278
Cyclopean eye, 243
Cyclopean lateral inhibition, 267–268
Cyclopean level of cortex, 243
Cyclopean size, 269–272
Cyclopean stereopsis, 239–243
Cyclopean upper disparity limits (CUDL), 275, 278
Cycloplegia, 142, 143, 146, 630, 685
Cyclovergence, 11, 210–212, 673, 674, 693–695

Dark focus of accommodation, 36–38, 42–46, 48, 65
Dark vergence, 32–39, 42, 45–46, 48–50, 61–67
Deep amblyopia, 154, 163
Defocus effects, 111
Demand line, 442–444
Depth aftereffect, 252
Depth constancy, 287
Depth cues, 344–346
Depth movement, 262–264
Depth of field, 181
Depth of focus, 105, 450, 452
Depth orientation specificity, 279–281
Depth perception, 270, 285–287
  cortical processing of, 665
  and diplopia, 237–238
  and discrimination level, 238–239
  and disparities, 204, 205, 236–238
  and proximal vergence, 92
  See also Stereopsis

Depth planes, 251–252, 257
Depth tilt, 259, 261
Derivative controller, 362, 363, 367, 370–371
Development, 26–27, 41–42, 133, 583–584
Deviation, 581–582, 586
Diagnosis
  criteria for, 449–461, 517–540
  and kinematics, 561–563
  for strabismus, 579–603
  and proximal vergence, 94
  of true and pseudovergence anomalies, 678–679
Dia-stereopsis, 252, 273
Diazepam (Valium), 677
Dichoptic stimulation, 200–201, 230–235
Diffrequency, 259–261. *See also* Spatial frequency
Diplopia, 17, 237–238, 448, 467
  adaptations to, 587
  forme fruste, 687
  neurological causes of, 675
  physiological, 218–220, 640–641
  and Random Dot Stereogram (RDS), 249–250
  and relative accommodation, 409–410
  and sensory fusion, 200
  in strabismus, 144
  stress-induced, 30
  in superior oblique myokymia, 694
  surgery for, 565, 576
  and vertical disparities, 205
Direction, and horopter, 200–205
Directional convergence, 450. *See also* Proximal convergence
Direction sensitivity, 261–264
Direction shifts, 385–397
Discrimination level, 238–239
Disjunctive eye movements, 299–300, 377–381, 404
Disparities, 261–262, 332, 484, 485, 486
  and blur-break ranges, 406–409
  course/fine separation of, 249, 251–253
  cyclopean/noncyclopean separation of, 249
  and fusional vergence, 58–60, 298
  local/global separation of, 249–251
  orientational, 259
  processing of, 199–295, 236–238, 253–254, 663–665
  psychophysical, 298–300
  and receptive field size, 257–258
  and stereopsis, 235–239, 243–244
  Upper Disparity Limit (UDL), 268, 269–272
  and vergence, 118, 176, 303–306
  See also Horizontal disparities; Vertical disparities
Disparity detectors, 218, 244, 247, 309–312, 331, 663–664
Disparity limits, 269–272, 274–275
Disparity modulation, 223–227, 262, 265–268, 270–271
Disparity phase lag, 324
Disparity presentations, 319–326, 336–341
Disparity processing centers, 161
Disparity vergence, 9, 177, 178, 180, 193, 197–400
  and accommodation, 389
  and accommodative vergence, 308–309
  characteristics of, 300–303
  feedback model of, 182–183, 301–303
  and fixation distance of, 309–310
  measurement of, 351–353
  modeling approaches to, 353–354
  sensory stimulus to, 300, 309–313
  target influences on, 306–309
  and tonic vergence, 18
  training of, 618
  See also Fusional vergence
Disparity vergence controller, 175, 181, 190–191, 301–303, 313–315, 358–371
Disparity vergence gain, 303–304, 323–324
Disparity vergence profiles, 304, 312–313
Disparity vergence system, 350–351, 365
  model of, 349–371
Disparometer, 521–523, 525, 535
Dissociated phoria, 179, 471, 495, 498–499
Dissociated vertical divergence (DVD), 691–692
Distance horopters, 204
Distance perception, 36–38, 48–50, 60–67
Distance phoria, 403, 451
Distance phoria technique, 125, 128, 134, 135, 139–140
Distance shifts, 385–397
Divergence, resting position, 26–27
Divergence amplitude and range, 674, 675
Divergence control, 673
Divergence dysfunction, 686–689
Divergence excess, 88–89, 154–155, 688–689
Divergence insufficiency, 686–688
Divergence mechanism, active, 29
Divergence paralysis, 687
Divergence paresis, 678–679, 688
DNA molecule, stereogram of, 272
Dominance, 201, 218, 231–234
Donder's law, 428, 545
Donder's line, 442–444
Double parallelogram model, 451–452
Drugs
  effect on AC/A ratio, 140–143
  effect on vergence, 30–32, 677–678
  therapy with, 683, 685
  See also specific drugs
Duane-White classification, 19
Dynamic optometers, 113, 193
Dynamic retinoscopy, 146

Eccentric fixation, 143, 144–145, 210, 594
Eccentricity, 38–40, 112–114, 144, 220–221, 239, 474–476
Echothiophate iodide, 143
Electrooculography (EOG), 118, 122, 351
Empirical horopter, 204, 212–220
Empty-field accommodation level, 110
Endocrine exophthalmos, 569
End-point nystagmus, 419
Epicanthal folds, 580
Equal components proposition, 381, 385–396
Eserine, 419
Esofixation disparity, 473, 476, 483, 501–504
Esophoria, 21, 27, 30–32, 461
  and fixation disparity, 468–469, 530, 531–536,
  orthoptics for, 537, 627
  surgery for, 139
Esotropia, 30, 42, 580, 630–631, 683, 678–679, 686–687
  and ARC, 589, 637
  prognosis for, 581, 598
  surgery for, 139, 565, 568–569, 570, 576
Ethanol, 140
Eucatropine, 142
Even-error, 102
Evoked potential. *See* Visual evoked potential
Excyclotorsion, 555
Excyclovergence, 673
Exofixation disparity, 473, 476, 483, 501–504
Exophoria, 21, 27, 30–32, 139, 457–458, 461
  and fixation disparity, 468–469, 530–536
  orthoptics for, 537, 627
Exotropia, 88–89, 580, 631, 678–679, 688
  prognosis for, 581, 586, 591–592, 598, 637
  surgery for, 565, 576
Extorsion, 211–212, 214
Extrafoveal stimulation, 329–330
Extraocular muscles
  innervation of, 549–563, 650–655
  modeling of, 354–358
  surgery for, 139, 565–577
  types of, 653–655
Eye alignment, 617–618
Eye movements
  amblyopic, 146
  anomalous fusional, 493
  conjugate, 299–300, 377–381, 404
  cyclofusional, 330–331, 332, 337, 411
  disjunctive, 299–300, 377–381, 404
  fusional hypothesis of, 216, 217, 410, 411
  and Hering's law, 373–381, 385–397, 404
  horizontal, 354, 655, 656
  measurements of, 381–397
  micromovements, 102
  modeling of, 354–358, 378–379, 544–546, 548
  neural circuitry for, 655, 656
  and stereopsis, 245–246, 253, 282–287
  See also Vergence eye movements
Eye position, and motoneuron firing rate, 651
Eye rotations, 544–563

Facilitation, 227–230, 243–244, 253
False torsion, 547–548, 557
Far point of eye, and accommodation, 112
Fast fusional vergence, 58, 484–491, 512–513
Feedback control, 176, 302, 359, 369
Fick system, 546
Fincham's theory, 178–181
Fine/course disparity, 249, 251–253
Fine-focus-control hypothesis, 111
Fine guide of accommodation, 111
First-order system, 359
Fixation, 205–207
  orthoptics for, 635
Fixation disparity, 31, 32, 36, 38, 42
  and accommodative vergence, 501–506
  and adaptations, 465–516
  and diagnosis, 494–501, 529–530, 535–536
  functional significance of, 467–468
  and fusional vergence, 58–60, 90, 472–474
  future studies of, 163
  measurement of, 466–467, 521–530
  model of, 485–491
  Proximal Convergence Distance Ratio (PCT) derived from, 87, 89
  and prisms, 55–60, 615, 616
  x axis intercept, 554–529, 531–536
  y axis intercept, 524–528, 531–537
Fixation disparity AC/A method, 128–129, 137, 178
Fixation disparity curves (FDC), 525–537
Fixation distance, disparity vergence and, 309–310
Fixation reflex, 16
Flipper test, 623
Flick, 467
Flom swing technique, 637–639
Forced duction fixation disparity curve, 476–477, 481, 489, 491, 494, 495, 499
Foveal fusion, 425, 475
Foveal tag, 635–636

Free-space measures, 80, 81, 82, 87, 639–642
Frequency of deviation, 582
Frequency response
accommodation, 106–107, 111, 126
accommodative vergence, 115
disparity vergence, 300, 303, 323, 359, 361–362
in amblyopia, 148
Fusion, 216–230, 566, 583–585. *See also* Motor fusion; Sensory fusion
Fusional aftereffect, 138
Fusional vergence, 672
and AC/A ratio, 134, 135, 137
and accommodation, 406–409
and accommodative vergence, 155–163
and adaptation, 55–60, 65–67
conditioned, 137
and cyclofusional response, 344–346
and disparity detectors, 663–664
effect of drugs on, 140, 141
and fixation disparity, 472–474
and fixation distances, 64
and graphical analysis, 424–427, 450–451
initiation and sustaining phases of, 315
histograms of, 607
Maddox and early views of, 16–17, 19, 27, 179–180
models of, 93, 485–491
and orthoptics, 88, 512–513, 676
and proximal vergence, 90–91
relaxation time, 477–480
in strabismus, 155–163, 591–593
symmetric, 120
and tonic vergence, 16–17, 27
and triad convergence, 413–415
and vergence final common pathway, 118
See also Disparity vergence; Fast fusional vergence; Panum's area; Slow fusional vergence
Fusional vergence amplitude, 480
Fusional vergence deficiency, 627–628
Fusional vergence dysfunction, 607–610, 675, 695–696
Fusional vergence gain, 498
Fusion field, 425
Fusion-free position, 43
Fusion horopter, 205, 221
Fusion limit, 220–227, 237, 249–250
Fusion range, 89–90, 675, 676
Fusion reflex, 424–427
Fusion reserves, 30–32, 55–56, 521
Fusion response, testing of, 595
Fusion system, 184, 205, 264

Gaze direction
and horopter, 211–212, 556–559
and Listing's law, 545–553, 559–563
and proximal vergence, 91
stability of, and illusory motion perception, 51–54
torsion, and convergence, 554, 561–562
Ghost images, 314
Glissades, 7
Global bandwidth limitation, 269
Global hysteresis, 273–274
Global lateral inhibition, 264–265
Global processing, stereopsis, 245, 264–282
Gradient AC/A ratio, 125, 128, 131, 135, 139–140
Gradient CA/C ratio, 511
Graphical analysis, 126, 403–437, 439–464, 499, 505–506, 521
Grating aftereffects, 161

Haidinger brush, 594
Haplopic images, 298, 310, 314
Haploscope, 107, 115
and AC/A ratio, 126–129, 136, 137
and accommodation, 417
and disparity vergence, 310–311
and voluntary convergence, 420–421
Harmonious ARC (HARC), 588–590
Head-motion technique, 47–48, 53–54
Helmholtz shear, 206
Helmholtz system, 546
Hering's law, 3, 7, 118, 300, 319, 341, 346, 373–381, 404, 494, 545
misinterpretations of, 375–376
Heterophoria
and fixation disparity, 468–471
measurement of, 19–20, 517–521, 611
and prism prescription, 616
signs and symptoms of, 625–626
treatment of, 614–615, 626–627
Hillebrand hyperbola, 384, 385–397
Hirshberg test, 595
Homeomorphic model, 181
Horizontal disparity, 204, 205, 223–227, 297–316, 319–323
Horizontal eye movements, 354, 655, 656
Horizonal fixation disparity, 472–474, 484, 491
Horizontal fusion response, 346
Horizontal oculomotor disorders, 517–540
Horizontal rectus muscles, 554–555
Horopter, 201–205, 212–220, 556–559
Hung-Semmlow vergence model, 92, 93
Huntington's chorea, 676
Hypercyclopean perception, 245, 248, 275–276, 281–282
Hypercyclopean specificity, 276–279
Hyperopia, 584–585, 624
Hypertropia, 561, 581, 690, 692

Hypoxia, 30–32, 40
Hysteresis, 273–274

Illumination. *See* Luminance
Inclination, 216, 259, 261
Incomitance. *See* Comitance
Incyclovergence, 673
Infantile strabismus, 566–567
Infrared eye monitor, 120–121, 126, 155, 610
Inhibition, 232–233, 264–265. *See also* Suppression
Innervation, 374–375, 380–381, 568. *See also* Hering's law
Instruction set, 111
Instrument convergence, 87
Instrument myopia, 113, 417
Instrument space measures, 80–82, 87
Integral controller, 181, 183, 325, 361–363, 367, 370–371, 484–491
Integrator controller, 184, 325, 359, 361
Internuclear opthalmoplegia (INO), 677
Interpupillary distance, 442, 443, 444–447

Jampel center, 411–416, 420
Jump duction exercise, 620

Kenyon effect, 11
Kinematics, of normal and strabismic eyes, 5, 543–564
Kittens, dark-reared, 555
Knowledge of nearness, 18, 27, 75

Laser optometer, 110, 147
Latency. *See* Frequency response
Latent accommodation, 418–419
Latent zone, accommodation, 106
Lateral inhibition, 264–268
Lateral motion, 261–262
Lateral phoria, 448
Lateral rectus muscles, 29, 571, 653, 657, 658
Lazy lag of accommodation, 105, 182, 505, 511
Leaky integrator, 182, 183, 468, 485–491
Lens dioptic power, 176, 178
Lens gradient technique, 125, 128, 131, 135
Lens therapy, 508, 537–538, 616–618, 630–631
Lenticular sclerosis, 106
Linear regression analysis, 147
Listing's law, 545–564
Listing's plane, 545, 560–561, 562–563
Local sign hypothesis, 216, 217
Local stereopsis, 244–245, 249–264

Longitudinal horopter, 204–205, 298
Low-pass filter, 147
Luminance, 223, 271
  effect on vergence, 32–67, 304, 306
  and luster, 234–235
Luster, 234–235, 243

Macular degeneration, 330
Maddox rod technique, 129
Maddox vergence, 15–21, 27–29, 177
Malingering, 678
Manifest zone, of accommodation, 104–105
Mallett unit, 525, 615
Mathematical models, 349–350
Maxwell spot, 594
Medial longitudinal fasciculus (MLF), 657–658, 676–677
Medial rectus motoneurons, 653, 657, 659
Meter angle, 440
Micromovements, 102
Microstrabismus, 467
Microtropia, 592
Midbrain
  control by, 118, 665, 666, 672
  lesions of, 658–659, 676–677
Minimal interocular apparent movement, 214
Mirror stereoscope, 641–642
Modeling, 353–354, 365–367, 488–491
Models
  bioengineering, 5
  accommodation, 148–149, 181
  ball and membrane, 544–546, 548
  disparity detection, 310
  disparity vergence, 58–60, 313–315, 349–371
  homeomorphic, 181
  near triad response, 181–192
  prism adaptation and fixation disparity, 485–488
  stereopsis, 244–249
  system plant, 354–358
  vergence, 29–30, 92–94
Modified estimated method (MEM), 511
Moire fringes, 216
Monkey, visual cortex of,
  Jampel center in, 412
  single-unit studies in, 253–254, 651, 653, 659–665
Monocular accommodative vergence, 178–180
Monocular adaptation, 65
Monocular flipper test, 623
Monocular kinematics, 559–563
Monocular neurons, 218–220, 227–230
Monocular perception, 268
Monofixational phoria, 592
Monofixation syndrome, 467, 468

Morgan's clinical norms, 518–521, 606, 627
Motion, 51–54, 261–264
Motoneurons, 555–556, 651–653, 655, 659–663
Motor adaptation, 55–60
Motor alignment, 580–586, 617–618
Motor control, 175–195, 498–499
Motor controller signal, 351
Motor fusion, 672, 689
 cyclofusional, 330, 334–336, 339, 341, 343, 344, 346
 disorders of, 675, 678, 695–696
 orthoptics and, 619, 639–642
 vertical, 319–323, 326, 329
Mueller accommodative vergence experiment, 3
Mueller paradigm, 120, 122–124
Muscle insertions, 571–575
Muscle tension curves, 570
Myopia, and AC/A ratio, 137. *See also* Instrument myopia; Night myopia

Narrow-band masking paradigm, 276
Near center, 178
Near-far jumps, 620–622
Near-far tracking, 620
Near phoria technique, 125, 128, 134, 135, 139–140
Near point of accommodation, 140, 141, 674
Near point of convergence, 30–32, 140–141, 449, 459–460, 673–674, 676
Near reflex, 675, 678
Near triad response, 7–11, 118, 175–195, 403, 427
 and AC/A ratio, 137
 cortical processing of, 664, 665–666
 modeling of, 181–192, 359, 367
 neural mechanisms in, 661
Negative feedback loop, 484, 486
Negative fusional convergence (NFC), 403, 404, 410, 452, 456–457
Neural channels, 263–264, 276
Neural circuitry, 655, 656
Neural classes, 253–254, 255
Neural control, 111, 132–133, 175, 549–553, 663–665
Neural control centers, 175, 184
Neural integrators, 485–491
Neural processing, of stereopsis, 243–249
Neural triad center, 411–413
Neurological chart, 441
Neuronal arrays, 246
Neurons
 abducens internuclear, 655–659
 binocular and monocular, 218–220, 227–230
 and binocular anomalies, 163
 disparity-specific, 261–264
 special-purpose, 246–247, 663–665
 Visual Evoked Potential (VEP) response of, 227–230
 See also Motoneurons
Night myopia, 45–46
Noncyclopean limits, 274–275
Nonharmonious ARC (NHARC), 589–590
Nonius alignment, 32, 36, 466
Nonius horopter, 213, 214
Nonlinearities
 in disparity vergence system, 365
 modeling of, 181, 182, 186
Normal retinal correspondence (NRC), 157, 589–590, 598
Nystagmus, 53, 565, 570

Object constancy, hypercyclopean, 281–282
Oblique muscles, 560–561, 574
Occlusion, 583–584, 588–589, 597, 634–635
Ocular center of rotation, 442
Ocular dominance columns, 663
Ocular drift, 145
Oculinum, 576–577
Oculomotor adaptation, 48, 54–67, 183, 276
Oculomotor adjustments, and illumination, 36–38
Oculomotor interaction, of accommodative vergence, 118–125
Oculomotor map, 377
Oculomotor nucleus, 659
Oculomotor pathology, peripheral, and Listing's law, 559–563
Oculomotor pathways, disorders of, 676
One-and-a-half syndrome, 677
One-turn helix model, 209, 221
Open-loop response
 accommodation, 106–107, 503–504, 509–511
 convergence, 509–511
 disparity vergence, 303–304, 324–326, 359, 363
 near triad, 184
Operating point, 529
Opponent-process model, 29–30
Ophthalmograph, 425
Optokinetic nystagmus (OKN), 51, 52
Optometric extension program (OEP), 518–521
Optometric vision training, 21
Orientation, 229, 280–281
Orientation disparity, 259, 330–346, 345–346
Orientation-sensitive cortical units, 552
Orientation specificity, 258, 278–281

Orthophoria, 469
Orthophoria line, 442–444
Orthophorization, 55, 492
Orthoptics, 87–88
  and AC/A ratio, 132–138
  for accommodation, 106, 624
  for accommodation vergence, 507–511
  for amblyopia, 149, 636–637
  and biofeedback, 642–644
  and center of symmetry, 500
  for convergence, 676, 682
  cure rate with, 598
  for cyclovergence, 693
  for divergence, 686
  for fusional vergence, 628
  future directions in, 163, 164
  and graphical analysis, 462
  for heterophoria, 627
  and prism adaptation, 469, 495–498
  for proximal vergence, 89–90
  and sensory and motor fusion, 639–642
  for strabismus, 596–597, 629, 676
  and vergence dynamics, 612–614, 618–622
Ortho-rater, 131

Palsy, 597–598, 676, 693
Panum's area, 200, 216, 309, 310, 341
  disparity detection in, 331–332
  and fixation disparity, 38, 42
  and stimulus size and complexity, 327–329
  temporal aspects of, 224
  variable size of, 220–227, 467, 474–476
Panum's limiting case, 311, 389, 393–394, 409
Panum-Wheatstone limiting case, 389
Paradoxical fixation disparity, 495–498
Parallel systems, 287–288
Paralysis, 677, 678
Paramedian pontine reticular formation (PPRF), 655, 672, 677
Parameter sensitivity study, 189
Paresis, 677, 678–679
Parinaud's syndrome, 676, 685
Parisian inch, 439
Parkinson's disease, 676
Patching, 634. *See also* Occlusion
Patent stereopsis, 238
Pattern reversal, 233
Perceived depth. *See* Depth perception
Perceived inclination, 216
Perception
  accommodation, 113
  hypercyclopean, 275–276
  in strabismus, 91
  and tonic vergence, 46–54, 60–67
Percival's criteria, 461, 521, 531–534, 537, 627–628
Peripheral accommodation, 112–113, 389
Peripheral fusion, 157, 425, 475
Peripheral stimulation, 38–42, 326–329, 341–344
Phase lag, 106, 118
Phoria, 492
  for asthenopia, 531–536
  diagnosis of, 536
  differentiated from strabismus, 586
  effects of stress on, 32
  and fixation disparity, 529–530
  in graphical analysis, 447, 448
  measurement of, 517–521
  oculomotor adaptations to prisms and, 55–60
  surgery for, and AC/A ratio, 139
  See also specific phorias
Phoria line, 462
Phoria method, to measure AC/A ratio, 125, 128, 134, 135, 139–140
Phoria position, 178
Photocell technique, 122, 351–352
Physiological correlates, tonic vergence, 69
Physiological resting position, 26–27, 30, 32, 34–38
Plant model, 351, 354–358
Plasticity
  of AC/A ratio, 132
  of tonic convergence, 26, 27, 29
Pleoptics, 635
Plus lens
  gradient technique with, 125, 128
  oculomotor adaptations to, 55
Point horopter, 204, 205–212
Positive fusional convergence (PFC), 403, 404, 451, 458–459
Positive relative convergence, 137
Power spectrum analysis, 106
Predictive smooth pursuit, 124
Predictor operator, 106, 117, 365–367
Preprogrammed movement, 124
Presbyopia, 91, 106, 131–132, 427, 428
Pretectum, 665–666
Primary direction of regard, 545–553, 560–561
Prism adaptation, 55–60, 67, 469, 476–488, 501, 616
  effect on convergence accommodation, 506–507
  excessive, 476, 495
  and exposure duration, 481–484
  functional significance of, 492–494
  influence on curve type, 480–481, 512–513
  model of, 485–488
  therapy for disorders of, 507–511

Prism blur-break ranges, 403, 406–409, 421–424, 451–454, 461
Prism diopter, 440
Prism dissociation, 448, 451
Prism distortion, 616
Prism duction tests, 38, 40, 55–57
Prism effectivity, 442
Prism neutralization, 524–527. *See also* Associated phoria
Prism prescription, 494–501, 508, 537–538, 615–616, 631–632
  for divergence, 686, 688
  fusional vs. triad response with, 413
  for heterophorias, 626–627
  for strabismus, 576
  for vergence, 21, 29, 689–690
Proportional controller, 181, 182, 468
Proportional integral controller, 361, 369–371
Proximal accommodation, 94
Proximal convergence, 90–94, 450, 672, 673
  and AC/A ratio, 125, 126, 135, 140
  and accommodation, 128–129
  and graphical analysis, 416–417
  and Jampel center,
  in modeling, 93–94
Proximal Convergence
  Distance Ratio (PCT) 77–82, 86–91
Proximometer, 418
Pseudo-derivative controller, 364, 367, 371
Pseudointegral controller, 363, 371
Pseudomyopia, 624
Psychiatric disorders, 675, 678, 685
Psychic convergence, 450. *See also* Proximal convergence
Psychophysical disparity, 298–300
Pupillary light reflex, 666
Pupillary response, 7–11, 307, 427. *See also* Near triad response
Pupillary size, 129, 138, 176, 411–416, 450
Purkinje images, 416, 594–595
Pursuit. *See* Smooth pursuit
Pykno-stereopsis, 251, 273

Radial symmetry, 545–548, 552
Random dot stereograms (RDS), 239–243
  Cyclopean Upper Disparity Limit (CUDL) for, 278
  depth averaging with, 251–252, 257
  and luster, 234
  and object constancy, 281
  and orientation, 258
  and receptive field size, 258
  to study stereopsis, 251–253, 264–268
  vergence in perception of, 283–287
  and Visual Evoked Potentials (VEP), 254

Receptive field
  corresponding, 218
  disparity, 218, 257–258, 269–272
  direction specificity, 261–264
  hypercyclopean, 275
  orientation disparity and specificity of, 258–261
  size of, 256–258, 269–272
  wiring of, 253
Receptor ambylopia, 145
Recession, 568
Reciprocal innervation, 355, 434–435
Recovery, 447–448, 518–519, 531–534
Rectus muscles, 69, 571–575, 653. *See also specific muscle types*
Red lens-prism technique, 639–640
Redundancy, 176
Reflex accommodation, 111, 503–504
Reflex fusion, 18, 675. *See also* Fusional vergence; Near triad response
Reflex fusion recovery test, 610–612, 617–618
Refraction, 126–128, 430, 440, 629–630
Relative accommodation, 20, 406, 409–410
Relative convergence, 422–424, 672. *See also* Fusional vergence
Resection, 568–569
Response AC/A ratio, 125–128, 131–132, 134–138
Response zones, 104–106
Resting position, 26–27, 30–32, 66
Resting state of accommodation, 114
Retinal cones, 102, 147
Retinal correspondence. *See* Anomalous retinal correspondence; Corresponding retinal points
Retinal disparity. *See* Disparity
Retinal eccentricity. *See* Eccentricity
Retinal motion, 263
Retinal region, and fusion response, 329–330, 341–344
Retinal shear, 205–207
Retinal slip, 466. *See also* Fixation disparity
Retinoscopy, 146, 429, 511
Rivalry, 231–234, 261, 273–274

Saccades, 7, 11, 148
  motoneuron activity during, 652
  theories of, 384–385, 389, 392–397
Saccadic control, 301, 358, 551
Scheiner optometer, 406
Scheiner principle, 406
Scotoma, 146–147
Search coil technique, 659
Sensitometric refraction, 430
Sensory adaptations, 586–593
Sensory delay, in amblyopia, 148

Sensory fusion, 56, 199–295, 309, 319–346, 351
  disorders of, 512, 675, 678, 695, 696
  orthoptics for, 618–619, 639–642
  and stimulus, 310–313, 328–329
Sheard's criterion, 461, 521, 531–534, 615, 627–628
Sheard's "demand" and "reserve," 461
Single-unit studies, 651–653, 659, 663
Sinusoidal gratings, 107, 147, 265, 267
Size specificity, 257–258
Skew deviation, 690
Skiascope, 429
Sleep, divergence in, 30
Sliding vergence training, 619
Slope, 529, 531–535, 537, 538
Slow fusional vergence, 58–60, 477, 484–491, 513
Smooth pursuit, 51–54, 123–124, 384–397, 653, 654
Snellen letters, 415
Soft saturation transition zone, 105
Space perception, 47, 285–287
Spatial frequency
  in amblyopia, 147
  of disparity modulation, 270, 271
  effect on accommodation, 107–112
  effect on VEP, 229
  hypercyclopean, 276–278
  See also Diffrequency
Spatial limits, fusion, 221–227
Specific distance tendency, 47–50
Spectacle plane, 440, 442
Spike, 413, 417–421
Square-wave gratings, 110
Squint. *See* Strabismus
Static accommodation response, 112
Stay-sutures, 575
Steady-state error, 359, 468, 488–489
Step response, 359, 360–365, 385–397, 613–614, 620
Stepwise discriminant analysis, 531–534
Stereoacuity, 239, 283–284
Stereograms, 271–272, 414–415. *See also* Random dot stereograms
Stereograting, 265, 267, 276–278
Stereomovement, 264, 281–282
Stereoperimetry, 214
Stereopsis, 199, 200, 235–244, 268, 282–287
  bandwidth limitation of, 256–257
  interaction with fusion, and cyclofusional response, 344–346
  models of, 249–287
  physiological basis of, 243–244
  processing levels of, 245
  and Random Dot Stereograms (RDS), 243
  and strabismus, 593
  theoretical framework for, 244–249
Stereoscope, 381–382
Stereoscopic depth interval, 309
Stereoscopic learning, 284–285
Stereothreshold disparity, 309
Stimulus AC/A ratio, 125–135, 138
Stimulus characteristics
  and cyclofusion, 331, 333–336
  and eye movements, 389
  and fixation disparity, 467–468
  and fusion, 222–227, 326–329
  and VEP, 229–230
Stimulus deprivation, 36–38
Strabismus, 11, 42
  AC/A ratio in, 115, 133–134, 153
  accommodation in, 143–153
  accommodative vergence in, 143–145, 149, 153–163
  and age, 566–567, 583–584
  and amblyopia, 581, 583–586, 593
  animal studies of, 161–163
  anomalies associated with, 161–163
  and ARC, 588–590, 637–644
  biofeedback and, 642–644
  classification of, 579–586
  diagnosis of, 541–646
  differentiated from phoria, 586
  distance perception in, 86, 87
  etiologies of, 584–585
  functional cure criteria for, 642
  and fusion, 157, 161, 591–593
  and graphical analysis, 461–462
  incidence and prevalence of, 143, 579, 605, 664
  and instrument convergence, 87
  intermittent, 582–583
  kinematics of, 549–563
  muscle forces in, 569
  lens therapy for, 617
  and orthoptics, 676
  perceptual effects of, 90
  and prism adaptation, 493, 513
  and prism prescription, 616
  prognosis for, 541–646, 637–644
  relation to performance, 593
  sensory adaptations in, 586–593
  and suppression, 587–588
  surgery for, 565–578, 596–597
  and symmetric vergence, 158
  testing of, 593–595
  tonic vergence in, 55
  treatment of, 89–96, 541–646
  See also specific types
Stress, 30–32, 40
  and convergence spasm, 684–685
  and fixation disparity, 60, 467–468
  and fusional vergence, 484
  and voluntary convergence, 678
Sudden-blur technique, 630
Superior colliculus, 665
Superior oblique myokymia, 674, 693

Supplementary accommodation, 404
Suppression
  antisuppression training, 618–619
  Brock string and beads technique for, 640–641
  development of, 201
  from diplopia, 144
  vs. disparity detector hypothesis, 664
  in divergence excess, 688
  foveal, 587–588, 593
  and fusion, 216–218, 231–234, 587–588, 593
  intermittent, 147
  and prism adaptation, 495–498
  stereomovement, 264
  in strabismus, 161
  treatment of, 597
Surgery
  for convergence excess esotropia, 683
  for cyclovergence insufficiency, 693
  for divergence insufficiency, 686
  effect on AC/A ratio, 139–140
  risks, 576–577, 599
  for strabismus, 565–578, 596–597
Suture improvements, 575
Sylvian aqueduct syndrome, 676
Symmetric convergence, 3, 158, 207–208, 221
Symmetric disparity error, 120, 122
Symmetric presentations, 319–321, 323–326, 336–339
Synergy, fusional, 216–217
Synkinesis, 101, 114–115, 118, 144–145, 501, 672. *See also* Near triad response
Synoptophore, 673
System analysis, 106, 181, 182, 350
System plant model, 351, 354–358

Target influences, on disparity vergence, 306–309
Test distance, 442, 443, 444–447
Test-retest variability, 135
Tilt aftereffect paradigm, 278–281
Time dissection technique, 180
Tonic convergence, 477, 672, 673
  and accommodation, 42–46, 404
  and age, 42
  cells specific for, 661
  effects of prism adaptation on, 61–64
  evidence for, 30–46
  future studies of, 69
  individual differences and plasticity of, 26, 27, 29
  insufficiency, 20
  Maddox view of, 16, 18, 27–29
  in modeling, 93
  and oculomotor adaptations, 54–67
  perceptual correlates of, 46–54
  perceptual and motor consequences of, 25–74
  in proximal, 23–97
  in relation between accommodation and convergence, 404
  under stress and reduced illumination, 32–38, 40
Tonic innervation, 25
Tonic muscle fibers, 653–654
Torsion, 543, 561–563
  and gaze direction 554
  and horopter, 210–212, 556–559
Torsional disparities. *See* Orientation disparity
Torus, 221
Transfer function, 358
Transient response, 367
Transposition operations, 572–575
Triad center, 411. *See also* Jampel center; Near triad response
Triad convergence, 413–415
Tropia, 451, 559–560
Tropia line, 462
Twitch muscle fibers, 653–654
Two-components proposition, 381–385

Unidirectional model, 29–30
Upper disparity limit (UDL), 268–272

Voluntary Vergence Accommodation Ratio (VD/A), 132
Vectograms, 525, 591, 615
Vergence, 3–11
  and abducens internuclear neurons, 657–659
  and accommodation, 36–38, 42, 99–105, 404–416
  for asthenopia, 531–536
  blur- and disparity-driven, 176, 177, 178
  diagnosis, 536
  distance range in darkness, 34–38
  errors of, 465–466
  final common pathway of, 118
  and fixation disparity, 465–516, 529–530
  innvervation, 374–375, 380–381
  interactions, 118
  latency, 611
  Maddox view of, 1–21
  measurements derived from, 19–20
  measurement of, 517–521
  motoneuron activity during, 653
  no-target response, 362–363
  peripheral, 38–42
  response, 175, 177
  in stereopsis model, 245–246, 282–287
  tracking rate, 613–614

Vergence (cont.)
triadic role of, 7–11
under stress and low illumination, 30–38
and version, 373–400
See also Convergence
Vergence ability, 673–676
Vergence accommodation. *See* Convergence accommodation
Vergence adaptation, 465–516
Vergence amplitude, 121–122, 124, 303–306, 674, 675
Vergence angle, 201, 286, 287, 659–663
Vergence anomolies, 304–305, 678–679
Vergence asymmetries, 304–305
Vergence control, 3–5, 29–30, 175, 663, 671–672
Vergence controller, 125, 140, 184, 303, 509–510, 665, 666,
Vergence dysfunction, 3–13, 536–538, 614–615, 605–646, 678–696
Vergence eye movements
and corpus callosum, 664
development of, 41–42
and disparity, 176, 205
and Listing's law, 553–559
modeling of, 354–358
neurologic aspects of, 647–703
neurophysiologic correlates of, 649–670
Vergence facility, 610–612
Vergence signals, 655–659, 666
Vergence system, 92–94, 182–183, 671–703
Veridical depth perception, 238
Version, 354, 373–400, 611, 655–659
Vertical disparity, 205, 223–227, 319–323
Vertical fixation disparity, 317–348, 473, 484, 491
Vertical horopter, 214–216
Vertical muscles, 560–563
Vertical vergence, 673, 674, 689–693
Vestibuloocular reflex (VOR), 51–54, 551
Vieth-Müller circle, 207, 212–220, 298, 378, 384–397
Vision training, 21, 126, 134–135, 462, 537, 576. *See also* Orthoptics
Visual cortex, 218, 663–666. *See also* Cortex
Visual direction, 201–205
Visual evoked potential (VEP), 227–230, 233–234, 254–255, 262
Visual imagery, 89–90
Visual noise, 256, 259, 261
Voluntary accommodation, 111, 113–114
Voluntary convergence, 18, 27, 420–421, 678, 682. *See also* Proximal vergence
Voluntary dominance control, 231
von Graefe method, 137

Wheatstone stereoscope, 591

Zero disparities, 200, 203, 304
Zero velocity response, 302
Zone of clear single binocular vision, 178, 409, 426–427, 447, 451, 452, 460, 461, 606–607